Springer

Milano
Berlin
Heidelberg
New York
Barcelona
Hong Kong
London
Paris
Singapore
Tokyo

A. Gullo (Ed.)

Anaesthesia, Pain, Intensive Care and Emergency Medicine - A.P.I.C.E.

Proceedings of the

13th Postgraduate Course in Critical Care Medicine
Trieste, Italy - November 18-21, 1998

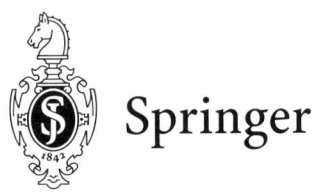 Springer

Prof. ANTONINO GULLO, M.D.
Head, Department of Anaesthesiology and Intensive Care
Trieste University School of Medicine
Trieste, Italy

Library of Congress Cataloging-in-Publication Data: Applied for

© Springer-Verlag Italia, Milano 1999

ISBN 88-470-0051-3

Printed: Tipografia-Litografia «Moderna» - Trieste

SPIN 10707109

Table of Contents

X

Authors Index

Adrogué H.J.
Dept. of Medicine and Renal Section, Veterans Affairs Medical Centre, Houston, Texas (U.S.A.)

Aitkenhead A.R.
Dept. of Anaesthesia, Queen's Medical Centre, University Hospital, Nottingham (U.K.)

Alberti A.
Dept. of Haemodynamics, Ca' Granda-Niguarda Hospital, Milan (Italy)

Alberti C.
Dept. of Anaesthesia and Intensive Care, Saint-Louis Hospital, Paris (France)

Allaria B.
Dept. of Anaesthesia and Intensive Care, National Institute for Cancer Research, Milan (Italy)

Alvisi R.
Dept. of Anaesthesia and Intensive Care, University of Ferrara, Ferrara (Italy)

Atlee J.L.
Dept. of Anaesthesiology, Froedtert Memorial Lutheran Hospital East, Milwaukee, Wisconsin (U.S.A.)

Auler J.O.C.
Dept. of Anaesthesiology, Institute of Cardiology, São Paulo University School of Medicine, São Paulo (Brazil)

Barvais L.
Dept. of Anaesthesiology, Free University of Brussels, Erasme Hospital, Brussels (Belgium)

Baue A.E.
Dept. of Surgery, St. Louis University Health Sciences Centre, St. Louis, Missouri (U.S.A.)

Baue R.D.
Dept. of Surgery, St. Louis University Health Sciences Centre, St. Louis, Missouri (U.S.A.)

Berkenstadt H.
Dept. of Anaesthesia and Intensive Care Medicine, Sackler School of Medicine, Tel Aviv University, Sheba Medical Centre, Tel Hashomer (Israel)

Bobbio Pallavicini F.
Dept. of Anaesthesia and Intensive Care, S. Andrea Hospital, La Spezia (Italy)

Boyd O.
Intensive Care Unit, Royal Sussex County Hospital, Brighton, West Sussex (U.K.)

Böhm S.H.
Dept. of Anaesthesiology, Erasmus University, Rotterdam (The Netherlands)

Brazzi L.
Dept. of Anaesthesia and Intensive Care, Maggiore Hospital - IRCCS, Milan (Italy)

Burchardi H.
Dept. of Anaesthesiology, Emergency and Intensive Care Medicine, University of Göttingen, Göttingen (Germany)

Cafiero T.
Dept. of Anaesthesiology and Intensive Care, Federico II University, Naples (Italy)

Candiani A.
Dept. of Anaesthesia and Intensive Care, University of Brescia, Brescia (Italy)

Capogna G.
Dept. of Anaesthesia, Fatebenefratelli Hospital, Rome (Italy)

Carmona M.J.C.
Dept. of Anaesthesiology, Institute of Cardiology, São Paulo University School of Medicine, São Paulo (Brazil)

Celleno D.
Dept. of Anaesthesia, Fatebenefratelli Hospital, Rome (Italy)

Chambrin M.C.
INSERM, University of Lille II, Lille (France)

Chopin C.
Dept. of Anaesthesia and Intensive Care, R. Salengro Hospital, Lille (France)

Coriat P.
Dept. of Anaesthesia, Pitié-Salpêtrière Hospital, Paris (France)

Dei Poli M.
Dept. of Anaesthesia and Intensive Care, National Institute for Cancer Research, Milan (Italy)

Di Renzo G.C.
Perinatal Medicine Centre, Perugia University, Perugia (Italy)

Donati L.
Perinatal Medicine Centre, Perugia University, Perugia (Italy)

Fábregas N.
Dept. of Anaesthesia and Intensive Care, University Hospital, Barcelona (Spain)

Faletra F.
Dept. of Haemodynamics, Ca' Granda-Niguarda Hospital, Milan (Italy)

Falke K.
Dept. of Anaesthesiology and Intensive Care, Humboldt University Hospital, Berlin (Germany)

Favaro M.
Dept. of Anaesthesia and Intensive Care, National Institute for Cancer Research, Milan (Italy)

Ferraro P.
Dept. of Emergency Medicine, San Paolo Hospital, Naples (Italy)

Fierro B.
Dept. of Neuropsychiatry, Palermo University, Palermo (Italy)

Fieschi C.
Dept. of Neurological Sciences, La Sapienza University School of Medicine, Rome (Italy)

Fruhwald S.
Dept. of Anaesthesiology and Intensive Care Medicine, Graz University, Graz (Austria)

Gattinoni L.
Dept. of Anaesthesia and Intensive Care, Maggiore Hospital - IRCCS, Milan (Italy)

Gollo E.
Dept. of Anaesthesiology and Intensive Care, S. Anna Hospital, Turin (Italy)

Goulon M.
Professor Emeritus of Paris V University, Paris (France)

Gries M.
Dept. of Anaesthesiology and Intensive Care Medicine, Graz University, Graz (Austria)

Gudi F.
Electronic Engineering Dept., University of Florence, Florence (Italy)

Guyatt G.
Dept. of Medicine and Dept. of Clinical Epidemiology and Biostatistics, McMaster University, Hamilton, Ontario (U.S.A.)

Hammerle A.F.
Dept. of Anaesthesia and General Intensive Care Medicine, University of Vienna (Austria)

Hillered L.
Dept. of Clinical Chemistry, Uppsala University Hospital, Uppsala (Sweden)

Iammarino G.
Perinatal Medicine Centre, Perugia University, Perugia (Italy)

Ickx B.
Dept. of Anaesthesiology, Free University of Brussels, Erasme Hospital, Brussels (Belgium)

Inghilleri G.
Immunohaematologic and Transfusional Centre, G. Pini Orthopaedic Institute, Milan (Italy)

Jaeschke R.
Dept. of Medicine, McMaster University, Hamilton, Ontario (Canada)

Jonson B.
Dept. of Clinical Physiology, University Hospital of Lund, Lund (Sweden)

Kim Y.K.
Division of Respiratory Medicine, Mount Sinai Hospital, Toronto University, Toronto (Canada)

Klugmann S.
Dept. of Haemodynamics, Ca' Granda-Niguarda Hospital, Milan (Italy)

Kunst P.W.A.
Dept. of Pulmonary Medicine, Academic Hospital, Free University, Amsterdam (The Netherlands)

Lachmann B.
Dept. of Anaesthesiology, Erasmus University, Rotterdam (The Netherlands)

Langer M.
Dept. of Anaesthesia and Intensive Care, Maggiore Hospital - IRCCS, Milan (Italy)

Latronico N.
Dept. of Anaesthesia and Intensive Care, University of Brescia, Brescia (Italy)

Le Gall J.R.
Dept. of Anaesthesia and Intensive Care, Saint-Louis Hospital, Paris (France)

Lohbrunner H.M.
Dept. of Anaesthesiology and Intensive Care, Humboldt University Hospital, Berlin (Germany)

Lumb P.D.
Dept. of Anaesthesiology, Penn State University College of Medicine, Hershey, Pennsylvania (U.S.A.)

Lyons G.
Dept. of Obstetric Anaesthesia, St. James's University Hospital, Leeds (U.K.)

MacIntyre N.R.
Respiratory Care Service, Duke University Medical Centre, Durham, North Carolina (U.S.A.)

Mahla E.
Dept. of Anaesthesiology and Intensive Care Medicine, Graz University, Graz (Austria)

Margaria E.
Dept. of Anaesthesiology and Intensive Care, S. Anna Hospital, Turin (Italy)

Marn Pernat A.
Institute of Critical Care Medicine, Palm Springs, California (U.S.A.)

Mastronardi P.
Dept. of Anaesthesiology and Intensive Care, Federico II University, Naples (Italy)

Mathieu D.
Dept. of Respiratory Emergency, Resuscitation and Hyperbaric Medicine, Calmette Hospital - CHRU, Lille (France)

Meade M.
Dept. of Medicine, McMaster University, Hamilton, Ontario (Canada)

Meduri G.U.
Dept. of Medicine, Division of Pulmonary and Critical Care, The University of Tennessee, Memphis, Tennessee (U.S.A.)

Melloni C.
Dept. of Anaesthesia and Intensive Care, Lugo Hospital, Lugo (Italy)

Mercuriali F.
Immunohaematologic and Transfusional Centre, G. Pini Orthopaedic Institute, Milan (Italy)

Metzler H.
Dept. of Anaesthesiology and Intensive Care Medicine, Graz University, Graz (Austria)

Möllhoff T.
Dept. of Anaesthesia and Intensive Care, Wilhelms University, Münster (Germany)

Montenero A.S.
Dept. of Cardiology, Sacro Cuore University, Gemelli Hospital, Rome (Italy)

Moro M.L.
Dept. of Medicine and Public Health, University of Bologna, Bologna (Italy)

Muchada R.
Dept. of Anaesthesia and Intensive Care, E. André Hospital, Lyon (France)

Naeije R.
Dept. of Intensive Care, Erasme University Hospital, Free University of Brussels, Brussels (Belgium)

Østergaard D.
Dept. of Anaesthesiology, Gentofte University Hospital, Copenhagen (Denmark)

Paladino F.
Dept. of Emergency Medicine, San Paolo Hospital, Naples (Italy)

Pandin P.
Dept. of Intensive Care, Erasme University Hospital, Free University of Brussels, Brussels (Belgium)

Parpaglioni R.
Dept. of Anaesthesia, Fatebenefratelli Hospital, Rome (Italy)

Perel A.
Dept. of Anaesthesia and Intensive Care Medicine, Sackler School of Medicine, Tel Aviv University, Sheba Medical Centre, Tel Hashomer (Israel)

Pernat A.
Institute of Critical Care Medicine, Palm Springs, California (U.S.A.)

Persson L.
Dept. of Neurosurgery, Uppsala University Hospital, Uppsala (Sweden)

Petrovitch C.T.
Dept. of Anaesthesiology, Providence Hospital, Washington, District of Columbia (U.S.A.)

Povoas H.P.
Institute of Critical Care Medicine, Palm Springs, California (U.S.A.)

Putensen C.
Dept. of Anaesthesiology and Intensive Care, University of Bonn, Bonn (Germany)

Rampoldi A.
Dept. of Haemodynamics, Ca' Granda-Niguarda Hospital, Milan (Italy)

Ravagnan I.
Dept. of Anaesthesia and Intensive Care, Maggiore Hospital - IRCCS, Milan (Italy)

Rhodes A.
Intensive Care Unit, St. George's Hospital, London (U.K.)

Righini E.R.
Dept. of Anaesthesia and Intensive Care, University of Ferrara, Ferrara (Italy)

Roncati Zanier E.
Dept. of Neurosurgical Intensive Care, Maggiore Hospital - IRCCS, Milan (Italy)

Rossi A.E.
Dept. of Anaesthesiology and Intensive Care, Federico II University, Naples (Italy)

Rossi S.
Dept. of Neurosurgical Intensive Care, Maggiore Hospital - IRCCS, Milan (Italy)

Rupreht J.
Dept. of Anaesthesiology, Erasmus University, Rotterdam (The Netherlands) and University of Ljublijana (Slovenia)

Safar P.
Safar Centre for Resuscitation Research and Dept. of Anaesthesiology and Critical Care Medicine, Pittsburgh University, Pittsburgh, Pennsylvania (U.S.A.)

Sanfilippo M.
Dept. of Anaesthesia and Special Odontostomatologic Anaesthesia, University of L'Aquila, L'Aquila (Italy)

Savettieri G.
Dept. of Neuropsychiatry, Palermo University, Palermo (Italy)

Scandella R.
Hyperbaric Institute, Zingonia, Bergamo (Italy)

Schiraldi F.
Dept. of Emergency Medicine, San Paolo Hospital, Naples (Italy)

Segal E.
Dept. of Anaesthesia and Intensive Care Medicine, Sackler School of Medicine, Tel Aviv University, Sheba Medical Centre, Tel Hashomer (Israel)

Shoemaker W.C.
Dept. of Anaesthesiology and Surgery, University of Southern California School of Medicine, Los Angeles, California (U.S.A.)

Slutsky A.S.
Dept. of Respiratory Medicine, Mount Sinai Hospital, Toronto University, Toronto, Ontario (Canada)

Sortino G.
Dept. of Anaesthesiology and Intensive Care, S. Anna Hospital, Turin (Italy)

Stewart T.E.
Division of Respiratory Medicine, Mount Sinai Hospital, Toronto University, Toronto (Canada)

Stocchetti N.
Dept. of Neurosurgical Intensive Care, Maggiore Hospital - IRCCS, Milan (Italy)

Stüber F.
Dept. of Anaesthesiology and Intensive Care, University of Bonn, Bonn (Germany)

Sutcliffe A.J.
Dept. of Anaesthesia and Intensive Care, University Hospital Birmingham NHS Trust, Birmingham (U.K.)

Tatschl C.
Dept. of Anaesthesia and General Intensive Care Medicine, University of Vienna (Austria)

Toller W.
Dept. of Anaesthesiology and Intensive Care Medicine, Graz University, Graz (Austria)

Torres A.
Dept. of Pneumology and Respiratory, University Hospital, Barcelona (Spain)

Tortoli P.
Electronic Engineering Dept., University of Florence, Florence (Italy)

Tosi P.
Dept. of Anaesthesia and Intensive Care, I.R.C.C.S. San Matteo Hospital, Pavia (Italy)

Verbrugge S.J.C.
Dept. of Anaesthesiology, Erasmus University, Rotterdam (The Netherlands)

Verde G.
Dept. of Anaesthesia and Intensive Care, I.R.C.C.S. San Matteo Hospital, Pavia (Italy)

Verdi M.K.
Dept. of Anaesthesia and Special Odontostomatologic Anaesthesia, University of L'Aquila, L'Aquila (Italy)

Vilardi V.
Dept. of Anaesthesia and Special Odontostomatologic Anaesthesia, University of L'Aquila, L'Aquila (Italy)

Vincent J.-L.
Dept. of Intensive Care, Erasme University Hospital, Free University of Brussels, Brussels (Belgium)

Volta C.A.
Dept. of Anaesthesia and Intensive Care, University of Ferrara, Ferrara (Italy)

Wattel F.
Dept. of Respiratory Emergency, Resuscitation and Hyperbaric Medicine, Calmette Hospital - CHRU, Lille (France)

Weil M.H.
Institute of Critical Care Medicine, Palm Springs, and The University of Southern California School of Medicine, Los Angeles, California (U.S.A.)

Wollmer P.
Dept. of Clinical Physiology, Malmö University Hospital, Malmö (Sweden)

Wrigge H.
Dept. of Anaesthesiology and Intensive Care, University of Bonn, Bonn (Germany)

Yamaguchi H.
Institute of Critical Care Medicine, Palm Springs, California (U.S.A.)

Younes M.
Respiratory Medicine, University of Manitoba, Winnipeg (Canada)

Zakowski M.
Dept. of Anaesthesiology, Cedars-Sinai Medical Center, Los Angeles, California (U.S.A.)

Zhang H.
Division of Respiratory Medicine, Mount Sinai Hospital, Toronto University, Toronto (Canada)

Zimpfer M.
Dept. of Anaesthesiology and General Intensive Care, University of Vienna, General Hospital, Vienna (Austria)

Zingone B.
Dept. of Cardiac Surgery, Maggiore Hospital, Trieste (Italy)

Abbreviations

ACC, American College of Cardiology

ACE, angiotensin converting enzyme

ACLS, advanced cardiac life support

ADH, antidiuretic hormone

AE, air embolism

AF, atrial fibrillation

AHA, American Heart Association

ALI, acute lung injury

ALS, advanced life support

AMI, acute myocardial infarction

APACHE, acute physiology and chronic health evaluation

APRV, airway pressure release ventilation

ARDS, acute respiratory distress syndrome

ARF, acute respiratory failure

ASA, American Society of Anesthesiologists

BAL, bronchoalveolar lavage

BARS, basic anti-inflammatory response syndrome

BCM, body cell mass

BGA, blood gas analysis

BIPAP, biphasic positive airway pressure

BLS, basic life support

CABG, coronary artery bypass grafting

CAD, coronary artery disease

CARS, compensating anti-inflammatory response syndrome

CAST, cardiac arrhythmia suppression trial

CBF, cerebral blood flow

CI, cardiac index

CIP, critical-illness polyneuropathy

CK, creatine kinase

CL, lung compliance

CMRO$_2$, cerebral oxygen metabolism

CMV, controlled mechanical ventilation

CNS, central nervous system

CO, carbon monoxide

CO, cardiac output

COP, colloidosmotic pressure

COPD, chronic obstructive pulmonary disease

CPAP, continuous positive air pressure

CPB, cardiopulmonary bypass

CPCR, cardiopulmonary cerebral resuscitation

CPP, cerebral perfusion pressure

CPR, cardiopulmonary resuscitation

CQI, continuous quality improvement

CRI, cardiac risk index

CSF, cerebral spinal fluid

CT, computed tomography

cTNI, cardiac troponin I

cTNT, cardiac troponin T

DCA, dichloroacetate

DI, diabetes insipidus

DIC, disseminated intravascular coagulation

DKA, diabetic ketoacidosis

DNR, do not resuscitate

DO$_2$, oxygen delivery

DPH, dynamic pulmonary hyperinflation

E, elastance

EBM, evidence-based medicine

ECASS, European Cooperative Acute Stroke Study

ECF, extracellular fluid

ECG, electrocardiography

ECM, extracellular matrix

ECW, extracellular water

ED, emergency department

EDRF, endothelial-derived relaxing factor

EEG, electroencephalography

EELV, end expiratory lung volume

EIT, electrical impedance tomography

EMFATAS, European Multicenter Four-arm Trial in Acute Stroke

ETT, endotracheal tube

EVLW, extravascular lung water

FARS, functional anti-inflammatory response syndrome

FBI, focal brain ischaemia

FDP, fibrinogen degradation products

FEV$_1$, forced expiratory volume in one second

FFP, fresh frozen plasma

FiO$_2$, inspired oxygen

FRC, functional residual capacity

GBI, global brain ischaemia

GEDV, global end-diastolic volume

GI, gastrointestinal

GIT, gastrointestinal tract

GOS, Glasgow outcome score

HBOT, hyperbaric oxygen therapy

HBsAg, hepatitis B surface antigen

HDR, host defense response

HPA, hypothalamic-pituitary-adrenal

HPV, hypoxic pulmonary vasoconstriction

HR, heart rate

HSP, heat shock protein

ICF, intracellular fluid

ICP, intracranial pressure

ICU, intensive care unit

ICW, intracellular water

IFN-γ, interferon-γ

IMPRV, intermittent mandatory release ventilation

IMV, intermittent mandatory ventilation

iNOS, inducible NO synthase

IRV, inverse ratio ventilation

ITBV, intrathoracic blood volume

ITTV, intrathoracic thermal volume

LIP, lower inflection point

L-NAME, N^G-nitro-L-arginine methyl ester

L-NMMA, N^G-mono-methyl-L-arginine

L-NNA, N^ω-nitro-L-arginine

LPS, lipopolysaccharide

LV, left ventricular

LVEF, left ventricular ejection fraction

MAC, minimal alveolar concentration

MAP, mean airway pressure

MAP, mean arterial pressure

MARS, mixed anti-inflammatory response syndrome

MB, methylene blue

MCA, middle cerebral artery

MD, microdialysis

MEG, mercaptoethylguanidine

MET, metabolic equivalent

MH, malignant hyperthermia

MI, myocardial infarction

MIGET, multiple inert gas elimination technique

MLC, myosin light chain

MOD, multiple organ dysfunction

MOSD, multiple organ system dysfunction

mP$_{crit}$, mean critical pressure

MPM, mortality probability model

MV, mechanical ventilation

NIC, neurointensive care

NO, nitric oxide

NOS, nitric oxide synthase

OR, operating room

P(A-a)O$_2$, alveolar-arterial gradient for oxygen

PAC, pulmonary artery catheter

PaCO$_2$, arterial carbon dioxide pressure

PACU, post-anaesthesia care unit

PAI-1, plasminogen activator inhibitor-1

PAR, postanaesthesia recovery

PAV, proportional assist ventilation

Paw, airway pressure

PAWP, pulmonary artery wedge pressure

PBV, pulmonary blood volume

PCA, patient controlled analgesia

PCO$_2$, carbon dioxide pressure

PCV, pressure controlled ventilation

PEEP, positive end-expiratory pressure

PEFR, peak expiratory flow rate

Pel-V, elastic pressure-volume

PET, positron emission tomography

PGI$_2$, prostacyclin

pHi, intramucosal pH

PIE, pulmonary interstitial emphysema

PIP, positive inspiratory pressure

PKA, prekallikrein activator

PLS, prolonged life support

PMI, perioperative myocardial infarction

PMNL, polymorphonuclear leukocytes

Ppa, pulmonary artery pressure

PPF, plasma protein fraction

Pra, right atrial pressure

Prv, right ventricular pressure

PSVT, paroxysmal supraventricular tachycardia

PT, prothrombin

PTCA, percutaneous transluminal coronary angioplasty

PtcO$_2$, transcutaneous oxygen tension

PTH, parathyroid hormone

PTT, partial thromboplastin time

PVB, premature ventricular beat

PVRI, pulmonary vascular resistance index

PVS, persistent vegetative state

PVS, protective ventilatory strategy

Q, blood flow

R, resistance

RAAS, renin-angiotensin-aldosterone-system

Raw, airway resistance

RCP, retrograde cerebral perfusion

RER, respiratory exchange ratio

RTA, renal tubular acidosis

RVEDVI, right ventricular end-diastolic volume index

RVEF, right ventricular ejection fraction

SAG, serum anion gap

SaO$_2$, arterial oxygen saturation

SIADH, inappropriate secretion of ADH

SIRS, systemic inflammatory response syndrome

SMR, standard mortality ratio

SMT, S-methylisothiourea sulfate

SNAP, S-nitro-N-acetyl-penicillamine

SpO$_2$, pulse oximetry

SPT, suppurative pelvic thrombophlebitis

SPV, systolic pressure variation

SV, stroke volume

SVI, stroke volume index

SvO$_2$, venous oxygen saturation

SVR, systemic vascular resistance

SVV, stroke volume variation

TBI, traumatic brain injury

TBW, total body water

TCI, target controlled infusion

TD, thermodilution

TE, expiratory time

TEE, transoesophageal echocardiography

THAM, tromethamine

TI, inspiratory time

TIMI, thrombolysis in myocardial infarction

TIVA, total intravenous anaesthesia

TNI, troponin I

TNT, troponin T

TOF, train of four stimolation

tPA, tissue plasminogen activator

TQM, total quality management

TSS, toxic shock syndrome

UA, urine anion

UAG, urine anion gap

UIP, upper inflection point

V̇, gas flow

V̇$_A$, alveolar minute ventilation

VA, volume assist

VAP, ventilator-associated pneumonia

VCV, volume controlled mechanical ventilation

V̇$_E$, minute ventilation

VF, ventricular fibrillation

VMA, vanillyl-mandelic acid

V̇O$_2$, oxygen consumption

VT, tidal volume

VT, ventricular tachycardia

WARS, whole anti-inflammatory response syndrome

WPW, Wolf-Parkinson-White syndrome

ZEEP, zero end-expiratory pressure

PROGRESS IN CRITICAL CARE

A Life in Critical Care

M. GOULON

For French-speaking countries "Réanimation" is the equivalent of critical care or intensive care in English-speaking countries. This new field aims at monitoring the internal functions of an incapacitated patient during the critical time of his or her acute disease. Hence, its field has a broader scope than resuscitation, the goal of which is to bring life back to an apparently dead person. As early as 1954, at the Claude Bernard Hospital in Paris, we French doctors adopted this new term for lack of another as simple and expressive. Today it is widely used in France.

During this presentation, I intend to focus on the following issues, based on my personal experience:
- origin and development of the intensive care concept
- implementation of new techniques
- ethical issues
- current status and international co-operation
- expected future development.

Origin and development of the intensive care concept

In the past, there were many attempts to remedy acute respiratory and circulation diseases arising from various conditions. Our predecessors were many, often creative. For example, the mouth-to-mouth technique was introduced by Réaumur as early as 1740 and by Buchanan in 1759, the positive pressure-breathing technique through a bellows by Hunter in 1776. Despite their outstanding reputation throughout Europe at their time, other attempts, like smoke exhalation in the rectum of drowned persons, fail to convince us.

External cardiac massage codification dates only from 1960 by Kouwenhoven. Long before, however, internal cardiac massage was used, first on animals by Schiff in 1874, then by d'Halluin in 1904. They practised tracheotomy and the insertion of tracheal cannula for suffocating dyspnea via diphteric laryngitis; due, however, to baro-traumatic incidents resulting from excessive inspiration pressures, the ventilation by the endotracheal passage that used to be practised in the 19th century was no longer endorsed in the first half of the XX century. External artificial breathing by means of steel lungs and cuirasses was recommended instead.

In 1878 the French doctor Woillez, way ahead of Drinker, invented an external breathing machine that he named the "spirophore", ancestor to the iron lung. This artificial breathing technique was immensely useful but had its limitations in the case of difficulties in swallowing.

In 1956, during a severe poliomyelitis epidemic in Argentina, I went there with J.J. Pocidalo to introduce and apply the technique of intermittent positive breathing via the endotracheal passage. At that time our American colleagues still used only the iron lung.

A new generation of therapeutic tools needed creating. Hence the birth of intensive care. It is this aspect of the history of modern intensive care that I will recount, having been one of its actors since its inception.

It was poliomyelitis, today an almost extinct disease thanks to vaccination, that kindled an interest in intensive care. In France, poliomyelitis annually caused several thousand cases and dozens of deaths by paralysis of the respiratory muscles. In 1953 Lassen and Ibsen, well versed in modern anaesthetic techniques, conceived the idea of applying them to patients suffering respiratory disorders due to poliomyelitis. The life saving results were conclusive; respirators were invented, the most famous – for its performance, reliability and sturdiness – being the Engström 150.

On September 1, 1954, at the Claude Bernard Hospital (an old institution of several buildings dating back to 1871, erected on the ancient fortifications of Paris and dedicated to infectious diseases) Professor Mollaret seized the initiative. A severe poliomyelitis epidemic was underway. Everything needed to be done: upgrade and adapt the premises; acquire respirators; set up a round-the-clock medical team, which required that one of its members be constantly present in the intensive care unit.

For its day, this was a novelty. At the beginning, we were only three. Coming from different specialities, we had first to learn the handling of the respirators. That's why in August 1954, we spent night and day practising on anaesthetised dogs under artificial respiration by means of the Engström apparatus. We also needed to acquire a better grasp of the physiopathology of respiratory, circulatory and metabolic disorders, as well as master the degree of electrolytes and of gas in the blood in order to understand better the relationship between clinical and biological realities.

Nothing was easy. You will certainly understand the anxieties and fears that constituted our daily bread until we finally hit our first successes. Critical cases of poliomyelitis were cured and are, despite severe consequences, still happily living today. Rapidly, we realised that our working method was also valid for other pathologies.

Out of the vast field of applications that opened to us, I would only cite a few examples.

Tetanus

At that time, tetanus was still a common disease, despite vaccinations by Ramon's anatoxin, compulsory in the army since 1936 and in schools since 1942. In its general manifestations with paroxysms, death was almost certain. We had the idea of using curare on these patients after they had been tracheotomised and respiratorily assisted. We sought to reverse the neuro-intoxication. In our first paper published in 1955, we reported three out of four tetanus patients cured. Year after year, performance improved and cases of tetanus declined. Out of the two hundred and ten cases observed in my intensive care unit in the Raymond Poincaré Hospital, the mortality rate declined to 24.7%.

Polyradiculonevritis

Primary critical polyradiculonevritis, observed by Guillain and Barré in 1916 and often considered benign, is in fact terrible in its general manifestation, due to the respiratory paralysis and dysautonomic disorders it induces. Life expectancy has been greatly enhanced thanks to the endotracheal respiration, and further improved thanks to plasmatic exchanges and/or gammaglobuline injections, which we were among the first to prescribe at the Raymond Poincaré Hospital in Garches.

Myasthenia gravis (MG)

Another immunology disease, myasthenia gravis, also benefited from intensive care procedures involving plasmatic exchanges, gammaglobulines and immunosuppressors such as azathioprine and cyclosporine, which we were among the first to promote.

I would like to underline the diagnostic errors associated with MG, often mistaken for either ophthalmic or rhino-pharyngitic diseases, or confused with myopathies.

Bronchio-pulmonary diseases

Those are too well known to necessitate the relation of my personal experience.

Intoxications

A great number of entries in critical care are due to various forms of intoxication. The kidney extra-epuration, specific antibody injections (for example in digitalic intoxication), antidote intakes and respiratory assistance have transformed the prognosis for intoxications.

I will illustrate this with the barbituric intoxication more frequent in past years than today. Until 1954, one used to treat this intoxication by the injection of large doses of strychnine, in fact by a second intoxication. The Claude Bernard team showed in 1956 that in addition to ventilation assistance, it was sufficient to give generous intravenous perfusions of slightly alkaline serum to obtain a recovery without adverse consequences. Several years later, we designated cases of severe intoxication, a condition to be strictly distinguished from *coma dépassé*, as "coma avec sidération végétative d'évolution favorable".

Metabolic, endocrine and hydro-electrolytic disorders

They cause many problems, and I will just tell you the following story about them: a thirty-year-old man, a heavy alcoholic, is hospitalised in a psychiatric hospital where, because of his potomania, he is allowed to drink as much water mixed with liquorice powder as he wants. He becomes quadriplegic and is sent to my intensive care unit for poliomyelitis. In fact, he was suffering from hypokaliemic paralysis, which we cured. Twenty years later, he murdered somebody and his lawyer called me to inquire if this episode could not mitigate his responsibility. I of course denied it; the man had remained an alcoholic.

Another instructive story concerns a Vietnamese man suffering from quadriplegia by hypokaliemia, related to an hyperthyroidy. There was complete recovery after a thyroidectomy, and even today, after thirty years, the man remains in good health.

Implementation of new techniques

I will mention only two of them: the membrane oxygenators (ECMO) and the hyperbaric oxygenotherapy (OHB).

ECMO

This technique gave rise to hope in the Eighties for efficiently curing critical respiratory disorders resistant to traditional treatment. With membrane oxygenators manufactured by Rhône-Poulenc, we treated eleven patients who remained anoxemic under respirators with positive pressure expiration. Nine died, five of them under ECMO; two were alive eight months later but with a slight restrictive syndrome (one by viral pneumopathy; the other one by azote dioxide intoxication).

We decided to abandon the ECMO for the following reasons: mediocre results, excessive risk of iatrogenic complications (specially of infectious origin), no specific treatment of alveolar lesions, too consuming of highly qualified staff at other patients' cost, too expensive.

OHB

On the other hand, OHB has been a growing success. One has to remember a book by Paul Bert published in 1878, "La pression barometrique", for which there was a renewed interest during the Second World War.

In 1964, I acquired for my hospital a Vickers pressure chamber, since replaced by a room. Our first publications date from 1965 in Durham, North Carolina. The applications are so numerous it is impossible to name them all: decompressing diving accidents with professional as well as amateur divers, gaseous gangrene, gaseous embolism, monoxide carbonic intoxication, etc.

I will make only two remarks:

– despite safety guidelines, CO intoxications remain too frequent due to misuse of defective gas-fueled hot-water heaters;
– with coelioscopic surgery development, there is a rise in gaseous embolisms.

Ethical issues

Critical care gives rise to many ethical issues:

– the frequent impossibility of obtaining informed consent from the patient or his relatives, hence an increased responsibility for doctors;
– medical refusal to use intensive care procedures when the patient's condition seems irremediable;
– termination of respiratory and even feeding assistance for chronic vegetative conditions (passive euthanasia is not accepted in France);
– maybe tomorrow the utilisation of cells, tissues and xenogenic organs.

Among these ethical issues, cerebral or brain death is one of the most acute. During the first months of my intensive care practice, I observed that patients placed under artificial respiration were in deep coma: spontaneous respiration and brain stem reflexes cancelled, EEG flat. But for these patients, other organs were still functioning for a while. I remember having asked to my collaborators the following question: "Where is this patient's soul?".

We waited, Professor Mollaret and myself, to collect twenty-three observations before publishing in 1959 a paper, the first in the world, on "coma dépassé", which was later renamed cerebral death.

At this time, we requested that four fundamental criteria be observed during a minimum time of 24 hours (today reduced to eight hours), in the absence of hypothermia and intoxications, before concluding that cerebral death had occurred:

– coma
– disappearance of spontaneous respiration
– brain stem abolition
– flat EEG.

This new concept of death despite the presence of a beating heart ("mort à coeur battant"), was a revolution. Its description preceded the implementation of organ transplants, which nowadays are increasing, although they still remain inferior to need.

Intensive care current status and international co-operation

The critical care concept was born in 1954. Since then, its expansion has been remarkable and the number of patients who have benefited from it is impossible to gauge. In Paris, the first center was the Claude Bernard Hospital, the second was the Raymond Poincaré Hospital in Garches. Today, there is at least one center in each department of France.

Developed in the field, this speciality is today fully recognised as a discipline in hospitals as well as universities. Emergencies are centralised at the regional SAMU centers. The Francophone Critical Care Society was founded in 1971. French publications are numerous:

– books such as "Réanimation et Médecine d'urgence", published in 1968, with an annual re-edition; "Abregé de Réanimation" and "Les urgences";
– Synopses of "Critical Care" and "Emergency Care", published since 1984;
– a journal entitled "Réanimation et Urgences".

A development just as important has occurred in other industrialized countries as well as in emerging ones. To coordinate research projects and organize international meetings, we proposed the creation of the "World Federation of Critical Care" during the second International Congress of Critical Care in Paris in 1977. I was one of its founding members, along with Ledingham, Gilston, Beurzstein and Perret.

The "WFIC Care" Council is currently presided by Professor Gattinoni, our eminent Italian intensive care specialist. Our common goal is to save lives. Once this goal is reached, patients still need to be offered a modus vivendi compatible with their handicap. It is to this end that associations for home respiratory assistance have been created; there are thirty-three in France, including the ADEP for the Ile-de-France region. Thousands of patients enjoy the benefit of this medico-social progress.

Expected future developments

For the last half century progress, inconceivable in 1950, has been accomplished. Emulation has involved not only doctors but also nurses and physiotherapists. The efficiency, but also the costs of treatment have been constantly rising. Some therapies were dismissed for lack of proven efficiency. Problems such as nosocomial infections have emerged and need to be addressed. Evaluation scores have been established but poor score results should not prompt the interruption of justified care.

In comparison with what we have done, which may seem easy today but I can assure you it was not, improvements will be more difficult to obtain, but progress will be constant.

What terrific luck it was to have been part of this modern medical epic!

Clinics, Technology, Ethics, and Humane Patient-Physician Relationships and Critical Care
(Monitoring, Diagnosis, Intervention Strategies)

R.D. Baue, A.E. Baue

Professor Gullo has given us a topic so broad that we can say almost anything about anything and that is exactly what we intend to do. First, let us join in the celebration of forty years of critical care medicine. Professor Gullo, you have gathered together the "Old Boys' Club" in intensive care – Safar, Weil, Shoemaker, Gattinoni, and Vincent. They are pioneers, friends and colleagues.

Peter Safar and one of us (AEB) have been on programs together way back in the past. Max Weil discussed a paper of mine at the Trauma Society Meeting in 1967. Will Shoemaker is a member of the Alexander Pope Club. It was Pope who said "The proper study of mankind is man". He was one of the pioneers studying sick surgical patients along with Francis Moore, George Clowes, Louis DelGuercio, John Siegel, and Stanley Levinson. It was also our pleasure to publish some of his provocative papers when I was editor of the Archives of Surgery. What has been more provocative than supernormal values of oxygen transport and consumption? There are others. Shoemaker and we also lived through the days when physiologists and biochemists would not vote to support studies in our ICUs. They said that it is not research, it is patient care. Now these basic scientists can't wait to get their latest molecular biological molecule into a clinical trial.

In 1958 one of us (AEB) was a surgeon in the United States Air Force based in the Philippine Islands and we shared that experience. We had a recovery room only. In 1961, when we were in the residency program and AEB was chief resident on the surgical service at the Massachusetts General Hospital, there was no intensive care unit. An anesthesiologist colleague named Henning Pontoppidan convinced Henry Beecher, the Chair of Anesthesiology at Harvard, and Henrik Bendixen, to set aside four beds in a special unit to care for difficult respiratory problems.

The first patient in that unit was a trauma patient of ours with a severe pulmonary contusion and a torn superior vena cava. We repaired the vena cava and, of course, the patient required ventilatory support afterward. Over the next several days the patient had at least 12 cardiac arrests, each of which occurred while he was being suctioned. From this we learned a lesson: that a ventilator-dependent patient requiring a high FiO_2 would become hypoxic during prolonged suctioning. Limiting suctioning to one pass and 15 seconds eliminated that problem. Who would have thought that becoming disconnected from a ventilator could be a fatal problem? It occurred in the early years without adequate monitoring and one-on-one nursing care.

Ethics and the ICU

This is a particularly important time in our professional lives to consider communication, concern for our patients and ethics in the intensive care unit. The high cost of health care, concerns over how it should be paid for, and insurance programs have all depersonalized the relationship between patient and doctor. This can be particularly true in intensive care where you were not the patient's original or primary physician and you may not be familiar initially with the patient's family and social and religious background.

Ethics (medical originally - now called bioethics) has exploded around the world. There have now been four world congresses of bioethics. There is the American Association of Bioethics, the International Association of Bioethics, an International Bioethics Summit Meeting, and a European society, as well, we are sure. There is East Asian Bioethics, Hispanic Bioethics, feminist approaches to bioethics, nursing ethics, research ethics, etc. Where did they all come from? Most of this has nothing to do with us. The ethics that has to do with us you know about. Every issue of Critical Care Medicine, the Journal of Intensive Care Medicine, JAMA, and NEJM has articles about health care ethics. Now the AMA has an EPEC Project - Education for physicians on end-of-life care which is sponsored by their Institute for Ethics. The purpose is to "train physicians in the basic knowledge and skills they need to appropriately care for dying patients" [11]. I would have thought that this would be part of any residency program but perhaps it isn't. We are inundated with ethics and ethical dilemmas. Even so there are important considerations related to our work.

Physicians are professionals, and the highest professional ethical standard places the welfare of the professional's patients first and foremost. Problems involved with intensive care and organ failure exemplify both the high cost of health care and poor or limited prognosis of terribly sick patients in combination with concern about privacy, dignity, the primacy of the individual, and the right to die peacefully with one's loved ones close at hand. No respectable physician prolongs life by mechanical or artificial means when it is unnecessary, unqualitative, or futile. But how does one determine necessity or quality or futility? Ethical discussions abound; living wills attempt to control one's fate, and legal battles continue.

We believe that ethical, concerned, compassionate physicians and nursing staffs, in consultation with the family, can resolve matters of futility, necessity, and quality. Such combined effort allows patients to make decisions quietly, progressively, and morally. Although concern about litigation is given as a reason to continue support for a patient when benefit is unlikely, no malpractice judgments have been made when life support systems for the terminally ill have been discontinued as a result of carefully documented professional care. Physicians are mandated legal responsibility to care for their patients in consultation with the patient's family [1].

Patients with multiple organ failure are treated in ICUs. Ontologists are persons who consider the nature and qualities of being. Who is the ontologist in the ICU when the patient is wired, ventilated, irrigated, restrained, and tubed in three or more orifices? Who is the ontologist in the ICU environment of bright lights, beeping monitors, constant television, and large ticking clocks? Is there an ontologist who decides whether medications are necessary, palliative, experimental, controlling, or restraining? Does anyone monitor the patient's privacy and dignity? Did, or would, the person-patient choose to be there [1]?

ICU ethics must presuppose a relationship among the staff, the patient, and the patient's family that is based on trust, honesty, and a genuine concern for the patient as a person. Physicians, residents and nurses must weigh their decisions and actions by applying the lessons of the past, the common sense of the moment, and the potential consequences of actions taken. ICU staff must be as adept with ethical imperatives as with technical qualifications. Neither the patient nor the patient's family is in the ICU because the ICU is pleasant or comfortable, therefore the conscientious care of the staff may have to be its own reward [2].

Admitting a patient to the ICU is admitting a person to the arena of the extraordinary means that require informed consent. Informed consent is not the same as being truly informed, and informed consent is rarely obtained from a patient with multiple organ failure. The onus of responsibility usually falls on the family, in consultation with the physician; thus the physician has a responsibility to delineate ethical boundaries. Two ethical lines that physicians are in danger of crossing in the care of such a patient are 1) experimentation versus treatment and 2) hopeless heroic measures. Each action of the physician must be balanced against the part of the Hippocratic Oath that states: "I will come for the benefit of the sick, remaining free of all intentional injustice, of all mischief". The 1980 Principles of Medical Ethics of the American Medical Association expanded the intent of the Hippocratic Oath: "As a member of this profession, a physician must recognize responsibility not only to patients, but also to society, to other health professionals, and to self". The Hippocratic Oath has been reinforced by the Nuremberg Code, which provides directives to prevent heinous medical crimes such as those committed by German National Socialists physicians.

Ethical care

The intrinsic quality of the ethical care that health professionals deliver depends on the prior development of their professional and personal ethics and an understanding of, and concern for, the ethics of others and their faith traditions. In addition, understanding the economic and political climate that forges both the treatment and the ethics of treatment has become important for health care professionals [3, 4].

Health care professionals need to be cognizant of relevant religious traditions. Knowledge of both the patient's and the physician's religious persuasions can assist a medical team and a patient's family when the patient cannot be responsible. In the final analysis, however, religious considerations may not prove to be as great an ethical factor as are the resources of the particular hospital and the composition of the board of governors. Ethics committees also need to be aware of the potential hazards of ethical decisions by majority rule. Although perfectly correct ethical expression may emanate from a majority opinion, that, in itself, cannot be an ethical criterion [5].

The leap from ethical theory to the treatment of a particular person with multiple organ failure, in which extraordinary and costly measures are deemed necessary, may not be short or easy. Despite the plethora of courses, books, and seminars on medical ethics, there are no definitive or permanent solutions. To study medical ethics by examining case studies is not difficult; to ask the correct questions and to find the correct answers in a given clinical situation may be extremely difficult. *Arete*, the Greek word frequently translated as virtue but more accurately translated as excellence, provides the shortest leap from theory to bedside. The first element of compassionate ethical treatment is to do the right thing; the next is to be able to do the right thing very well.

In support of patient preference, Knaus recently stated that "there is a tragic mismatch between the health care many seriously ill and dying patients want and what they get" [6]. Knaus was commenting on a study carried out by the SUPPORT principal investigators who described a controlled trial of improved care for seriously ill hospitalized patients. The study revealed that many physicians did not know when their patients preferred to avoid cardiopulmonary resuscitation [7]. Do not resuscitate orders were written within two days of death. A large number of patients who died spent at least ten days in an intensive care unit, and 50% of unconscious patients died in the hospital, suffering moderate to severe pain at least half the time. These problems were not improved by a Phase 2 intervention attempt; thus, the study confirmed substantial shortcomings in the care of seriously-ill, hospitalized adults. In an editorial review, Lo had several suggestions for future investigation of care near the end of life [8]: 1) do not project our own concept of a good death onto patients; 2) gather preliminary data on promising interventions; 3) quality improvement requires organizational changes; 4) constraints and incentives may be needed to reduce inappropriate interventions; 5) discussions should be improved with patients about the decisions at the end of life.

To incorporate patient's preferences into medical decisions is another important matter, particularly in the intensive care unit where families and patients should actively participate in what *is* being done, and what *should* be done [9].

The quality of life after treatment in intensive care unit has increasingly been studied. Konopad et al. reviewed the quality of life measures before and one year after admission to an intensive care unit [10]. She found that patients admitted to intensive care units tended to have a decrease in the level of activity of daily living for a year after their stay, although most patients returned home. Quality of life outcome has become increasingly important, particularly in the elderly, where many emphasize quality of life over duration of life [11, 12].

Must a physician provide care that he or she believes is unreasonable or futile for the patient even though the patient and/or the family members insist upon it? In certain circumstances CPR is believed to be futile [13]. A futility rationale has been used, along with do not attempt resuscitation orders [14]. The issue of physician refusal of requested care has not been resolved by law or legal statute. It is supported by ethical principles. Luce writes that physicians are not ethically required to provide futile or unreasonable care, especially to patients who are either brain dead, vegetative, or critically or terminally ill, or unlikely to benefit from resuscitation [15]. Civetta reviews this area in a practical approach to futile care and states that "in reality, the ideal case is resolution of conflict between the family and providers before any outsiders need to be involved" [16].

Significant debate exists over whether or not to continue established therapy or to try to institute new and unproven therapy. Evidenced-based medicine has now become the buzz-word for the future. In addition, aspects of monitoring have become important. We also recognize the errors or mistakes made in the care of our patients in intensive care units, and it behooves all of us to make decisions to provide fail-safe symptoms as best we can.

All of our institutions have broad-based committees involved in reviewing research proposals and other facets of intensive care unit ethics. It is important to point out, however, that there is both informed consent and informed refusal. A patient may refuse to accept therapy based upon his or her own beliefs and approach to life. We must as physicians, also be willing to accept "refusal".

Let us think again about the first circular sentence in Book I of the *Nicomachean Ethics*, which epitomizes Aristotle's entire work as well as our own mandate for ethical action: "Every craft and every investigation, and likewise every action and decision, seems to aim at some good; hence the good has been well described as that at which everything aims".

Observations

We will make some observations based on a shared 44-year career in surgery – observers of the passing scene who are becoming progressively apoptotic.

As stated by Barrett-Connor and Stuenkel, "Everyone dies too early or too late". How do you define dying at the right time? [17]. Older patients rarely die of a single cause. This makes therapy trials in older patients a problem. Therapy against which cause?

If a patient is declared "Do not resuscitate" (DNR) postoperatively, could this have been done preoperatively and thus avoid the entire technical exercise? If a surgeon knows that he can treat a problem operatively, such as a perforated duodenal ulcer, must he do so if the patient has end-stage Alzheimer's disease and has not been in contact for some time? We can therefore – we must – is not a sound approach to patient care in today's world. This has been referred to as the "technological imperative". I will come back to that again.

Patients may be afraid of dying a high-technology death but many, when the time comes, are also afraid of dying. What does refusal of treatment mean? – medically, morally, religiously – and can it be legally safeguarded? Paul Ramsey wrote "If the sting of death is sin, the sting of dying is solitude – the chief problem of the dying is how not to die alone" [18].

Johnson et al. reported that a major complaint of families of ICU patients is lack of continuity of nursing care (not having the same nurse every day) and changes in attendings (rotations off-service, laboratory time, etc.) [19]. Other important factors for families include family sleeping rooms adjacent to the waiting area or within the medical center complex and regarding families as family, not visitors. Remember that the family and the patient did not select you. They were not referred to you prospectively. You were assigned or assigned yourself. Thus, you must get to know them, their wishes, their problems, their family associations. Harvey described a comment of William Osler as follows: "Perhaps it is more important to know what kind of patient has a disease than what kind of disease the patient has" [20].

There are major differences in ICUs, depending on the medical specialty. I have observed that, if an ICU is staffed by internists, pulmonologists, cardiologists, or neurologists, then the family doctor or primary care physician pulls back and the ICU physician takes over. The family doctor may stop by to say hello, more of a social call, but that is all. Some surgical ICUs may be staffed by surgical intensivists and/or anaesthesiologists, but the primary surgeon stays actively involved – seeing the patient every day, writing orders, talking to the family, etc.

However, it is hard, if not impossible, for a general surgeon in practice who is five to ten years out of his residency to be capable of managing all aspects of an ICU patient. If the surgical ICU does not have a full-time intensivist, then care in the unit is provided by a parade of consultants – pulmonologists, cardiologists, nephrologists, etc. The most common ICU surgeons are trauma surgeons who are not required to be in the operating room every morning. Therefore, they can manage an ICU for trauma and general surgery patients. Neurology and neurosurgery patients are frequently managed jointly in their ICU. Cardiac surgeons frequently staff their own ICUs with or without help from anaesthesiology.

As medical care continues to evolve, so will our specialties. Emergency physicians treat urgencies and emergencies of all kinds. Anaesthesiologists provide anaesthesia and monitoring for operations, pain control and intensive care. Intensivists monitor and treat very sick people, unstable patients, patients with complications and those after big operations. Therapy in an ICU is to support organ function and treat the iatrogenic complications. Thus, the focus is on being very sick and not on specific diseases. This has advantages in terms of expertise – monitoring and organ support – but it has the hazard of lumping all sick people together based on how sick they are. I will speak more about this tomorrow.

This lumping together of all patients who are sick enough to be in an ICU leads to concepts such as SIRS and MODS. These and MOF are not diseases, they are not even syndromes. They are simply classifications of being sick and how sick. An example is shown in Fig. 1. Another example is the acronymania that comes from the proposal of CARS and CHAOS (Table 1) [21]. An absurdity would be recommendations for the treatment of SIRS (Table 2). In intensive care conferences, congresses and jamborees, there is a great tendency – in fact, an overwhelming thrust – to lump everything together. ARDS is not broken down into causes. ARDS also is not a disease, it is not a syndrome, it is lung failure from a multitude of causes. They include those shown in Table 3.

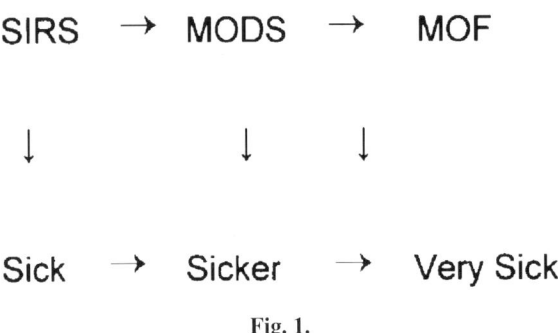

Fig. 1.

The recent report by Dellinger and colleagues, on a randomized trial of the use of inhaled nitric oxide in patients with significant ARDS, showed improvement in some patients and not in others [22]. I predict that, if this is broken down, it will be found that certain causes of ARDS will respond to NO and others will not. Thus, we have to be specific. A recent report by Mathisen of the use of nitric oxide inhaled by patients with pulmonary failure after a thoracic operation showed improvement in all such patients [23]. The survival rate also seemed to be increased although it was not a randomized trial. This is encouraging. In contrast to this, internists and surgeons are increasingly becoming what has been called SODs (single organ doctors).

Table 1. Acronymania

Basic anti-inflammatory response (BARS)
Compensating anti-inflammatory response (CARS)
Functional anti-inflammatory response (FARS)
Mixed anti-inflammatory response (MARS)
Whole anti-inflammatory response (WARS)
All of these may lead to CHAOS

Table 2. Early treatment of SIRS

Temperature
a) If low, warm patient with warming blankets, extracorporeal warming circuit, warm i.v. fluids, irrigate peritoneal cavity with warm saline
b) If high, use external cooling, cool bath, rectal aspirin, etc.
Rapid heart rate: slow with calcium channel blockade, rapid-acting digitalis, etc.
Rapid breathing: i.v. morphine, other sedation, intubation, paralysis, and controlled ventilation
For a low WBC: give G-CSF
For a high WBC: consider chemotherapeutic agents to control bone marrow

Table 3. Different causes of lung failure - ARDS

1. End-stage COPD
2. After cardiac surgery
3. After thoracic surgery
4. After general surgery
5. Pneumonia
6. Infection elsewhere
7. Severe trauma and pulmonary contusion
8. Severe trauma and MOF

Possible moves in intensive care

There are moves that we detect as observers of critical or intensive care that are good and/or needed. First, improved communication with family about the condition of the patient, possibilities for the future, and decisions about end-of-life matters. We call this "working it through" – the process is important – do not resuscitate or withdrawal of life support decisions take days to work through with the family and/or the patient.

There is greater involvement of nurses with families and in decisions. The nurse who is encouraged to keep a patient alive takes time to adjust to a reversal of that approach. There is also an increased tendency to talk to the patient and with the patient on rounds and at other times even if the patient is intubated or comatose or seemingly unresponsive. The provision of sleeping quarters for families near the ICU is becoming much more common to allow greater access of families to their family member patient.

There is now an honest, nonpunitive approach to error in the ICU – medications, nursing, physicians so as to systematize to decrease error [24]. Demming, the industrial consultant, once commented about a five per cent error rate that was thought to occur in health care. He said that such an error rate in air travel would lead to two 747 airline crashes a day at JFK Airport.

Where will critical care medicine be in the future – critical care and emergency medicine, critical care and anaesthesia, critical care and internal medicine, critical care and trauma surgery, or critical care alone as an independent specialty? What will the Euro do to critical care?

Finally, where will we all be when we accept integrated biology and nonlinearity with CHAOS theory? Percy points out that "Science can tell us nothing about an individual" [25]. According to Goodwin, the contribution of CHAOS theory to the practice of medicine "... has been the simple but profound negative statement: traditional science cannot predict complex systems. Complete understanding should be abandoned as a goal" [26]. We may well be facing a revolution, not evolution, in the way we think about sick patients and their scientific problems. Thus, the future is not what it used to be. More about this comes later.

Are we making progress?

The mortality rate in ICUs has changed little over the years. Attempts to document such progress have been few and have been difficult to carry out.

Zimmerman et al. compared risks and outcomes for intensive care unit patients with organ system failure from 1982 to 1990 [27]. They found that the incidence of organ system failure of 48 per cent among patients treated from 1988 to 1990 was similar to the 44 per cent occurrence rate in patients from 1979 to 1982. An identical proportion, 14 per cent, developed multiple organ system failure during both time periods. They found significant improvement, however, in hospital mortality for patients with three or more organ system failures on day four or later in the intensive care unit. In spite of this, overall hospital mortality rates from MOF were not different over this eight-year period. The most important predictor of death in the hospital was the severity of physiological disturbance on the initial day of organ failure. Christou et al. provided a 20-year follow-up of 4,292 surgical patients in which they studied the delayed type hypersensitivity (DTH) skin test [28]. They found that overall hospital surgical mortality fell over the year due to improved preoperative, intraoperative and postoperative care. However, there was no change in mortality of patients who required intensive care. Offner et al. reviewed the post-injury MOF incidence and outcomes over the past five years in a trauma center in Denver [29]. They found that the annual incidence of post-injury MOF and MOF case mortality did not change significantly over the five-year period. The incidence of MOF was 17 per cent with an overall mortality in those patients of 37 per cent. Again, the question must be raised as to whether more seriously ill patients are surviving in order to develop MOF and thus overall patient mortality may be improving, although it is not demonstrated in this kind of study.

Are there clinical problems which are decreasing in frequency?

Regel et al. described a decrease in renal failure and ARDS in trauma patients in recent years [30]. Other problems which are no longer severe threats to survival or represent improvements are shown in Table 4. Christou et al. documented a decreased mortality rate for elective surgery in recent years [28]. The development of trauma centers and trauma teams has improved results for trauma victims. This has been well documented in the literature. There are other examples which could be cited. The threat of GI stress bleeding has decreased. This may be due to better general patient care. Prophylaxis, which seems better with Sucralfate or Omeprazole is still used commonly in severely ill or sick ICU patients. Ranitidine may increase infectious complications in trauma patients. Methods to control GI bleeding by nonoperative endoscopic means have also improved. How do we document these improvements? The only documentation is from reports of clinical experience. ARDS had been frequent in elderly patients with hip or long bone fractures treated by bedrest and traction. There was a revolution in patient care when early or immediate fixation or joint replacement was carried out. Patients could get out of bed [31]. They didn't need ventilator support. They were much better off. Then it was learned that reaming a long bone fracture in order to put in a nail damaged the lung. Thus, reaming was stopped. Also, with pulmonary contusions from trauma, early fixation was not as well tolerated [32].

Intra-abdominal and liver abscesses have decreased in frequency. When they do occur, it is much more likely that they can be drained percutaneously without operation, by CT guided control of catheter insertion. Resuscitation after injury is often initiated in the field and is much more vigorous in the hospital. Complete resuscitation cannot be completed until sites of blood loss are controlled.

Thromboembolism prophylaxis by mini-dose heparin and/or calf compression has reduced the likelihood of pulmonary emboli. Better monitoring techniques such as right ventricular function measurements, venous oxygen and other measurements are helpful. Finally, minimal surgical procedures decrease the metabolic and neuroendocrine stress response to operations that improve safety and decrease risk. Anaesthesia techniques, such as epidural anaesthesia, also decrease the response to injury, improve comfort and help to get patients well faster.

Table 4. Advances in clinical procedures which promote survival

Advances	
Recognition of the abdominal compartment syndrome	
Methods for reexploration for generalized peritonitis	
Abbreviated laparotomy for trauma patients	
Early fixation of femur and pelvic fractures without reaming	
Microcirculatory blood flow measurement and correction (pHi)	
Minimal surgical procedures	
The widespread use of epidural anaesthesia and other adjuncts	
Recombinant human growth hormone in patients with short bowel syndrome	
Ventilatory support	
Pressure controlled inverse ratio ventilation	Nitric oxide inhalation
Permissive hypercapnia with tracheal gas insufflation	Steroids for late ARDS
Partial liquid ventilation with perfluorocarbons	Opening up partially collapsed lungs
Prone position	

These clinical advances may be difficult to document by improvement in overall mortality. In fact, a patient may avoid some of these problems only to survive longer and develop other complications. This could actually increase the incidence of MOF.

Some clinical advances seem to contribute to better patient care and then fall into disuse or are never used extensively simply because they did not make enough difference. There are a number of examples of this such as low molecular weight dextran, tris-hydroxy-methoaminomethane, 2,3-diphosoglycerate (2,3 DPG), $NaHCO_3$ and others. Some of these represent modern clinical controversies such as driving oxygen, transport and consumption to supernormal values, selective gut decontamination and vasoactive agents – which one, when and why? Hypothermia does not protect trauma patients. Maintaining normal temperature intraoperatively seems to decrease wound infections.

There are many concepts that are still clinically relevant in 1998. First of all, septic patients are more likely to survive if there are surgically amenable sources present. Prevention of MOF should be the goal. A return to basic surgical principles for injured and operated patients is critical so that there are no anastomotic leaks, no wound dehiscences, and no other complications such as bleeding, thromboembolism, gastroduodenal problems, persistent stasis haematomas, etc. Finally, we must have clean body cavities and intact, functioning organs. Thus, prevention of complications in all ICUs, from physician and nursing errors in medication, monitoring and therapy are critical.

Clinical advances which seem to be important and have benefitted some patients but may not have demonstrated a decrease in mortality

There are therapeutic contributions which make good sense clinically but the evidence is divided over their worthwhile effects. This may help in some patients with specific problems but not in others. Some of these are shown in Table 5.

Table 5. Potential improvements in patient care

Delaying secondary operations until inflammation has subsided (avoid an early second hit)
Preventing ischaemia/reperfusion injury in trauma patients by antioxidants and free radical scavengers
Whole gut washout for severe sepsis or selective decontamination
Omeprazole or sucralfate to prevent stress-mucosal damage
Immunostimulation or modulation with indomethacin, thymopentin, ranitidine and others
Measurement of right heart function
Low molecular weight heparin
Immunomodulating enteral feeding formulas
Aggressive fluid resuscitation to restore not only BP and CO but also regional or microcirculatory flow (is it volume needed or time to correct flow?)
Inhaled NO

The idea, proposal or hypothesis that a single agent which is not specific for the entire clinical problem and is given after a complex insult will reduce mortality is preposterous.

Unsolved problems

There are a number of unsolved problems in critically ill patients with injury, operation and inflammation. These are listed but not discussed. They should be a challenge to young investigators.

1. Is there a clinical pH and oxygen paradox with ischaemia/reperfusion?
2. Is there an ischaemia/reperfusion injury (I/RI) after shock in the entire patient. Certainly there is regional I/RI (lower part of the body with aneurysm operations) and isolated organ I/RI (heart, intestine, transplanted organs)?
3. There seems to be biologic self destruction from an overwhelming inflammatory response (the Horror Autoxicus). How? Why?
4. Can we control the inflammatory process which is necessary for healing without doing harm to the patient?
5. Biologic conundrums with serious inflammation – cytokines are necessary and cytokines are destructive.

6. Harbingers of doom – predictors of disaster. Are these critical measurements (i.e. IL-6) or events which predict a bad outcome?

7. Immunosuppression – why? What is its clinical relevance?

8. Innate or genetic resistance – is it important? Non-responders – why? "Give us this day our daily germs". Thus, there may be a cytokine imbalance state (tendency toward TH_2 cells) and an uneducated T-cell regulation state (limited prior exposure of T-cells to foreign antigens).

9. The capillary leak syndrome – acute/ARDS, chronic – the oedematous ICU patient. What can be done about it?

10. The major accomplishments in improving the health of mankind have been through public health measures which prevent disease – nutrition, sanitation, communicable disease eradication, vaccines. Can we prevent MODS and MOF by better organ support, better immunization for patients to increase resistance, and a better understanding of the various disease processes?

Integrative or nonlinear biology

A new concept in biology has been described which will have a great impact on how we take care of patients and how we approach an inflammatory response. Stanley Schultz [33], in the Claude Bernard lecture to the American Physiological Society entitled "Homeostasis, Humpty Dumpty and Integrative Biology", described integrative biology. He stated that, "in biology, the parts are dynamic or plastic. They can change shape when they are brought together – that's what nonlinearity means!". The shape of the "whole" cannot be predicted by knowing only the shapes of the "separated parts". If you substitute function for shape we can see that the function of the whole cannot be predicted by knowing only the functions of the separate parts. This seems to be where we are now in trying to determine pro-inflammatory mediators, antiinflammatory mediators, and whatever. Schultz goes on to say that molecular biology provides parts of a puzzle – "putting them together is the problem". He reviewed Cannon's homeostasis concept and believed that homeodynamics would have been a jazzier and technically more correct expression. Tim Buchman stated, "if nested, nonlinear models are better representatives of human physiology than Cannon's collection of negative feedback servomechanisms, then therapy should be redirected toward transitions to a basal range – not therapeutically manipulating things such as cytokines or nitric oxide [34]". Focusing on the phases of inflammation (pro-anti, etc.) would be Walter Cannon's approach. Blocking one mediator may change not only the effects of that mediator but may disturb other mediators and the entire system. As Buchman has also said, we are "prolonging lives far beyond the limited capacity of intrinsic physiologic responses".

Lewis Thomas was referred to earlier in his thoughts about the lack of integration in the response system [35]. His description should be of interest to us because he had great insight into the inflammatory process. The question is – did Thomas see the beginning of nonlinearity in the new physiology or the new pathophysiology in human disease?

Sir Karl Popper in his Medawar Lecture in 1986 to the Royal Society in London said that "biology cannot be reduced to physics because biochemistry cannot be reduced to chemistry. Reductionism is not possible in biologic systems. An organism cannot be reduced to a series of systems". Weiss and Miller question: "How can mammals develop and maintain such a lethal defense system without ultimately harming themselves?". Many are studying this question. They state that "excessive or unrestricted use of this arsenal can result in injury to the host as can occur in autoimmune diseases, toxic shock syndrome and food poisoning" [36]. It is interesting that they do mention or discuss the problems of overwhelming trauma and sepsis. The relationship of cytokines and inflammatory cells can be: 1) an interaction which is successful in host defense; 2) unsuccessful in immune deficiency problems; 3) inappropriate in autoimmunity and allergy; 4) perhaps inappropriate also with severe illness and injury.

I can - Therefore I must

In recent years we have observed with our residents the care of patients with surgical emergencies. On occasion an elderly patient confined to a nursing home with severe senile deterioration or an any age patient with severe Alzheimer's disease is brought to the emergency ward with a surgical emergency such as a perforated ulcer, perforated diverticulitis, acute cholecystitis or a perforated colon cancer. The patient is seen by a surgeon who performs an operation which corrects the acute problem. After the operation, and with the patient in ICU, the patient's family and the surgeon agree on a "do not resuscitate" order (DNR), order to be placed in the patient's chart. We have raised the question – why not a DNR order preoperatively? If the patient has not been in contact with his or her family or with the outside world and is in a chronic vegetative state, is it necessary to do an operation because there is a urgent medical problem which can be corrected surgically? We believe it is not necessary. If the quality of life is not improved and the patient will be returned to institutional, custodial care, then the patient is not helped. On occasion a patient's family insists procedures, operations or support techniques be done even when the judgement of the physician may be different. The family may say: "Do everything you can". The reason for a family's insistence may be based on a number of factors, one of which is guilt. If the family has not been very attentive to the patient they may feel that in a crisis they must do something positive for their relative. One of us (AEB) once had a patient who died and I hoped to get an autopsy to determine the cause of death. The responsible family member was a son who had not seen his father for 10 years. When he arrived and learned that his father was dead he insisted that nothing further be done. He was going to protect his father from further suffering and there would be no autopsy.

DNR means – do not carry out cardiac resuscitation for a cardiac arrest – do not intubate and ventilate for respiratory failure. Could it also mean do not operate for a perforated ulcer? The argument has been given that the operation helps the patient be more comfortable. No major operation helps a patient be more comfortable. A vegetative state patient with a perforated ulcer can be kept comfortable with pain medication. Is a perforated ulcer as a way of dying different from a cardiac arrest? If a patient is not to be resuscitated then perhaps they should not be operated upon in the first place.

These considerations have been called problems of a technological imperative. The term was first used by an economist named Fuchs in 1968 to indicate that doctors work on the premise that "we should do everything we can do – that consists of all that is possible" [37]. Fox and Lipton described the pressure to perform a procedure because it can be done [38]. Moser later attributed the driving power of technology and health care to a concept which he termed "intellectual imperative" [39]. He referred to the pursuit of new ideas – no matter what. Barger-Lux and Heaney reviewed these concepts and authors in writing about "for better and worse". The development of medical or health care ethics has helped us confront these concepts more realistically. No longer do most physicians ascribe to the aspect of the technological imperative as described by Barger-Lux and Heaney as "the prolongation of life i.e. death prevention as the deciding factor, purpose or goal of health care" [40].

Fortunately we have learned about the moral domain, the rights of patients, the needs of patients and their families and an ethical approach to technological and intellectual imperatives. We are sure there are many such approaches and decisions to be made by all of you in intensive care medicine and anaesthesiology and other related disciplines.

Conclusions

If we are serious about decreasing mortality in our hospitals and ICUs we must focus on prevention – prevention of MOF but also prevention of illness and injury by healthy lifestyles, prevention of obesity, elimination of tobacco, immunization for all, prenatal care for all to decrease prematurity, decreased speed limits, elimination of drunken drivers, strict gun control and decreasing violence and drug-related injury or crime.

References

1. Baue RD (1990) The patient as a person: Ethical considerations of patients with multiple organ failure. In: Baue AE (ed) Multiple organ failure: Patient care and prevention. Mosby-Year Book, St. Louis, pp 512-514
2. Baue AE, Baue RD (1996) Ethics in critical care medicine. Medical decision making in critical care - a patient as a person. In: Gullo A (ed) Anaesthesia, pain, intensive care and emergency medicine. Springer, Berlin Heidelberg New York, pp 969-974
3. Harron F, Burnside J, Beauchamp T (1983) Health and human values: a guide to making your own decisions. Yale University, New Haven
4. Levine H (1986) Life choices: confronting the life and death decisions created by modern medicine. Simon & Schuster, New York
5. Bulger RJ (1987) On the drinking of hemlock: Socrates, Semmelweis, and Barbara McClintock; Erikson EH: The Golden Rule and the cycle of life; Pellegrino ED: Toward an expanded medical ethics: the Hippocratic ethic revisited. In: Bulger RJ (ed) In search of the modern Hippocrates. University of Iowa, Iowa City
6. Compiled-from News Services (1995) Patients' care seldom matches their wishes: Efforts to prolong life cause suffering for dying, Study finds, St. Louis Post-Dispatch, 22 November
7. Connors AF Jr, Dawson NV (1995) A controlled trial to improve care for seriously ill hospitalized patients: The study to understand prognoses and preferences for outcomes and risks of treatment (SUPPORT). JAMA 274(20):1591-1598
8. Lo B (1995) Improving care near the end of life: Why is it so hard? JAMA 274(20): 1634-1636
9. Kassirer JP (1994) Incorporating patients' preferences into medical decisions. N Engl J Med 330(26):1895-1896
10. Konopad E, Noseworthy TW, Johnston R et al (1995) Quality of life measures before and one year after admission to an intensive care unit. Crit Care Med 23(10):1653-1659
11. Eiseman B (1995) Independence, pain relief rated top therapeutic goals: Elderly emphasize quality of life over duration. General Surgery & Laparoscopy News, p 1
12. Testa MA, Simonson DC (1996) Assessment of quality-of-life outcomes. Curr Concepts 334(13):835-840
13. Alpers A, Lo B (1995) When is CPR futile? JAMA 273(2):156-158
14. Curtis R, Park DR, Krone MR et al (1995) Use of the medical futility rationale in do-not attempt-resuscitation orders. JAMA 273(2):124-128
15. Luce JM (1995) Physicians do not have a responsibility to provide futile or unreasonable care if a patient or family insists. Crit Care Med 23(4):760-766
16. Civetta JM (1996) A practical approach to futile care. Bull Am Coll Surg 81(2):24-29
17. Barrett-Connor Y, Stuenkel CA (1998) Questions of life and death in old age. JAMA 279: 622-623
18. Ramsey P (1995) Quoted by Farley MA in the Santa Clara Lectures. Santa Clara University, Santa Clara 1:1-15
19. Johnson D, Wilson M, Cavanaugh B et al (1998) Measuring the ability to meet family needs in an intensive care unit. Crit Care Med 26:266-271
20. Harvey MA (1998) Evolving toward – but not to – meeting family needs. Crit Care Med 726:206-207
21. Bone RC (1996) Sir Isaac Newton, sepsis, SIRS, and CARS. Crit Care Med 24;7:1125-28
22. Dellinger RP, Zimmerman JL, Taylor RW et al (1998) Effects of inhaled nitric oxide in patients with acute respiratory distress syndrome. Results of a randomized phase II trial. Crit Care Med 26:15-23
23. Mathisen DJ, Kuo EY, Hahn C et al (1998) Inhaled nitric oxide for adult respiratory distress syndrome following pulmonary resection. Ann Thorac Surg (in press)
24. Leape LL (1994) Error in medicine. JAMA 212:1851-57
25. Percy W (1997) Quoted by Goodwin in CHAOS and the limits of modern medicine. JAMA 278:1399-1400

26. Goodwin JS (1997) CHAOS and the limits of modern medicine. JAMA 278:1399-1400
27. Zimmerman J, Knaus W, Wagner D et al (1996) A comparison of risks and outcomes for patients with organ system failure: 1982-1990. Crit Care Med 24:10:1633-1641
28. Christou N, Meakins J, Gordon J et al (1995) The delayed hypersensitivity response and host resistance in surgical patients 20 years later. Ann Surg 222(4):534-548
29. Offner P, Moore F, Sauaia A, Moore E (1998) Temporal trends in postinjury MOF incidence and outcome. J Trauma (in press)
30. Regel G, Lobenhoffer P, Grotz M et al (1995) Treatment results of patients with multiple trauma: An analysis of 3406 cases treated between 1972 and 1991 at a German level I trauma center. J Trauma 38(1):70-78
31. Trentz O, Oestern HJ, Hempelmann G et al (1978) Kriterien für die Operabilität von Polytraumatisierten. Unfallchirurg 81:451-458
32. Pape HC, Kolk M, Paffrath T et al (1993) Primary intramedullary femur fixation in multiple trauma patients with associated lung contusion – a cause of post-traumatic ARDS. J Trauma 43:574-580
33. Schultz SG (1996) Homeostasis, Humpty Dumpty and integrative biology. News Physiol Sci 11:238-246
34. Buchman TG (1996) Physiologic stability and physiologic state. J Trauma 41(4):599-605
35. Thomas L (1970) Adaptive aspects of inflammation. Third Symposium International Inflammation Club. Excerptia Medica 107, Upjohn Co, Kalamazoo
36. Weiss A, Miller LJ (1998) Halting the march of the immune defenses. Science 280:179
37. Fuchs VR (1968) The growing demand for medical care. New Engl J Med 279:192
38. Fox M, Lipton HI (1983) The decision to perform cardiopulmonary resuscitation. New Engl J Med 309:607
39. Moser RH (1983) The intellectual imperative and its prodigious progeny. J Chron Dis 36:414
40. Barger-Lux MJ, Heaney RP (1986) For better and worse: The technological imperative in health care. Soc Sci Med 22(12):1313-1320

Cerebral Resuscitation 2000 A.D.

P. SAFAR

As the brain is the most vulnerable vital organ, the clinical and socioeconomic importance of cerebral resuscitation is obvious. After the global brain ischaemia (GBI) of cardiac arrest (CA), the focal brain ischaemia (FBI) of stroke, or traumatic brain injury (TBI), we must aim for "good outcome" in terms of CPC 1 (cerebral performance category 1) (normal) or CPC 2 (moderate disability). In addition, we must learn to prevent long-term survival with "poor" outcome, i.e., CPC 3 (severe disability but conscious), CPC 4 (coma, persistent vegetative state), or CPC 5 (brain death or death). Thus, we must differentiate between overall and cerebral performance categories (OPC 1-5 vs CPC 1-5) [1].

Cerebral protection-preservation by hypothermia (Hth) during elective circulatory arrest for heart or brain surgery has been researched since the 1950s. We extended in 1961 the cardiopulmonary resuscitation (CPR) system to the cardiopulmonary cerebral resuscitation (CPCR) system [1], and began in 1970 with systematic cerebral resuscitation research for CA [2]. All 3 phases of CPCR, basic-, advanced-, and prolonged life support (BLS, ALS, PLS), need to be oriented toward preservation and resuscitation of the brain [1, 2]. The discoveries around 1970 by Hossmann and by Safar initiated cerebral resuscitation research by an increasing number of investigators [2]. Hossmann noted that the majority of cat brain neurons can recover after GBI of 1 h [3]. Safar [4, 5] found that after prolonged GBI in monkeys or CA in dogs, brain-oriented extracerebral life support [1, 2, 4] and cerebral blood flow (CBF) promoting measures [5] and other measures of brain-oriented extracerebral life support can improve outcome. Results in GBI and CA models have led to renewed research efforts into neuron-saving measures also after FBI [6] and TBI [7]. The encephalopathy after ischaemic or traumatic insult is multifactorial, which requires novel multifaceted therapies [2].

We must differentiate between *protection* (treatment initiated before the insult) and *preservation* (treatment during the insult), vs *resuscitation* (treatment to reverse the insult and support recovery). Treatment effects may differ between the temporary complete GBI of CA, as opposed to the incomplete GBI of shock, the permanent incomplete FBI of stroke, or the many different types of TBI. Studies in small animals (e.g., gerbils, rats) which are low on the phylogenetic scale give less relevant results than studies in large animals (e.g. monkeys, dogs, pigs) in which long-term control of extracerebral organ function after co-ma-inducing insults is possible [2, 8]. Prolonged, post-insult intensive care is crucial, because after CA, FBI or TBI, the encephalopathy matures slowly, over several days. Differences in details of animal models can give different outcome results.

In clinical trials of novel resuscitation methods, we must differentiate be-tween studies designed to evaluate feasibility and side effects, which are essen-tial after positive animal outcome studies, and studies aimed at statistically de-termining in patients effects on outcome of different treatments. Randomized clinical outcome studies of novel emergency resuscitation methods have given unconvincing results because of numerous uncontrollable factors effecting re-covery of the brain [2]. This brief review will focus on cerebral recovery in terms of outcome after cerebral ischaemia or trauma.

Global brain ischaemia (GBI)

Until recently, the temporary complete GBI of normothermic CA – longer than 5 min of VF or exsanguination-induced no-flow or 2 min of asphyxia-induced no-flow [9] – followed by restoration of spontaneous normotension with CPR, has invariably resulted in varying degrees of brain damage, in spite of prolonged standard life support. During arrest, ATP stores become exhausted in 5 min and complicated chemical cascades set the stage for later cell death. Anoxia induces glutamate release, intracellular calcium loading, and activation of proteases and other destructive enzymes. This sets the stage for even more complicated cas-cades during reperfusion-reoxygenation, which include production of destruc-tive free radicals [10]. This sequence results in necrosis or apoptosis of selec-tively vulnerable neurons [2, 8, 11]. Restoration of cerebral blood flow (CBF) after prolonged CA seems hampered by a no-reflow phenomenon only when reperfusion is with low pressure. After CA and normotensive or hypertensive reperfusion, transient diffuse cerebral hyperemia is followed at 1-2 h by pro-tracted multifocal hypoperfusion, i.e., it is accompanied by a return of cerebral oxygen metabolism ($CMRO_2$) to or above baseline, creating a supply/demand mismatching [12-14]. The morphologic damage matures over several days (15-18), resulting in functional partial or complete recovery, persistent vegetative state (PVS), or brain death. Permanent brain damage can be predicted by three days after CA and seems certain after 1 week [19, 20].

Animal and patient data since the 1970s have led to the conclusion that even without specific cerebral resuscitation measures, permanent post-CA brain dam-age is less likely to occur if arrest time and CPR (low flow) times are short; if standard external CPR resistant cases are reperfused with the physiologically more potent open-chest CPR [21-24] or emergency (portable) cardiopulmonary bypass (CPB) technique [25, 26]; if accidental spontaneous mild Hth is not re-versed by rewarming [27]; and if during coma brain-oriented extracerebral life support is applied [1, 2, 5, 28, 29]. The latter includes control of normal (or mildly low) temperature, and normal MAP, PaO_2, $PaCO_2$, pHa, electrolyte balance and blood glucose [30, 31].

Thiopental loading, after some promising data in animals [32-35] and patients [36], was evaluated in the first randomized clinical CPCR outcome study, the multicenter international brain resuscitation clinical trial I (BRCT I) (1979-1984) [37]. The barbiturate treatment did not statistically increase the overall proportion of patients with good cerebral outcome, but a subgroup of severely insulted patients showed numerical benefit from thiopental.

Calcium entry blocker therapy with lidoflazine after CA improved cerebral outcome in dogs [38]. In the BRCT II (1984-1989) [39], there was again no statistically significant difference in the overall proportion of patients who achieved good cerebral outcome with vs without lidoflazine. Retrospective analysis, however, of only those patients without post-CA hypotension or rearrest, found the lidoflazine group with significantly more survivors with good cerebral outcome than the control group [40]. Similarly, after the calcium entry blocker nimodipine showed benefit in monkeys after GBI [41], it demonstrated no statistical overall improvement in a clinical trial [42], but a subgroup showed benefit of nimodipine. It seems impossible to identify patients within the therapeutic window. Proof of no or only moderate benefit in some cases seems impossible with randomized clinical outcome studies of CA patients. A breakthrough effect would be so obvious that randomly withholding the novel treatment raises questions of ethics. CA-outcome studies in reproducible large animal models with intensive care, should be accepted as "clinical trials" and be followed by feasibility and side effect studies in sick humans, before general use.

Other drugs were evaluated in incomplete forebrain ischaemia rat models [43, 44], the asphyxial cardiac arrest rat model [45], GBI models in monkeys [8, 16, 34, 35, 41] and the clinically most relevant CA models in dogs with intensive care and outcome evaluation [8, 25, 38, 48]. Drugs which showed no significant improvement in outcome included lidocaine, antioxidant (free radical scavenger) cocktails, the excitatory amino acid receptor blocker MK-801, and a neuron specific omega calcium entry blocker [2]. Some drugs which caused reduced hippocampal damage in rat models showed no benefit in dog CA models. Exploration of physical cerebral resuscitation after CA has been more promising.

CBF promotion with hypertension, haemodilution and/or heparinization, normalized post-CA CBF [46, 47] and improved cerebral outcome [4, 48]. A brief hypertensive bout (spontaneously as the result of epinephrine given during CPR, or induced by a vasopressor) improved cerebral recovery in dogs [48]. In patients, hypotensive reperfusion was associated with worse and hypertensive reperfusion with improved cerebral outcome [49, 50]. A brief hypertensive bout during or after restoration of spontaneous circulation should be part of standard CPCR [4, 46-50]. Normalizing global CBF in patients after CA in relation to global $CMRO_2$ would be possible by titrating arterial pressure, haematocrit and

$PaCO_2$ to normalize superior jugular bulb (cerebral venous) PO_2 (normal value is ≥ 30 mmHg).

Mild resuscitative Hth is the second physical treatment documented recently as highly effective [2]. Hth should be induced as soon as possible, ideally during CPR steps A-B-C; the optimal duration remains to be clarified. Mild Hth (T 33-36°C), is best after CA, but for protection-preservation during CA, moderate (28-32°C), deep (11-27°C), profound (5-10°C), or ultra profound Hth (< 5°C) is increasingly more effective. In the 1950s, moderate Hth (30°C) was introduced to protect-preserve the brain during circulatory arrest of open-heart or neurologic surgery [51]. Uncontrolled observations with resuscitative (post-CA) moderate Hth were followed by abandonment of this treatment because of difficulty in cooling adults, arrhythmias, and pulmonary infection with prolonged moderate Hth. In 1987, Safar and his associates discovered in outcome data of dog studies that after prolonged CA, protective-preservative accidental mild Hth correlated with good cerebral outcome [25, 27]. This was followed by 5 controlled resuscitative (post-arrest) mild Hth trials in dogs, which all documented the outcome benefit of mild cooling early post-arrest [52-56]. Simultaneously and independently, other investigators documented protective-preservative as well as resuscitative benefit from mild Hth in incomplete forebrain ischemia rat models [57, 58]. The best outcome so far achieved in dogs has been after normothermic VF CA of 11 min using a combination of mild Hth from restoration of spontaneous circulation to 12 h, plus promotion of CBF. This resulted in complete functional recovery and histology near-normal [56]. These result were better than with each treatment alone in historic comparisons [55]. A multicenter clinical study of mild Hth after CA has been initiated by F. Sterz (Vienna, Austria). The mechanism by which mild Hth saves neurons after GBI is multifactorial. Reduction in $CMRO_2$ is minimal [59]. There is synergism of preserved ATP, reduced lactacidosis, reduced free fatty acid production, improved glucose utilization, mitigation of abnormal ion fluxes; tightening of membranes; and decreased excitotoxicity, deleterious enzyme reactions, and free radical reactions [2, 52]. Induction of Hth can be by a variety of means, in this order of rapidity: intracarotid cold flush, CPB, peritoneal cold irrigation, veno-venous or arterio-venous external blood cooling, whole body ice water immersion (impractical), external head-neck-trunk cooling with cooling garments or ice bags [2, 60, 61].

Uncontrolled accidental Hth, with shivering, vasoconstriction and sympathetic discharge, can be deleterious. Controlled mild Hth under poikilothermia (induced by insult or drugs), is easy to induce and safe. For trauma patients in hypovolemic shock, there is a discrepancy between accidental uncontrolled Hth correlating with poor outcome in patients and increased survival time and rate in animals with controlled mild or moderate Hth during shock [62, 63]. The most vulnerable organs in shock, the vasoconstricting abdominal viscera, seem protected by Hth [62, 63]. The previously healthy brain protects itself with vasodilation. In prolonged normothermic haemorrhagic shock with MAP 30-40 mmHg for about 1 h, experiments in rats [64] and monkeys [65] have shown no evidence of even subtle brain damage.

Suspended animation (SA) for delayed resuscitation, a concept introduced by Safar and Bellamy in 1984, has been under investigation at the University of Pittsburgh since 1988 [66], now with a multicenter laboratory study, coordinated by Safar and Tisherman, supported by the U.S. Department of Defense. SA is "protection-preservation of the whole organism, during 1 h or longer of clinical death, for transport and resuscitative surgery (or otherwise infeasible elective surgical repair) without pulse, followed by delayed resuscitation to complete recovery without brain damage" [66]. We are working on a method which allows induction of SA in the field within seconds, with a combination of mild Hth and a still to be determined drug cocktail, flushed via an aortic balloon catheter [67] into brain and heart [68]. The flush-SA would then be followed, as soon as possible, by profound hypothermic circulatory arrest [69], induced and reversed with portable emergency CPB [70]. Using the latter, with brain T at 5-10°C, we have so far achieved complete functional and histologic brain recovery of dogs after 1 h of severe normothermic haemorrhage shock, followed by 1 h of profound hypothermic no-flow [69].

Focal brain ischaemia (FBI)

Acute embolic or thrombotic FBI is common in the elderly. The traditional observation-rehabilitation-only attitudes towards stroke are giving way to a resuscitative approach. There are, however, problems with clinical outcome trials in stroke patients. Neuron-saving possibilities of limited efficacy have been observed in experimental or clinical sudden obstruction of the middle cerebral artery (MCA). The goal is to increase regional CBF in the partially ischaemic penumbra zone, thereby trying to reduce infarct size and neurologic deficit. Some are exploring the use of iv tissue plasminogen activator (tPA) therapy [71, 72]; thrombolysis directly into the MCA; and emergency infarctectomy to prevent focal swelling of dead tissue to cause herniation. Arterial bypass surgery is controversial [73]. The threshold for energy failure threatening viability of neurons is about 1/5 of normal CBF (namely a regional CBF reduction from about 50 to 10 ml/100 g/min). The necrotic focus depends on the first 20 min; revascularization should be attempted within 1 h; some neurons can still be saved in the penumbra zone within 6 h. Treatments which reduced infarct size in experimental temporary or permanent MCA occlusion include: induced hypertension [74-78] (if induced late may provoke haemorrhage); haemodilution [79, 80]; barbiturate [81-86]; calcium entry blocker [87, 88]; isofluorane [86, 89]; and hypothermia [90, 91]. The aminosteroid Trilazad is under investigation. There might emerge around 2000 A.D. novel aggressive tissue saving efforts, begun in the prehospital arena, and continued via emergency room and radiology to the ICU. For rehabilitation of chronic post-stroke disability, the University of Pittsburgh's transplant programs recently conducted the first transplant of engineered human neurons into stroke tissue sites.

Traumatic brain injury (TBI)

Brain tissue responds to a variety of multifocal or global mechanical insults first with low regional CBF and then with brain swelling as a result of oedema and perhaps hyperemia [7, 92, 93]. That can lead to brain herniation, apnea, and intractable hypotension. TBI induces primary necrosis in the focus and can cause distant cells to undergo apoptosis. The secondary derangements in the brain can include any of the molecular and cellular tissue reactions identified for CA above. In addition, there is rupture of cell membranes and blood brain barrier, free heme which is neurotoxic, and more inflammatory response [7]. Molecular and cellular mechanisms are now being studied predominantly in rat models of cortical contusion [7]. Early decision on emergency craniotomy for removal of haematomas and dead tissue is crucial.

Resuscitation from TBI-induced coma should start in the field by a bystander immediately providing airway control (moderate head tilt plus jaw thrust) and exhaled air ventilation for "impact apnea" [94]. Then, field rescuers should provide the comatose TBI patient with rapid intubation [95] (without causing bucking), and prevention of hypotension, hypoxaemia, hypercapnia, hyperthermia, seizures, and aspiration – and start inducing mild Hth. In the ICU, delayed brain swelling and herniation can often be prevented by ICP monitoring (by intraventricular catheter) and ICP control [96] below the 20-25 mmHg threshold. Presently recommended is a sequence of CSF drainage, head elevation, paralysis, controlled ventilation (brief hyperventilation, otherwise normocapnia), osmotherapy, seizure control, barbiturate, and hypothermia.

Resuscitative Hth for TBI is based on the studies of Rosomoff in the 1950s in dogs. Lethal ICP rise from brain swelling can best be prevented by moderate Hth [92]. Large animal outcome models allowing ICP control are needed to conquer ICP rise during rewarming. After loss of outcome models in monkeys [97], the long-term outcome model of TBI in dogs is available [98, 99]. In that dog model, moderate Hth was found more effective than mild Hth to keep ICP normal [98], but if prolonged to 48 h can be associated with coagulopathy and pulmonary problems [99]. In comatose TBI patients, moderate Hth for 24 h was used without complications and was associated with a significant improvement in outcome in a single center study [100]. This study has led to a multicenter study, the results of which are now being analyzed.

Conclusions

Currently, the measures available for cerebral resuscitation from CA, with proven efficacy in animal models and suggestive positive data in humans, are: 1) brain oriented extracerebral life support; 2) CBF promotion with hypertensive bout followed by titrated mild hypertension, haemodilution and $PaCO_2$ controls; and 3) mild Hth started as early as possible and continued for at least 12 h.

These measures I recommend for clinical use. Searches for additional efficacy enhancing drug treatments continue.

References

1. Safar P, Bircher NG (1988) Cardiopulmonary-cerebral resuscitation, guidelines by the World Federation of Societies of Anaesthesiologists (WFSA), 3rd edn. WB Saunders, London
2. Safar P (1977) Resuscitation of the ischemic brain. In: Albin MS (ed) Textbook of neuroanesthesia with neurosurgical and neuroscience perspectives. McGraw-Hill, New York, pp 557-593
3. Hossmann KA, Sato K (1970) Recovery of neuronal function after prolonged cerebral ischemia. Science 168:375-376
4. Safar P (1975) Resuscitation of the arrested brain. In: Safar P (ed) Advances in CPR. Springer, New York 27-29:177
5. Safar P, Stezoski SW, Nemoto EM (1976) Amelioration of brain damage after 12 minutes of cardiac arrest in dogs. Arch Neurol 33:91-95
6. Gelabert HA, Moore WS (1994) Occlusive cerebrovascular disease. Medical and surgical considerations. In: Cottrell JE, Smith DS (eds) Anesthesia and neurosurgery. CV Mosby, St. Louis, pp 448
7. Kochanek PM, Clark RSB (1998) Pharmacologic augmentation of endogenous neuroprotective responses after traumatic brain injury. In: JL Vincent (ed) Yearbook of intensive care and emergency medicine. Springer, Berlin, pp 679-687
8. Safar P, Gisvold SE, Vaagenes P et al (1982) Long-term animal models for the study of global brain ischemia. In: Wauquier A et al (eds) Protection of tissues against hypoxia. Elsevier, Amsterdam, pp 147-170
9. Safar P, Paradis NA (1996) Asphyxial cardiac arrest. In: Paradis NA, Halperin HR, Nowak RM (eds) Cardiac arrest. The science and practice of resuscitation medicine vol. 39. Williams and Wilkins, Philadelphia, pp 702-726
10. Traystman RJ, Kirsh JR, Koehler RC (1991) Oxygen radical mechanisms of brain injury following ischemia and reperfusion. J App Physiol 71:1185-1195
11. MacManus JP, Linnik MD (1997) Gene expression induced by cerebral ischemia: An apoptotic perspective. J Cereb Blood Flow Metab 17:815-832
12. Lind B, Snyder J, Safar P (1975) Total brain ischemia in dogs. Cerebral physiologic and metabolic changes after 15 minutes of circulatory arrest. Resuscitation 4:97-113
13. Sterz F, Leonov Y, Safar P et al (1992) Multifocal cerebral blood flow by Xe-CT and global cerebral metabolism after prolonged cardiac arrest in dogs. Reperfusion with open-chest CPR or cardiopulmonary bypass. Resuscitation 24:27-47
14. Oku K, Kuboyama K, Safar P et al (1994) Cerebral and systemic arteriovenous oxygen monitoring after cardiac arrest. Inadequate cerebral oxygen delivery. Resuscitation 27:141-152
15. Brierley JB, Meldrum BS, Brown AW (1973) The threshold and neuropathology of cerebral anoxic-ischemic cell change. Arch Neurol 29:367-37
16. Nemoto EM, Bleyaert AL, Stezoski SW et al (1977) Global brain ischemia: A reproducible monkey model. Stroke 8:558-564
17. Radovsky A, Safar P, Sterz F et al (1995) Regional prevalence and distribution of ischemic neurons in dog brains 96 hours after cardiac arrest of 0 to 20 minutes. Stroke 26:2127-2134
18. Radovsky A, Katz L, Ebmeyer U et al (1997) Ischemic neurons in rat brains after 6, 8, or 10 minutes of transient hypoxic ischemia. Toxicol Pathol 25:500-505
19. Mullie A, Buylaert W, Michen N et al (1988) Predictive value of Glasgow coma score for awakening after out-of-hospital cardiac arrest. Lancet i:137-140

20. Edgren E, Hedstrand U, Kelsey S et al (1994) Assessment of neurological prognosis in coma-
    tose survivors of cardiac arrest. Lancet 343:1055-1059
21. Del Guercio LRM, Feins NR, Cohn JD (1965) A comparison of blood flow during external
    and internal cardiac massage in man. Circulation 31 [Suppl 1]:171-180
22. Bircher NG, Safar P (1985) Cerebral preservation during cardiopulmonary resuscitation. Crit
    Care Med 13:185-190
23. Bircher N, Safar P (1984) Open-chest CPR: an old method whose time has returned. Am J
    Emerg Med 2:568-571
24. Hachimi-Idrissi S, Leeman J, Hubloue Y et al (1997) Open chest cardiopulmonary resuscita-
    tion in out-of-hospital cardiac arrest. Resuscitation 35:151-156
25. Safar P, Abramson NS, Angelos M et al (1990) Emergency cardiopulmonary bypass for re-
    suscitation from prolonged cardiac arrest. Am J Emerg Med 8:55-67
26. Tisherman SA, Safar P, Abramson N et al (1991) Emergency cardiopulmonary bypass for re-
    suscitation from CPR-resistant cardiac arrest: Preliminary report on clinical feasibility study.
    Prehosp Disaster Med 6:206 (abstract)
27. Safar P (1988) Resuscitation from clinical death: Patho-physiologic limits and therapeutic po-
    tentials. Crit Care Med 16:923-941
28. American Heart Association (1992) Guidelines for cardiopulmonary resuscitation and emer-
    gency cardiac care. JAMA 268:2171-2302
29. European Resuscitation Council (1998) Advanced life support working group of the Euro-
    pean Resuscitation Council. Brit Med J 316:1863-1869
30. Sieber FE, Traystman RJ (1991) Special issues, glucose and the brain. Crit Care Med 20:
    104-114
31. Katz, Wang Y, Ebmeyer U et al (1995) Dextrose plus insulin after cardiac arrest (CA) im-
    proves cerebral outcome in rats. Acad Emerg Med 2:381 (abstract)
32. Yatsu FM, Diamond I, Graziana C et al (1972) Experimental brain ischemia: protection from
    irreversible damage with a rapid-acting barbiturate (methohexital). Stroke 3:726-732
33. Smith AL, Hoff JT, Nielson SL et al (1974) Barbiturate protection against cerebral infarction.
    Stroke 5:1-7
34. Bleyaert AL, Nemoto EM, Safar P et al (1978) Thiopental amelioration of brain damage after
    global ischemia in monkeys. Anesthesiology 49:390-398
35. Gisvold SE, Safar P, Hendrickx HHL et al (1984) Thiopental treatment after global brain is-
    chemia in pigtailed monkeys. Anesthesiology 60:88-96
36. Breivik H, Safar P, Sands P et al (1978) Clinical feasibility trials of barbiturate therapy after
    cardiac arrest. Crit Care Med 6:228-244
37. Brain Resuscitation Clinical Trial I Study Group (1986) Randomized clinical study of
    thiopental loading in comatose survivors of cardiac arrest. N Engl J Med 314:397-403
38. Vaagenes P, Cantadore R, Safar P et al (1984) Amelioration of brain damage by lidoflazine
    after prolonged ventricular fibrillation cardiac arrest in dogs. Crit Care Med 12:846-855
39. Brain Resuscitation Clinical Trial II Study Group (1991) A randomized clinical study of a
    calcium-entry blocker (lidoflazine) in the treatment of comatose survivors of cardiac arrest. N
    Engl J Med 324:1225-1231
40. Abramson N, Kelsey S, Safar P et al (1992) Simpson's paradox and clinical trials: What you
    find is not necessarily what you prove. Ann Emerg Med 21:1480-1482
41. Steen PA, Gisvold SE, Milde JH et al (1985) Nimodipine improves outcome when given after
    complete cerebral ischemia in primates. Anesthesiology 62:406-414
42. Roine RO, Kaste M, Kinnamen A et al (1990) Nimodipine after resuscitation from out-of-
    hospital ventricular fibrillation: A placebo controlled, double-blind randomized trial. JAMA
    3171-3177
43. Smith ML, Bendek G, Dahlgren N et al (1984) Models for studying long-term recovery fol-
    lowing forebrain ischemia in the rat. A two vessel occlusion model. Acta Neurol Scand 69:
    385-401
44. Siesjo BK (1988) Mechanisms of ischemic brain damage. Crit Care Med 16:954-963

45. Katz L, Ebmeyer U, Safar P et al (1995) Outcome model of asphyxial cardiac arrest in rats. J Cereb Blood Flow Metab 15:1032-1039
46. Hossman KA, Lechtape-Gruter H, Hossman V (1973) The role of cerebral blood flow for the recovery of the brain after prolonged ischemia. J Neurol 204:281-299
47. Leonov Y, Sterz F, Safar P et al (1992) Hypertension with hemodilution prevents multifocal cerebral hypoperfusion after cardiac arrest in dogs. Stroke 23:45-53
48. Sterz F, Leonov Y, Safar P et al (1990) Hypertension with or without hemodilution after cardiac arrest in dogs. Stroke 21:1178-1184
49. Martin DR, Persse D, Brown CG et al (1993) Relation between initial post-resuscitation systolic blood pressure and neurologic outcome following cardiac arrest. Ann Emerg Med 33: 206 (abstract)
50. Spivey WH, Abramson NS, Safar P et al (1991) Correlation of blood pressure with mortality and neurologic recovery in comatose postresuscitation patients. Ann Emerg Med 20:453 (abstract)
51. Dripps RD (ed) (1956) The physiology of induced hypothermia. National Academy of Sciences, Washington DC
52. Leonov Y, Sterz F, Safar P et al (1990) Mild cerebral hypothermia during and after cardiac arrest improves neurologic outcome in dogs. J Cereb Blood Flow Metab 10:57-70
53. Sterz F, Safar P, Tisherman S et al (1991) Mild hypothermic cardiopulmonary resuscitation improves outcome after prolonged cardiac arrest in dogs. Crit Care Med 19:379-389
54. Weinrauch V, Safar P, Tisherman S et al (1992) Beneficial effect of mild hypothermia and detrimental effect of deep hypothermia after cardiac arrest in dogs. Stroke 23:1454-1462
55. Kuboyama K, Safar P, Radovsky A et al (1993) Delay in cooling negates the beneficial effect of mild resuscitative cerebral hypothermia after cardiac arrest in dogs: A prospective, randomized, controlled study. Crit Care Med 21:1348-1358
56. Safar P, Xiao F, Radovsky A et al (1996) Improved cerebral resuscitation from cardiac arrest in dogs with mild hypothermia plus blood flow promotion. Stroke 27:105-113
57. Busto R, Dietrich WD, Globus MY et al (1989) Postischemic moderate hypothermia inhibits CA 1 hippocampal ischemic neuronal injury. Neurosci Lett 101:299-304
58. Coimbra C, Drake M, Boris-Moller R et al (1996) Long-lasting neuroprotective effect of postischemic hypothermia and treatment with an antiinflammatory/antipyretic drug. Evidence for chronic encephalopathic processes following ischemia. Stroke 27:1578-1585
59. Oku K, Sterz F, Safar P et al (1993) Mild hypothermia after cardiac arrest in dogs does not affect postarrest multifocal cerebral hypoperfusion. Stroke 24:1590-1598
60. Tisherman S, Safar P, Sterz F et al (1991) Methods for rapid induction of resuscitative cerebral hypothermia. Prehosp Disaster Med 6:207 (abstract)
61. Safar P, Klain M, Tisherman S (1996) Selective brain cooling after cardiac arrest. Crit Care Med 24:911-914
62. Kim SH, Stezoski SW, Safar P et al (1997) Hypothermia and minimal fluid resuscitation increase survival after uncontrolled hemorrhagic shock in rats. J Trauma 42:213-222
63. Takasu A, Stezoski SW, Stezoski J et al (1998) Mild or moderate hypothermia, but not increased oxygen breathing, increases long-term survival after uncontrolled hemorrhagic shock in rats. Acad Emerg Med 5(5):470 (abstract)
64. Carrillo P, Takasu A, Safar P et al (1998) Prolonged severe hemorrhagic shock and resuscitation in rats does not cause subtle brain damage. J Trauma (in press)
65. Bar-Joseph G, Safar P, Saito R et al (1991) Monkey model of severe volume-controlled hemorrhagic shock with resuscitation to outcome. Resuscitation 22:27-43
66. Bellamy R, Safar P, Tisherman SA et al (1996) Suspended animation for delayed resuscitation. Crit Care Med 24[Suppl]:S24-47
67. Safar P, Stezoski SW, Klain M (1995) Portable and modular cardiopulmonary bypass apparatus and associated aortic balloon catheter and associated method. Patent 5,383,854
68. Woods R, Takasu A, Tisherman S et al (1998) Hypothermic aortic arch flush for cerebral preservation during prolonged exsanguination cardiac arrest in dogs. Abstract submitted to J Trauma for EAST meeting 1999

69. Capone A, Safar P, Radovsky A et al (1996) Complete recovery after normothermic hemorrhagic shock and profound hypothermic circulatory arrest of 60 minutes in dogs. J Trauma 40:388-394
70. Safar P, Stezoski SW, Klain M (1994) Portable and modular cardiopulmonary bypass apparatus and associated aortic balloon catheter and associated method. Patent 5,308,320
71. Meyer JS, Gilroy J, Barnhart MI et al (1964) Anticoagulants plus streptokinase therapy in progressive stroke. JAMA 189:373
72. The National Institute of Neurological Disorders and Stroke, rt-PA Stroke Study Group (1995) Tissue plasminogen activator for acute ischemic stroke. New Engl J Med 333: 1581-1587
73. EC/IC Bypass Study Group (1985) Failure of extracranial-intracranial arterial bypass to reduce the risk of ischemic stroke: Results of an international randomized trial. New Engl J Med 313:1191-1200
74. Hayashi S, Nehls DG, Kieck CF et al (1984) Beneficial effects of induced hypertension on experimental stroke in awake monkeys. J Neurosurg 60:151-157
75. Hope DT, Branston MM, Symon L (1977) Restoration of neurological function with induced hypertension in acute experimental cerebral ischemia. Acta Neurol Scand [Suppl]64:506-507
76. Wise G, Sutter R, Burkholder J (1972) The treatment of brain ischemia with vasopressor drugs. Stroke 3:135-140
77. Hoff JT (1986) Cerebral circulation. J Neurosurg 65:579-591
78. Muizelaar JP, Becker DP (1986) Induced hypertension for the treatment of cerebral ischemia after subarachnoid hemorrhage. Direct effect on cerebral blood flow. Surg Neurol 25:317-325
79. Heros RC, Korosue K (1989) Hemodilution for cerebral ischemia. Stroke 20:423-427
80. Kusunoki M, Kimura K, Nakamura M et al (1981) Effects of hematocrit variations on cerebral blood flow and oxygen transport in ischemic cerebrovascular disease. J Cereb Blood Flow Metab 1:413-417
81. Michenfelder JD, Milde HJ, Sundt TM (1976) Cerebral protection by barbiturate anesthesia. Use after middle cerebral artery occlusion in Java monkeys. Arch Neurol 33:345-350
82. Selman WR, Spetzler RF, Roessmann UR et al (1981) Barbiturate-induced coma therapy for focal cerebral ischemia, effect after temporary and permanent MCA occlusion. J Neurosurg 55:220-226
83. Hoff JT, Nishimura M, Newfield P (1982) Pentobarbital protection from cerebral infarction without suppression of edema. Stroke 13:623-628
84. Nussmeier NA, Arlund C, Slogoff S (1986) Neuropsychiatric complications after cardiopulmonary bypass: Cerebral protection by a barbiturate. Anesthesiology 64:165-170
85. Gelb AW, Floyd D, Lok P et al (1986) A prophylactic bolus of thiopental does not protect against prolonged focal cerebral ischemia. Can Anaesth Soc J 33:173-177
86. Warner D et al (1995) Low-dose pentobarbital reduces focal ischemic infarct volume in a magnitude similar to burst suppression. J Neurosurg Anesth 7:303 (abstract)
87. Allen GS, Ahn HS, Prezioso TJ et al (1984) Cerebral arterial spasm - A controlled trial of nimodipine in patients with subarachnoid hemorrhage. N Engl J Med 308:619-624
88. Gelmers HJ (1988) A controlled trial of nimodipine in acute ischemic stroke. N Engl J Med 318-203
89. Warner DS, Zhou JG, Ramani R et al (1991) Reversible focal ischemia in the rat: Effects of halothane, isoflurane and methohexital anesthesia. J Cereb Blood Flow Metab 11:794-802
90. Rosomoff HL (1957) Hypothermia and cerebral vascular lesions. II. Experimental middle cerebral artery interruption followed by induction of hypothermia. Arch Neurol Psychiatr 78:454-464
91. Morikawa E, Ginsberg MD, Dietrich WD et al (1992) The significance of brain temperature in focal cerebral ischemia: Histopathological consequences of middle cerebral artery occlusion in the rat. J Cereb Blood Flow Metab 12:380-389
92. Rosomoff HL, Kochanek PM, Clark R et al (1996) Resuscitation from severe brain trauma. Crit Care Med 24[Suppl]:S48-56

93. White RJ, Likavek MJ (1992) The diagnosis and initial management of head injury. N Engl J Med 327-1507

94. Levine JE, Becker DP (1979) Reversal of incipient brain death from head injury apnea at the scene of accident. N Engl J Med 301-109

95. Stept WJ, Safar P (1970) Rapid induction/intubation for prevention of gastric content aspiration. Anesth Analg 49:633-636

96. Bullock R, Chestnut RM, Clifton G et al (1996) Guidelines for the management of severe head injury. Joint Section on Neurotrauma and Critical Care. New York, The Brain Trauma Foundation. Eur J Emerg Med 3:109-127

97. Gennarelli TA et al (1982) Physiological response to angular acceleration of the head. In: Grossman RG, Gildenberg PL (eds) Head injury, basic and clinical aspects. Raven, New York, pp 129-140

98. Pomeranz S, Safar P, Radovsky A et al (1993) The effect of resuscitative moderate hypothermia following epidural brain compression on cerebral damage in a canine outcome model. J Neurosurg 79:241-251

99. Ebmeyer U, Safar P, Radovsky A et al (1998) Moderate hypothermia for 48 hours after temporary epidural brain compression injury in a canine outcome model. J Neurotrauma 15: 323-336

100. Marion DW, Penrod LE, Kelsey SF et al (1997) Treatment of traumatic brain injury with moderate hypothermia. N Engl J Med 336:540-546

Early Goal-Directed Invasive and Noninvasive Monitoring of High Risk Postoperative and Septic Surgical Patients Improves Outcome

W.C. SHOEMAKER

Circulatory assessment by invasive monitoring for high risk postoperative patients

Diagnosis of shock at the very earliest time may be difficult because shock is routinely recognized by imprecise signs and subjective symptoms that are observer-dependant. By contrast, shock is easy to recognize in the late stages when therapy may be ineffective. If shock could be recognized earlier and treated more vigorously to physiologic endpoints, improved outcome might be anticipated. A major problem is that shock is routinely recognized by unstable vital signs such as falling blood pressure and tachycardia plus altered mental status, cold clammy skin, weak thready pulse, and other subjective signs and symptoms. However, it is not until after the patient reaches the ICU that haemodynamic measurements are made.

Invasive pulmonary artery Swan-Ganz catheter (PAC) was reported to improve outcome in the early postoperative period of high risk elective surgical and severely injured patients. However, Conners et al. [1] recently reported lack of effectiveness of the invasive monitoring shortly after ICU admission in critically ill late stage medical and surgical patients with organ failure; they found higher mortality with PAC in the initial care of a large series of high mortality medical patients with ARDS or multiple organ failure. Previous studies using physiologic targets in patients with myocardial infarction [2-4] and recent randomized controlled studies by Hayes et al. [5] and Gattinoni et al. [6] primarily on surgical patients admitted to ICUs after developing organ failures failed to show improved outcome or had worse outcome with invasive PAC. Conners et al. [1] did not have a plan of therapy. Improved outcome can not be expected if monitoring is done without changing therapy. If you order X-rays but don't see them or change therapy, does it improve patient care?

Therapy targeted at physiological goals given early [7-18], or prophylactically [8], was previously demonstrated to reduce mortality and organ failure. These differences in results are due to: a) definitions of the term "early", which to some mean early after ICU admission, to others early means shortly after the patient develops a potentially lethal organ failure, b) differences in the nature of circulatory dysfunction or failure in medical and surgical patients, and c) therapeutic aggressiveness in medical versus surgical problems. Fluid excess occurs in medical patients with peripheral and pulmonary oedema, chronic cardiac, pulmonary, and renal diseases, but the major problem in surgical patients is early recognition of hypovolaemia and titration of fluid therapy.

Recently a consensus conference [19] found insufficient evidence to fully determine whether PA catheter-guided therapy significantly alters outcome, but they recommended more prospective randomized clinical trials should be undertaken. This consensus conference was made of like-minded persons; those who disagreed, having done major work in early monitoring of trauma and high risk surgical patients, were eliminated. The consensus conference arrived at an ambiguous evaluation because they did not properly consider time factors but mixed early and late studies together. However, in a more insightful meta-analysis, Boyd and Bennett [20] found no outcome improvement in seven prospective randomized studies of patients who entered the ICU after organ failure or sepsis had occurred, but they noted significant outcome improvement in seven other randomized studies when PAC-directed therapy was given early or prophylactically [7-12, 18]. They concluded improved outcome is unlikely when ICU admission for PAC is delayed until organ failure occurs [20]. The ineffectiveness of monitoring or optimal therapy in the late stages after appearance of organ failure is not unexpected. Clearly time factors, which have been largely ignored, are the major unresolved issue. If these crucial time factors continue to be ignored, the next consensus conference may evaluate outcome effects of antibiotics sprinkled on a corpse.

Statement of the problem

Unresolved issues largely revolve around indications for monitoring, the definition of what is physiologically and clinically "early," and description of therapy. Indications and time limitations for PAC monitoring of critical illness, and for initiating, titrating, or discontinuing therapy have not been adequately evaluated nor widely accepted. Because invasive monitoring requires a critical care environment, early haemodynamic patterns are missed when the patient is admitted to the ICU late in the course of his illness. Understandably, considerable thought and discussion may influence the decision to use PAC; often decisions are made to observe, adjust medication dosages, or wait and see if there will be sufficient improvement to avoid invasive monitoring. When monitoring is started after periods of delay or after organ failure occurs, it is relatively late in the course of illness when oxygen debt is irreversible. Organ failures and death from oxygen debt after shock and trauma have been related to delays in correcting circulatory and perfusion deficiencies [21, 22].

Since early recognition and prompt therapy are crucial to outcome, the obvious answer is to develop methods and concepts for noninvasive monitoring that can be applied anywhere in the hospital including the emergency department (ED) as well as in the operating room (OR), hospital floors, and prehospital areas OR, and hospital floors. A multicomponent noninvasive haemodynamic monitoring was developed and tested for use within minutes of admission to the ED as an alternative to invasive monitoring. We found noninvasive monitoring systems: a) give similar information to that of the invasive monitoring with thermodilution catheters; b) provide continuous on-line real time displays of physiologic data; c) allow early recognition and correction of circulatory dysfunction; and d) provide for an integrated approach to cardiac, pulmonary, and tissue oxygenation. They are clinically acceptable alternatives for use when invasive monitoring is unavailable or as the front end of invasive monitoring. In the early stage of acute illness, both methods identified reversible low flow and poor tissue perfusion that were greater in nonsurvivors.

Multicomponent noninvasive monitoring

Noninvasive cardiac output combined with pulse oximetry and transcutaneous O_2 and CO_2, may be used for early warning of the three major circulatory components: cardiac, pulmonary, and tissue perfusion functions. They were used throughout the hospital including the emergency department (ED), operating room (OR), postanaesthesia recovery unit (PAR), intensive care unit (ICU), step-down units, and hospital floor; they provide continuous display of data that facilitates prompt recognition of circulatory abnormalities and allow titration of therapy. Earlier diagnosis allows therapy to be initiated sooner when time factors are crucial [23].

Noninvasive cardiac output monitoring

A new thoracic electrical bioimpedance device for continuous noninvasive cardiac output based on recently available hardware and software innovations was devised by Wang et al. [24, 25] and developed for clinical application (Renaissance Technology, Newtown PA). The noninvasive disposable prewired hydrogen electrodes were positioned on the skin and three ECG leads were placed across the precordium and left shoulder [24-28]. A 100 kHz, 4 mA alternating current was passed through the patient's thorax by the outer pairs of electrodes and the voltage was sensed by the inner pairs of electrodes; the voltage sensed by the inner electrodes captured the baseline impedance (Zo), the first derivative of the impedance waveform (dZ/dt), and the ECG. The ECG and bioimpedance signals were filtered with an all-integer-coefficient technology to decrease computation and signal processing time. The digital signal processing used time-frequency distributions to increase signal-to-noise ratios [25].

Comparison of bioimpedance and thermodilution cardiac outputs

Simultaneous measurements of cardiac output by thermodilution and the new bioimpedance method were compared in 2192 instances; the regression formula was $y = 0.85x + 0.50$; r was 0.85; r^2 was 0.73; and $p < 0.001$ [26-28]. The precision and bias was $-0.124 + 0.75$ L/min/m^2. The average difference between the bioimpedance and thermodilution estimations was $16 + 14\%$ of their average value. Initial studies demonstrated reasonable reliability in the absence of severe pulmonary oedema or marked expansion of the extracellular fluid by massive crystalloid infusions. In these cases, occurring in about 8% of our patients, we found the baseline impedance (Zo) to be < 16 ohms and the height of impedance waveform (dZ/dt) to be < 0.3 ohms. We therefore accepted impedance values when Zo values > 16 ohms and dZ/dt values > 0.3 ohms. Values below these numbers were observed to track and trend thermodilution values, but were not considered sufficiently reliable to base therapeutic decisions; this is a major limitation of impedance methods. Using Zo > 15 ohms and dZ/dt values > 0.3 ohms as criteria in 214 simultaneous pairs of thermodilution and impedance cardiac output measurements during the past 10 months, we found the correlation, r was 0.93, $r^2 = 0.87$; bias and precision was $-0.14 + 0.54$ L/min/m^2 and the average difference was $9.8\% + 6.7\%$ [28].

Measurement of tissue perfusion and oxygenation

PtcO$_2$ has been used for several decades to track PaO$_2$ in neonates; it uses the Clark polarographic O$_2$ sensor to measure O$_2$ tension in a local segment of heated skin [29-35]. This is not necessarily the same as in other peripheral tissues; because the skin is most sensitive to peripheral vasoconstriction from the adrenomedullary stress response, it provides an earlier warning than SvO$_2$ and $\dot{V}O_2$ [29, 31]. The transcutaneous oxygen electrode accurately measures the oxygen tension of the heated skin surface. Previous studies demonstrated the capacity of transcutaneous oxygen tensions to track tissue oxygen tension [32]. Transcutaneous oxygen tension (PtcO$_2$) has been shown to reflect the delivery of oxygen to the local area of skin; it also parallels the mixed venous oxygen tension except under late or terminal conditions where peripheral shunting leads to high mixed venous hemoglobin saturation (SvO$_2$) values [29]. Obviously, the oxygenation of a skin segment does not reflect the state of oxygenation of all tissues and organs, but it has the advantage of being the most sensitive early warning tissue, since vasoconstriction of the skin is one of the first stress responses of shock syndromes. PtcO$_2$ closely tracked oxygen consumption ($\dot{V}O_2$) values in shock and resuscitation in the initial baseline period, the nadir, and the postresuscitation values; the changes were significant ($p < .05$), but not necessarily synchronous; the PtcO$_2$ values decreased first in most patients [28].

Abnormal circulatory values in trauma patients

Table 1 summarizes the observed variables, their normal values, criteria for each variable indicating circulatory deficiency, and the mean of each variable at its minimum (nadir) or maximum when abnormal. Of 139 trauma patients, cardiac index decreased to a mean of 1.83 + 0.69 (SD) L/min/m² at its nadir; hypotension averaged 58 + 1.8 mmHg; low arterial saturations averaged 84.8 + 1.4%, reduced transcutaneous oxygen tension averaged 31.6 + 2.6 torr; high transcutaneous CO_2 values averaged 77.5 + 1.8 torr; oxygen consumption measurements at their low averaged 91.5 + 3.8 mL/min/m². Most patients had two or more abnormalities.

Table 1. Variables, units, normal values, values indicating circulatory deficiency, number and percentage of patients with abnormal values, and means of the abnormal values at their nadirs

Variable	Units	Normal values	Abnormal values	N (%) of abnormal	Mean + SD at nadir
CI	L/min/m²	3.2 ± 0.2	< 3.0	38/75 (51%)	1.83 ± 0.69
MAP	mmHg	85 ± 3	< 80	30/75 (40%)	58 ± 1.8
POx	%	97 ± 1	< 90	12/65 (18%)	84.8 ± 1.4
$PtcO_2/FiO_2$	–	> 250	< 150	40/75 (53%)	31.6 ± 2.6
$PtcCO_2$	torr	50 ± 3	> 60	35/75 (47%)	77.5 ± 1.8
$\dot{V}O_2$	mL/min/m²	130 ± 10	< 110	18/32 (52%)	91.5 ± 3.8

CI, cardiac index; MAP, mean arterial pressure; POx, pulse oximetry; $PtcO_2$, transcutaneous oxygen tension; $PtcCO_2$, transcutaneous carbon dioxide tension; $\dot{V}O_2$, oxygen consumption

Patterns in medical (nontrauma) patients

Patients with cardiac problems including acute myocardial infarction, hypertensive crisis, and chronic congestive heart failure with acute exacerbation, neurologic failure, drug overdose, and haemorrhage initially had low cardiac index which then decreased further along with tissue perfusion as reflected by $PtcO_2$; with resuscitation, the cardiac index and $PtcO_2$ values of the survivors usually increased above normal values, but the responses of nonsurvivors were less pronounced. Patients with sepsis, septic shock, community acquired pneumonia, and stress-related disorders started with higher than normal cardiac index values, but these values deteriorated along with $PtcO_2$ as the shock syndrome progressed. With resuscitation, these values increased above their baseline control levels in survivors but not in nonsurvivors.

Haemodynamic and oxygen transport patterns in septic shock

Time relationships for postoperative patients are easily marked by the time of onset or the end of the surgical operation. Sepsis, by contrast, has a more subtle and insidious onsets. Time relationships are obscure, and progression from localized infection to generalized infection with systemic manifestations, to the septic syndrome, to the septic shock, and to death may be gradual and not readily apparent. The progress of the disorder may not be recognized until advanced stages; the fulminating form of sepsis may have a cataclysmic deterioration and rapid demise [33, 34].

Septic shock is also difficult to understand because of the heterogeneity of patients affected; that is, widely different clinical manifestations occur in postoperative, post-traumatic, urologic, general internal medicine patients, and those with respiratory failure. Sepsis may be the primary disorder, or it may be a complication. Sepsis also may be the expected consequence in patients with obstruction to the normal flow of biologic fluids (urine, bile, or gastrointestinal fluids), immunodeficiencies, and late-stage malignancies.

Sequential haemodynamic and oxygen transport patterns of survivors and nonsurvivors were described in a series of 378 consecutive internal medicine and surgical septic shock patients to differentiate primary from secondary and tertiary events and to evaluate possible underlying mechanisms and their therapeutic implications [33, 34]. Because of the gradual transitions between the stages of septic shock and variations in the duration of each stage, specific physiologic criteria were used to define the following stages: 1) an early period that began with the first recorded increase in cardiac output; 2) a middle period, which was the time 48 hours before and after the maximum metabolic activity, defined as the period characterized by the highest recorded rate of oxygen consumption; and 3) a late period, which was the time 48 hours before death or recovery; the last of these was defined as the time when the patient had recovered sufficiently to allow discontinuation of measurements and the removal of the catheters.

The earliest haemodynamic changes were increased heart rate, CI, and DO_2. Early transient reductions in $\dot{V}O_2$ that preceded the temperature elevations and hypotension were observed in both survivors and nonsurvivors. Subsequently, in the early and middle periods, progressive increases in CI, DO_2 and $\dot{V}O_2$ were noted. These increases were greater in the survivors than in the nonsurvivors at comparable time periods.

Although 84% of the patients with sepsis were consistently hyperdynamic, transient hypodynamic episodes, defined as CI < 2.5 L/min·m², were seen in approximately 10% of the measurements. Also, in 8% of the nonsurvivors, transient preterminal hypermetabolic periods, defined as $\dot{V}O_2$ > 200 mL/min·m², were also observed; these usually occurred 18 to 72 hours prior to death and were followed by a progressive downhill course. In the terminal period of nonsurvivors, MAP, CI, DO_2, and $\dot{V}O_2$ fell abruptly. Thus, early increases in CI and

DO_2 represent physiologic compensations for circulatory deficiencies that limit body metabolism and compromise survival.

Hankeln and associates [15] reported that postoperative and cardiac patients with ARDS who did survive had supranormal CI and DO_2; in their series, non-survivors had lower values than did survivors. Abraham and colleagues [35] demonstrated further increases in DO_2 and $\dot{V}O_2$ after fluid loading with colloids in patients with septic shock from peritonitis. Others have corroborated the increased CI, DO_2 and $\dot{V}O_2$ in septic shock patients given fluids or inotropes [36-38]. Edwards and colleagues [37, 38] took the concept one step further by driving DO_2 and $\dot{V}O_2$ to optimal supranormal values with the administration of fluids and dobutamine; using this approach, they demonstrated improved survival rates in severely ill septic shock patients. In prospective randomized studies on medical patients with septic shock, Tuchschmidt and coworkers [12] showed reduced mortality when CI was driven to 6 L/min·m² with fluids and dobutamine. In the late stage after organ failures develop, however, this approach is not effective.

Pathophysiology of postoperative ARDS

The hypothesis for the pathogenesis of ARDS is that cytokines and other mediators are produced in the anoxic acidotic endothelium of the peripheral microcirculation; on reperfusion, they are washed out of peripheral tissues into the venous blood, which goes directly into the pulmonary circulation (the first capillary network encountered), where they produce ARDS and other organ failures. The corollary hypothesis is that ARDS and perhaps other organ failures can be prevented by rapid restoration and maintenance of both overall flow as well as tissue perfusion/oxygenation [22]. The assumption is that this may be accomplished by adequate fluids that stay in the intravascular space without expanding the interstitial space.

Can early monitoring and optimization prevent ARDS?

The incidence of postoperative ARDS was reduced to 10% of that of the control patients in a prospective randomized series of elective high risk patients [7]. In randomized series of severe trauma patients, Bishop et al. [9] reduced the incidence of ARDS in the protocol group to less than half of that of the control group. The basis of prevention or reduction of the incidence of ARDS lies in the maintenance of peripheral perfusion beginning with the onset of acute illness, trauma, or high risk surgery. By maintaining tissue perfusion/oxygenation intraoperatively with a complex protocol involving adequate fluids (mostly colloids) and nitroglycerine carefully titrated to correct uneven flow from vasoconstriction, Thangathurai et al. [22] reported no postoperative ARDS in 179 high risk surgical cases maintained on the protocol compared with 6/24 (17%) in control patients who developed ARDS. While many proposals for resuscitation of high risk elective and severe trauma patients exist, none have taken explicit concern for achieving physiological goals at the earliest point in time, i.e., the immediate period after admission to the ER. Although physiologic therapeutic goals based on survivors' values have been proposed for the trauma victim in the postoperative ICU period, they are not used in the initial resuscitation, primarily because invasive Swan-Ganz catheter studies are not usually available in the Emergency Department (ED) or OR.

Integrated approach to circulatory dysfunction and shock

The conventional approach is a one-at-a-time search for defects; after the first defect is documented and corrected, the search continues for the next defect, then the next, and so on. This leads to an uncoordinated sometimes contradictory therapeutic plan. Alternatively, circulatory problems may be addressed by an integrated systematic approach to circulatory function that optimizes the three major circulatory components: cardiac, pulmonary, and tissue perfusion functions [39, 40]. Rather than addressing each sign, symptom, or deranged circulatory variable by itself as an independant problem, continuous on-line, real time display of physiological data by the three noninvasive monitoring systems allow an integrated systematic approach to cardiac, pulmonary, and tissue perfusion/oxygenation functions. The deficiencies of each of these three systems are not just corrected or normalized but optimized early or when possible prophylactically.

The advantage of this noninvasive systematic approach is that it provides a visual image of the status of each circulatory component, displays the deficiencies, defines the optimal therapeutic goals, identifies interacting problems, and allows titration of specific therapy to improve outcome.

Conclusions

A major assumption was that early circulatory deficiencies that ultimately lead to shock, organ failure, and death begin with or shortly after onset of haemorrhage, surgery, trauma, or sepsis. Insertion of a pulmonary artery catheter requires about 20-30 minutes that may not be available except in the ICU, but the noninvasive electrodes can be applied in < 2 minutes on ED admission almost as easily as ECG electrodes. If noninvasive systems are being used in an inner city county hospital emergency conditions, they could be used almost anywhere. Despite the exigencies of emergency situations, noninvasive data provided useful information for physiologic evaluation at the bedside to allow earlier recognition of circulatory dysfunction. They are easier, safer, less expensive, as sensitive, and more cost effective than invasive monitoring. More importantly they provide the means to titrate therapy to appropriate predetermined therapeutic goals. Their primary advantage is to enable the clinician to recognize circulatory problems earlier and to provide objective physiologic criteria for titration of therapy to achieve optimal physiologic goals. The basic hypothesis of this study is that earlier recognition and identification of circulatory problems leads to more prompt administration of therapy and improved outcome.

References

1. Conners AF Jr, Speroff T, Dawson NV et al (1996) The effectiveness of right heart catheterization in the initial care of critically ill patients. JAMA 276:899-997
2. Gore JM, Goldberg RJ, Spodick DH et al (1987) A community-wide assessment of the use of pulmonary artery catheters in patients with acute myocardial infarction. Chest 92:721-727
3. Zion MM, Balkin J, Rosenmann D et al (1990) Use of pulmonary artery catheters in patients with acute myocardial infarction: analysis of experience in 5841 patients in the SPRINT registry. Chest 98:1331-1335
4. Blumberg MS, Binns GS (1994) Swan-Ganz catheter use and mortality in myocardial infarction patients. Health Care Financ Rev 15:91-103
5. Hayes MA, Timmins AC, Yau EHS et al (1994) Elevation of systemic oxygen delivery in the treatment of critically ill patients. New Engl J Med 330:1717-1722
6. Gattinoni L, Brazzi L, Pelosi P et al (1995) A trial of goal-oriented hemodynamic therapy in critically ill patients. N Engl J Med 333:1025-1032
7. Shoemaker WC, Appel PL, Kram HB et al (1988) Prospective trial of supranormal values of survivors as therapeutic goals in high risk surgical patients. Chest 94:1176-1186
8. Boyd O, Grounds M, Bennett D (1993) Preoperative increase of oxygen delivery reduces mortality in high risk surgical patients. JAMA 270:2699-2704
9. Bishop MH, Shoemaker WC, Kram HB et al (1995) Prospective randomized trial of survivor values of cardiac index, oxygen delivery, and oxygen consumption as resuscitation endpoints in severe trauma. J Trauma 38:780-787
10. Berlauk JF, Abrams JH, Gilmour IJ et al (1991) Pre-operative optimization of cardiovascular hemodynamics improves outcome in peripheral vascular surgery. Ann Surg 214:189
11. Yu M, Levy MM, Smith P et al (1993) Effect of maximizing oxygen delivery on mortality and mortality rates in critically ill patients: A prospective randomized controlled study. Crit Care Med 21:830-838
12. Tuchschmidt J, Fried J, Astiz M et al (1992) Evaluation of cardiac output and oxygen delivery improves outcome in septic shock. Chest 202:216
13. Scalea TM, Simon HM, Duncan AO et al (1990) Geriatric blunt multiple trauma: Improved survival with early invasive monitoring. J Trauma 30:129-136
14. Moore FA, Haemel JB, Moore EE et al (1992) Incommensurate oxygen consumption in response to maximal oxygen availability predicts postinjury oxygen failure. J Trauma 33:58-62
15. Hankeln KB, Senker R, Schwarten JN et al (1987) Evaluation of prognostic indices based on hemodynamic and oxygen transport variables in shock patients with ARDS. Crit Care Med 15:1
16. Creamer JE, Edwards JD, Nightingale P (1990) Hemodynamic and oxygen transport variables in cardiogenic shock secondary to acute myocardial infarction. Am J Cardiol 65:1287
17. Rady MY, Edwards JD, Rivers EP et al (1993) Measurement of oxygen consumption after uncomplicated acute myocardial infarction. Chest 103:886-895

18. Schultz RJ, Whitfield GF, LaMura JJ et al (1985) The role of physiologic monitoring in patients with fractures of the hip. J Trauma 25:309-316
19. Taylor RW and the Pulmonary Artery Catheter Consensus Conference (1997). Pulmonary Artery Catheter Consensus Conference. Crit Care Med 25:910-925
20. Boyd O, Bennett D (1996) Enhancement of perioperative tissue perfusion as a therapeutic strategy for major surgery. New Horiz 4:453-465
21. Shoemaker WC, Appel PL, Kram HB (1992) Role of oxygen debt in the development of organ failure, sepsis, and death in high risk surgical patients. Chest 102:208-215
22. Thangathurai D, Charbonnet C, Wo CCJ et al (1996) Intra-operative maintenance of tissue perfusion prevents ARDS. New Horiz 4:453-465
23. Shoemaker WC, Wo CCJ, Demetriades D et al (1996) Early physiologic patterns in acute illness and accidents. New Horiz 4:395-412
24. Wang X, Van De Water JM, Sun H et al (1993) Hemodynamic monitoring by impedance cardiography with an improved signal processing technique. Proc IEEE Eng Med Biol 15:699
25. Wang X, Sun HH, Van De Water JM (1995) Time-frequency distribution technique in biological signal processing. Biomed Instr Technol 203-212
26. Shoemaker WC, Wo CCJ, Bishop MH et al (1994) Multicenter trial of a new thoracic electric bioimpedance device for cardiac output estimation. Crit Care Med 22:1907
27. Wo CCJ, Shoemaker WC, Bishop MH et al (1995) Noninvasive estimations of cardiac output and circulatory dynamics in critically ill patients. Curr Opin Crit Care 1:211-218
28. Shoemaker WC, Belzberg H, Wo CCJ et al (1998) Multicenter study of noninvasive monitoring as alternative to invasive monitoring in early management o acutely ill emergency patients. Chest (in press)
29. Tremper KK, Waxman K, Shoemaker WC (1979) Effects of hypoxia and shock on transcutaneous PO_2 values in dogs. Crit Care Med 7:526-530
30. Tremper KK, Shoemaker WC (1981) Transcutaneous oxygen monitoring of critically ill adults with and without low flow shock. Crit Care Med 9:706-709
31. Lubbers DW (1981) Theoretical basis of the transcutaneous blood gas measurements. Crit Care Med 9:721-33
32. Tremper KK, Waxman K, Bowman R (1980) Continuous transcutaneous oxygen monitoring during respiratory failure, cardiac decompensation, cardiac arrest, and CPR. Crit Care Med 8:337
33. Shoemaker WC, Appel PL, Kram HB et al (1993) Temporal hemodynamic and oxygen transport patterns in medical patients in shock. Chest 104:1529-1536
34. Shoemaker WC, Appel PL, Kram HB et al (1993) Sequence of physiologic patterns in surgical septic shock. Crit Care Med 21:1876-1887
35. Abraham E, Bland RS, Cobo JC et al (1984) Sequential cardiorespiratory patterns associated with outcome in septic shock. Chest 85:75-81
36. Haupt MT, Gilbert EM, Carlson RW (1985) Fluid loading increases oxygen delivery and consumption in septic patients with lactic acidosis. Am Rev Respir Dis 131:912-918
37. Edwards JD, Brown GCS, Nightingale P et al (1989) Use of survivors values as therapeutic goals in septic shock. Crit Care Med 17:1098-1103
38. Edwards JD (1991) Oxygen transport in cardiogenic and septic shock. Crit Care Med 19: 658-663
39. Shoemaker WC, Appel PL, Kram HB (1989) Incidence, physiologic description, compensatory mechanisms, and therapeutic implications of monitored events. Crit Care Med 17:1277
40. Shoemaker WC, Appel PL, Kram HB (1992) Role of oxygen debt in the development of organ failure, sepsis, and death in high risk surgical patients. Chest 102:208-215

Postresuscitation Myocardial Dysfunction

H. Yamaguchi, M.H. Weil

The ultimate goal of cardiopulmonary resuscitation (CPR) for the nearly 500,000 victims of sudden death in the United States is to return the victims to long-term and functional survival. Yet of the approximately 39% of victims who are initially resuscitated successfully, as few as 3% represent hospital survivors [1, 2]. This large fall off in survival reflects what we now recognize as two discrete stages of cardiac resuscitation. The first stage is that of initial resuscitation with re-establishment of a spontaneous circulation. The second is the management of postresuscitation arrhythmias and myocardial failure including a high incidence of recurrent cardiac arrest. We suggest the term postresuscitation myocardial dysfunction for this second stage [3]. These two discrete stages of cardiac resuscitation may therefore call for two distinct therapeutic goals. The first is to restore spontaneous circulation. The second is to secure the effective pumping function of the heart and especially the moderation of dysrhythmic events and myocardial failure.

Experimental studies

Initial studies on postresuscitation myocardial dysfunction were performed by our group on isolated, perfused rat hearts. After successful resuscitation from ventricular fibrillation (VF), myocardial compliance was reduced together with contractile dysfunction. The slope of the diastolic pressure-volume relationship shifted superiorly and to the left [3] (Fig. 1). In pigs [4], myocardial contractility was strikingly reduced after resuscitation from electrically induced VF. The stroke volume index was decreased to 70% of the baseline, and the left ventricular ejection fraction was reduced from 41% to 20% (Fig. 2). Myocardial mechanical impairment was characterized by decreased systolic and diastolic functions. Electrical dysfunction was also documented. It was characterized by ectopic ventricular rhythms. The severity of both dysfunctions was increased, 1) after increasing duration of untreated cardiac arrest, 2) after administration of β-adrenergic agonist and specifically epinephrine during CPR, 3) when CO_2 tension in the myocardium exceeded a threshold value during global myocardial ischaemia, and 4) when large electrical energies were delivered to the heart prior to successful defibrillation [5-7].

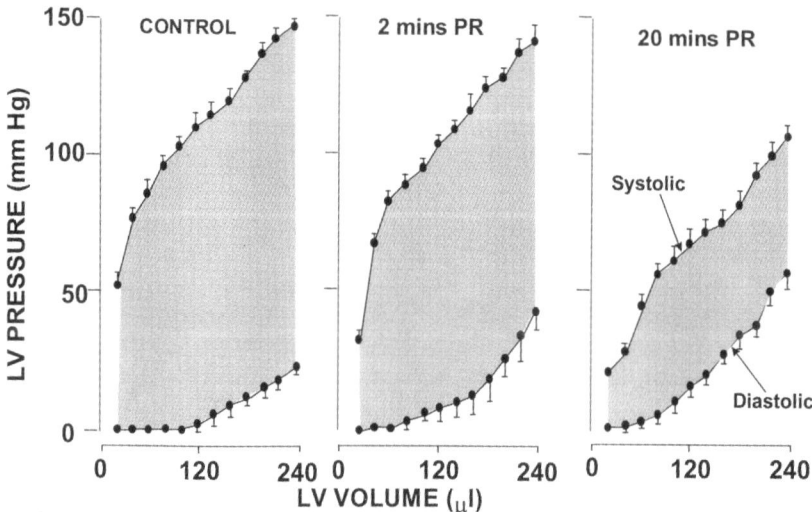

Fig. 1. Pressure-volume relationship after successful resuscitation. Effects on the generated ventricular systolic and diastolic pressure are shown in hearts harvested at 2 mins after resuscitation (2 mins PR) and 20 mins after resuscitation (20 mins PR). LV, left ventricular; PR, postresuscitation. Values are mean ± SD. (Modified from Wanchun T et al. Progressive myocardial dysfunction after cardiac resuscitation. Crit Care Med 1993;21:1046-1050)

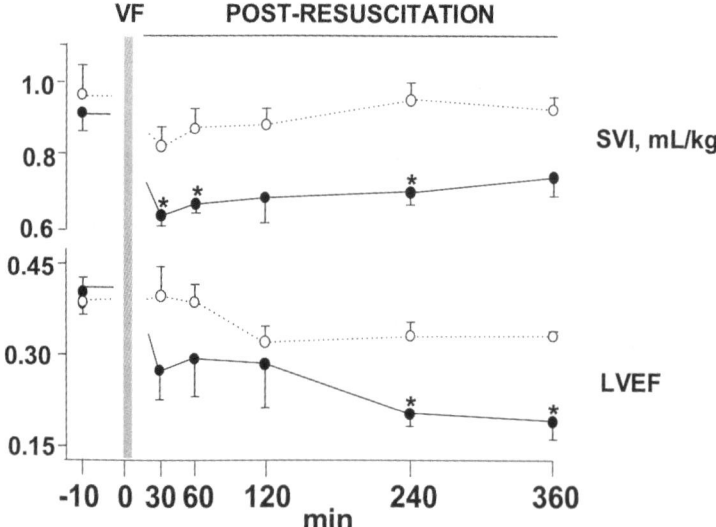

Fig. 2. Stroke volume index (SVI) and left ventricular ejection fraction (LVEF) after successful resuscitation. Measurement were obtained 10 mins before cardiac arrest and during a 6-hr interval after successful resuscitation. Values are mean ± SEM. VF, ventricular fibrillation. *$p < .001$ vs sham. Open circles, sham control; solid circles, resuscitation animal. (Modified from Raul G et al. Myocardial dysfunction after successful resuscitation from cardiac arrest. Crit Care Med 1996;24: 992-1000)

Clinical significance

Postresuscitation myocardial dysfunction has been implicated as one of the major causes of in hospital death following initial successful resuscitation. In a study of 301 patients who had prehospital ventricular defibrillation, 101 (34%) victims were resuscitated and these patients survived long enough to be hospitalized. A majority (57%) manifested ventricular arrhythmias during the initial 24 hours and 75% of these patients died within 7 days after initial successful resuscitation. Less than one half, namely 40%, died on the first day after admission [8]. In a multicenter study that enrolled 1280 victims of out-of-hospital cardiac arrest, 407 patients (32%) were initially resuscitated and hospitalized, approximately 171 hospitalized patients (42%) died during the first 72 hours. Arterial hypotension and fatal ventricular arrhythmias preceded death. Only 57 patients (4.5%) were discharged alive from the hospital [9]. In another multicenter study in which 650 patients were enrolled, only 132 patients (20%) were initially resuscitated, and only 26 patients (4%) were discharged alive from the hospital [10]. A collaborative study included 520 victims representing 24 hospitals in eight countries, 322 of successfully resuscitated patients (62%) died within 7 days [11]. Each of these reports proves the importance of post-resuscitation complications.

Postresuscitation myocardial injury is typically reversed after hours or days following successful resuscitation. In pig models of cardiac arrest due to untreated VF of 4 min duration, normal heart rate, mean aortic pressure, cardiac index and stroke volume were restored within 48 hours after successful cardiac resuscitation. A study by Kern B.K. et al. [12] on pigs confirmed full recovery at 48 hours after successful resuscitation. There is currently less data on human patients. Three patients were successfully resuscitated from VF within 3, 10, or 30 min after onset of cardiac arrest. Ventricular function returned to normal after 2 weeks in each instance [13]. Among 301 victims of pre-hospital cardiac arrest due to VF, 101 patients (34%) survived to be hospitalized. However, only 42 of these patients (14%) were discharged alive from the hospital. A majority of these patients, namely 25 (60%) were returned to pre-arrest function including employment [8]. Accordingly, we recognize an opportunity for increasing meaningful survival and recovery by appropriate management of postresuscitation myocardial dysfunction.

Mechanisms

The pathophysiology of postresuscitation myocardial dysfunction is as yet not well understood. Postischaemic myocardial dysfunction may reflect intracellular calcium overloading with generation of oxygen-derived free radicals [14-20]. Calcium overload reduces the capability for actin-myosin bridging. Accordingly, myocardial contractility of such ischaemic or "stunned" myocardium is reduced [20]. Calcium overload also impairs mitochondrial function. Free radicals are generated during reperfusion. These attack virtually all cellular components. Swelling and disruption of mitochondria, blebbing of the sarcolemma, and breaks within the sarcolemmal membrane are identified in myocytes [21, 22].

Electrical defibrillation is also implicated as a cause of postresuscitation myocardial dysfunction. The electrical current generates free radicals. High-energy defibrillation of itself increases the severity of postresuscitation myocardial dysfunction. Increases in intramyocardial temperature generated during defibrillation also have been impaired [6, 23, 24]. These mechanisms are illustrated in Fig. 3.

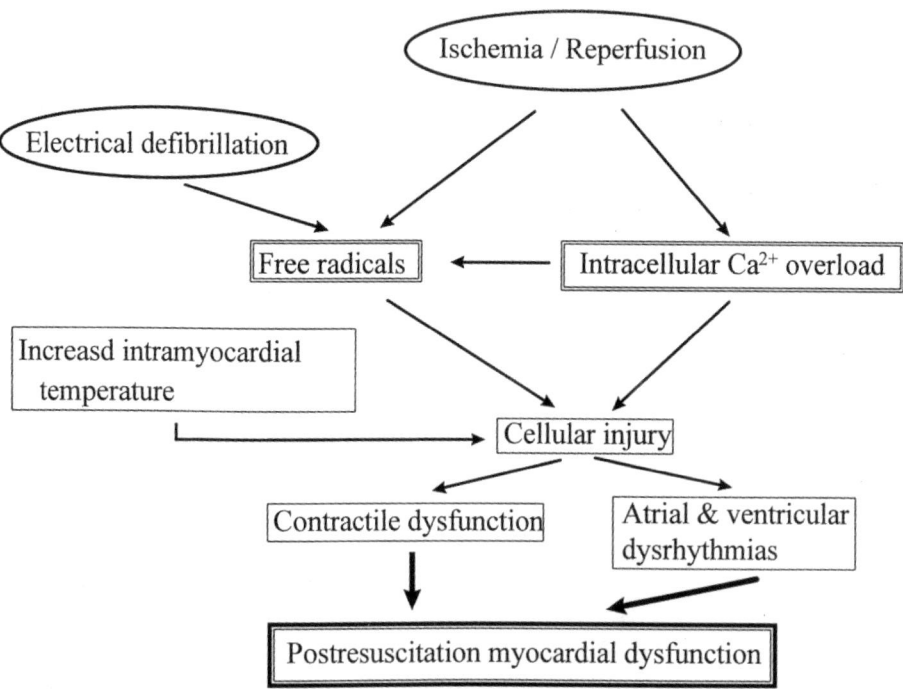

Fig. 3. Current concept of the mechanisms accounting for postresuscitation myocardial dysfunction

Diagnosis

After successful resuscitation, a combination of haemodynamic abnormalities characterize postresuscitation myocardial dysfunction (Table 1). They all reflect reduced work capability of the left ventricle. There is spontaneous reversal of postresuscitation myocardial dysfunction after hours or days.

Table 1. Diagnosis of postresuscitation myocardial dysfunction

1. Increased heart rate
2. Reduced cardiac output
3. Decreased arterial pressure
4. Ventricular dilation
5. Dysrhythmias; supraventricular and ectopic ventricular arrhythmias

Management

No controlled studies are currently available that would objectively document specific therapeutic interventions for either myocardial failure or dysrhythmias. For haemodynamic management, current routines include optimization of preload and afterload to assure optimal cardiac output and to reverse heart failure. The goal is to improve myocardial systolic and diastolic function and thereby increase stroke volume. Concurrently, immediate life threatening arrhythmias have been treated with drugs, electrical pacing and override pacing, or electrical cardioversion of supraventricular tachycardia, ventricular tachycardia, and recurrent VF. Pharmacologic agents include inotropic agents, vasopressor agents, and preload and afterload reducing agents, including angiotensin-converting enzyme inhibitors. Though each of these agents is included as part of the American Heart Association Guidelines, their ultimate benefits are not established.

Dobutamine stimulates both β_1- and β_2-adrenergic receptors. It therefore acts as a mild vasodilator to reduce systemic vascular resistance, increase cardiac output and stroke volume by its inotropic actions, and improve systemic and coronary flow in part by increasing heart rates. Increases in myocardial oxygen requirements produced by dobutamine may however increase the risks of myocardial ischaemic injury in settings of continuing myocardial ischaemia. In doses of between 5 and 10 μg/kg/min of dobutamine, administrated within 15 minutes of successful resuscitation, stroke volume and ejection fractions were increased and pulmonary occlusive pressure was decreased [25].

Dopamine stimulates α-, β- and dopaminergic-receptors. At dosages of 5 μg/kg/min or less, dopamine stimulates dopaminergic receptors directly and such produces relatively selective vasodilation of splanchnic and renal arterial beds. Accordingly, renal blood flow and glomerular filtration are improved. With larger doses, dopamine enhances norepinephrine release, resulting in both increased β-adrenergic receptor and peripheral vasoconstriction. Accordingly, in postresuscitation settings, dopamine would best be reserved for management of life-threatening hypotension.

Phosphodiesterase inhibitors such as amrinone and milrinone exert both inotropic and arterial vasodilator actions such that systemic vascular resistance is reduced and cardiac output is increased.

Nitrates, including nitroglycerin and nitroprusside, act by generating nitric oxide which produces venous and arterial vasodilation. Such reduces both ventricular preload and afterload. These effects are theoretically appropriate in settings of postresuscitation myocardial dysfunction but still of unproven ultimate benefit.

For the management of postresuscitation ventricular dysrhythmias, lidocaine remains the drug of first choice. Adenosine may be an appropriate drug for treatment of supraventricular tachycardia and AV junctional tachycardias although electrical cardioversion or overdrive pacing are more predictable. Electrical options for management of bradycardia include initial transcutaneous and subsequently temporary transvenous pacing. Procainamide and bretylium are secondary options but we presently have little enthusiasm for their use in these settings. Atropine is routinely administered for the initial treatment of sinus or atrial bradyarrhythmias, but its ultimate efficacy is doubtful. Both hypokalaemia and hypomagnesaemia are best corrected for they will contribute to both rhythm and contractile defects, especially recurrent VF, and especially Torsade de Point.

Mechanical ventilation is likely to be of benefit when cardiac output and both systemic and coronary blood flows are reduced because it allows for sedation, narcosis, and even neuromuscular blockade and reduces the energy cost of breathing. Pulmonary complications and, most importantly, aspiration may require endoscopic interventions and more selective management of the airway. Increases in the FiO_2 and mild positive end-expiratory pressure are appropriate routines in setting of hypoxaemia. For all of these interventions, however, secure proof that they improve outcomes is still needed.

We have summarized current options of management in Table 2.

Table 2. Current options for management of postresuscitation myocardial dysfunction

1. Pharmacological intervention	
Drug	*Indication*
A) For myocardial dysfunction	
Dopamine, norepinephrine	Life-threatening hypotension
Nitrates	Ventricular preload and afterload adjustment
Dobutamine	Inotropic, increase stroke volume
Phosphodiesterase inhibitor	Reduce systemic vascular resistance and increase cardiac output
B) For postresuscitation dysrhythmia	
Adenosin	Supraventricular and A-V junctional tachycardias
Atropine	Sinus or atrial bradycardias
Lidocaine	Ventricular ectopy, tachycardias
Procainamide, bretylium	Ventricular ectopy, tachycardias
2. Electrical mechanical intervention	
Electrical cardioversion	Tachycardia, predominantly ventricular
Override pacing	Tachycardia, predominantly supraventricular
Mechanical ventilation	Hypoxia, hypercapnia, reduce energy cost of breathing
Temporary transvenous pacing	Bradycardia, heart block

References

1. McGrath RB (1987) In-house cardiopulmonary resuscitation - After a quarter of a century. Ann Emerg Med 16:1365-1368
2. AHA Medical / Scientific Statement (1991) Improving survival from sudden cardiac arrest: The "Chain of Survival" concept. Circulation 83:1832-1847
3. Tang W, Weil MH, Sun S et al (1993) Progressive myocardial dysfunction after cardiac resuscitation. Crit Care Med 21:1046-1050
4. Gazmuri RJ, Weil MH, Bisera J et al (1996) Myocardial dysfunction after successful resuscitation from cardiac arrest. Crit Care Med 24:992-1000
5. Sun S, Weil MH, Tang W et al (1996) Effect of buffer agents on postresuscitation myocardial dysfunction. Crit Care Med 24:2035-2041
6. Xie J, Weil MH, Sun S et al (1997) High-energy defibrillation increases the severity of postresuscitation myocardial dysfunction. Circulation 96:683-688
7. Tang W, Weil MH, Sun S et al (1995) Epinephrine increases the severity of postresuscitation myocardial dysfunction. Circulation 92:3089-3093
8. Liberthson RR, Nagel EL, Hirschman JC et al (1974) Prehospital ventricular defibrillation. N Engl J Med 291:317-321
9. Brown CG, Martin DR, Pepe PE et al (1992) High-Dose Epinephrine Study Group. A comparison of standard-dose and high-dose epinephrine in cardiac arrest outside the hospital. N Engl J Med 327:1051-1055
10. Stiell IG, Hebert PC, Weitzman BN et al (1992) High-dose epinephrine in adult cardiac arrest. N Engl J Med 327:1045-1050
11. Brain Resuscitation Clinical Trial II Study Group (1992) A randomized clinical study of calcium-entry blocker (lidoflazine) in the treatment of comatose survivors of cardiac arrest. N Engl J Med 324:1225-1231
12. Kern BK, Hilwig RW, Rhee KH et al (1996) Myocardial dysfunction after resuscitation from cardiac arrest: An example of global myocardial stunning. J Am Coll Cardiol 28:232-240
13. DeAntonio HJ, Kaul S, Lerman BB (1990) Reversible myocardial depression in survivors of cardiac arrest. Pacing Clin Electrophysiol 13:982-985
14. Kloner RA, Przyklenk K, Whittaker P (1989) Deleterious effects of oxygen radicals in ischemia/reperfusion. Circulation 80:115-1127
15. Figueredo VM, Dresdner KP, Wolney AC et al (1991) Postischemic reperfusion injury in the isolated rat heart: effect of ruthenium red. Cardiovasc Res 25:337-342
16. Bagchi D, Wetscher GJ, Bagchi M et al (1997) Interrelationship between cellular calcium homeostasis and free radical generation in myocardial reperfusion injury. Chem Bio Int 104:65-85
17. Bolli R (1988) Oxygen-derived free radicals and postischemic myocardial dysfunction ("stunned myocardium"). J Am Coll Cardiol 12:239-249
18. Murphy JG, Marsh JD, Smith TW (1987) The role of calcium in ischemic myocardial injury. Circulation 75:V-15
19. Marban E (1991) Myocardial stunning and hibernation. The physiology behind the colloquialisms. Circulation 83:681-688
20. Opie LH (1989) Reperfusion injury and its pharmacologic modification. Circulation 80:1049-1062
21. Burton KP, McCord JM, Ghai G (1984) Myocardial alterations due to free-radical generation. Am J Physiol 246:H776-H783
22. Burton KP (1988) Evidence of direct toxic effects of free radicals on the myocardium. Free Radical Biol Med 4:15-24
23. Doherty PW, McLaughlin PR, Billingham M et al (1979) Cardiac damage produced by direct current countershock applied to the heart. Am J Cardiol 43:225-232
24. Caterine MR, Spencer KT, Pagon-Carlo LA et al (1996) Direct current shock to the heart generates free radicals: An electron paramagnetic resonance study. J Am Coll Cardiol 28: 1598-1609
25. Kern KB, Hilwig RW, Berg RA et al (1997) Postresuscitation left ventricular systolic and diastolic dysfunction: Treatment with dobutamine. Circulation 95:2610-2613

Telemedicine: Steps into the Future

M. ZIMPFER

In a world which is daily confronted with recognition of the complexity of natural and technological processes, innovation rarely happens in an isolated setting. In fact, cooperation and communication have become the pillars of innovation, and scientists connect with one another in an increasing variety of ways. Of course, there are the regular meetings of the specialty with the numerous reports from studies carried out at individual institutions. Our department, for one, has experienced a remarkable increase since the early '90s in the number of papers presented at these meetings (Fig. 1). Worldwide, in every medical discipline, fellowships foster the exchange of new ideas and new directions in research. So, in our department, too, we have made a point of sending promising staff members abroad (see Fig. 2 for destinations in the United States) to absorb the latest currents of thought, techniques and approaches. However, although it is unlikely that regular professional specialty meetings and personal contact can ever be fully replaced by other modes of communication, the time pressures on physicians are growing to such an extent that more and more opt to attend fewer and fewer meetings. And where is the physician who can attend the meeting of another specialty?

In response have come the various ways of bringing information to the individual physician. Videoconferencing, for example, has become an efficient, time-sparing method of facilitating the exchange of specifically needed information. Using our department as an example once again, our videoconference link with a major East Coast American university has enabled us to benefit from discussion of complicated cases, in which we exchange the patient history along with laboratory reports, X-rays, CT and NMR scans, and even transoesophageal echocardiography sequences in motion (Fig. 3). Telemedicine – the transmission and exchange of delayed and real time medical data via telecommunication networks – has been developing with increasing acceleration, in step with the advances in communications technology, for decades. It is now a major tool for the exchange of medical information. In a further development, the delivery of continuing medical education has for the first time turned to the tool of telecommunications, with the launch last year of the Health Channel of Baylor College of Medicine in Houston/USA, which will be discussed later in this paper.

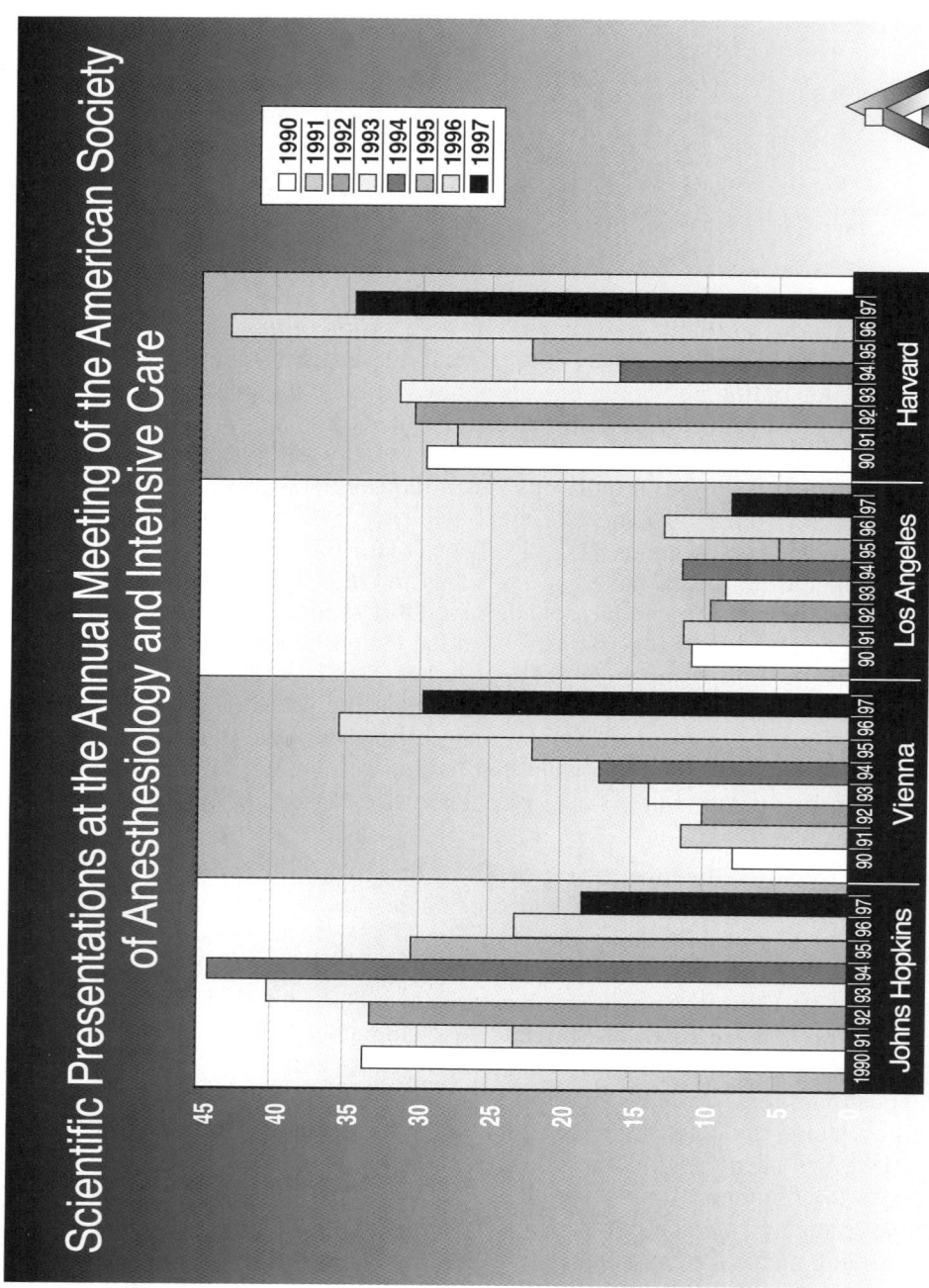

Fig. 1. Major medical centers provide a large number of reports at the annual meetings of the American Society of Anesthesiologists. The contribution of the University of Vienna has grown strongly during the decade of the 1990s

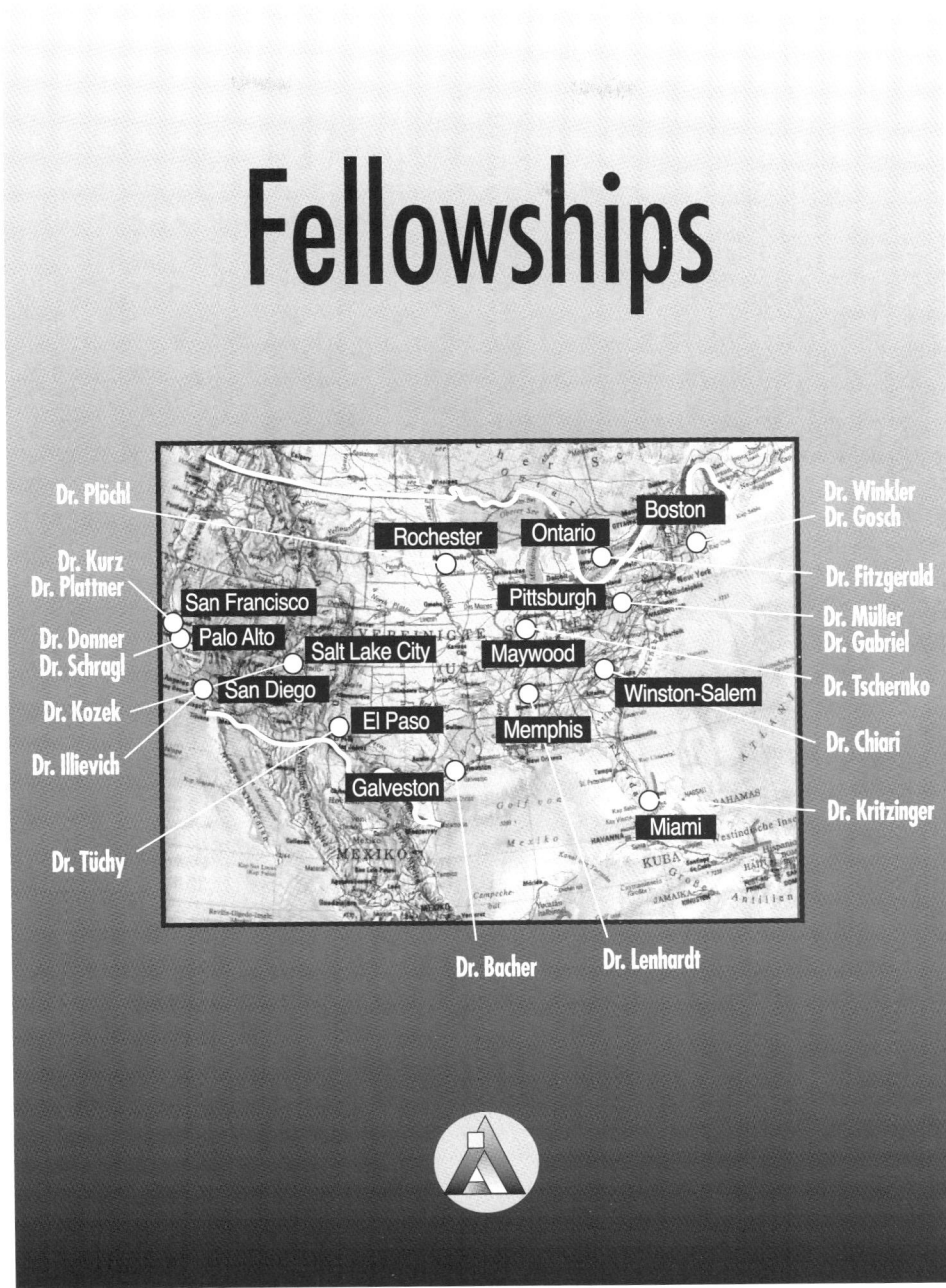

Fig. 2. Advantages accrue to the institution that provides fellowships for international study for promising staff members

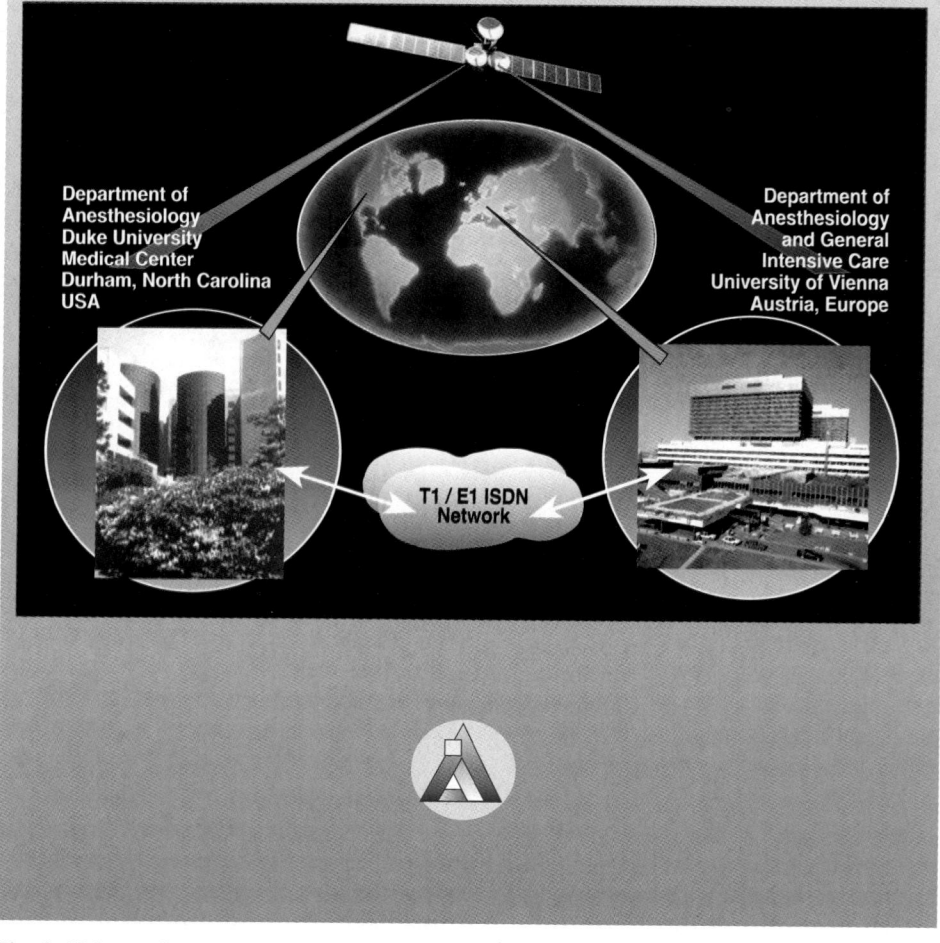

Fig. 3. Videoconferencing links with medical centers of outstanding international repute provide the invaluable opportunity of exchanging expertise on a real-time basis, particularly in complicated cases

Telemedicine

Telemedicine is the use of telecommunications technologies for the purpose of improving patient care. In the broadest sense, it includes the use of long-familiar telephones or fax machines. In more complicated applications, information is transmitted by video, in certain circumstances via a computer network.

Although the enormous interest in telemedicine of the last 4-5 years creates the impression that this is a totally new development, in fact some applications have been in use for over 30 years. Thus, physiological data were first transmitted telemetrically in the '60s, simultaneously with the development of manned space flight. Subsequently, the establishment of communications satellites facilitated not only the establishment of telemedical applications, but, above all, their availability to the civilian health system.

One of the earliest applications of telemedicine for civilian use was a project to provide medical care to the Papago Indian Reservation in Arizona, USA, in 1972. The provision of medical expertise to the reservation population was made possible by a mobile out-patient service, with EKG, radiology and transmission units connecting to each of two hospitals. Other early examples of telemedical applications include psychiatric consultation via television in the state of Nebraska in 1955, an audiovisual channel from Massachusetts General Hospital to Logan Airport in Boston to provide medical assistance to both airport personnel and travellers in 1967, a provider network among 26 user sites in Alaska in 1971, as well as a network in Australia in 1984. In Finland radiologists developed and completed a "teleradiology" system during the decade of the 1970s.

According to estimates of the Centers for Health Policy Research in Denver/USA, approximately 30 telemedical systems were in use in 1994, with 50 new programs under development that year. It is assumed that telecommunications technology could revolutionize medical communications to the same extent that the introduction of fax machines revolutionized business communications. With regard to the medical specialties at present best served by this technology, radiographic processes best traverse the long distances. The evaluation of pathological specimens will require high-resolution equipment, which has to a large extent yet to be developed. Other favorable areas of medicine include dermatology, cardiology, internal medicine, obstetrics and gynecology, and surgery.

Although the provision of telemedicine to outlying areas may be considered to be most beneficial to thinly populated areas, it is certainly feasible that in more densely populated Central Europe, a network connecting university clinics, community hospitals, doctors in private practice, and medical laboratories could be established to retrieve specialized information or a particular test result (e.g., X-ray) when required. With a high-density network, the number of patient transfers and repeated tests could be reduced, and, in emergency cases, a significant amount of time would be saved in calling up existing test results. For reasons such as these, health insurance coverage for telemedical consultations is available in the states of Georgia, Kansas, and Montana in the U.S. However, the growing expansion of telemedical applications brings in its wake demands with regard to data protection ("intranet-gate-keeping") that need to be taken seriously.

Physicians in outlying areas are by necessity generalists. Teleconsulting with specialists in distant medical centers thus represents help and support for them. It also offers them the possibility of increasing their own specialized knowledge through direct conversations with their specialist colleagues. Often it is precisely young doctors with relatively little practical experience who, out of a sense of social obligation, work in outlying areas. In acute cases, it is of the essence to decide whether the patient needs to be transferred to a specialized center or can be cared for locally. Teleconsulting can reduce the risk of a wrong decision, can improve the quality of local care, and help avert the unnecessary strain of an avoidable patient transfer.

Mobile patient monitoring is another interesting application of telemedicine. The core function is the continuous monitoring of a patient's physiological parameters (e.g., with the help of miniaturized biosignal amplifiers) and their transmission via mobile radio networks to the treating physician. The patient remains ambulatory, i.e., can move around freely both indoors or out without losing contact with the care-giving physician. The advantages here are patient observation under everyday conditions, the avoidance of long hospital stays, and the optimization of diagnosis and treatment.

Global earth-observation data can be linked with regional data via telecommunications systems to improve early earning systems and to facilitate wherever possible the prevention of situations damaging to health. Thus, at present there are international programs in place to observe the ozone gap. If these observations are linked with regional and super-regional data on climatic changes and the increasing UV-B radiation reaching the earth, then long-term predictions and preventive measures will be made possible.

Telemedicine is used in different ways in different countries, but all to the same end – the dissemination of medical knowledge. In the United States, the institutions that actively use telemedicine range from the National Aeronautics and Space Administration, through the National Institutes of Health, the National Library of Medicine, the Department of Veterans Affairs, the Department of Health and Human Services, to the U.S. Army. It is estimated that total expenditures came to more than $100,000,000 in 1994. Internationally, NATO, the World Health Organisation, as well as the European Union support telemedical projects. The word "telematics" originated with the World Health Organisation, which defines telemedicine as a special area of "health telematics" (health-related activities which make use of information and communications technologies). In the context of its "health-for-all-strategy for global health development", WHO is, in fact, extremely interested in the development of these new technologies, is studying their benefits and risks, and is working to develop a telematics policy. The organization's aim is patient-oriented technical development and even-handed accessibility. The EU's "Health Telematic Application Programme" at the present time consists of 8 different areas of interest, which are concerned chiefly with the setting of standards, improved cooperation and exchange of scientific information, more inclusive networks, better consultation services, and patient information. EU projects in the area of health telematics are put out for bid (total budget 130 million ECU). So also the Group of 7 has agreed on cooperation in a number of telecommunications projects in health care, ranging from information networks, databases and reference centers to round-the-clock multilingual telemedicine surveillance and emergency service.

The Health Channel

While the newly-formed Health Channel, a venture of Baylor College of Medicine in Houston, is an educational channel and thus not strictly an instrument of telemedicine as such, its development is highly relevant to the future delivery of medical knowledge and our understanding of telemedicine. Baylor, an internationally eminent medical school, initiated the Health Channel (http://www.the-healthchannel.org) in response to two realities: the obligation of American physicians to earn continuing medical education credits in order to maintain certification and the rapid spread of managed care as a mode of health-care delivery in the United States. Under the assumptions of managed care, primary care physicians are expected to diagnose and treat patients who would have been quickly referred to specialists in the past. There is, therefore, an existing need for knowledgeable and experienced delivery of the latest medical know-how. Medical conferences do not meet the needs of a great number of doctors, because of the demands on their time and, in the managed care system, the pressures on their income. Baylor's solution is a direct response to the pressures that are being felt by academic institutions and physicians alike, by offering the teaching expertise of its experienced faculty in a form that reaches its intended audience efficiently, simply and economically. In creating the Health Channel Baylor turned to the familiar, easily accessible technology of television. The Health Channel offers its programs by digital satellite broadcast to subscribing physicians, nurses, and allied health care professionals. Programs cover every medical specialty and subscribers can participate in interactive sessions. At present broadcasting only in the United States, the Health Channel plans to expand to reach an international audience. As part of that plan, the Vienna General Hospital, through the Department of Anesthesiology and General Intensive Care, participated in the launch of the Channel (Fig. 4) and is the first non-American institution to provide programming content.

In our department we greeted the Health Channel as a logical development in medical communications because of our highly favorable experiences with videoconferencing. We expect that through our participation in the work of the

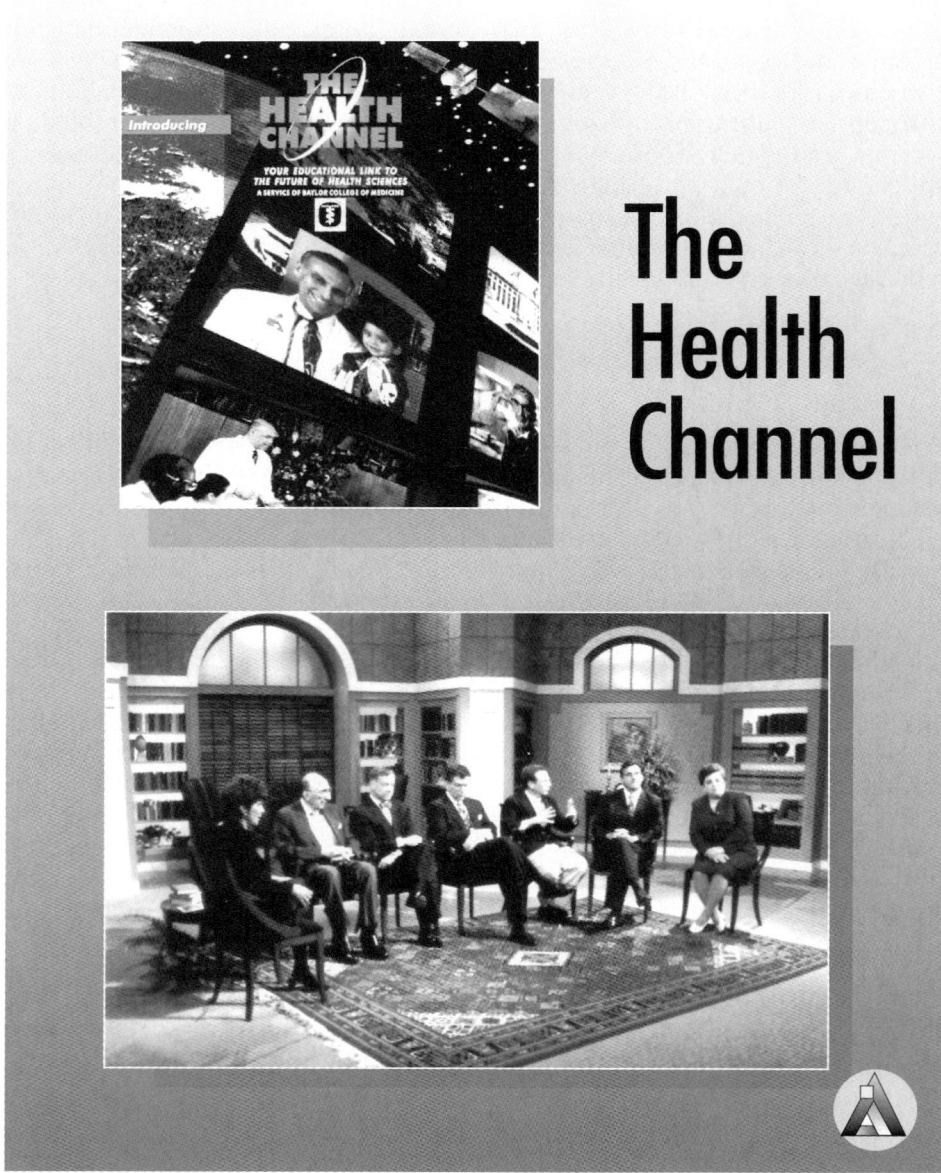

Fig. 4. Participants at the televised panel discussion launching the Health Channel in Houston, Texas. From left to right: Ellen Kingsley, moderator; Michael E. DeBakey, MD, Chancellor Emeritus, Baylor College of Medicine; Dr. Arthur Garson, Jr., MD, Dean of Academic Operations, Baylor; Mark C. Rogers, MD, Senior Vice President, Perkin-Elmer Corporation; Robert M. Johnson, VP for Administration, Baylor; the author; and Nancy W. Dickey, MD, President-Elect, American Medical Association. By videoconference: C. Everett Koop, MD, former U.S. Surgeon General

Health Channel well-informed practitioners will learn how far they can go in their own practices and how quickly – or not at all – to refer patients for in-house, specialist care. The Health Channel will surely lead to a productive increase in cooperation and understanding between medical centers and practitioners.

Internationally organized continuing education programs, for instance such as we have instituted in our department with anesthesiologists from selected Eastern European countries, profit greatly from these communications technologies. They offer much-needed support for ongoing contact and follow-up in internationally organized research projects and field studies. These programs may require some re-thinking on the part of the profession and they certainly presuppose a wish to communicate. Sometimes, however, these machines, like the ubiquitous mobile telephones, may have to be turned off so that we can think in silence; and we will have to give some thought to such matters as the legal aspects of mistakes transmitted internationally, the protection of patient data, and the possibly wrong reading of medical information by lay people. We in the medical profession have an obligation to be watchful to ensure that our patients are protected from possible errors and misuse arising from these more powerful tools of communication and that the great promise of these technologies, the more even provision of a high general level of medical expertise, is realized.

Evidence-Based Medicine in the ICU

R. Jaeschke, G. Guyatt, M. Meade

On the challenges of being an intensivist

In daily routine work clinicians of all specialties must make a variety of decisions, including whose needs and problems to address first, what diagnostic tests to order, what treatments to recommend or institute, how to measure the results of those treatments interventions, how to predict the fate of the patients, and when to stop the diagnostic or therapeutic process. Those challenges and questions are particularly concentrated in the setting of an intensive care unit where the time to make decisions is limited by the acute nature of the underlying diseases, where available information is commonly incomplete, and where the consequences of decisions are frequently of immediate and major importance to the patients. Resuscitating, providing life support, and providing intensive monitoring in a setting of advanced diagnostic and therapeutic technology requires clinicians to rapidly decide who should receive such care, what are the potential alternative management strategies, and what are the risks, benefits and costs of each alternative. In making a final management decision clinicians must also consider patients and relatives' values and preferences, as well as the societal, cultural, religious, moral, and legal implications of their choices.

Recent fiscal pressures add an additional dimension to decision-making in the ICU because it consumes a significant portion of a hospital budget, and frequently provides care during the last few days or weeks of life. Advancing technologies, aging population, and increasing societal expectations on the one side, and fiscal constrains on the other are likely to provide intensivists with increasing challenges in their future work.

Each health care system, each hospital, each ICU, and every clinician tries to deal with these sometimes conflicting demands in their own way. Our goal is to review one of the tools which, we believe, can help clinicians and health managers make optimal decisions on the level ranging from the care of individual patients to directions and priorities of the health care system.

What is evidence-based practice?

In 1990, a group of clinicians at McMaster University began to use the term "evidence-based medicine" to describe a particular philosophy of medical practice [1]. The principles of evidence-based medicine (EBM) apply equally well to other disciplines of health care, including nursing, respiratory therapy, physiotherapy, occupational therapy, and so on. The principles also apply equally well to the care of individual patients and to decisions concerning allocation of health care resources and are therefore highly relevant to health managers, purchasers, administrators and other health policy-makers. Thus the wider terms, evidence-based clinical practice (for care of individual patients) or evidence-based health care (for construction of health policies) have been introduced. The main goal of evidence-based medicine is to facilitate rapid and accurate application of evidence from sound clinical research to clinical practice.

One definition suggests that evidence-based medicine is the process of making health care decisions while using, in a conscientious and judicious way, the current best evidence from clinical research. Conscientious means that evidence is applied consistently and carefully to each patient. Judicious use requires considering the risks and benefits of diagnostic tests and alternative treatments, taking into account their clinical circumstances and preferences. The role of all crucial elements of this decision making process – evidence, clinical experience and values – is thus explicitly recognized in the EBM model. While EBM focuses clinicians' attention on evidence, if they fail to understand that evidence does not dictate decisions in isolation from patients', clinicians', and societal values, experiences, and expectations they are likely to misunderstand EBM and find its application disappointing.

Why do we need evidence-based practice?

What has led to the rise of the evidence-based medicine? First, use of weak study designs in assessing health care interventions has proved misleading when compared with the results of randomized trials (observational studies yield systematically larger estimates of treatment effect than randomized trials [2], concealed randomization results in smaller apparent treatment effects than open randomization, and double-blind studies produce smaller treatment effects than unblinded studies [3]).

Second, physiological rationale has failed to consistently predict the results of randomized trials. For example, trials of patients with heart failure demonstrated that angiotensin-converting enzyme inhibitors reduce mortality, whereas other promising vasodilators have had marginal or no effect [4] and some agents with vasodilator and inotropic properties actually increased mortality [5]. Promising cerebrovascular surgical procedures have had no effect or have increased stroke morbidity [6], while others have proved dramatically effective in reducing stroke [7]. Antiarrhythmic agents can obliterate non-lethal cardiac arrhythmias while increasing mortality [8].

Studies demonstrating that physicians manage similar patients very differently have provided a third impetus to the rise of evidence-based health care. In results unexplained by differences in patient characteristics, rates of common surgical procedures have varied up to seven-fold among countries [9], and rates of coronary artery bypass surgery have varied more than three-fold among Canadian provinces [10]. Possible explanations of this phenomenon included delay in the dissemination of new, valid information [11], and the lack of understanding of what the information means [12]. That some of these variations might lead to additional costs without additional benefit have made the dilemma more pressing and underlined the fourth major stimulus to evidence-based practice: the need to apply limited resources for health-care delivery in the most beneficial way.

Evidence-based practice and traditional approaches

Knowing some of the factors that have led to its high profile, we can better understand evidence-based medicine by focusing on how it differs from traditional approaches. One can view these differences as fundamental or revolutionary, or evolutionary. The former view contends that EBM represents a shift in the underlying paradigm of health-care delivery and notes changes in the associated assumptions, while the latter sees evidence-based medicine as a fine-tuning of approaches and ideas that were already in wide use.

The revolutionary concept of EBM identifies and questions the appropriateness of the assumptions behind the traditional practice of medicine, where clinical experience is considered a valid way to gain information; where physiologic principles constitute an appropriate guide for clinical practice; where the ability to assess evidence is acquired through usual medical training and common sense; and where uncertainty can be resolved by relying on experts.

According to the old paradigm clinicians sort out clinical problems they face by reflecting on their own clinical experience, on the underlying biology, by going to a textbook, or asking a local expert. When clinicians use the original literature to address a patient problem, the introduction and discussion are the main areas of interest. The old paradigm puts a high value on scientific authority and adherence to standard approaches.

Proponents of the new paradigm of evidence-based practice readily acknowledge that clinical experience, and the development of clinical instincts (particularly with respect to diagnosis), are necessary parts of becoming a competent physician. Many aspects of clinical practice cannot be adequately tested because of ethical or situational considerations. Clinical experience is again particularly important in these situations. Evidence-based practice, however, emphasizes that systematic attempts to record observations in an unbiased fashion markedly increase the confidence we have in knowledge about patient prognosis, the value of diagnostic tests, and the efficacy of treatment. In the absence of systematic observation, clinicians must be cautious in interpreting information derived from clinical experience and intuition, for it may be misleading.

Second, evidence-based medicine supporters have observed that inferences about the usefulness of diagnostic and therapeutic interventions that follow from pathophysiologic principles may lead to inaccurate predictions (vide treatment of ventricular arrhythmias [8]). A third principle is that the assessment of evidence requires knowledge of the rules governing the validity (believability) of such evidence, knowledge not taught in traditional medical curricula. Finally, EBM practitioners expect content and clinical experts, advisors, and teachers to refer to the available systematic evidence, thus avoiding confusing opinions with evidence, and distinguishing frequent scientific uncertainty [13] from unfamiliarity with the topic.

It follows that clinicians working in the new paradigm will regularly consult the original literature (including the "Methods" and "Results" sections) in solving clinical problems. Proponents of the new paradigm will gain the skills to make independent assessments of evidence, and thus evaluate the credibility of opinions being offered by experts [14].

This dramatic distinction between "new" and "old" paradigms is not only attractive and catches attention, but also generates controversy and antagonisms. An alternative conceptualization of evidence-based medicine sees it as an evolutionary process. While clinicians have always used the health care literature to solve patient problems, evidence-based practitioners acknowledge an explicit hierarchy of evidence ranging from a systematic review of randomized trials of interventions, through randomized trials of relevant management strategies, to high quality observational studies. If the literature is altogether barren, they will fall back on the underlying biology, and on their own and colleagues' clinical experience.

Both concepts of EBM emphasize, what is likely clear to all ICU practitioners, that the ultimate decision that clinicians make will not flow directly from the evidence, but includes tradeoffs, preference or value judgements about the alternatives involved [15, 16]. Ideally, the values and preferences for decisions about individual patient care will come from the patients themselves. Some patients, or their families, will prefer the traditional model of care in which the health worker makes decisions on the patients' behalf. In other situations patients or their representatives will insist on a more active role [17].

Practicing evidence-based medicine

Whether one finds the revolutionary or evolutionary conceptualization of evidence-based practice more appealing, they both imply a number of steps in clinical decision-making. Both models imply that to solve individual patient's or more general health care problems the practitioner (manager) must acquire skills that are not traditionally part of health-care training. These steps and skills, aimed at explicit identification and incorporation of evidence into decision making process include: defining a patient problem in a precise, answerable terms; deciding on what information is required to solve the problem; conducting an efficient search of the literature, which involves skilled use of computerized data bases; selecting the best of the relevant studies, which requires thorough knowledge of the rules of evidence required to determine their validity; extracting the clinical message; applying it to the patient problem; and preserving the content of the whole exercise, including the strengths, weaknesses, and clinical implications of the evidence, for future use. Practitioners need these skills when they must confront conflicting opinions, new findings, general uncertainty about how to proceed, and the clinical dilemma is important enough to spent time and effort to resolve. This does not imply that every clinical decision requires such a rigorous process (no astute clinician will search the literature to decide whether to give a rapid-acting diuretic to a patient in pulmonary oedema). Rather, practitioners should be equipped with the skills to answer dilemmas that arise in their clinical practice.

Life of EBM practitioner made easier

Clinicians can call on a wide variety of resources to learn the skills necessary to become efficient evidence-based practitioners. These include a series of articles published in JAMA [18] and a small, practically-oriented book [19]. These publications include strategies for defining clinical questions in ways that allow the clinician to seek their solution through the medical literature. They outline how computer searching can efficiently locate the best evidence, the software programs available, and search strategies for maximizing the comprehensiveness of the search without identifying an excessive number of irrelevant or methodologically weak articles.

Original journal articles can usefully be classified according to the clinical problem they address [20]. Primary articles provide original data regarding issues in treatment [21], diagnosis [22], harm [23] and prognosis [24]. Clinicians can apply a set of simple rules to decide whether a particular study is likely to be biased or unbiased in estimating the impact of treatment, the power of a diagnostic tests, or the likelihood of harm from a particular exposure (Table 1). For instance, if one finds a randomized trial addressing a treatment issue, and that trial is double-blind with complete follow-up of all patients, it is very likely that the study will yield an unbiased assessment of the treatment effect.

Clinicians may find many studies that address a clinical question and all may provide reasonably unbiased estimates of treatment benefit and harm, patient

Table 1. Guides for selecting articles that are most likely to provide valid results: Primary Studies

Therapy	Was the assignment of patients to treatments randomized and patients analyzed in the groups to which they were allocated?
	Was follow-up sufficiently complete?
Diagnosis	Was there an independent, blind comparison with a reference standard?
	Did the patient sample include an appropriate spectrum of the sort of patients to whom the diagnostic test will be applied in clinical practice?
Harm	Were there clearly identified comparison groups that were similar with respect to important determinants of outcome (other than the one of interest)?
	Were outcomes and exposures measured in the same way in the groups being compared?
Prognosis	Was there a representative patient sample at a well-defined point in the course of disease?
	Was follow-up sufficiently complete?

prognosis, or a diagnostic test's power. For each individual clinician appraising and summarizing these studies is prohibitively time-consuming. Thus, evidence-based practitioners are increasingly turning to integrative studies that combine results across a number of primary studies. These integrative studies include systematic reviews, decision analyses, practice guidelines, and economic analyses. These types of articles are as subject to systematic distortion from the truth (bias) as the primary research on which they are based, and clinicians must be able to distinguish between integrative studies with high and low likelihood of bias. For this they can apply an equally straightforward set of rules to make this differentiation (Table 2). Evidence-based clinicians should refrain from an uncritical acceptance of expert-based practice guidelines, economic analyses, and decision analyses to guide clinical practice. Principles of evidence-based practice suggest clinicians should critically evaluate any guidelines they consider adopting (Table 2) [25], and carefully consider individual patient circumstances in their application.

Once they have found the best evidence regarding the patient problem before them, and have determined the likelihood of bias, clinicians must extract the message from the paper. Treatment effects can be summarized by reductions in relative risk (treatment reduces the likelihood of death by a quarter, a third, or a half) or reductions in absolute risk (the risk of dying drops from 10% to 7.5%). Inevitably, a study's estimate of the treatment effect will involve some imprecision (measured by confidence intervals): in general the larger the sample size of a valid study, the more confident we can be that the truth lies somewhere near the study estimate. Finally, patients at high and low risk will differ according to the impact of treatment. In general, higher risk patients will receive more benefit. Evidence-based practitioners can integrate this information to help decide on optimal recommendations to offer to the patient [26].

Table 2. Guides for selecting articles that are most likely to provide valid results: Integrative Studies

Overview	Were the criteria used to select articles for explicit and appropriate?
	Was the search strategy comprehensive?
Practice guidelines	Were the options and outcomes explicit and appropriate?
	Did the guideline use an explicit process to identify, select and combine evidence?
Decision analysis	Did the analysis faithfully model a clinically important decision?
	Were the baseline probabilities and utilities based on valid data?
Economic analysis	Were two or more clearly described alternatives compared?
	Were the expected consequences of each alternative based on valid evidence?

The biggest challenge to evidence-based practice involves considerations of efficiency. Searching for and evaluating the evidence required to solve a clinical problem takes time. Fortunately, tools to help evidence-based practitioners become more efficient are increasingly available. More and more journals use structured abstracts that provide most of the methodologic information required to decide on the likelihood of bias, the applicability of the findings, and a quantitative estimate of their impact. The *American College of Physicians Journal Club* and *Evidence-Based Medicine* summarize the high-quality emerging literature by applying a methodologic screen to articles from a wide variety of journals and publishing structured abstracts of relevant articles that meet the criteria. "Best Evidence" provides a cd-rom and floppy disc version of these journals.

We are witnessing an explosion of integrative articles that avoid bias in their summary of the available information. This effort is spearheaded by the Cochrane Collaboration, a world-wide multidisciplinary network of clinicians, methodologists, and policy-makers whose goal is to provide systematic reviews for the approximately 250,000 randomized trials that have tested health care interventions, and to organize these reviews in a clinician and patient-friendly fashion. The results, the Cochrane library, is available both on disk and online. Finally, computer technology is allowing clinicians faster and more efficient access to all these sources of information.

Objections to evidence-based practice

Not everyone has greeted evidence-based health care with enthusiasm. Most of the doubts and disagreements come, we believe, from misunderstandings of the nature of evidence-based practice. EBM specific skills are a supplement and not a replacement of traditional clinical skills. The application of evidence to solve patient problems will be useless unless guided by clinical judgement that flows from both an expert knowledge of underlying physiology and a large experience of dealing with similar patient problems. Clinical skills, clinical experience, and understanding of physiology remain at the core of clinical assessment and management.

At the same time, clinical research, the domain of main interest for EBM practitioners, does not compete with basic research, but rather it heavily depends and builds on it. In this spirit we believe that application of EBM does not tie clinicians' hands and does not preclude them from using gray zone interventions [13, 27]. On the contrary, by allowing clinicians to grade the strength of evidence, it facilitates acknowledgement that decisions are made with uncertainty and distinguishing opinions from evidence. Last but not least, being able to evaluate the strength of evidence helps to direct to this areas of weak evidence warranting the attention of researchers and granting agencies.

The dangers to avoid in practicing and teaching EBM arise from misinterpretations of what EBM is and what it is not. The include: 1) indiscriminate rejection of clinical experience, physiological principles and common sense from the decision making process; 2) rigid dismissal of non-RCT derived clinical evidence (i.e. equating evidence with RCTs' results); 3) expecting the evidence to "make decisions" in isolation from clinical experience and the system of values operating in a particular setting; 4) equating lack of valid evidence of efficacy with the evidence of lack of efficacy; 5) excessive scepticism about generalizing results to patients other than those eligible for particular studies; 6) neglecting direct patient care while concentrating on learning critical appraisal skills, and 7) using rules of evidence selectively to support preconceived ideas. Finally, 8) avoiding decision making under conditions of uncertainty is a direct contradiction to the actual term "evidence-based medicine", which implies weighing the pros and cons of particular decisions under such conditions. If any of the above misconceptions was actually part of EBM philosophy, criticism of EBM would be fully justified. While some of these misconceptions may have their advocates, it would be however both inappropriate and dangerous to confuse them with the philosophy of evidence-based care.

Barriers to practicing EBM include the time and effort involved in critical appraisal, the threatening nature of evidence-based practice in the face of rudimentary critical appraisal skills, and that sense of futility that may arise when evidence is weak. The strategies to introduce EBM principles in medical decision making and daily medical practice include explicit recognition that EBM-specific skills are a supplement and not a replacement of traditional clinical skills, that critical appraisal exercise should be conducted only in a clinically relevant settings, and that the rules and hierarchy of evidence have to be few and simple.

Finally, even appropriate use of research evidence will not provide optimal care unless applied in a humane and compassionate manner.

Conclusion

Evidence-based medicine and health care has direct implications for critical practice. Its main strength is in empowering clinicians to explicitly recognize the role of evidence, experience, and values in clinical decision making, to recognize the quality of available evidence, and to distinguish lack of knowledge from scientific uncertainty. Evidence-based practice allows more precise communication among patients, clinicians, and administrators. It facilitates assessment of proven and potential benefits, especially associated with the introduction of new diagnostic and therapeutic ICU interventions and technologies. Evidence-based care requires rigorous testing of new diagnostic and therapeutic technologies. This evaluation should result in estimates of the benefits to patients, and leave us confident that the resources devoted to application of the technology are not better spent elsewhere. The standards may seem onerous, but they are necessary if we are to enhance the quality and efficiency of critical care delivery.

References

1. Guyatt GH (1991) Evidence-based medicine [editorial]. Ann Internal Medicine 114[Suppl 2]
2. Sacks HS, Chalmers TC, Smith H Jr (1983) Sensitivity and specificity of clinical trials. Randomized versus historical assignment in controlled clinical trials. Arch Intern Med 143: 753-755
3. Schulz KF, Chalmers I, Hayes RJ, Altman DG (1995) Empirical evidence of bias. Dimensions of methodological quality associated with estimates of treatment effects in controlled trials. JAMA 273:408-412
4. Mulrow CD, Mulrow JP, Linn WD et al (1988) Relative efficacy of vasodilator therapy in chronic congestive heart failure. JAMA 259:3422-3426
5. Packer M, Carver JR, Rodeheffer RJ et al (1991) Effect of oral milrinone on mortality in severe chronic heart failure. N Engl J Med 325:1468
6. The EC/IC Bypass Study Group (1985) Failure of extracranial-intracranial arterial bypass to reduce the risk of ischemic stroke. N Engl J Med 313:1191-1200
7. North American Symptomatic Carotid Endarterectomy Trial Collaborators (1991) Beneficial effect of carotid endarterectomy in symptomatic patients with high-grade carotid stenosis. N Engl J Med 325:445-453
8. Echt DS, Liebson PR, Mitchell LB et al (1991) Mortality and morbidity in patients receiving encainide, flecainide, or placebo. The Cardiac Arrhythmia Suppression Trial. N Engl J Med 324:781-788
9. McPherson K (1990) Why do variations occur? In: Anderson TF, Mooney G (eds) The challenges of medical practice variations. Macmillan, London, pp 16-35
10. Anderson GM, Lomas J (1989) Regionalization of coronary artery bypass surgery: effects on access. Med Care 27:288-296
11. Antman EM, Lau J, Kupelnick B et al (1992) A comparison of meta-analyses of randomized trial and recommendations of clinical experts: Treatment of myocardial infarction. JAMA 268:240-248
12. Fahey T, Griffiths S, Peters TJ (1995) Evidence based purchasing: understanding results of clinical trials and systematic reviews. BMJ 311:1056-1060
13. Naylor CD (1995) Grey zones of clinical practice: Some limits to evidence-based medicine. Lancet 345:840-842

14. Chalmers I (1983) Scientific inquiry and authoritarianism in perinatal care and education. Birth 10:151-164
15. Hayward R, Wilson MC, Tunis SR et al and the Evidence-Based Medicine Working Group (1995) Users' guides to the medical literature. VIII. How to use clinical practice guidelines. Part A. Are the recommendations valid? JAMA 274:570-574
16. Guyatt GH, Sackett DL, Sinclair J et al (1995) Users' guides to the medical literature. IX. A Method for grading health care recommendations. JAMA 274:1800-1804
17. Hope T (1995) Evidence based patient choice. Report to the Anglia and Oxford Health Authority into the use of evidence based information for enhancing patient choice. Anglia and Oxford Regional Health Authority, Oxford
18. Guyatt GH, Rennie D (1993) Users' guides to the medical literature: Editorial. JAMA 270: 2096-2097
19. Sackett DL, Richardson WS, Rosenberg W, Haynes RB (1997) Evidence-based medicine. Churchill Livingston, New York
20. Oxman AD, Sackett DL, Guyatt GH for the Evidence-based Medicine Working Group (1993). Users' guides to the medical literature. I. How to get started. JAMA 270:2093-2095
21. Guyatt GH, Sackett DL, Cook DJ for the Evidence-based Medicine Working Group (1993) Users' guides to the medical literature. II. How to use an article about therapy or prevention. Part A. Are the results of the study valid? JAMA 270:2598-2601
22. Jaeschke R, Guyatt GH, Sackett DL for the Evidence-based Medicine Working Group (1994) Users' guides to the medical literature. III. How to use an article about a diagnostic test. Part A. Are the results of the study valid? JAMA 271:389-391
23. Levine M, Walter S, Lee H et al for the Evidence-based Medicine Working Group (1994) Users' guides to the medical literature. IV. How to use an article about harm. JAMA 271: 1615-1619
24. Laupacis A, Wells G, Richardson S, Tugwell P for the Evidence-based Medicine Working Group (1994) Users' guides to the medical literature. V. How to use an article about prognosis. JAMA 272:234-237
25. Wilson MC, Hayward R, Tunis SR et al for the Evidence-Based Medicine Working Group (1995) Users' Guides to the medical literature. VIII. How to use clinical practice guidelines. B. What are the recommendations and will they help me in caring for my patients? JAMA 274:1630-1632
26. Guyatt GH, Sackett DL, Cook DJ for the Evidence-based Medicine Working Group (1994) Users' guides to the medical literature. II. How to use an article about therapy or prevention. Part B. What were the results and will they help me in caring for my patients. JAMA 271: 59-63
27. Kilbourn RG (1997) Evidence based medicine in critical care: Will it takes us over the cutting edge? Crit Care Med 25:1448-1449

ETHICS AND QUALITY CONTROL IN THE ICU

The Problem of Informed Consent in Critically Ill Patients

H. Burchardi

The special situation in intensive care medicine

In intensive care medicine decisions are characterised by: uncertainty of diagnosis, urgency of treatment, continuous change of situation, and high costs of interventions. Specific pressure is caused by the "technologic imperative" which means:

1. the need to do everything, regardless of outcome, potential effects or costs, particularly when patients are likely to die without aggressive treatment and when patients cannot make their own decision;

2. strict legal demands for liability and claims for damages promote defensive medicine and high level of measures for diagnosis and therapy: invasive (e.g. pulmonary artery catheter) as well as expensive (e.g. Labs, CT scans) diagnostics and treatments (e.g. operations, organ function replacement).

Altogether, ICU physicians seem to be more procedure-oriented and to look less after quality-of-life-factors of their patients. However, our professional ethics must prevent the ICU physicians from performing unreasonable or undesirable activism. This is mandatory for ethical reasons and not because of economical arguments. Nevertheless, the cut down of economical resources may accelerate the need.

The policy for admission to the ICU varies considerably throughout Europe as an international survey has demonstrated [1], in particular according to the availibility of ICU beds in the different European countries. Despite limited beds two third of the respondents did admit patients even whith little or no hope of survival.

In a society in which everybody has a legal claim for full medical service, I am strongly convinced that admission to the ICU should not be restricted even if chances for a favourable result is limited: "everybody should get a chance"! In this case, however, also withholding and withdrawing treatment must be possible and feasible in daily practice. But this decision is extremely difficult in patients generally unconscious when it is difficult to protect their autonomy.

The uncertainty of the conditions

Futility - inappropriateness - inadvisability

From a review from literature Luce [2] concluded that physicians are not ethically required to provide futile or unreasonable care to patients who are brain dead, vegetative, critically or terminally ill with little chance of recovery, and unlikely to benefit from CPR. The issue of the physician's refusal of requested care has not been resolved by case law or legal statute, but it is supported by the ethical principles.

According to the SCCM Consensus Report [3] futile treatments should never be offered. However, futility is a rare situation in intensive care medicine and needs further specification. Therefore, the "Ethics Committees" of the SCCM [4] defined these conditions more specifically:

> Treatments should be defined as futile only when they will not accomplish their intended goal. Conflicts arise when there are disagreements about whether the desired goal is appropriate and whether the probability of success is sufficiently great... Since these conflicts are typically about differences in values rather than disagreements about facts, clinicians should be very cautious about labelling these therapeutic options as futile. Seen in this context, treatments may be classified into four categories: a) treatments that have no beneficial physiologic effect; b) treatments that are extremely unlikely to be beneficial; c) treatments that have beneficial effect but are extremely costly; and d) treatment that are of uncertain or controversial benefit. Treatments that fall into the first category..., should be labelled as *futile*. Treatments that fall into the other three categories may be considered *inappropriate and hence inadvisable*, but should not be labelled futile.

Thus, the concept of futility is generally not useful in establishing policies to limit treatment. Futile treatments, as defined above, are rare, and are not usually offered or disputed. On the other hand, there are many treatments that have extremely unlikely, extremely costly, or extremely marginal benefit. These are *inappropriate or inadvisable treatments*. A judgement that a treatment is inadvisable should occur only after completing a process that ensures respect and consideration of all relevant viewpoints (i.e. all medical and non-medical factors) [4]. And such a decision should not be made under pressure of time.

Prognosis of near death

Scoring systems are not developed for individual prognosis. Their use as a sole guide for decisions whether to initiate or continue to provide intensive care is therefore inappropriate.

In a retrospective analysis from two large data bases (USA) the prognostic power of APACHE III to predict the factual death in individuals one week and one day before was determined (Table 1).

Table 1. Prognoses of seriously ill patients few days before death

Retrospective analysis of two large studies:
- SUPPORT: 9.105 patients with one of nine selected serious illnesses:
             2.360 died in hospital
             4.537 died within 180 days (5 hospitals, 4 yrs data collection)
- APACHE III: 16.622 patients in 40 hospitals:
             2.750 patients died

Predicted chance of survival for 2 months:
             1 week before death: 51% (resp. 45%)
             1 day before death: 17% (resp. 14%)

Modified from [8]

There were large variations among the different diseases. This indicates that death mostly remains unpredictable, even just days before death!

Nevertheless, scoring systems may be a valuable argument when discussing probability of survival and, thus, may help to estimate the appropriateness of treatment in individual patients.

Who decides? Autonomy and surrogates for patient's decision

Definitions [5]

Informed consent: for an autonomous consent, legal competency, decision making competency, adequate information, true understanding, voluntary decision, and free choice are mandatory. Consent should be given in writing, orally, or at least by participation.

Anticipated consent: consent by the patient before he becomes disabled for instance by sedation.

Consent by proxy: in some countries it has become practice (and accepted by Law) that another person, especially the spouse or a near relative, is given the power of attorney in health care.

Consent by guardian: a legal representative ("guardian") of a child or a mentally handicapped adult is able to consent officially for the person to treatment decisions.

Presumed consent: in unconscious patients (often the case in intensive care medicine) it can be presumed that the patient would allow all medical interventions and decisions in his favour, unless otherwise stipulated.

Informed consent and its problems

Patient's autonomy has the highest priority. This means that it is the patient who has to decide after informed consent what he wants to be done. It is doubtful whether completely informed consent is ever possible, there may be various degrees from poorly to completely which also depends on the benefit/risk relationship. But, even when the patient is competent and fully informed, there is always the possibility of dependency to the treating physician. Thus, even for the competent patient the fully informed consent may be regarded more as an ethical ideal rather than an unlimited demand. And patient's autonomy can certainly not be an acceptable argument for the physician to withdraw from his professional responsibility.

Information of patients and/or proxies is necessarily incomplete. In a recent investigation [6] on the effect of a 30 minutes preoperative information for a simple diagnostic procedure (bronchoscopy) in 80 patients a large majority was satisfied by the information and had no further request. However, more than one third was unable to remember one out of the nine risks mentioned to them. Nevertheless, the oral dialogue apparently created a certain degree of relief and confidence, whereas, written information was regarded as frightening. It demonstrates that the dialogue between the physician and his patient can be regarded as a vehicle for confidence rather than for information; furthermore, the patient (or his relatives) primarily want to trust rather than to decide. Often such a dialogue ends with the question: "Doctor, how would you decide in my situation?".

In intensive care medicine most patients (at least those for whom foregoing decisions becomes necessary) are unconscious. Possible surrogates in this situation are (Table 2): a patient's advanced directive (rarely specific enough), a legal representative appointed by court (rarely attendant in acute diseases typically in ICM), family members or friends (= assent). However, the surrogate for consent/assent by family members is not allowed in some West-European countries (e.g. in Germany).

Table 2. Informed consent and surrogates

Autonomy ("informed consent"): highest legal and ethical priority

Patient's advanced directive: mostly regarded as not specific and sufficiently actual;
    in Germany accepted only as indication for patient's request (Bundesärztekammer 1993)

Legal representative (appointed by court, "guardian"): decision needs approval by court
    (except in urgency), no definite regulations (legal uncertainty!)

Family: in Germany no decision-making power, accepted only as a source of information about
    patient's preferences

Physicians, ICU team: advocate for patient's "best interest", compassion (danger of paternalism!),
    decision based on presumed consent of the patient

In some countries (e.g. in Germany) the *presumed consent* of the patient may be taken as a surrogate in case of unconsciousness and lack of other surrogates. The presumed consent can be inquired from members of the family or close friends. However, this always remains questionable, as it is difficult for physicians to transmit the complete information of the situation to the relatives. Furthermore, it is difficult to separate the wishes and motives of the patient from those of the relatives. Different motives (such as a sense of guilt, a supposed moral obligation, or the instinctive fright of reproaches by family members or neighbours) may prevent from an honest decision. Also, death is rarely a topic of discussion between humans under normal conditions (which count for the acute situations in intensive care). And, last but not least, it often seems not to be acceptable to burden the family with the merciless end-of-life decision.

To inform or not to inform: the reality

A questionnaire was sent to 1272 western European intensivists, 504 completed questionnaires from 16 countries could be analyzed [7]: 25% of respondents said that they always give complete information to a patient (or the family), although 35% felt they should. 32% would give complete details of an iatrogenic incident, but 68% felt they should. 75% would accept the right of a patient to refuse treatment, but 19% would carry out the procedure against the patient's wishes. There was a significant difference between countries in these attitudes with a tendency to less autonomy from North to South (influenced perhaps also by religious backgrounds).

Conclusion: Doctors are often not completely honest with their patients regarding their diagnosis or prognosis. However, most doctors will respect a patient's right to refuse treatment.

A proposal

Planning end-of-life in intensive care medicine is a real dilemma [8]: there is no satisfactory definition of terminal illness. There are no parameters for prognosing death even few days before. Terms like "terminally ill" or "merely mortal" are unavoidable arbitrary.

Thus, planning for end-of-life care must occur while the patient still has a considerable chance of survival. In clinical practice a "combined management" is needed: seeking (and fighting) for survival, while already acknowledging the likelihood of death. This is a continuous process, trying to gain confidence of the patient (if conscious) and/or the relatives.

1. In the acute, life-threatening situation admission to intensive care should not be limited. Effective and intensive treatment needs to be initiated quickly.

2. However, if the presumed result of the treatment is not achieved in a reasonable period of time, the further decisions should be faced. This needs honest discussion and confident information of relatives about the patient's views and belief and his personal objectives.

3. The final decision, however, must be taken by an experienced, reliable physician. It is an individual decision closely linked to our medical professional ethic, it can never be handed over to e.g. a committee (an ethics committee, however, can offer valuable support and advice).

Accepted decisions of withholding and withdrawal treatment can only be based on a profound confidence between the physician and the family – and this is an ongoing process (Table 3).

Table 3. Talking about withdrawal life support

Talk with and seek unanimity among the various members of the healthcare team
Solicit the patient's views regarding life support or (if the patient is unable to participate decision-making) seek any available evidence of the patient's wishes
Be patient, and work toward a unanimous decision
Establish time-limited goals
Allow the patients (and relatives) the opportunities to express feelings of anger or mistrust
Be understanding and avoid becoming defensive
Seek facilitators, especially when conflict arises

From Guidelines of the Stanford University Medical Centre [9]

References

1. Vincent JL (1990) European attitudes towards ethical problems in ICM: Results of an ethical questionnaire. Crit Care Med 16:256-264
2. Luce JM (1995) Physicians do not have a responsibility to provide futile or unreasonable care if a patient or family insists. Crit Care Med 23:760-766
3. Task Force on Ethics of the Society of Critical Care Medicine (1990) Consensus report on the ethics of foregoing life-sustaining treatments in the critically ill. Crit Care Med 18:1435-1439
4. The Society of Critical Care Medicine Ethics Committee (1992) Attitudes of critical care medicine professionals concerning forgoing life-sustaining treatments. Crit Care Med 20:320-326
5. Deutsch E (1997) Clinical studies in the intensive care unit: ethical and legal aspects. In: Burchardi H (ed) Current topics in intensive care, vol 4. WB Saunders, London Philadelphia Toronto, pp 265-280
6. Bieda K, Meran JG, Wagner TOF et al (1997) Aufklärung zwischen rechtlicher Forderung und Patientenwunsch. Forum Deutsche Krebsgsellschaft 12:112-116
7. Vincent JL (1998) Information in the ICU: Are we being honest with our patients? The results of a European questionnaire. Intensive Care Med (in press)
8. Lynn J, Harrell F, Cohn F et al (1997) Prognoses of seriously ill hospitalized patients on the days before death: implications for patient care and public policy. New Horiz 5:56-61
9. Ruark JE, Raffin TA, Stanford University Medical Center Committee on Ethics (1988) Initiating and withdrawing life support: Principles and practice in adult medicine. N Engl J Med 318:25-30

Progress in Scoring Systems, Safety and Quality of Care in the ICU

J.-R. Le Gall, C. Alberti

Probability models derived from scoring systems are used to evaluate the performance of ICUs [1-5]. The comparison of observed versus expected mortality or standard mortality ratio (SMR) is said to be reproducible and related to the efficacy of the units.

Of course, the efficacy of intensive care is a major economic and ethical problem in the world. The costs of intensive care are indeed high, more than 10% of a given hospital's expenditures. In addition, the efficacy, i.e., the usefulness of intensive care, can be determined only by comparing the observed with the predicted mortality rate because a randomized clinical trial would be unethical.

Using the Acute Physiology and Chronic Health Evaluation (APACHE) II [3] or III [1], the SMR varies from 0.59 to 1.58 from the "best" to the "worst" ICU. Using the Mortality Probability Model (MPM) II in 25 ICUs [6], 21 ICUs were found to lead clinical performance index between −1 and +1 SD. The best performing unit had an index 1.57 SDs above the mean and the worst an index 3.55 SDs below.

However, when looking at subgroups of patients, it appears that the calibration of the probability models is very poor. In obstetric patients in the ICU, the observed mortality rate is 6.9%, whereas mortality predicted by 16.6% [7].

The MPM is not well calibrated when applied to patients in the United Kingdom and Ireland [8]. Applied to 1292 Japanese patients [9], the APACHE II system shows a lower observed mortality than expected, especially for the more severe patients and for males (SMR, 0.88). The role of case mix variations in these differences is not clear.

Using the APACHE II in 1973 patients from Hong Kong [10], the global predicted (38%) and observed (36%) death rates were close, but calibration was better for surgical patients. In the risk ranges between 0.35 and 0.55 differences of 10% to 32% exist between the observed and expected death rates. In another study of 656 patients from one ICU, the SMR by APACHE II was 0.99 for medical patients and 0.49 for surgical patients [11].

The calibration of APACHE II for 2061 patients in a surgical ICU in Switzerland was very poor [12]. The discriminant power in this study was worse for elective patients.

It is difficult to compare the SMR of two units if the proportion of elective, surgical emergency, and medical patients is not known. Multiple diagnoses are frequent in intensive care patients, and it may be difficult to choose a principal diagnosis [13], which will influence the expected death rate. The diagnosis weight depends on the influence of this diagnosis on mortality in the original database. Nevertheless, variables other than those chosen for the database may be influential. For instance, in patients whit acute renal failure the presence of anuria and sepsis and the time of the onset have a prognostic role [6]. In the original data base in which the diagnoses are not precisely defined these parameters are not taken into account.

Whether a patient is from the emergency or another ward, the operating room, or another hospital will influence the prognosis, but these parameters are difficult to control from one country to another [14, 15]. What can we do to resolve these issues? The first method is to look at the results in one specific disease that occurs with high frequency (e.g., chronic obstructive pulmonary disease, drug overdose). The published probability models must be checked and customized if necessary. The second method is to compare the performances of the units, taking into account all patients. In fact, the difference in observed versus expected mortality may be due only to the difference in case mix. Also, the method by which a principal diagnosis is chosen when the probability model includes multiple diagnoses must be the same for all users.

Routinely measuring performance of an ICU based on the SMR is impossible without accurate data collection and analysis. Guidelines for definition of variables and application of methods were until now either absent, not provided in sufficient detail, or not objective enough to ensure standardization of data across centers. Some variables are easy to standardize: age, diuresis, and presence of AIDS using precise criteria. Some are more difficult: what is the Glasgow coma score of a sedated patient? Due to the variability of the case mix over time within the same ICU and the even higher variability between ICUs, the sample size must be sufficient to assess the performance of any given scoring system.

We must be very careful when analyzing the SMR [16]. When the observed mortality is different from the expected by more than two SDs, an analysis of case mix, recruitment protocols, organization, and resources is necessary before a difference in clinical efficacy can be supposed [6].

Problems exist with data collection for most case mix adjustment methods. Guidelines for applications of adjustment methods must be standardized and published. Before judging the performance of an ICU based on its SMR, many improvements of the predictive ability of the probability models must be made.

A recent position paper has been published by Teres et al. [17]. Most of the following text has been inspired by this work that we have taken part in. The tables have been reproduced from the original article.

Risk-adjusted severity-of-illness measurements have gained widespread acceptance in general medical/surgical ICUs but have not successfully achieved field or external validation. Several practical questions arise regarding evaluation of quality of care across multiple institutions, including standardization of the time to start measuring the major critical episode and identifying which particular ICU admission should be counted. There are now problems using hospital discharge to decide vital status when ventilator-dependent patients are transferred to chronic or sub-acute care facilities.

Teres et al. propose (Table 1):

1. Defining a set of simple rules to systematize a time to trigger the clock to start measurements.
2. Measuring a standardized mortality ratio based on a target patient sample of 300 consecutive evaluable patients twice per year. For high volume ICUs this would translate into two three-month data collection efforts. ICUs with smaller patient volume may need an extended time to reach the target sample size, or a minimum of 200 patients.
3. Establishing a fixed time interval of ninety days after the first major ICU admission to determine the predicted and observed mortality of the acute episode of care.
4. Generating a simple weighted hospital or care scale to measure resource consumption as a cost proxy over the same ninety day time period.

They feel that the risk adjusted outcomes approach combining clinical performance and resource consumption is preferable to structural, organizational, or procedural approaches to defining a high performance system. The severity-adjusted methodology, uniquely available in critical care, is inherently simple and powerful and provides benchmark data for future comparisons.

They define a high-performance ICU as one standard deviation better than the benchmark for both clinical and resource measures at ninety days post-acute ICU episode of illness. They suggest collaboration among national and international critical care societies to study, criticize, evaluate, and pre-test our definition, rules, and methodology and then to organize the initiative through local-regional business-community hospital coalitions.

Table 1. Standardized mortality ratio (observed mortality/mean predicted mortality)

Advantages
    Measure performance pre-ICU and post-ICU discharge (System Performance)
    Need large sample size
    Show confidence interval
    Show goodness-of-fit table
Problems
    When does ICU care start?
    What does hospital discharge mean?
    What about multiple admissions?

(From: Teres D, Higgins T, Steingrub J et al (1998) Defining a high-performance ICU system for the 21st century: a position paper. J Int Care Med 13:195-205. With permission)

New focus on the acute episode of critical illness

Teres et al.'s approach to refining severity models for the 21st century is to take into account changes in medical practice, and to focus on the acute episode of critical illness. They want to maintain the general integrity of the severity of illness models as much as possible. It has been repeatedly demonstrated that simple physiology and conditions do correlate with patient mortality following acute critical illness. Lead-time bias has been recognized in a comparison of medical patients admitted directly or through an emergency department. The APACHE III system does have a factor for lead time bias but does not reflect the complexity of the issues (Table 2).

Table 2. General ICU severity models for adult patients

APACHE II/III @ 24 hours
SAPS II @ 24 hours
MPM II at presentation and 24 hours
Post-operative cardiac surgery models
Multi-organ failure @ 24 hours

Teres et al. support intermittent rather than continuous data collection because of the costs associated with maintaining high quality data over an extended time period. They recommend a target population of 300 evaluable patients would allow calculation of SMR plus confidence interval (Table 3).

Table 3. Suggested definition of a high performance ICU

- • Low severity adjusted mortality 90 days after first major ICU experience at highest level hospital*
- • Low severity adjusted resource use 90 days after first major ICU exposure including ICU stay, hospital stay, and skilled nursing facility stay
- • Among patients who die 72 hours after ICU admission, low percentage of terminal CPR
- ◦ Low severity adjusted mortality at hospital discharge
- ◦ Low percentage of monitor patients
- ◦ Low re-admission rate
- ◦ Low re-intubation rate
- ◦ Low percentage of resistant nosocomial infections
- ◦ High satisfaction score from patients and/or families
- ◦ High level of provider satisfaction

• Recommended measures
* Based on 300 consecutive, evaluable patients; for ICUs with smaller patient volume, the minimum would be 200 patients
◦ Associated with high performance ICU but not easily measured

(From: Teres D, Higgins T, Steingrub J et al (1998) Defining a high-performance ICU system for the 21st century: a position paper. J Int Care Med 13:195-205. With permission)

Recommendations and suggested rules for starting the clock

To minimize and simplify complex issues of lead time bias, Teres et al. suggest an arbitrary start time to be the first major admission to a critical care unit at the highest level hospital, even if the patient is subsequently transferred from a single organ ICU to a multi-disciplinary unit (Fig. 1).

Resource measures

Resource utilization costs can best be estimated by using a simple weighted hospital care day approach that includes post-acute hospital care. Teres et al.'s methodology is based on a proposal by Rapoport et al. using ICU and hospital days. The suggested weights for ICU, step-down, hospital and post hospital facilities are listed in Table 4.

Table 4. Suggested formula for resource use 90 days post first major ICU exposure*

ICU admission day (including re-admission):
= 14 units if on life support†
= 10 units if not on life support
Next 6 days in ICU:
= 12 units/day if on more than one life support†
= 10 units/day if on a ventilator
= 6 units/day if not on a ventilator
After 7 days in ICU:
= 8 units/day if on a ventilator
= 6 units each day not on a ventilator
Intermediate/step-down:
= 4 units each day
General ward:
= 2 units each day
High level rehabilitation unit (including ventilator unit):
= 2 units each day
Nursing home or extensive home care:
= .5 unit each day
Full support chronic care facility:
= 2 units each day

---

* Arbitrary scale, generally reflecting physician (including consultants), nurse, support staff and mid level care provider differences among levels of care: needs testing, including sensitivity analysis.
† e.g., mechanical ventilation, acute dialysis, or vasopressors

(From: Teres D, Higgins T, Steingrub J et al (1998) Defining a high-performance ICU system for the 21st century: a position paper. J Int Care Med 13:195-205. With permission)

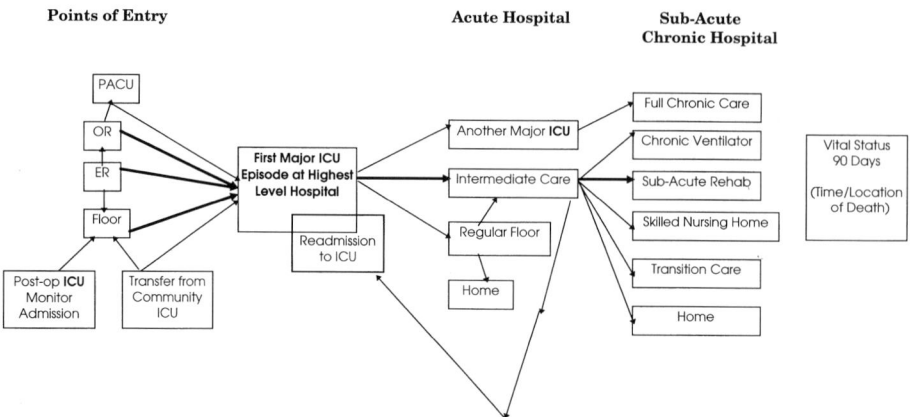

Fig. 1. Episode of critical illness (when to start the ICU clock)

New definition of a high performance ICU system

A high performance ICU system has a low observed to mean expected mortality ratio at ninety days after the first major ICU admission, and a low severity adjusted resource utilization including post hospital care during the same ninety day period.

Table 5. Levels of care at 90 days

- Intensive care unit
- Step-down or ventilator unit in hospital
- Acute care hospital
- Ventilator unit in chronic care facility
- Level I subacute rehabilitation
- Level II skilled nursing facility
- Level III custodial facility
- Level IV rest home
- Home with home care support
- Independent living

(From: Teres D, Higgins T, Steingrub J et al (1998) Defining a high-performance ICU system for the 21st century: a position paper. J Int Care Med 13:195-205. With permission)

Summary

General ICU severity models have become accepted and are in widespread use, have an extensive published literature, and contain "simple" clinical values.

They are robust when used for outcome-based population analyses of large numbers of heterogeneous patients but do poorly in external field applications. Although there are recognized problems with using standardized mortality ratio as a measure of outcome, many can be minimized by the described rules on when to start and stop the clock. By adopting an "official" definition of the start of ICU care and using a ninety day observation period, the standardized mortality ratio (with confidence interval) can be used to compare quality of care among similar ICU systems for local, national, and international application.

It should be acknowledged that the SMR is not the sole measure of quality. However, other important outcomes need to be better defined. We propose measuring the rate of terminal DNR orders in the ICU, and the patient's location at 90 days as a proxy for functional outcome. A simple weighted resource scale also collected over ninety days will provide a proxy measure for the "costs" of the episode of critical illness. ICU systems with high clinical performance and low resource use should be identified (with documentation by external audit), recognized, acknowledged and studied. These ICU systems should be identified as medallion level I ICUs.

References

1. Zimmerman JE, Shortell SM, Knaus WA et al (1993) Value and cost of teaching hospitals: a prospective, multicenter, inception cohort study. Crit Care Med 21:1432-1442
2. Knaus Wa, Draper EA, Wagner DP, Zimmerman JE (1986) An evaluation of outcome from intensive care in major medical centers. Ann Intern Med 104:410-418
3. Zimmerman JE, Shortell SM, Rousseau D et al (1993) Improving intensive care: observations based on organizational case studies in nine intensive care units: a prospective, multicenter study. Crit Care Med 21:1443-1451
4. Le Gall JR, Lemeshow S, Saulnier F (1993) A new simplified acute physiology score (SAPS II) base on a European/North American multicenter study. JAMA 270:2957-2963
5. Loirat P (1995) Scores de gravité: évaluation des performances. Actualités en Réanimation et Urgences. Arnette, Paris 91-98
6. Rapoport J, Teres D, Lemeshow S, Gehlbach S (1994) A method for assessing the clinical performance and cost-effectiveness of intensive care: a multicenter inception cohort study. Crit Care Med 22:1385-1391
7. Lewinsohn G, Herman A, Leonov Y, Klinowski E (1994) Critically ill obstetrical patients: outcome and predictability. Crit Care Med 22 1412-1414
8. Rowan KM, Kerr JH, Major E et al (1994) Intensive care society's acute physiology and chronic health evaluation (APACHE II) study in Britain and Ireland: a prospective, multicenter cohort study comparing two methods for predicting outcome for adult intensive care patients. Crit Care Med 22:1392-1401
9. Sirio CA, Tajmi K, Tase C et al (1992) An initial comparison of intensive care in Japan and the United States. Crit Care Med 20:1207-1215
10. Oh TE, Hutchinson R, Short S et al (1993) Verification of the acute physiology and chronic health evaluation scoring system in a Hong Kong intensive care unit. Crit Care Med 21: 698-705
11. Marsh HM, Krishan I, Naessens JM (1990) Assessment of prediction of mortality by using the APACHE II scoring system in intensive care units. Mayo Clin Proc 65:4549-1557

12. Berger M, Marazzi A, Freeman A, Chiolera R (1992) Evaluation of the consistency of Acute Physiology and Chronic Health Evaluation (APACHE II) scoring in a surgical intensive care unit. Crit Care Med 20:1681-1687
13. Loirat P (1994) Critique of existing scoring systems: admission scores. Réanimation Urgences 3:173-175
14. Escarce J, Kelley MA (1990) Admission source to the medical intensive care unit predicts hospital death independent of APACHE II score. JAMA 264:2389-2394
15. Borlase BC, Baxter JK, Kenney PR (1991) Elective intrahospital admissions versus acute interhospital transfers to a surgical intensive care unit: cost and outcome prediction. J Trauma 31:915-918
16. Boyd O, Grounds RM (1993) Physiological scoring systems and audit. Lancet 341:1573-1574
17. Teres D, Higgins T, Steingrub J et al (1998) Defining a high-performance ICU system for the 21st century: a position paper. J Int Care Med 13:195-205

Is Mortality the Only Outcome Measure in ICU Patients?

J.-L. Vincent

Clinical trials, by definition, need to have an aim, an outcome measure. Indeed, there is no point conducting a trial if there is no endpoint in view. The choice of the outcome measure employed will vary according to the agent/technique being assessed but in intensive care medicine, the majority of clinical trials currently focus on the 28 day all-cause mortality rate. This measure may, however, not necessarily be the most appropriate, and we will discuss the reasons for this, and possible alternatives, in this paper.

Mortality as the outcome measure

Survival is determined by many factors including a patient's primary diagnosis and physiologic reserve (Fig. 1). The multiple factors involved in the death of a patient make it unlikely that we will be able to significantly alter survival with a single therapeutic strategy, and we are perhaps naive (or arrogant!) to believe this is possible. In conditions where the exact pathological mechanism of death is known and the proposed therapy has a direct action on that process, then mortality may be an appropriate measure [1]. However, such cases are rare, far more frequently we are unable to explain the exact process involved in patient death.

Another factor influencing mortality is the standard of patient care. Our advanced knowledge of disease processes, improved imaging techniques, increased range of available drugs, have all lead to high quality intensive care. This in turn means that any improvement in mortality by a proposed agent is likely to be small. We no longer have the possibility, as Lister did in the 1860s, of demonstrating a drop in mortality from 46% to 15% by the introduction of a new therapy (in this case, the application of antiseptic measures to patients following amputation). Our results are likely to be considerably less dramatic! Death as an outcome measure is, thus, neither sensitive nor specific, and the fact that a proposed new intervention has no effect on 28 day mortality in a particular group of patients does not necessarily indicate that the agent is not effective.

As a result of the factors discussed above, in order for any trial with mortality as an endpoint to be completed within a reasonable time frame, large numbers of patients must be enrolled. The pressure to show an improvement in 28

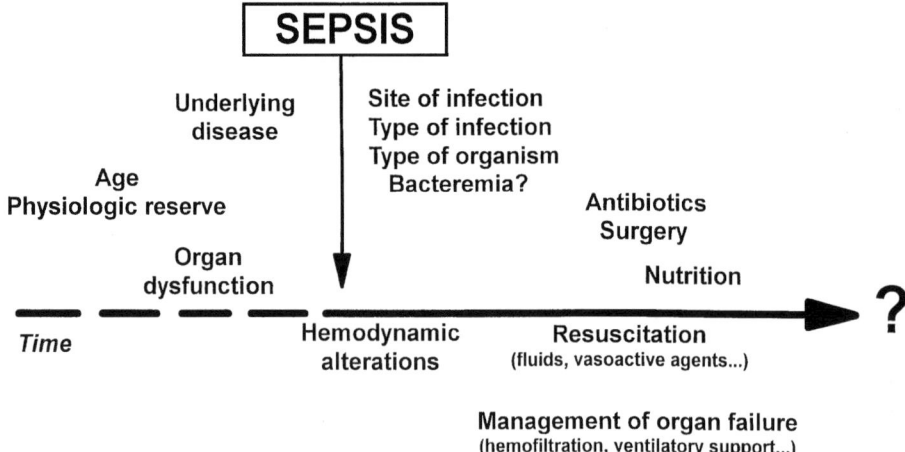

Fig. 1. Multiple factors involved in the outcome of sepsis. (From Vincent JL (1997) New therapies in sepsis. Chest 112:5330-5338. With permission)

day mortality has, thus, led to many studies of new therapeutic agents being conducted on heterogeneous patient populations. This carries its own problems, in that an intervention may be beneficial in some patients but not in others. For example, dexamethasone was shown to be effective at reducing mortality in patients with severe typhoid fever [2]. However, studies on corticosteroids in "sepsis syndrome" have given negative results [3]. Corticosteroids are highly effective agents (in many clinical situations) and it is likely that some patients will, in fact, have benefited from receiving corticosteroid therapy. However, these patients had no impact on the final outcome figures, either because they were lost in the overall analysis, for example, the use of penicillin in septic patients is only beneficial in some Gram-positive infections and studies of heterogeneous groups of patients with mixed infections may not necessarily reveal this fact even in large populations with careful post-hoc analysis, or, because the benefits offered to some patients were counterbalanced by the hurt done to others.

The time scale chosen for mortality may also be significant. Some interventions may have an effect on early mortality but no effect by 28-days but this finding could provide useful information about the pathophysiology of the disease process. Alternatively, the 28-day limit may be too short to provide any indication of the long-term effects of the agent.

Morbidity as the outcome measure

Morbidity may be a valid endpoint, but how does one assess morbidity? Until fairly recently, morbidity in septic patients was assessed simply on the basis of the presence or absence of organ failure. Newer scores, such as the MODS (multiple organ dysfunction score) [4] and the SOFA (sequential organ failure assessment, Table 1) [5] have been developed to enable us to measure degrees of organ failure, and changes in organ failure over time, thus offering a more accurate analysis of morbidity.

Table 1. The sequential organ failure assessment (SOFA) score

Organ system	SOFA score				
	0	1	2	3	4
Respiration					
PaO_2/FiO_2, mmHg	> 400	≤ 400	≤ 300	≤ 200 with respiratory support	≤ 100
Coagulation					
Platelets x $10^3/mm^3$	> 150	≤ 150	≤ 100	≤ 50	≤ 20
Liver					
Bilirubin, mg/dL	< 1.2	1.2-1.9	2.0-5.9	6.0-11.9	>12.0
(μmol/L)	(< 20)	(20-32)	(33-101)	(102-204)	(> 204)
Cardiovascular					
Hypotension	None	MAP < 70 mmHg	D ≤ 5 or Db (any dose) *	D > 5 or E ≤ 0.1 or N ≤ 0.1 *	D > 15 or E > 0.1 or N > 0.1 *
CNS					
Glasgow coma score	15	13-14	10-12	6-9	< 6
Renal					
Creatinine, mg/dL	< 1.2	1.2-1.9	2.0-3.4	3.5-4.9	> 5.0
(μmol/L)	(< 110)	(110-170)	(171-299)	(300-440)	(> 440)
or urine output				< 500 ml/d	< 200 ml/d

PaO_2, partial pressure of arterial oxygen; FiO_2, fraction of inspired oxygen; MAP, mean arterial pressure; D, dopamine; Db, dobutamine, E, epinephrine; N, norepinephrine

* Adrenergic agents administered for at least 1 hour (doses given in μg/kg per minute)

Another problem with the use of morbidity as an endpoint is that on its own it is not sufficient. Theoretically, one could have a drug that improves lung function and hence morbidity, but is highly nephrotoxic, and thus worsens mortality. No one would say that such an agent was of benefit to patients. One therefore needs to employ a combination of endpoints; morbidity and mortality. Reduced morbidity is only an acceptable endpoint if it is associated with a trend towards reduced mortality.

However, a problem with the combination of these two endpoints is that it is difficult to evaluate organ failure in non-survivors. Obviously in any trial in septic patients, there are going to be four groups of patients; survivors with no organ failure; patients with organ failure who survive; patients with organ failure who die; and some patients who die so early that they do not have time to develop organ failure. In this latter group, how does one assess morbidity? There is no effective way of dealing with this issue: some may count the number of days alive without organ failure; others apply an arbitrary multiple organ failure score to those who die early, but in this case, how do you select the score, as too low a figure will underestimate the mortality, and too high a score will lead us back to a situation of mortality as the primary endpoint.

Conclusions

Mortality is, undoubtedly, a very important endpoint in clinical trials of new therapeutic modalities in intensive care patients. However, improved mortality rates are not the only aim. Indeed, many would not classify a treatment as successful if it leaves a patient alive but in a permanent vegetative state or profoundly handicapped. One cannot talk about survival without mentioning quality of life. With today's technology, many patients can be kept "alive" for prolonged periods of time, but with what quality of life? Indeed, the majority of deaths in the ICU are now the result of withdrawing/withholding therapy [6, 7], as it is realized that these patients will have a very poor quality of life if life-sustaining treatment is continued.

Improving morbidity is thus an important outcome measure. For health management purposes also, a focus on improving morbidity is useful, as the patient who dies early is unlikely to use much of the ICU budget, but the patient requiring mechanical ventilation, haemodialysis, etc., i.e., the patient with organ failure, will be a large financial burden. The ability to reduce morbidity and hence length of ICU stay and costly interventions, is thus a relevant aim in today's cost-conscious health care systems.

The debate over the "best" outcome measure will continue with some advocating mortality [8] and others preferring morbidity [1]. I would propose that a combination of morbidity with a trend to improved mortality will enable us to obtain the most relevant data from trials of new therapeutic agents. Indeed, as recommended by a recent consensus conference on clinical trials for the treatment of sepsis [9, 10], future trials should:

1. consider mortality as an important endpoint but not restrict it to the 28-day window;
2. regard the reduction or reversal of organ failure as a valid efficacy endpoint;
3. consider quality of life as an endpoint.

References

1. Petros AJ, Marshall JC, van Saene HKF (1995) Should morbidity replace mortality as an endpoint for clinical trials in intensive care? Lancet 345:369-371
2. Hoffman SL, Punjabi NH, Kumala S et al (1984) Reduction of mortality in chloramphenicol-treated severe typhoid fever by high-dose dexamethasone. N Engl J Med 310:82-88
3. The veterans administration systemic sepsis cooperative study group (1987) Effect of high-dose glucocorticoid therapy on mortality in patients with clinical signs of systemic sepsis. N Engl J Med 317:659-665
4. Marshall JC, Cook DJ, Christou NV et al (1995) Multiple organ dysfunction score: A reliable descriptor of a complex clinical outcome. Crit Care Med 23:1638-1652
5. Vincent JL, Moreno R, Takala J et al (1996) The SOFA (sepsis-related organ failure assessment) score to describe organ dysfunction/failure. Intensive Care Med 22:707-710
6. Sprung CL, Eidelman LA (1996) Worldwide similarities and differences in the forgoing of life-sustaining treatments. Intensive Care Med 22:1003-1005
7. Prendergast TJ, Luce JM (1997) Increasing incidence of withholding and withdrawal of life support from the critically ill. Am J Respir Crit Care Med 155:15-20
8. Decruyenaere J, De Deyne C, Poelaert J, Colardyn F (1995) Morbidity or mortality as endpoint for clinical trials in intensive care (letter). Lancet 345:986-987
9. Sibbald WJ, Vincent JL (1995) Round table conference on clinical trials for the treatment of sepsis. Brussels, March 12-14, 1994. Intensive Care Med 21:184-189
10. Vincent JL (1997) New therapies in sepsis. Chest 112:S330-S338

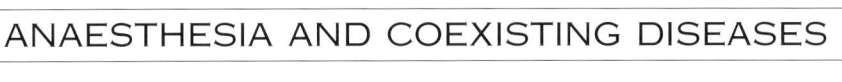

ANAESTHESIA AND COEXISTING DISEASES

Perioperative Care: Physiology and Practicality

P.D. Lumb

Anaesthesiologists and critical care practitioners are increasingly responsible not only for satisfactory clinical outcomes following surgery, but also for insuring appropriate utilization of the resources involved. Indeed, clinical pathways have provided a powerful tool to track patients' progress, and early intervention stimulated by physiological deviation from the expected course may prove beneficial and decrease total length of hospital stay despite the possibility of increasing time in the ICU. To accommodate these responsibilities, physicians must hone traditional clinical skills while learning the new behaviors associated with integrating business practices into medical care. Certainly, the art as well as the science of medicine are still alive, but the understanding of medicine as a business is a reality that clinicians ignore at their peril. The following discussion will focus on two traditional areas of perioperative care. It will conclude by introducing a third arena in which physician interest and direction will dictate future success.

Respiratory monitoring

Assessment of the respiratory system and associated airway management is a frequent requirement of the anaesthesiologist and critical care practitioner. These techniques are usually associated with intubated and mechanically ventilated patients, but application of these skills in ambulatory and non-ICU applications is becoming increasingly important. The clinician must recognize and respond appropriately to any patient with compromised respiratory function. Usually, the situation will require urgent action, but occasionally assessment will permit expectant observation with close monitoring to prevent undetected deterioration. Notwithstanding adequate assessment and facilities for close patient observation, the clinician must always remember that the secured airway is usually the most appropriate, especially if support personnel and facilities are available for its management.

Clinical observation is the most important aspect of respiratory assessment, and the alert clinician will often control a compromised patient electively, preventing deterioration and emergency management. Uncompromised ventilation is characterized by negative observations: breathing is silent, unhurried and non-labored; diaphoresis, cyanosis and agitation are absent; cognitive function is intact. *The patient who is observed to be breathing is in respiratory distress until proven otherwise.* Clinical tests may be valuable in further assessing the compromised patient, and a rule of "tens" can be defined by asking the patient to count out loud on exhalation following a deep inhalation. A healthy adult can count well beyond fifty without difficulty; a compromised patient counting beyond twenty is probably safe being observed carefully in a non-ICU setting; ability to count beyond ten but less than twenty represents an individual requiring close observation in a carefully controlled environment; individuals unable to reach ten should be intubated immediately and managed in an ICU. Obviously, this assessment fails in those patients with chronic disease processes and respiratory compromise, but in the acute patient these values are useful clinical signposts that may indicate urgent intervention.

Following a decision to intubate, the clinician must evaluate the patient's cognitive state and determine the requirements for pharmacological intervention prior to airway manipulation. Although use of sedation and muscle relaxants is seductive and appropriate in many situations, gentle technique, careful explanation and judicious use of topical anaesthesia may be appropriate in many situations, thereby avoiding the potential disadvantages of sedation and paralysis. Prior to initiating any therapeutic intervention, the clinician must confirm a thorough inventory of necessary equipment. Continuous monitoring of haemodynamic and respiratory function is essential during this period, and pulse oximetry, EKG and non-invasive blood pressure should be available. Additionally, in the absence of capnography, a litmus determination of exhaled carbon dioxide (E_TCO_2) should be available to confirm endotracheal intubation. Initiation of mechanical ventilation is not without hazard, and continuous assessment of haemodynamic stability must be initiated concomitantly.

In order to assure safe and efficient mechanical support, the patient-ventilator interface requires continuous monitoring. Important clinical information can be obtained by paying careful attention to pressure and volume information readily obtainable from ventilator outputs. Calculations focused on work of breathing, pulmonary compliance and the mean airway pressure generated during the respiratory cycle may provide important, early diagnostic clues to either deterioration in pulmonary status or appropriate response to therapeutic intervention. Additionally, the clinician will require this information to assess the patient's appropriateness for weaning from mechanical ventilatory assistance. Coupled with metabolic data, nutritional support can be targeted appropriately to meet the patient's unique needs based upon actual requirements; this may eliminate the dangers associated with excess caloric support.

In summary, clinically useful aspects of respiratory monitoring that facilitate rapid intervention and provide mechanisms to assure appropriate support levels that minimize complications associated with airway management and mechanical ventilation have been discussed. Clinicians must concentrate on those aspects of monitoring that provide a reasoned approach to managing the patient-ventilator interface in elective and critical situations.

Haemodynamic stability: assessing resuscitation

Man is an aerobic creature. Resuscitation must either preserve or restore global oxygen delivery. Rapid restoration of haemodynamic stability with associated adequacy of peripheral perfusion and end organ function has been used to judge the effectiveness of therapeutic regimens. These techniques are crude and do not help clinicians modify treatment effectively and rapidly. Interventional medicine's rise paralleled the technologic capacity of the microchip computer and space industries. Rapidly, haemodynamic assessment expanded to include determinations of cardiac output (CO) and the associated calculations of haemodynamic performance. Although useful, these measurements did not assess oxygen delivery (DO_2), and their integration with arterial and mixed venous blood gas data became commonplace in an attempt to define acceptable resuscitation targets. Fiberoptic bundles were incorporated into pulmonary artery catheters, and continuous measurement of mixed venous oxygen saturation (SvO_2) became possible. Early attention was focused on measuring CO continuously from SvO_2, but their non-linear relationship, except in low output states, and technical problems relating to accuracy confounded the attempt and delayed acceptance of the measurement. Non-invasive measurement of arterial oxygen saturation (SaO_2) with pulse oximetry (SpO_2) became a mandated measurement in anaesthesiology, and attention shifted to assessing the ability of cardio-respiratory capacity to support oxygen delivery. Although independently useful, if combined, pulse and venous oximetry data may provide insight about the adequacy of resuscitation; more importantly, by displaying information derived from multifactorial physiologic relationships, therapeutic responses may be accelerated. This discussion will focus on technologic advances in haemodynamic monitoring that provide continuous, clinically relevant information that may help direct therapy in specific situations.

Airway patency, cardiac stability and adequate circulating fluid volume are the hallmarks of cardiopulmonary resuscitation. Cardiac and trauma life support courses focus on restoring these components of oxygen transport hierarchically. Once achieved, subsequent resuscitation and maintenance targets are less well defined. Confusion exists because the physiologic abnormalities associated with critical illness are seldom confined to a single organ, and maintenance of adequate oxygen transport requires knowledge of both delivery and utilization. Therapeutically useful relationships between DO_2 and oxygen consumption ($\dot{V}O_2$) – oxygen flux, (F^*O_2) – are often theorized based on results obtained from exercise physiology or controlled haemorrhage experiments and irrelevant to the clinical situation. Sepsis and associated multiple organ system dysfunction (MOSD) provides the major intellectual challenge for the intensivist, but in post-surgical critical care units, therapeutic choices should be based on haemorrhage models because of their similarity to many clinical situations. The validity of this approach will be established, and common errors in application will be discussed. Integrating F^*O_2 and haemodynamic assessment is instrumental to guide rapid, effective resuscitation efforts for surgery and trauma patients.

Theoretically and clinically, the assessment of oxygenation provides an interesting challenge for the clinician. No single measurement provides the requisite information, although individual values may indicate global delivery inadequacy. For example, although SaO_2 of 92% may be physiologically normal for some individuals and provide adequate oxygenation for activities of daily life, this value may be grossly inadequate when the same individual is faced with unexpected physiologic challenge such as surgery, sepsis or other critical illness. Equally, SaO_2 of 80% would be recognized as inadequate for long term survival, irrespective of the individual's chronic status. Quantification of the deficit, and perhaps more importantly, identification of the threshold at which critical oxygen delivery is reached remains elusive. For this reason, attention has focused on a number of technologies that measure multiple biopsies of oxygenation status. When diagnosed and assimilated, the results can provide a detailed view of the patient's acute metabolic response within the physiologic context of his/her chronic health condition and any additional disease related co-morbidity. Therapeutic interventions may be evaluated based upon global changes in F^*O_2, the assumption being that positive trends in this value are beneficial. Oxygen is not a benign drug, and although attention is focused on preventing irreversible hypoxaemia and anaerobiasis, appropriate interventions will minimize the delivered inspired oxygen concentration (FiO_2) to that which is necessary.

The amount of oxygen carried by haemoglobin (oxygen content, CO_2) is expressed by the following equation:

$$CO_2 = 1.39 * Hb * SaO_2 + 0.0031 * PaO_2$$

CO_2 can be measured in arterial and venous blood across any organ or the whole organism, and this assessment is valuable in manipulating clinician controlled variables to improve F^*O_2. Early measurements were cumbersome and requisite calculations difficult; therefore, results were available intermittently and clinicians did not use this information routinely in managing patients. SvO_2 measurement is required to evaluate global oxygen delivery, and it is only recently that available technology has provided the integrated approach necessary to evaluate the determinants of oxygen supply and consumption. In order to evaluate F^*O_2, the determinants of DO_2 and $\dot{V}O_2$ must be measured and the results analyzed:

$$DO_2 = CO * CaO_2$$

and

$$\dot{V}O_2 = CO * D(a-v)O_2$$

where $D(a-v)O_2$ is the difference between the oxygen contents in the arterial and venous circulations. For global DO_2 assessment, the venous content value used is that from the pulmonary artery termed "mixed" venous oxygen content. However, if an individual organ is analyzed, then its $F*O_2$ is measured by evaluating the CO_2 difference between the arterial input and venous effluent.

From the above, it will be noted that CO_2 is dependent upon the haemoglobin concentration (Hb) and SO_2. In order to assess delivery, integration of cardiac output was necessary. This permits $F*O_2$ to be described by the ratio:

$$F*O_2 = \dot{V}O_2 /DO_2 = \text{oxygen utilization}$$

The relationship between oxygen content and oxygen saturation is fundamental to assessing the functional components of oxygen delivery and the interdependence of the cardiovascular and respiratory systems.

A fundamental question is posed between the effectiveness of arterial oxygen saturation versus oxygen tension measurements in the evaluation of pulmonary function. Because of the nature of the measurements and the physiology of cardiorespiratory function, situations exist that favor each measurement in different pathologic conditions. Effective arterial oxygenation requires matched pulmonary function and cardiac output. The relationship between alveolar ventilation (V_A) and oxygen delivery and related blood flow (perfusion, Q) is termed the ventilation/perfusion ratio (V/Q). When either wasted ventilation or perfusion exists, efficiency of the lung decreases; arterial hypoxaemia may develop when some areas of the lung have decreased ventilation with relatively increased perfusion. The hypoxaemic effect of low V/Q lung areas is exacerbated by decreased FiO_2. In order to assess true intrapulmonary shunt (Q_{SP}/Q_T), patients breathed 100% oxygen in order to mask the effect of low V/Q areas. However, because of the non-linear nature of the oxy-haemoglobin dissociation curve, as PaO_2 exceeds 150 torr, inevitably, SaO_2 is maximum at 100%. Obviously, arterial oxygen continues to climb at higher oxygen tension, and the measurement of true shunt requires availability of mixed venous blood and the calculation of both arterial and mixed venous oxygen contents. On the venous side, the oxy-haemoglobin saturation curve at physiologic oxygen tensions is nearly linear; thus, so is the relationship between saturation and tension. It may be beneficial, within safe physiologic limits of SaO_2, to utilize a decreased FiO_2 in patients requiring supplemental oxygen or mechanical ventilatory support. Although this exacerbates the hypoxaemic effect of low V/Q areas, it may reduce the PaO_2 sufficiently to re-establish its linear relationship to SaO_2. If PaO_2 and SaO_2 are maintained in the physiologic range of the oxyhaemoglobin dissociation curve where reciprocal, linear changes in saturation and tension occur, qualitatively similar information can be determined by following saturation alone rather than the more complex evaluations involving either oxygen tension or calculation of total arterial and venous oxygen contents [1].

Pulmonary shunt is a valuable indicator of oxygenation because it depends on several factors, all of which are variably deranged in critical illness. Increased Q_{SP}/Q_T can be caused by either: a) diffusion impairment caused by thickened or damaged capillary endothelial membrane, b) V/Q abnormalities, or c) atelectasis, consolidation and pulmonary oedema [2]. The relevant formula for Q_{SP}/Q_T is:

$$Q_{SP}/Q_T = Cc'O_2 - CaO_2/Cc'O_2 - CvO_2$$

where $Cc'O_2$ is end capillary oxygen content and is derived in the following manner:

$$Cc'O_2 = Hb * 1.39 * Sc'O_2 + .0031 * Pc'O_2$$

but, since $Sc'O_2$ cannot be measured, it is either: a) arbitrarily set to 1, b) estimated by subtracting the measured dys-haemoglobins in the arterial blood gas sample and subtracting this value from 1, or c) calculating a value from the modified Severinghaus equation [3]. Likewise, $Pc'O_2$ is assumed equal to alveolar oxygen tension and estimated from the alveolar air equation in the following manner:

$$PaO_2 = FiO_2 (P_B - P_{H_2O}) - PaCO_2/RER$$

where P_B = barometric pressure, P_{H_2O} = saturated water vapor pressure at the measured body temperature, and RER = the respiratory exchange ratio which is estimated at 0.8 for individuals eating a normal diet in the unstressed state. RER can be measured with a metabolic cart.

An evaluation of the mathematical operations and measurements required to evaluate the individual components of the shunt equation associated with the assumptions necessary to complete its calculation do not make it a readily available measurement of pulmonary function. However, a number of recent authors have revised these concepts and created a useful simplification that is dependent upon the continuous measurement of arterial and mixed venous oxygen saturation integrated with a microprocessor to perform the calculations required to complete the evaluation [2, 3]. To understand the use of continuous arterial and venous oximetry (dual oximetry) in assessing cardio-respiratory function, the following expansion of the previously described $F*O_2$ or O_2 utilization has been formulated:

$$
\begin{aligned}
F*O_2 &= \dot{V}O_2/DO_2 \\
&= CO * C_{(a-v)}O_2/CO * CaO_2 \\
&= C_{(a-v)}O_2/CaO_2 \\
&= 1 - C_vO_2/CaO_2 \\
&= 1 - [Hb * 1.39 * SvO_2 + PvO_2 * .0031/Hb * 1.39 * SaO_2 + PaO_2 * .0031 \\
&= 1 - SvO_2/SaO_2
\end{aligned}
$$

From this, Nelson inferred that mixed venous oxygen saturation accurately represents total body oxygen utilization [4], and other investigators have contended that SvO_2 more accurately predicts the ratio between $\dot{V}O_2$ and DO_2 than does CO, PaO_2, DaO_2, $\dot{V}O_2$ or any other variable suggested for determining the adequacy of whole body oxygenation [5]. SvO_2 is dependent upon the following four variables: Hb, CO, metabolic rate (as reflected in $\dot{V}O_2$) and SaO_2. If SvO_2 is used to estimate oxygen utilization, complete saturation of arterial blood oxyhaemoglobin is mandatory, but this requirement is eliminated with continuous integration of SpO_2 data into the calculations. With this assumption, Downs suggests the use of an oxygen extraction ratio O_2EI that incorporates all of the above arguments and is expressed as:

$$O_2EI = 1 - (SpO_2\text{-}SvO_2)/SpO_2$$
$$= 1 - SvO_2/SpO_2$$

The information derived from the measurement of arterial and mixed venous blood gases has long been used to evaluate the oxygenation status of critically ill patients. Modern technology permits the continuous assessment of oxyhaemoglobin saturation in these locations, and the preceding discussion provides a theoretic basis on which this information may be used to monitor the effects of therapeutic options designed to augment oxygenation continuously. Unlike intermittent "snapshots", this approach may provide clinicians with a rapidly responsive monitor that will improve the application of combination therapies that modulate cardiac and respiratory effects independently. Dual oximetry provides continuous, instantaneous estimates of pulmonary gas exchange and peripheral tissue oxygenation [6]. Application of this technique may improve the efficiency with which clinicians are able to manage critically ill patients.

Moss et al. postulated that resuscitation from acute haemorrhage has three phases: 1) asanguineous volume expansion; 2) restoration of the red cell mass; and 3) replacement of clotting factors [7]. This approach is helpful in assigning resuscitation priorities, and Shoemaker has argued that "supranormal" oxygen transport values are necessary to insure survival with minimum morbidity [8, 9]. Additionally, Levy described an experimental model in which the oxygen extraction ratio provides a valuable indicator of transfusion requirement in animals with limited cardiac reserve [10]. Integration of oxygen transport data with measurements of cardiac efficiency provides clinicians with important information to evaluate resuscitation efficiency and effectiveness. By utilizing the measurements of oxygen transport and related indices of cardio-respiratory efficiency, therapeutic interventions to restore $\dot{V}O_2$ rapidly and in proportion to deficit can be made in the hope of augmenting patient survival.

Cost reduction initiatives: the working process

This discussion will attempt to provide members of the Critical Care community with necessary information to structure initiatives and provide methodology to initiate cost awareness and reduction programs in their institutions. Some of the ideas presented and conclusions are surprising and probably do not conform to the bias of practitioners unit staff members.

The top three areas for initiatives in cost containment are:

Introduction of Continuous Quality Improvement programs into ICUs in order to formulate and refine standards of care

Total Quality Management (TQM) programs, re-introduced into the United States from Japan, have become increasingly recognized and are gaining popularity in non-industrial applications. [A focus of JCAHO surveys in 1995 and beyond will be review of each institution's Quality Management initiatives and the staff's understanding of and participation in them]. A key component of the quality management process is the empowerment of the employee to initiate change following the collection, analysis and prospective interpretation of targeted data. Unlike the scientific enterprise that attempts to collect and analyze data to describe the physical or existential reality of an object or process under investigation, TQM attempts to utilize data to change the described situation. The change is anticipated to be beneficial and defined by consensus, although in early initiatives, management should anticipate controlling its direction. If the program is enacted successfully, there is little intellectual doubt that processes can be improved; and, if the target of cost reduction without quality decay is established, it is likely that the desired result will be achieved. The key will be the corporate "buy-in" and dedication through empowerment of the process owners, in this case ICU physicians and other staff members.

In order to recognize change, it is imperative to define the base state from which deviation is tracked. In the absence of strict protocols, it is unlikely that effective behavioral modification can occur, especially if an iterative process is envisioned. In accepting "In my experience..." the critical care team loses an important yardstick against which therapeutic efficacy can be tracked. Certainly, the use of protocols to direct care should not be viewed as eliminating or restricting physician prerogative; rather, when used appropriately, it should supplement the capability of the physician and his/her unit to meet or exceed targeted performance standards.

Unfortunately, this sophistication does not exist in most critical care environments, and indeed it is one that is foreign to medical practice. Therefore, it is appropriate for educational fora such as this to disseminate information about the techniques to critical care unit directors and hospital administrators. The involvement of industry partners in the CQI process makes the importance of the information compelling. Behavioral change is not well translated into lectures, and the success of the process in a number of sophisticated applications may mitigate anticipated physician skepticism. However, the potential benefits expand beyond the theoretical and concentrate the traditional morbidity and mortality or case conference methodology of Quality Assurance into a more uniformly applicable data base that should minimize the occurrence of iatrogenic complications by identifying problem areas early. This will be accomplished through the facilitation of communications within the institution and unit to improve awareness at all levels of the process. Additionally, the perceived "ownership" of the process empowers the employee to consider him/herself responsible for implementing change and avoiding error. In order to accomplish these goals, inefficiencies can not be hidden, and participants experience intellectual satisfaction and honesty through manipulating their job tasks responsibly.

Potential benefits of the quality improvement process will be to increase the participation of all members of the critical care team, thus reducing staff "burnout" and the associated costs of retraining and down time. Targeted reductions in costly resource and charge items can be accomplished by improving the processes through which they are ordered or consumed. Certainly, behavioral modification will be necessary to accomplish the changes, but it is hoped that the encumbrances of past bias will be lost in the adoption of a new, egalitarian leadership style. The introduction into medical practice will be difficult initially because therapeutic decisions no longer flow from the primary attending. However, this perception changes as sophisticated practitioners are unburdened and able to focus on more important issues while recognizing that entitling procedures will slowly evolve and improve. The education of the physician participants will require a collegial approach to practice that crosses not only specialty lines, but also traditional lines of prerogative. However, once initiated, the process works well and quality improvement becomes an anticipated norm rather than a pleasant surprise. Certainly, alterations in medical staff practice associated with early extubation protocols following certain cardiac surgical procedures has highlighted the effectiveness of the team approach to patient management in a number of ICU's. Indeed, cost reeducation has been noted from a variety of different areas that, heretofore, may have been ignored.

Once the baseline has been established, cost reduction in a cost-effective fashion becomes possible. Without process, the benefits of one therapy over another will never be analyzed adequately to guarantee the expected result. An example of a potentially successful program, the impact of which depends upon the institutional environment, is that of Patient Controlled Analgesia (PCA). Certainly, the administration of analgesics to patients in pain by an automated, safe, self-controlled device has a great deal of appeal. However, true success is often measured either by a real reduction in cost of service or by demonstrating an improved patient outcome. Results in hospitals in which nursing staff take ownership of the program and become involved in targeting patients for earlier mobilization and discharge have seen benefit from program initiation. These are not matched in those hospitals in which the program remains tightly controlled, and lacks therapeutic empowerment and general ownership of the process. There is no staff vesting to earlier patient discharge, and the new technology merely increases cost without altering outcome. Product line management will be an area in which the process will become valuable, and this may be the easiest in which to introduce CQI efforts because the realities of patient flow and treatment are, of necessity, cross departmental and service.

Critical care managers must take a leadership role in informing practitioners of the importance of a new philosophy that accentuates process, accelerates progress, empowers employees, leads to measurable improvements in process (hopefully translated into improved patient outcome), and solidifies the leadership role of the physician in a collegial, not dictatorial, manner. Indeed, it comes as close as possible to providing an environment in which the usually incompatible states of consensus and idealism can coexist.

Educational initiatives

The importance of peer review and intellectual honesty is not only to recognize the current status of knowledge about any given subject, but also to recognize the limits of that knowledge and the profoundly greater depths of our ignorance. Not only is the current problem of reducing the cost of critical care service delivery daunting, but also it is complicated by the lack of a systematic data base that facilitates cost data transfer and knowledge. Cost center shifting is common and logical for a number of reasons. The result in medicine, perhaps the last of the barter economies, has been to confuse the issue and allow non-uniform application of complex reimbursement formulas that differ by state and regions within states. Ultimately, the true cost of most equipment, pharmaceuticals, services, etc. is unknown, and any analysis is based upon the ubiquitous surrogate, cost/charge ratio. This ignorance has condoned the emergence of a fiscally ignorant practice in which the cost of any item (disposable, diagnostic test, labor-consuming activities) is seldom factored into the medical decision. Traditional advocates support this as appropriate because it should provide the best care, unencumbered by theoretical restrictions if cost limits choice or access. In countries in which nationalized plans exist, there is little evidence to support this belief, although the systems are not perfect and exhibit enormous waste and abuse leading to cost overruns. However, while these populations perceive their health care to be acceptable, nonetheless, there exists in the United States a system in which access is potentially limited by ability to pay, there are a number of individuals whose insurance is inadequate or lacking entirely, and there is increasing apprehension about the cost of providing a service that is no longer regarded as providing the most appropriate care in all cases. Certainly, primary care is lacking for many, and although an unusual thought for ICU based practitioners, some of the cost reduction slated for short term accounting may in fact be an appropriate long term investment by improving the population's general health through increased access to preventive care.

Therefore, critical care physicians must develop a cost-conscious attitude to the quality of care. The emphasis must be on cost-effective delivery rather than a simplistic approach that implies that decreasing individual pharmaceutical or equipment charges will lead to cost reduction. The recognition that more expensive agents may provide cost savings will be realized only when effective cost accounting systems are in place and used. Does this imply that progress must await technologic support before effective action can be taken? No, but the recognition of change may be more difficult to document and realize.

An adjunct to effective reduction of critical care costs is to decrease the provision of unnecessary or inappropriate care. Although presentations of this nature usually exclude a discussion of ethics, nonetheless, it recognized that a public education program to define the risks and benefits of critical care delivery is mandatory. Public expectation of critical care medicine's efficacy is inflated, partially because the advertising, entertainment and malpractice industries have spawned unrealistic images of success. Death is sanitized or overwhelmingly final, and cure with unusual or fabricated therapy abounds. It is not surprising that expectation exceeds reality, and public demand overwhelms medical capability. Any attempt to curtail services is met with suspicion, and the ICU's capacity is compared to the perceived reality of the success in Star Trek's *Enterprise's* sick bay. Parenthetically, Captain Picard's lack of command decisions contrasts with the original Kirkian approach, but the perception of a quality management system in place is perpetuated by the recognition that the success rate of the continuing mission has been enhanced. So too will the transition occur in medical practice; public education will concentrate awareness on individual responsibility for remaining healthy and partnership in the "wellness" continuum. Unrealistic expectations will be reduced and the realities of Do Not Resuscitate (DNR) orders and living wills/advanced directives will be accepted, rather than resisted, by health care providers and institutions. It is likely that reimbursement changes will reduce the perceived inducements to continuing futile care.

Alternate delivery sites and use of health care extenders may reduce significantly the costs of chronic care, but their implementation awaits a public and professional awareness and acceptance that is lacking today. Critical care physicians should take a leadership position in providing educational materials that support alternative decisions and improve the technologies of chronic, supportive care. Cost awareness will play a role in the transition from current practice modes, but so too will educational and advertising programs aimed at integrating the realities of catastrophic illness with the capabilities of an empowered critical care delivery system.

Technology: threats and opportunities

Generally advertised and perceived as escalating costs, technologic advances have not received the critical analysis required to assess their impact that they deserve. Many technologic and pharmaceutical advances provide short-term gain in attaining discrete goals that have no impact on survival. Outcome research has become a popular descriptor against which future cost-effective hospital acquisition may be targeted. In the absence of standardized care, it is unlikely that this approach will improve outcome or reduce cost. Critical care practitioners are in a unique position to advocate responsible technology assessment. SCCM established a Technology Assessment Task Force to address this issue. Guidelines for assessment have been produced and promulgated, and the Society and its members should take a leadership position in this area.

Without integrated data acquisition and analysis, cost-effective ICU management is impossible; cost information must be available to and resource conservation by all members of the health care team demanded.

Conclusions

Industrial success with Total Quality Management programs and the present trend to adapt these processes to non-industry applications has been discussed, and a definite future focus for critical care practitioners will be the rational incorporation of these practices into their units. Creating protocols to direct various aspects of care must concentrate heavily on the iterative and integrated nature of the process that depends upon empowerment at all levels of the care delivery network. The appropriate integration of new information management technology into this arena will facilitate success.

Available cost data is inadequate. Effective policies to reduce true cost require integrated information and demand behavioral change from providers. Detailed information on current cost will be required to evaluate the impact of new pharmacological and technologic advances. Pharmacoeconomic data will become increasingly utilized in an attempt to understand waste and apportion expenses appropriately. Education of the provider, vendor and consumer will be necessary to create a milieu in which reduction in cost will be accomplished without erosion of quality or access.

Research initiatives will remain a key component of future critical care. Centers of evaluation established to generate and refine treatment protocols may define future initiatives. Can successful protocols be transported from one environment into another without benefit of institutional "cultural" development? Behavioral change, the use of care-extenders in non-traditional environments and multi-center research based on stable methodology will be key components to future progress.

Appropriate use of current resources can be maximized by administrative innovations such as product line management and critical path scheduling. Initiatives that cut across traditional specialty and department lines will force improved utilization of scarce resources. Modification of services within an institution into acuity based units that, when appropriate, transfer patients to more or less specialized areas may provide economies. The example usually flows from ICU to step down to routine care and discharge, but the concept may also be successful in surgical areas by transferring complex, long term patients from short-term 'recovery' to multi-disciplinary, hospital based units. Aggregation of care, not regionalization may be an important future concept.

The future foundation for progress is based on outcome research, protocol-generated care, and iterative ICU management. Advances in pharmacology and technology will parallel, and to some extent drive, those in the clinical arena and the value of industrial partnerships with academic institutions will be recognized as therapeutic need is met by innovation. This contrasts criticisms that equate increased costs to irresponsible incorporation and exploitation of new, costly technology.

Critical Care directors should focus their attention and the activities of their institutions in the following areas:

1. CQI/Standards of Care
2. Education
3. Technology
4. Administration
5. Research

A natural partnership exists between critical care providers and hospital administration. Responsible reduction of costs will require careful collaboration between all components of the health care delivery team, the definition of which must be expanded. Educational programming must be provided to all providers to demonstrate the finite capacity of medical care and the infinite ability of the human organism to challenge it.

References

1. Civetta JM (1998) Bedside use of arterial and venous oximetry. In: Monitoring: Practical applications, pp 313-324
2. Sutter PM, Fairley B, Schlobohm D (1975) Shunt, lung volume and perfusion during short periods of ventilation with oxygen. Anesthesiology 43
3. Bongard FS, Leighton TA (1992) Continuous dual oximetry in surgical critical care: Indications and limitations. Ann Surg 216(1):60-68
4. Nelson LD (1983) Continuous venous oximetry in surgical patients. Ann Surg 203:349-352
5. Mitchell LA, Downs JB, Dannemiller FJ (1975) Extrapulmonary influences on (A-a) DO_2 following cardiopulmonary bypass. Anesthesiology 43:583-586
6. Rasanen J, Downs JB, Malec DJ et al (1988) Real-time continuous estimation of gas exchange by dual oximetry. Intensive Care Med 14:118-122
7. Gould SA, Rice CL, Moss GS (1984) The physiologic basis of the use of blood and blood products. Surg Annual 16:13
8. Shoemaker WC, Appel P, Bland R (1983) Use of physiologic monitoring to predict outcome and to assist in clinical decisions in critically ill postoperative patients. Am J Surg 146:43-49
9. Hayes M, Yau EHS, Timmins AC et al (1993) Response of critically ill patients to treatment aimed at achieving supranormal oxygen delivery and consumption: Relationship to outcome. Chest 103(3):886-895
10. Levy PS, Chavez RP, Crystal GJ et al (1992) Oxygen extraction ratio: A valid indicator of transfusion need in limited coronary vascular reserve? J Trauma 32;6:769-774

Coagulation Disorders

C.T. Petrovitch

In reviewing the many causes of bleeding disorders, it is easiest to categorize the bleeding disorders according to which component of the haemostatic mechanism is affected, the blood vessels, platelets, or the clotting factors. Bleeding disorders may be further classified as to whether the disorder is inherited or acquired. However, practically speaking it is probably best for anaesthesiologists and critical care physicians to focus on the diagnosis and treatment of acquired bleeding disorders since most patients with a hereditary bleeding disorder are usually under the care of a haematologist from an early age.

The first process of the haemostatic mechanism, primary haemostasis, requires the proper interaction of blood vessels and platelets. Primary haemostasis can be defective when vascular integrity is disrupted as a result of surgical trauma or when the blood vessels are compromised by an immune or inflammatory process. Primary haemostasis may also be impaired when either platelet number and/or function are compromised. Too few platelets, or thrombocytopenia, is defined as a platelet count that falls below 150,000 mm^3 [1].

Thrombocytopenia

Quantitative acquired platelet deficiencies may result from five general causes: the platelets may be 1) inadequately produced by the bone marrow, 2) sequestered in the spleen, 3) consumed with massive tissue damage or peripheral consumption, 4) diluted by massive transfusions, or 5) destroyed by immune mechanisms.

Inadequate platelet production may occur if the patient's bone marrow is suppressed or destroyed. Radiation therapy or chemotherapy may lead to bone marrow hypoplasia and consequent thrombocytopenia. Many drugs and certain infectious agents may be toxic to the bone marrow and lead to bone marrow suppression and thrombocytopenia. Binge drinking of alcohol and prolonged administration of estrogens have both been implicated to cause bone marrow suppression [2]. Finally, invasion of the bone marrow by cancer cells or replacement by fibrotic tissue will lead to inadequate platelet production.

Splenomegaly may result in thrombocytopenia. Normally, approximately one third of the platelet pool is sequestered in the spleen [3]. With the development of splenomegaly, an increasing number of platelets are sequestered in the spleen and this may result in thrombocytopenia.

Platelets may be consumed by massive tissue damage. Whenever the vascular endothelium is denuded or disrupted, the natural process of primary haemostasis proceeds. Platelets adhere to the subendothelial collagen layers, aggregate, and form a platelet plug. With massive tissue damage, platelets may be rapidly consumed and thrombocytopenia may ensue. Such consumption of platelets occurs in patients with large body burns and in those patients with an extensive vasculitis such as occurs in preeclampsia of pregnancy. The initiation of cardiopulmonary bypass leads to thrombocytopenia as well. Once the bypass tubing is inserted into the patient's vascular tree, the platelets adhere to the nonendothelialized artificial surfaces and thrombocytopenia develops.

The patient's normal platelet pool may be diluted following massive transfusions with crystalloids or stored red blood cells which are deficient in viable platelets. Of course, such transfusions dilute the patient's platelet count in proportion to the volume transfused.

One of the most common immune causes of thrombocytopenia is idiopathic thrombocytopenia purpura (ITP). In this condition, platelets are destroyed prematurely by circulating platelet antibodies. Exposure to certain drugs such as heparin and quinine can lead to an immune-mediated thrombocytopenia [4]. Several autoimmune diseases such as systemic lupus erythematosus and rheumatoid arthritis lead to the formation of antigen-antibody complexes that lead to platelet destruction.

Platelet dysfunction

Acquired platelet defects may be the result of several medical conditions, including renal failure, liver disease, DIC, and cardiopulmonary bypass, which alter the milieu in which the platelet circulates. Patients who are uremic are found almost universally to have an acquired platelet function defect [5]. It is thought that certain toxic metabolites, guanidino succinic acid and hydroxy phenolic acid, accumulate in the patient's blood and prevent the platelets from exposing the phospholipid surface termed platelet factor 3 (PF3). However, dialysis improves this haemostatic defect since these two compounds are dialyzable. Other mechanisms for the platelet defect associated with uraemia have been proposed. Certainly, the platelet dysfunction produced by uraemia improves following treatment with DDAVP, estrogen compounds, and cryoprecipitate.

Acute and chronic liver disease is associated with platelet dysfunction. Chronic liver disease leads to an activation of the fibrinolytic process and the production of fibrin degradation products (FDPs). With hepatic insufficiency these FDPs accumulate to some extent in the blood and compromise platelet function by inhibiting the exposure of platelet factor 3 (PF3). This platelet phospholipid surface is critical to surface mediated reactions and the coagulation process that follows. In addition, it is thought that the FDPs coat the surface of the platelet and interfere with platelet aggregation. Disseminated intravascular coagulation (DIC), like liver disease, is associated with the accumulation of FDPs in the blood and consequently with platelet dysfunction. Chronic alcoholism produces a multi-factorial platelet defect as well. For the most part, the alcoholic patient with chronic liver disease can be presumed to have platelet dysfunction and may require platelet transfusions [6].

Platelet dysfunction is most commonly caused by drug administration. Drugs can interfere with platelet function by many mechanisms. Drugs may interfere with the platelet membrane function, platelet receptors, platelet prostaglandin synthesis, or they may inhibit phosphodiesterase activity [7]. Aspirin ingestion inhibits the cyclooxygenase enzyme which is important in the prostaglandin synthetic pathway. Aspirin poisons the platelet for the life of the platelet, interfering with the synthesis of thromboxane A_2. Non-steroidal antiinflammatory drugs only inhibit this synthetic platelet function temporarily.

Finally, platelets develop a storage defect due to a depletion of their energy stores when platelets are stored. The resulting platelet defect results in decreased platelet aggregation and may last up to 20 hours after transfusion. Acquired platelet defects occur following cardiopulmonary bypass for a multitude of reasons, but principally thought to be due to the traumatic effects of cardiotomy suction, the bypass circuit, the membrane oxygenator, and the effects of hypothermia. The platelets suffer through many stages of platelet activation. Many lose their surface receptors; others extrude the contents of their cytoplasmic granules, etc. resulting in platelets of varying functional capacity.

Autoimmune disorders, such as systemic lupus erythematosus, rheumatoid arthritis, and scleroderma are also associated with acquired platelet dysfunction [8].

Factor deficiencies

Acquired factor deficiencies result from liver disease, vitamin K deficiency, massive transfusions that dilute both the platelet count and the available clotting factors, and from disseminated intravascular coagulation (DIC).

Because the liver synthesizes most of the clotting factors (with the possible exception of factor VIII), liver disease produces a multi-factorial bleeding disorder. Of all of the clotting factors, factor VII, however, has the shortest half-life. This means that it will be the first clotting factor to be depleted with the onset of liver disease. As a result of the initial depletion of factor VII, the prothrombin time will be prolonged before there is any prolongation of the partial thromboplastin time. Over time, as further factor deficiencies develop, both pathways will be affected.

Vitamin K deficiency also produces a multi-factorial bleeding disorder. Four of the clotting factors, factors II, VII, IX, and X and the two anticoagulant proteins, protein C and protein S, require the presence of vitamin K for their proper synthesis in the liver. Vitamin K deficiency leads to the defective synthesis of these clotting factors. A deficiency of vitamin K may result from many causes. Vitamin K is obtained in our diet from leafy green vegetables. Dietary inadequacies can lead to vitamin K deficiency in a brief period of time. Because the vitamin K is fat soluble, biliary excretion is important for the vitamin's absorption in the jejunum; biliary obstruction can impair vitamin K absorption. Common bacterial flora in the gut also play an important role in converting the vitamin to its active form. For this reason, sterilization of the gut with antibiotics can impact vitamin K stores. Clinically, patients with malabsorption syndromes, pancreatic insufficiency, biliary obstruction or GI obstruction may all develop vitamin K deficiency and a bleeding disorder. Patients maintained on i.v. fluids alone may deplete their vitamin K stores in roughly one week. Treatment may require the administration of vitamin K (Aquamephyton) in doses of 10 to 20 mg.

Coumadin administration will produce the same bleeding defect as vitamin K deficiency. This is because the mechanism of action of coumadin is to compete with vitamin K for binding sites in the liver. The presence of coumadin displaces vitamin K and results in vitamin K-dependent factor deficiencies (II, VII, IX, and X). Factor VII is the first to be depleted and subsequently IX, X and then II (thrombin).

The administration of heparin also results in clotting factor deficiencies via heparin's action on antithrombin III. Antithrombin III is a natural anticoagulant that circulates in the blood and binds to the activated factors in the intrinsic pathway [9]. In the presence of heparin, the binding of antithrombin III is enhanced 100-1000 times.

Massive transfusions with crystalloids or with banked red blood cells may produce a bleeding disorder. The initial defect is usually due to dilutional thrombocytopenia, but with massive volume transfusions, clotting factors may be diluted as well. When a patient is massively transfused with stored red blood cells, the patient's blood begins to have the same characteristics of "banked blood". These stored red blood cells are deficient in 2,3-diphosphoglycerate (DPG), the activity levels of the labile factors, factors V and VIII, are deficient, and most of the platelets are non-viable [10]. The platelet count may not fall as precipitously as anticipated if some platelets are released from the spleen [11]. However, when the platelet count falls acutely below 75,000 mm^3, the patient will probably bleed [12].

The massively transfused trauma victim may develop a bleeding disorder due to other causes besides the dilution of platelets and clotting factors. These patients are compromised due to prolonged periods of hypotension, acidosis and hypothermia. The patient's degree of acidosis and hypothermia may help to predict outcome [13].

Review of a patient's chart may often suggest the cause of an acquired bleeding disorder. Patients with severe liver disease usually have a history of chronic alcoholism, cirrhosis of the liver, or some form of hepatitis. Patients who present clinically with many of the scenarios which produce vitamin-K deficiency may likewise be anticipated to have a bleeding disorder. Even more obvious is the diagnosis of a bleeding disorder due to massive transfusion with banked red blood cells or due to the administration of coumadin or heparin. However, an insidious cause of bleeding is that produced by disseminated intravascular coagulation, DIC. It is often overlooked until the patient is overtly bleeding. DIC is certainly a paradox. The patient who has uncontrolled coagulation, clotting throughout the vascular tree, may eventually "bleed" to death.

The syndrome of DIC may be precipitated by many different underlying causes but all lead to uncontrolled rampant coagulation and the circulation of excess thrombin [14]. In response, the fibrinolytic system is activated in an attempt to lyse the blood clots and restore blood flow. The result is the circulation of plasmin in the blood stream and the production of multiple fibrin degradation products (FDPs). These fibrin degradation products produce platelet dysfunction and contribute to the patient's bleeding diathesis. The patient bleeds due to thrombocytopenia, factor deficiencies and due to the actions of the FDPs which act as inhibitors of coagulation.

References

1. Chong BH (1994) Clinical aspects of thrombocytopenias. Australian Family Physician 23: 1463-1465
2. Watson C, Schultz A, Wikoff H (1947) Purpura following estrogen therapy with particular reference to hypersensitivity to dietylstilbestrol and with a note on the possible relationship of purpura to endogenous estrogens. J Lab Clin Med 606
3. Harker LA, Finch CA (1969) Thrombokinetics in man. J Clin Invest 48:963-974
4. Breddin HK, Radziwon P, Boczkowska-Radziwon B (1994) Laboratory monitoring of new antithrombotic drugs. Clin Lab Med 14:825-846
5. Bick R (1992) Hemostasis in liver and renal disease. In: Anonymous disorders of thrombosis and hemostasis: Clinical laboratory practice. ASCP, Chicago, p 239
6. Bick RL (1994) Disseminated intravascular coagulation. Objective laboratory diagnostic criteria and guidelines for management. Clin Lab Med 14:729-768
7. Triplett D (1978) Appendix C: Miscellaneous lists and forms. In: Triplett D (ed) Platelet function evaluation: Laboratory evaluation and clinical application. ASCP, Chicago, p 291
8. Rao AK, Walsh PN (1983) Acquired qualitative platelet disorders. Clin Haematol 12:201-238
9. Mehta JL, Kitchens CS (1987) Pharmacology of platelet-inhibitory drugs, anticoagulants, and thrombolytic agents. Cardiovasc Clin 18:163-179
10. Troianos CA, Ellison N (1991) Hematologic considerations in vascular surgery. In: Joel A, Kaplan MD (eds) Vascular anesthesia, 1st edn. Churchill Livingstone, New York, pp 549-563

11. Boral LI, Henry JB (1991) Transfusion medicine. In: Tomas RH, Henry JB (eds) Clinical & diagnosis management by laboratory methods, 18th edn. WB Saunders, Philadelphia, pp 930-975
12. Miller RD, Brzica SM Jr (1986) Blood, blood components, colloids and autotransfusion therapy. In: Miller RD (ed) Anesthesia, 2nd edn. Churchill Livingstone, New York, pp 1329-1367
13. Crosby ET (1992) Perioperative haemotherapy: i. indications for blood component transfusion. Can J Anaesth 39:695-707
14. Bick RL (1994) Disseminated intravascular coagulation: Objective criteria for diagnosis and management. Med Clin North Am 78:511-543

Neuromuscular Disorders and Anaesthesia

J. RUPREHT

Adequate muscle power and excellent co-ordination of muscles are essential for survival. Ventilation depends on muscle power so much that life is threatened within few minutes without the rhythmic and perpetual action of breathing muscles. Other muscles keep the airway open. Muscle power is required for protective reflexes without which life is also not sustainable. Furthermore, without muscle power a person cannot communicate with others.

Anaesthesia affects muscles and the co-ordination of muscles. Vital functions must artificially be sustained in an anaesthetised person. Several disorders of the musculo-skeletal system, peripheral nervous system, and of the central nervous system profoundly influence the outcome of the anaesthetist's drugs on the muscle system. In specific neuromuscular disorders some anaesthetic agents can provoke life-threatening reactions. Very often it is not known that the patient suffers from a neuromuscular disorder which makes the effect of anaesthesia more unpredictable. The response of muscles to anaesthetic agents may be abnormal, more profound, example being a myasthenic patient. The response may also be completely different, example being hyperpyrexic reaction.

Muscular diseases are often associated with many other abnormalities. Cardiac muscle may be affected as well as heart-conduction system. Respiratory insufficiency or infection is often present. Abnormal muscles are often seen in combination with abnormality of the skeletal system, like in kyphoscoliosis. Furthermore, metabolic derangements in patients with muscular disease may result in abnormal pharmacodynamic response to anaesthetic agents.

Classification of neuromuscular disorders

Classical neurological grouping of neuromuscular diseases (Table 1) usually gives information about the aetiology of the disorder and also indicates therapeutic possibilities as well as the outcome [1].

It is difficult to classify diseases like "Stiff Man Syndrome" which is a disorder of the brain but manifests itself by cramps of normal voluntary muscles. A more useful classification of neuromuscular diseases for an anaesthetist is whether the disease results in weakening of protective reflexes, in respiratory insufficiency or, whether the muscles may react abnormally to specific anaesthetic agents (Table 2).

Beside the awed disposition for malignant hyperthermia, the following musculoskeletal diseases most often influence management of anaesthesia: muscular dystrophy, myotonic dystrophy, myasthenia gravis, myasthenic syndrome (Eaton-Lambert), periodic paralyses and Guillain-Barré syndrome.

Malignant hyperthermia (MH) occurs in susceptible patients when triggering anaesthetic agents are administered: volatile anaesthetics, depolarising relaxants, phenothiazines, haloperidol, or antidepressants. The safe anaesthetic agents include intravenous anaesthetics, non-depolarising relaxants, local analgesic, opioids, nitrous oxide and benzodiazepines. If a hyperpyrexic reaction is promptly recognised and treated, the mortality is low; Dantrolene (1 mg/kg^{-1}, repeated as necessary) alongside with cooling and correction of metabolic derangement will usually save the patient but the suspected diagnosis must be verified later. Prophylactic use of dantrolene in susceptible individuals is controversial, partly because of side effects of the drug and because one can avoid MH by exclusion of triggering drugs.

Table 1. Conventional groups of neuromuscular diseases

Diseases of the neuromuscular junction
Muscular dystrophies
Myotonia
Metabolic muscle diseases
Inflammatory myopathies
Toxic myopathies
Periodic paralyses
Diseases of the motor neurons

Table 2. Classification of the neuromuscular diseases according to whether or not they involve the bulbar muscles

Bulbar weakness	No bulbar weakness
Myotonic dystrophy	X-linked dystrophies
Oculopharyngeal dystrophy	Periodic paralyses
Mitochondrial myopathies	Adult-onset nemaline rod disease
Myositis	Adult-onset acid maltase deficiency
Myasthenia gravis	Central core disease
Botulism	Distal myopathy
Guillain-Barré	Alcohol myopathy
Motor neuron disease	Steroid myopathy
Intoxication	Eaton-Lambert syndrome
Tetanus	

Muscular dystrophies comprise diseases like Duchenne's muscular dystrophy, fascioscapulohumeral dystrophy, Emery-Dreifuss disease, McArdle's disease, mitochondrial myopathy and nemaline rod myopathy. Common to all of these is generalised or local muscle wasting, often associated with abnormalities of myocardic and heart-conduction system. In general, one should carefully titrate induction agents while inducing anaesthesia. Cardiac performance must be closely monitored. Suxamethonium is better avoided in order to prevent hyperkaliaemic response of wasted muscles. Vigorous postoperative respiratory therapy may be indicated to prevent pulmonary infection. Prolonged postoperative monitoring is necessary for a few days because muscle weakness may relapse late after anaesthesia.

Myotonias are characterised by prolonged muscle contraction following a stimulus. Cold may be a trigger and all myotonic patients must be kept normothermic at all times. The most severe form is *myotonia dystrophica* which is associated with cardiomyopathy and arrhythmias. Anaesthetic agents must be titrated carefully, suxamethonium should be avoided. Low-dose non-depolarising relaxants are usually sufficient and should be followed by spontaneous recovery of muscle power. Neostigmine may worsen myotonia. Atracurium and cis-atracurium are certainly relaxants of choice, in reduced dose.

Functionally, myotonias end in muscle weakness and ventilatory postoperative support may be needed in advanced cases of the disease. Direct monitoring of muscle power by train of four stimulation (TOF) may indicate false recovery in the stimulated muscle while the whole body is still relaxed. Uterine atony often calls for emergency hysterectomy in myotonic parturients. Local anaesthetic blocks in patients with myotonic dystrophy are possible but preferential consideration should be given to general anaesthesia.

Myasthenia gravis is characterised by antibodies to the postsynaptic receptor and may be combined with other autoimmune disorders. The classical treatment may be thymectomy, nowadays performed at an earlier stage. Pyridostigmine and corticosteroids may be introduced. The pharmacologic treatment of myasthenia gravis should be continued until the scheduled operation. Postoperative ventilatory support is often indicated, especially in patients with a long-standing disease. Babies of myasthenic mothers may require respiratory support for several days. The muscle relaxant of choice is atracurium. Excessive use of sedatives is not advisable in myasthenic patients.

Myasthenic syndrome (Eaton-Lambert) is clinically similar to myasthenia gravis. However, this autoimmune disease does not react to cholinesterase inhibitors. Four amino-pyridine results in increased muscle power. During anaesthesia all depressants and relaxants should be sparingly titrated.

Familial periodic paralyses are characterised by intermittent muscle weakness based on defects of the membrane transport of potassium. The hypokaliaemic form requires correction of plasma potassium preoperatively and monitoring of cardiac rhythm during anaesthesia. Hyperkaliaemic muscle weakness requires normalization of serum potassium preoperatively. Suxamethonium should be avoided. Normothermia must be maintained. Similarly, continuous monitoring of potassium and cardiac rhythm, with required corrections, have been recommended for the normokaliaemic periodic paralysis [2]. Again, atracurium is the muscle relaxant of choice and muscle power should be allowed to recover spontaneously.

Polyradiculoneuritis (Guillain-Barré) is ascribed to viral infection a few weeks before weakness and paresthesias occur in legs. Paralysis spreads cephalad and may cause insufficiency of breathing and protective reflexes. Prolonged ventilatory support may be mandatory. Complicating factor for the anaesthetist is dystonia of the autonomic nervous system. Wide fluctuations of blood pressure and cardiac rhythm may be present. α- and β-adrenergic blockade may be required. During anaesthesia, cardiovascular function must be monitored all the time and manipulated, if needed. Suxamethonium should be avoided. Again, atracurium is a suitable muscle relaxant. Intensive postoperative care is usually needed.

Multiple sclerosis is a borderline disease between typical neuromuscular disorders and afflictions of the central nervous system. In some patients muscle weakness is very pronounced and ventilatory support may be required postoperatively. Protection with corticosteroids preoperatively may be advisable in hope of preventing a relapse. Hypotension must be avoided in the perioperative period. Patients with multiple sclerosis must be instructed that a relapse is possible following anaesthesia and surgery but that anaesthesia is not an exclusive provoking factor. When local or regional analgesia is performed, the lowest effective concentration of the local analgesic drug should be administered.

Other disorders affecting muscles

Hemiplegia, cerebral palsy, Parkinson's disease, tetanus, botulism, paraplegia, quadriplegia, amyotrophic lateral sclerosis and Friederich's ataxia may all severely, though secondarily, affect voluntary muscles. Whenever muscles have been denervated, there is danger of hyperkaliaemia following suxamethonium. Positioning of patients may present problems and care must be taken to prevent pressure damage. In some neurological disorders and in eclampsia magnesium sulphate is used. Such patients have diminished power in voluntary muscles and the required doses of non-depolarising relaxants are much lower.

Some practical considerations about anaesthesia and neuromuscular disorders

Several muscle disorders result in poor ventilation and retention of secretions, possibly combined with respiratory infection. As a rule, muscle power and ventilation should be optimized before surgery in order to minimise need for post-operative artificial ventilation. Prolonged clinical observation is needed because respiratory depression may occur one or two days after surgery. Postoperative analgesia must be optimal so that pain does not inhibit breathing and coughing. Sedatives should be avoided preoperatively whenever possible. In some neuro-muscular disorders local blocks are preferable, example being compensated myasthenia gravis. Whenever muscle relaxants are used, continuous TOF-guard-ing is mandatory and minimal dose of relaxant should be titrated to the effect. Suxamethonium should be avoided in most neuromuscular disorders. The good alternatives are atracurium or cis-atracurium. Their effect reliably wanes, inde-pendently of the patient's metabolic mechanisms. Also, neostigmine need not be administered, provided that sufficient time is allowed for Hoffmann's elimina-tion of atracurium.

In rare neuromuscular disorders sufficient time must be taken for specific preoperative measures and planning for conduct of anaesthesia and subsequent monitoring. All this has become very problematic in day-case surgery. The im-pact of anaesthesia may be greater than the operation itself. Furthermore, in-creased duration of anaesthesia is associated with more postoperative complica-tions in day-case surgery.

Smooth muscles are weakened in some neuromuscular disorders. Precau-tions should be taken in cases of gastric atony.

Not strictly neuromuscular disorders like crash-syndrome, prolonged immo-bilisation, hemiplegia or critical-illness neuropathy, all call for increased caution when anaesthesia is planned. Some acute infections and several intoxications al-so are characterised by dimished muscle power. Suxamethonium should be re-placed by a short acting non-depolarising relaxant and need for postoperative ventilatory support should be kept in mind.

References

1. Hopkins PM, Ellis FR (1996) Neuromuscular pathology and malignant hyperthermia. In: Prys-Roberts C, Brown Jr BR (eds) International practice of anaesthesia. Butterworth-Heinemann, Oxford, pp 1/92/1-7
2. Dierdorf SF (1992) Rare and coexisting diseases. In: Barash PG et al (eds) Clinical anesthesia (2nd edn). Lippincott, Philadelphia, pp 563-587

Anaesthesia and Coexisting Diseases: Chronic Obstructive Pulmonary Disease

R. Alvisi, E.R. Righini, C.A. Volta

Knowledge about the prevalence of chronic obstructive pulmonary disease (COPD) is still incomplete, especially in Italy. However, it is estimated that in USA 4 to 6% of adult white male population and 1 to 3% of adult white female population suffer from COPD [1]. Therefore, it is more than a possibility that COPD patients could develop a disease requiring surgery. Moreover, since COPD affects elderly which are more likely to develop diseases due to COPD itself and tobacco abuse, surgery can be associated with increased risk of morbidity and mortality.

Preoperative evaluation

Preoperative evaluation of COPD patients is a challenging process which involves the indications for surgery, the surgical site, the experience of the surgical team, the type of anaesthesia, the need for a postoperative ventilatory assistance and the degree of respiratory impairment [2, 3].

Respiratory impairment assessment

The approach to COPD would be greatly facilitated by a staging system which would allow standardized categorization of the heterogeneous population of patients suffering from this disease.

The staging of the disease severity should be based on the relationship of the sensation of breathlessness, impairment of airflow and derangement in gas exchange [4]. According to the ATS criteria on the interpretation of lung function, COPD can be classified on three stages of severity. Stage I includes the majority of patients. These patients have $FEV_1 \geq 50\%$ predicted, minimal impact on health-related quality of life and moderate abnormalities of gas exchange. Stage II includes patients with FEV_1 ranging between 35 to 49% predicted, significant impact on health-related quality of life, hypoxaemia and/or severe hypercarbia and they may require continuing care by a respiratory specialist. Stage III include a minority of patients with $FEV_1 < 35\%$ predicted, profound impact on health-related quality of life, severe abnormalities of blood gas exchange and continuing care by a respiratory specialist [5].

Patients with stage I (mild to moderate) have perioperative risks similar to general population and need no special approach [2]. On the other hand, careful attention to perioperative respiratory management of stage II and III COPD patients can improve the outcome and reduce the perioperative morbidity.

In addition to routine clinical history investigation and physical examination, for a complete assessment of the respiratory impairment, a battery of respiratory and cardiovascular tests should be considered (Table 1). Spirometry and quantitative scintigraphy are useful in patients with severe COPD undergoing lung resection surgery. Moreover, the routine use of preoperative spirometry was reported to be helpful in determining risks of postoperative complication in upper abdominal surgery [2].

Table 1. Tests for preoperative evaluation

Standard chest X-ray (AP and L)
ECG
Blood gas analysis
Spirometry (*)
Diffusing capacity (*)
Exercise tests (*)
Oesophageal echocardiography (*)
Quantitative ventilatory/perfusion scintigraphy (*)

(*) Useful for lung surgery

Since many COPD patients have other diseases associated with the age and with tobacco abuse, scheduling preoperative visit before the elective surgical procedure can allow the anaesthesiologist to collect and coordinate the inputs of a multidisciplinary team of consultants that includes the surgeon, a pneumologist, a cardiologist and a physiotherapist. Useful preoperative pulmonary therapy and measures in COPD patients are reported in Table 2 [3, 7].

Recently, it has been stressed out the role of perioperative aids to lung expansion such as incentive spirometry or continuous positive airway pressure (CPAP) and deep breathing exercises in reducing length of hospital stay [2, 3, 8].

Site of surgery

Upper abdominal surgery shifts the respiratory pump from the diaphragm to the accessory muscles. Moreover, other pathophysiological changes result from anaesthesia and surgery, such as mucus hypersecretion with the development of

Table 2. Preoperative intervention for COPD patients

Discontinue smoking (8 weeks at least)
Adjust pharmacological therapy (step-by-step):
selective β_2-agonists MDI aerosol
ipratropium MDI aerosol
oral theophylline and or slow release β_2-agonist
steroid MDI aerosol
Treat infection
Improve mobilisation of secretions:
hydration
huff coughing
chest percussion and drainage
mucokinetic agent
Graded exercise programs
Deep breathing exercise
Incentive spirometry
Treat malnutrition
Low-flow oxygen (when indicated)
Treat cor pulmonale:
oxygen supplementation
diuretics
digitalis

airway flow limitation, hyperinflation and increased lung and chest wall elastance [9]. All of them pose upper abdominal surgery at high risk of postoperative pulmonary complications (PPC), particularly among patients with COPD stage II or III. When predisposing factors, such as obesity, heart disease and old age coexist, morbidity may approach 80% and mortality rate is approximately 3 to 5%.

PPC include purulent bronchitis, atelectasis requiring bronchoscopy or respiratory therapy, pneumonia, pulmonary embolism, pulmonary oedema and cardiorespiratory failure.

In this connection it should be noted that laparoscopic procedure is considered an effective way to reduce these operative risks [10].

Lower abdominal surgery is associated with a lower risk to develop PPC. However, patients with $FEV_1 < 1$ L are at an increased risk for complications and may require postoperative intensive care [2, 6].

Cardiac surgical procedures and *major vascular surgery* routinely require admission to a postoperative intensive care unit for monitoring and ventilatory support. Weaning from mechanical ventilation should not be attempted until the patient's cardiovascular status is stable. Diaphragm dysfunction secondary to phrenic nerve injury during cardiac procedures can be an important cause of prolonged ventilatory dependency.

Approximately 80% of patients with lung cancer have concomitant COPD and 20 to 30% have severe pulmonary dysfunction.

Spirometry and diffusing capacity should be performed routinely before *lung surgery*. These tests, however, should not be used to reject patients from a potentially life-saving surgical procedure (this is the case of a resectable lung cancer), but they should be used to select those patients who require a regional physiological assessment of lung function.

This because, apart from the temporary decrement (up to 30%) of vital capacity for several month due to the thoracotomy, if the region that should be resected has no function, no further loss in respiratory function will result. Therefore, patients who cannot sustain wide lung volume resection could be candidate to smaller resections such as wedge resection, segmentectomy and lobectomy [11].

Quantitative ventilation/perfusion lung scintigraphy can give information on regional contributions to lung function. A simple formula can be applied to predict FEV_1 after lung resection (Postoperative FEV_1 = Preoperative FEV_1 x % function of residual lungs after resection): if the calculated FEV_1 after resection is greater than 40% of predicted based on patient age, sex and height, resection can be carried out with relative safety [12].

Recently, some surgical procedures have been developed to improve lung function. Resection of large bullae compressing more normal lung tissue can be helpful in relieving severe dysfunction and dyspnea. Several studies suggest that even with very low FEV_1 removal of compressive bullae is indicated [13]. It is fundamental, in preoperative assessment, to differentiate bullae from non compressive destructive emphysema in which surgery can produce devastating results. CT scan of the lung can be helpful in diagnostic. Preliminary reports are encouraging in the use of lung volume reduction to relieve dyspnea and improve FEV_1 and FVC in patients with severe nonuniform emphysema [14].

Intraoperative management

When possible, regional anaesthesia is considered an ideal choice in COPD patients [9]. Regional techniques are not feasible if patients refuse or if the site of operation does not permit them. However, a non negligible consequence of regional anaesthesia is the loss of expiratory muscle power [15], although the clinical relevance of this phenomena is still unclear in patient with severe degree of airway obstruction. Such patients may have added difficulties because of surgical positioning and the need for sedatives and analgesics.

Otherwise, general anaesthesia, with or without paralysis, causes profound changes in respiratory function. A first aspect is the effect of posture: with the subject in supine position, functional residual capacity (FRC) is about 1 litre less than in upright position. Induction of anaesthesia will further reduce FRC until it is close to the residual volume for the cephalad movement of the diaphragm following muscle tone relaxation [16]. This has various effects on lung function:

- in dependent parts of the lungs airway resistance increases for airway caliber reduction;
- because of the aforementioned reduction during anaesthesia, FRC may be less than closing capacity. This will result in airway closure, atelectasis of dependent parts of the lung, shunting and arterial hypoxaemia [17];
- anaesthesia results in a reduction of total lung capacity and respiratory system compliance. The major component of this change is the lung rather than the chest wall. The causes of this phenomenon are not immediately obvious. There is no general agreement on the effects of anaesthetics on the pulmonary surfactant and the reduced compliance might well be secondary to the reduced FRC (18).

Other changes in respiratory function during anaesthesia depend on the administration of pharmacological agents.

Inhaled anaesthetics have generally a bronchodilating effect that is dose-dependent and is the result of several sites of action of the drug: peripheral and central depression of bronchoconstriction reflexes, β-receptors stimulating action, direct action on the fiber involving the cyclic AMP mechanisms and Ca^{++} channels activity [19, 20].

At MAC > 1 halothane, enflurane, isoflurane and sevoflurane produce a similar decrease in airway resistance during bronchospasm, but at lower concentrations halothane results the most effective [21, 22].

Other important effects include depression of ventilation and ventilatory responsiveness to inhaled CO_2. In their study on the effect of anaesthesia on COPD patients Pietak et al. clearly showed the decreased ability of these patients to respond to increased $PaCO_2$ values [23]. Moreover, volatile anaesthetics also depress hypoxic responsiveness in humans at subanaesthetic concentrations. Thus, the ability of these patients to maintain adequate ventilation while breathing spontaneously may be severely impaired.

Intravenous non narcotic agents have various effects on respiratory function.

Thiopental depresses respiration in a dose-related manner. Responsiveness to CO_2 stimulation is markedly impaired, and, at least in animals, the response to hypoxia is altered [24].

The bronchoconstrictive response to thiopental has not been confirmed by convincing data. Part of the concern about bronchoconstriction with thiopental may be related to the fact that manipulation of the airway easily results in laryngospasm and bronchospasm at light levels of thiopental anaesthesia.

When used at anaesthetic doses, ketamine produces moderate respiratory depression but CO_2 responsiveness is maintained. In patients with reactive airway disease ketamine decreases airway resistance and bronchospasm [25, 26].

At anaesthetic doses propofol produces respiratory depression. In clinical studies it showed bronchodilating properties, but in a laboratory study propofol did not reduce airway responsiveness in canine sublobar segments [27, 28].

Clinical implications from these observations are questionable. The high incidence of PPC in patients with COPD stage II and III is well known. Studies of outcome with different anaesthetic agents are not specific enough to evaluate the role of anaesthetic drugs on postoperative morbidity.

Intraoperative management of ventilation

The need for positive pressure ventilation is unavoidable during general anaesthesia, but the approaches to mechanical ventilation in patients with airflow obstruction have been controversial.

Many investigators suggest that the appropriate approach to ventilation of patients with airway obstruction should be characterized by delivery of relatively low tidal volume (VT) with relatively high inspiratory flow; and a respiratory frequency low enough to allow adequate time to passive expiration [29]. The therapeutic goals are to avoid respiratory alkalosis, to ameliorate ventilation distribution between "slow compartments" and "fast compartments" of the lung and to minimize lung hyperinflation.

Parameters useful for ventilator setting could be preoperative $PaCO_2$ values and plateau pressure. Since an end expiratory airway occlusion cannot be easily performed with an anaesthesia ventilator, the presence of dynamic hyperinflation can be suspected looking at the flow trace [30].

Postoperative period

The immediate postoperative period is crucial in COPD patients for the high risk of developing PPC. The previously mentioned acute diaphragmatic dysfunction, which is particularly relevant after upper abdominal surgery, can further worsen the chronic impairment between the respiratory load, that is increased for the obstructive disease, and the ability to sustain this load that is usually decreased due to hyperinflation [31]. Moreover, intraoperative fluid management direct to improve splanchnic organs perfusion can deteriorate lung function as well. Since hypercapnic hypoxaemic respiratory failure can abruptly occur in the early postoperative period, an accurate monitoring including clinical examination, pulse oximetry, daily blood gas analysis, PVC measurement, urinary output, daily liquid input-output is required to recognize and treat hypoxaemia, acidaemia, retained secretions and hypoventilation.

Oxygen therapy should be instituted to prevent life-threatening tissue hypoxia. However, to preserve cellular oxygenation, the clinician should also consider the other oxygen transport variables, including haemoglobin, cardiac output and distribution of tissue perfusion.

The goal of oxygen therapy is the correction of hypoxaemia to obtain a SaO_2 > 90% [32]. Although the most common and inexpensive method for oxygen delivery is the dual prong nasal cannula, a nasal cannula or a Venturi mask should be preferred when an accurate and constant FiO_2 is required.

It is recommended to monitor $PaCO_2$ and pH while initial titration of the oxygen flow is required. In titration of the oxygen flow setting it must be remembered that it takes about 20-30 minutes to achieve a steady state in a COPD patient; therefore, blood gas analysis at closer intervals may be misleading.

In general, patients receiving oxygen able to rise SpO_2 to values up to 90% will not experience CO_2 retention or acidosis. If the patient is a chronic CO_2 retainer, a reasonable goal is to adjust the oxygen setting to correct the hypoxaemia and maintain CO_2 at a stable, albeit elevated, level. If adequate oxygenation is not achievable without progressive respiratory acidosis, then mechanical ventilation must be considered.

An adequate care of pain relief, fundamental for all the maneuvers that enhance lung expansion; a rationale approach to fluid management, nutritional support and continuation of the preoperatively prescribed antibiotics, bronchodilators, corticosteroids and theophylline represent other cornerstones of postoperative management.

Patients with COPD stage II and III undergoing major upper abdomen surgery, cardiac surgery or major vascular surgery may require routinely admission to a postoperative intensive care unit and mechanical ventilation.

Recently, in a controlled study carried out on 271 elderly patients (including COPD patients) undergoing non cardiac major surgery, we have shown that scheduled admission to a postoperative intensive care unit can significantly reduce major postoperative complications and ameliorate patients early outcome [33]. According to other authors, accurate gas exchange monitoring and mechanical ventilation seem to play a fundamental role in reducing PPC in critically ill patients undergoing major surgical procedures [34].

Mechanical ventilation in COPD patients

In early postoperative period the main goals of mechanical ventilation are the correction of hypoxaemia and respiratory acidaemia, the resting of ventilatory muscles and the reduction of respiratory workload impact on the cardiovascular system.

COPD patients are prone to develop dynamic pulmonary hyperinflation (DPH) which can adversely affect circulation, increase the risk of barotrauma, increase work of breathing and place the diaphragm and the inspiratory muscles in a condition of mechanical disadvantage.

Therefore, specific concerns of mechanical ventilation in obstructive lung disease are to minimize the thoracic volume about which the lungs are ventilated [35] and to avoid hyperventilation that can result in acute respiratory alkalaemia, especially in patients with chronic hypercapnia.

Knowledge about preoperative $PaCO_2$ value may be helpful in determining appropriate ventilatory settings; moreover, ventilator adjustments designed to minimize DPH should be geared toward lowering ventilator mean expiratory flow that is to lower VT and to increase expiratory time (TE). Adjustments in I:E ratio and reduction in machine rate are less effective than VT reduction. Recently we observed an effective reduction in DPH when the monitoring of mean expiratory flow (VT/TE) was used for ventilator adjustments in mechanically ventilated COPD patients.

At bedside, clinical patient's evaluation, deformations of the flow and airway pressure waveforms on ventilator screen, variations in frequency, volume and peak airway pressure are important to notice to better synchronize the ventilator to the patient flow demands [36]. To optimize machine-patient synchronization, it is crucial to remove, when possible, any cause of increasing ventilatory demand such as pain, fever, liquid overload and cardiac failure.

Weaning from mechanical ventilation should not attempted until the recovery of the ventilatory pump and lung function are verified and the patient's cardiovascular status has become sufficiently stable to tolerate assumption of the work of breathing. Thereafter patients are generally considered ready to start a discontinuation process when a significant resolution of the initial precipitating illness occurs.

Weaning strategies are various modes to graduate the patient and the ventilator contributions to work of breathing. The clear superiority of one of the weaning methods proposed has not been convincingly demonstrated if each method is properly used [37].

Although the subjective assessment of an experienced clinician remains the most reliable predictor of weaning success or failure, predictive indices, such as endurance indices which reflect both breathing capability and the amount of ventilatory load, can be helpful for the judgement because they provide important information regarding the patient's pathologic state.

References

1. Higgins MW, Thom T (1990) Incidence, prevalence and mortality: intra- and inter-county differences. In: Hensley MJ, Saunders NA (eds) Clinical epidemiology of chronic obstructive pulmonary disease. Marcel Dekker, New York, pp 23-43

2. Kroenke K, Lawrence VA, Theroux JF et al (1993) Postoperative complications after thoracic and major abdominal surgery in patients with and without obstructive lung disease. Chest 104:1445-1451

3. ATS Statements (1995) Standards for the diagnosis and care of patients with chronic obstructive pulmonary disease. Am J Respir Crit Care Med 152:S77-120

4. Mahler DA, Weinburg DH, Wells CK et al (1984) The measurement of dyspnea: contents, interobserver agreement and physiologic correlates of two new clinical indexes. Chest 85: 751-758

5. ATS statement Lung function testing (1991) Selection of reference values and interpretative strategies (statement). Am Rev Respir Dis 144:1201-1218

6. Celli BR, Rodriguez KS, Snider GL (1984) A controlled trial of intermittent positive pressure breathing, incentive spirometry and deep breathing exercises in preventing pulmonary complication after abdominal surgery. Am Rev Respir Dis 130:12-15

7. Benumof JL, Alfery DD (1986) Anesthesia for thoracic surgery. In: Miller RD (ed) Anesthesia 2nd edn. Churchill Livingstone, New York, pp 1371-1462

8. Hall JC, Tarala R, Harris J et al (1991) Incentive spirometry versus routine chest physiotherapy for prevention of pulmonary complications after abdominal surgery. Lancet 337:953-956

9. Ford GT, Rosenal W, Clergue F (1993) Respiratory physiology in upper abdominal surgery. Clin Chest Med 14:227-236

10. MacFadyen BV, Ponsky JL (1992) Laparoscopy for the general surgeon. Surg Clin N Am 72:997-1185

11. Marshall MC, Olsen GN (1993) The physiologic evaluation of the lung resection candidate. Clin Chest Med 14:305-320

12. Markos J, Mullan BP, Hillman DR et al (1989) Preoperative assessment as a predictor of mortality and morbidity after lung resection. Am Rev Respir Dis 139:902-910

13. Nickoladze GD (1992) Functional results of surgery for bullous emphysema. Chest 101: 119-122

14. Cooper JD, Trulock EP, Triantafillou An et al (1995) Bilateral pneumectomy (volume reduction) for chronic obstructive pulmonary disease. J Thorac Cardiovasc Surg 109:106-119

15. Paskin S, Rodam T, Smith TC (1969) The effect of spinal anesthesia of the pulmonary function of patients with chronic obstructive pulmonary disease. Ann Surg 169:35-40

16. Hewlett AM, Huilands GH, Nunn JF (1974) Functional residual capacity during anesthesia. II. Spontaneous respiration. Br J Anaesth 46:486-494

17. Nunn JF, Coleman AJ, Sachithanandan T (1965) Hypoxaemia and atelectasis produced by forced expiration. Br J Anaesth 37:3-12

18. Westbrook PR, Stubbs SE, Sessler AD (1973) Effects of anesthesia and muscle paralysis on respiratory mechanics in normal man. J Appl Physiol 34:81-86

19. Yamamoto K, Morimoto N, Warner DO (1993) Factors influencing the direct actions of volatile anesthetics on airway smooth muscles. Anesthesiology 78:1102-1111

20. Namba H, Tsuchida H (1996) Effect of volatile anesthetics with and without verapamile on intracellular activity in vascular smooth muscle. Anesthesiology 84:1465-1474

21. Durenil B (1996) Anesthesia et hyperreactivité bronchique. Encycl Med Chir (Elsevier Paris) Anesthesie et Reanimation 36-655-F10, p 8

22. Brown RH, Zerhouni EA, Hirshman CA (1993) Comparison of low concentrations of halothane and isoflurane as bronchodilators. Anesthesiology 78:1097-1101

23. Pietak S, Weenig CS, Hickey RF et al (1975) Anesthetic effects on ventilation in patients with chronic obstructive pulmonary disease. Anesthesiology 1975;42:160

24. Hirshman CH, McCullough RE, Cohen PJ et al (1975) Hypoxic ventilation drive in dogs during thiopental, ketamine or pentobarbital anesthesia. Anesthesiology 43:628

25. Zsigmond EK, Matsuki A, Kothary SP et al (1976) Arterial hypoxemia caused by intravenous ketamine. Anesth Analg 55:311
26. Cheng EY, Mazzeo AJ, Bosnjak ZJ et al (1996) Direct relaxant effects of intravenous anesthetics on airway smooth muscle. Anesth Analg 83:162-168
27. Conti G, Dell'Utri D, Vilardi V et al (1993) Propofol induces bronchodilatation in mechanically ventilated chronic obstructive pulmonary disease (COPD) patients. Acta Anesthesiol Scand 37:105-109
28. Mehr EH, Lindeman KS (1993) Effects of halothane, propofol and thiopental on peripheral airway reactivity. Anesthesiology 79:290-298
29. Gal TJ (1994) Bronchial hyperresponsiveness and anesthesia: physiologic and therapeutic perspective. Anesth Analg 78:559-573
30. Tuxen DV, Lane S (1987) The effects of ventilatory pattern on hyperinflation, airway pressures, and circulation in mechanical ventilation of patients with severe airflow obstruction. Am Rev Respir Dis 136:872-879
31. Rochester DF, Braun NMT (1985) Determinants of maximal inspiratory pressure in chronic obstructive pulmonary disease. Am Rev Respir Dis 132:42-47
32. Mithoefer JC, Keighley JF, Karetzky (1971) Response to arterial PO_2 to oxygen administration in chronic pulmonary disease: interpretation of findings in a study of 46 patients and 14 normal subjects. Ann Intern Med 74:328-335
33. Righini ER, Cocciolo F, Santini M et al (1994) La gestione postoperatoria del paziente anziano. Decorso postoperatorio, morbilità e sopravvivenza a breve termine. Minerva Anestesiol 60[Suppl]1:31-41
34. Cullen DJ, Nemeskal AR, Cooper JB et al (1992) Effect of pulse oximetry, age and ASA Physical Status on the frequency of patients admitted unexpectedly to a postoperative intensive care unit and the severity of their anesthesia related complications. Anesth Analg 74: 181-188
35. Slutsky S (1993) Mechanical ventilation. Chest 104:1833-1859
36. Marini JJ, Capps JS, Culver BH (1985) The inspiratory work of breathing during assisted mechanical ventilation. Chest 87:612-618
37. Marini JJ (1991) Weaning from mechanical ventilation. N Engl J Med 324:1496-1498

Optimization of the Perioperative Period in High-Risk Patients

A.F. Hammerle, C. Tatschl

Cardiovascular complications, respiratory events and allergic reactions represent the most frequent adverse events in patients undergoing surgery and anaesthesia [1, 2].

The increase in mean life expectancy has brought about a change in population structure. Today, more than 14 per cent of the US population are older than 65 years. It is expected, that the proportion of this age group will have expanded to more than 20 per cent by the year 2020. Age is associated with an increased prevalence of cardiovascular morbidities such as hypertension, congestive heart failure, and coronary artery disease. Several factors such as the underlying disease, physical status, and invasiveness of the surgical procedure [2] contribute to perioperative risk and to the development of cardiovascular compromise, many of which can be modified throughout the perioperative period.

Therefore, these risk patients constitute a growing challenge for the anaesthesiologist.

Cardiac risk

Assessment of risk

Risk scores

Several scores have been developed in order to quantify risk. Among these, the American Society of Anesthesiologists (ASA) physical-status-score and the Cardiac Risk Index (CRI) are most commonly applied.

The ASA score is a simple subjective means to assess the physical condition of the patient [3].

CRI was originally developed by Goldman et al., who investigated 1001 patients undergoing noncardiac surgery. In multivariate analysis, 9 variables were identified to predict the development of perioperative cardiac complications [4].

This index was modified by Detsky and colleagues, who incorporated severe angina and remote myocardial infarction as additional risk factors [5].

These scores have been directly compared in more than 16,000 patients. This study suggests specific combination of both modalities to increase predictive power [6].

Guidelines for the approach to the cardiac risk patient

The recognition of the importance of assessment and management of cardiac risk, along with the economic pressure has led to the development of guidelines for evaluation of the patient at risk [7-9]. These guidelines propose algorithmic approaches and give recommendations for the use of diverse preoperative testing strategies.

The approach includes risk stratification according to the modified CRI, determination of low-risk variables, definition of the severity of the surgical procedure, and evaluation of the patient's functional capacity, expressed by metabolic equivalent (MET) levels (i.e. the aerobic demands for specific activities).

Thereafter, the patient may directly proceed to surgery, or has to undergo further testing and risk factor modification, eventually leading to delay or cancellation of the operation.

Preoperative optimization of cardiovascular haemodynamics

Vascular patients constitute a group of people, who are at an increased risk of cardiovascular complications because of the high prevalence of comorbidities such as diabetes mellitus, congestive heart failure, and hypertension. These coexisting diseases are all known to jeopardize the patient's postoperative outcome.

Although there is controversy about the use of the pulmonary artery catheter, preoperative circulatory "tune-up" to optimize left ventricular function and oxygen transport seems to improve outcome in this patient population. In a prospective, randomized clinical trial, patients were treated preoperatively by fluid loading, after load reduction, or inotropic support to achieve a pulmonary artery wedge pressure (PAWP) ≤ 15 mmHg, a cardiac index (CI) ≥ 2.8 L/min/m^2, and a systemic vascular resistance (SVR) ≤ 1100 dyne-sec-cm^{-5}, end points that are known to have an impact on outcome. The patients, who were optimized with the use of a PA catheter, had significantly fewer adverse intraoperative events, a reduced postoperative cardiac morbidity, and a decreased risk of graft thrombosis [10].

The importance of perioperative volume optimization was confirmed in patients undergoing proximal femoral fracture repair [11]. In this prospective, randomized, controlled trial, volume optimization was guided by minimally invasive oesophageal Doppler ultrasonography. Protocol patients exhibited significantly greater changes in stroke volume than did those who received conventional intraoperative fluid management. Furthermore, protocol patients had a faster postoperative recovery.

Boyd et al. [12] randomized high risk surgical patients to either a control group or to receive dopexamine to increase oxygen delivery index to greater than 600 mL/min/m². The patients in the protocol group had a significant reduction in terms of mortality and complications.

Retrospective analysis of this study population revealed that this approach led to a marked reduction in hospital costs [13].

Perioperative sympatholysis

Activation of the sympathetic nervous system as a response to stress endangers the myocardium, because the increased metabolic demands often are no longer met by the amount of oxygen supplied. Ten years ago Roizen rose the question, whether we all should have a sympathectomy before surgery [14].

Data from the published literature now strongly suggest that the idea of dampening the adrenergic response may be correct during the entire perioperative period.

α2-adrenoceptor agonists

Clonidine

Clonidine is an α2-adrenergic receptor agonist, that is known to interfere with thermoregulation. Clonidine lowers the shivering threshold and vasoconstrictor threshold [15] and its utility for the prevention of postoperative shivering has been demonstrated in several studies [16, 17].

In addition, clonidine appears to be useful to maintain circulatory stability during the perioperative period. In a randomized placebo-controlled, double-blind study on patients undergoing aortic surgery, it could be demonstrated that administration of clonidine suppresses the increase in plasma catecholamines, reduces intraoperative blood pressure and improves stroke volume index. Patients in the protocol group required significantly less anaesthetic or circulatory interventions [18].

Another controlled trial on patients undergoing major non-cardiac surgery revealed that premedication with a transdermal clonidine system on the night before surgery and oral application shortly before anaesthesia resulted in a reduction of anaesthetic requirements, lower incidence of intraoperative tachycardia, and a reduction in the occurrence of myocardial ischaemia [19].

These favorable results were confirmed in a very recent study conducted by Quintin et al. In this trial vascular patients received clonidine as oral premedication and intravenously from aortic unclamping to skin closure. Anaesthetic, analgesic, and sedative requirements were reduced by approximately 40 per cent.

Hormones of the stress response (epinephrine, norepinephrine, plasma renin activity) were suppressed and the need for circulatory adjustment was diminished [20].

Mivazerol

Mivazerol is a new and selective α2-adrenoceptor agonist, developed to prevent adverse perioperative cardiac events in patients with coronary artery disease.

In the animal model it was demonstrated that mivazerol induces a dose related decrease in heart rate without significantly altering blood pressure. Perioperative treatment lead to the suppression of the cardiovascular response to surgical stress [21].

Furthermore, administration of mivazerol was demonstrated to suppress the catecholamine activation in the vasomotor center of the medulla and to decrease the incidence of tachycardia on emergence from halothane anaesthesia [22, 23].

It seems likely, that the sympathoinhibitory effects are mediated by central as well as peripheral mechanisms [24].

In a recent multicenter phase II trial, the potential beneficial effects of mivazerol were studied in a placebo-controlled, double-blind, randomized manner. Patients undergoing noncardiac surgery received either high or low dose mivazerol or placebo during surgery and for 72 hours in the postoperative period. The incidence of tachycardia and the number of patients requiring treatment for this event were significantly lower in the high dose group throughout the entire perioperative period. The occurrence of intraoperative hypertension was diminished by either dose of mivazerol. Perioperative bradycardia was observed more frequently in those patients receiving the study drug, but without an increased need for treatment. Furthermore, a significant reduction in myocardial ischaemia was found in the high dose group.

No rebound effect was demonstrated after withdrawal of the study drug [25].

β-adrenoceptor blocking agents

In a non-double-blind, prospective, randomized study mildly hypertensive patients undergoing surgery, who had not been given antihypertensive therapy before the trial period, were screened for the incidence of myocardial ischaemia during anaesthesia. Ischaemic episodes during intubation and during emergence from anaesthesia were observed frequently in these patients. The risk of myocardial ischaemia was significantly reduced by a single oral dose of a β-adrenoceptor blocking agent given along with premedication [26].

Mangano et al. investigated the impact of perioperative (throughout hospitalization) administration of atenolol on overall survival and cardiovascular morbidity in patients undergoing noncardiac surgery, who had or were at risk for coronary artery disease.

This group was able to demonstrate a reduction in mortality by 8 per cent in patients receiving atenolol. Rates of combined myocardial infarction, unstable angina, or congestive heart failure requiring hospital admission were reduced by 15 per cent. The beneficial effects of atenolol in reducing cardiovascular complications were observed for as long as two years [27].

The American College of Physicians deemed these results convincing enough to recommend the perioperative use of atenolol in patients who are at an increased cardiac risk (as defined in the study protocol by Mangano) as long as no serious contraindications such as asthma occur [8, 9].

A second study performed by the group of Mangano revealed that patients at risk for coronary artery disease, who were given atenolol for 1 week perioperatively, exhibited a marked reduction in in-hospital postoperative myocardial ischaemia. The decrease in postoperative ischemic episodes was associated with a reduction in the risk for death at 2 years [28].

Calcium channel blocking agents

The cardioprotective potential of the calcium channel blocker diltiazem was recently evaluated in patients undergoing elective coronary bypass surgery. Patients who received diltiazem had a lower number of ventricular premature beats, fewer and shorter transient ischaemic events, and lower levels of CK-MB and troponin T [29].

In such patients, diltiazem administration was demonstrated to be associated with a better preservation of left ventricular diastolic function in the post-cardiopulmonary bypass period, as assessed by transoesophageal echocardiography. Furthermore, no significant negative inotropic effect could be observed [30].

Myocardial protection also can be achieved with the combination of a β-blocking agent with the calcium channel blocker nifedipine. The combination of metoprolol and nifedipine proved to be useful in the attempt to prevent myocardial ischaemia and was able to reduce the incidence of reperfusion-induced arrhythmias. Significant negative inotropic effects were not produced by this combination [31].

Inhibitors of the angiotensin converting enzyme

The renin-angiotensin-aldosterone-system (RAAS) plays an important role in cardiovascular homeostasis.

In a recent study on patients undergoing coronary artery bypass grafting, clonidine, the phosphodiesterase III inhibitor enoximone, and the ACE inhibitor enalaprilat were evaluated for their potential to protect the myocardium from ischaemic injury.

Enalaprilat infusion was most effective in these patients, reflected by the smallest changes in the levels of serologic marker proteins of myocardial ischemia (troponin T, glycogen phosphorylase isoenzyme BB, and CK-MB).

Of interest, clonidine did not provide protective effects in this clinical setting [32].

Prevention of hypothermia

Unintended hypothermia occurs frequently in patients undergoing major surgery. Besides the cold environment in the operating room, anaesthesia-induced impairment of thermoregulation and fluid administration contribute to the decrease in body temperature.

It was shown that patients receiving routine thermal care often had core temperatures as low as 35.3°C on admission to the postanaesthetic care unit. When compared to patients being treated with forced-air-skin-surface warming, in whom mean core temperature was maintained at 36.7°C, patients with mild hypothermia had elevated norepinephrine levels immediately and 3 hours after surgery. In addition, mean, systolic, and diastolic blood pressure were significantly higher in these patients [33].

Furthermore, in patients in whom normothermia was maintained, less perioperative cardiac events such as unstable angina, cardiac arrest, or myocardial infarction occurred less frequently and the incidence of postoperative tachycardia was reduced. Multivariate analysis identified hypothermia as an independent predictor for morbid cardiac events, with a 55 per cent reduction of risk, when a patient was kept warm [34].

Ischaemic preconditioning

The term "ischaemic preconditioning" describes the possibility to delay lethal cell injury due to ischaemia by exposing the heart to a short interruption of blood flow before a subsequent sustained ischaemic insult occurs.

Murry et al. preconditioned dogs with four 5-minute ischaemic episodes before the coronary artery was occluded for a period of 40 minutes. This procedure of preconditioning paradoxically resulted in a decrease in infarct size to 25 per cent of that observed in control animals, in whom no preconditioning was performed [35].

The infarct limiting potential of preconditioning is a biphasic phenomenon. Kuzuya et al. found a significant reduction in infarction size when the sustained coronary artery occlusion was carried out immediately or 24 hours after preconditioning, whereas no such benefit could be demonstrated when the sustained occlusion was performed 3 hours of 12 hours after the preconditioning episode [36]. This late phase of the infarct limiting effect was designated as the "second window of protection".

Several observations support the notion that ischaemic preconditioning occurs in humans. It is well known, that many patients experiencing angina pectoris are able to exercise to the same extent without development of chest pain after pausing for a short period (warm up phenomenon).

In a clinical study, patients with severe stenosis of the left anterior descending artery performed two consecutive exercise tests, separated by a pause of 15 minutes. Exercise was tolerated significantly longer in the second test, and ST segment depression was less pronounced [37].

Deutsch et al. reported that during percutaneous transluminal coronary angioplasty, a second balloon occlusion was better tolerated and accompanied by less ST segment shift and lower mean pulmonary artery pressure [38].

Ischaemic preconditioning may also have contributed to the findings of the Thrombolysis in Myocardial Infarction (TIMI) 4 trial. Patients with acute myocardial infarction had a better in-hospital outcome, when they had a history of previous angina [38, 39].

Induction of ischaemic preconditioning with cycles of aortic cross clamping was also performed in humans. Patients undergoing open heart surgery, who were preconditioned by this regime, showed less leakage of cardiac enzymes, a reduction in ST-segment shift, enhanced myocardial contractility and a decreased need for inotropic support [40, 41].

The mechanisms involved in the generation of the beneficial effects of preconditioning are not fully understood. However, ATP dependent potassium channels and adenosine are most likely to be central mediators [42, 43].

In patients undergoing coronary artery bypass grafting, the addition of adenosine to cold blood cardioplegia resulted in a reduced postoperative need for dopamine and nitroglycerine. In addition, ejection fraction was higher when adenosine was added to cardioplegia [44].

Risk of perioperative pulmonary complications

Assessment of pulmonary risk

There is much less agreement concerning the factors that might predict the risk of pulmonary complications in the perioperative period. Several variables were proposed to be associated with an increased pulmonary risk, including age, impaired preoperative cognitive function, a history of recent smoking (see below), obesity, cancer, and incision site of the abdomen [45].

Furthermore, preoperative arterial partial oxygen pressure (PaO_2) and grading the severity of preoperative dyspnoea may add some information [46]. However, as stated in a recent detailed review regarding this topic, there is a need for randomized prospective trials with clear definitions of pulmonary complications to achieve progress in this field [47].

Asthma

Most patients with asthma may safely undergo surgery, especially if they are young and do not present with symptoms. The frequency of bronchospasm and laryngospasm appears to be very low in such patients, and in most cases do not lead to severe postoperative morbidity [48].

In addition, well controlled asthmatic children undergoing elective surgery do not exhibit a greater decrease in peak expiratory flow rate (PEFR) and FEV$_1$ following general anaesthesia than do healthy matched controls [49].

The low incidence of bronchospasm can also be depicted from the *American Society of Anesthesiologists closed claims study*. However, this database provides important information: 1) though rarely associated with serious pulmonary complications, bronchospasm does sometimes bring about adverse outcome. 88% of perioperative brochospasms resulting in claims were associated with brain damage or death; 2) half of the patients did not have a history of asthma, or chronic obstructive lung disease [50].

The main cause of bronchospasm is endotracheal intubation. This should be counteracted by the anaesthesiologist's choice of the anaesthetic technique such as the use of a laryngeal mask instead of endotracheal intubation.

Pizov et al. demonstrated the value of propofol for induction of anaesthesia in a randomized, double-blinded, prospective study. The incidence of wheezing, as assessed by a blinded observer auscultating the lungs 2 and 3 minutes postintubation, was lower in both asthmatic and nonasthmatic patients after induction with propofol than in those patients receiving a barbiturate [51].

Ketamine is another intravenous narcotic that is well tolerated by asthmatics. Hirota and colleagues evaluated the capacity of ketamine to produce bronchodilation by directly measuring bronchial cross-sectional area with a superfine fiberoptic bronchoscope in a canine model, in which bronchoconstriction was induced with histamine. Ketamine reversed histamine induced bronchospasm and significantly potentiated the relaxing effects of epinephrine [52].

In addition, its usefulness for postanaesthetic pain management was demonstrated in asthmatic patients, who received ketamine along with midazolam [53].

Smoking

Chronic obstructive pulmonary disease (COPD) and atherosclerosis are well known long term complications of tobacco smoking. However, there are also more acute implications of cigarette smoking. Increased sensitivity of the upper airway reflexes are found in cigarette smokers [54].

Furthermore, specific respiratory events such as re-intubation, laryngospasm, bronchospasm, aspiration, etc., have been demonstrated to occur more frequently in smokers than in non-smokers. Especially young smokers with chronic bronchitis exhibited a high relative risk (25.7) for the development of perioperative bronchospasm [55].

Cessation of smoking 8 weeks before surgery appears to be a rational basis to decrease the risk of perioperative pulmonary complications in smokers [45, 56].

Latex allergy

Although reactions to muscle relaxants are most commonly involved in adverse immunologic reactions during anaesthesia, latex hypersensitivity is now becoming recognized as a major potential hazard in the operating room. Latex is more often involved in allergic reactions than are hypnotics, benzodiazepines, opioids, colloids, or antibiotics [57].

The spectrum of symptoms that arise from latex hypersensitivity ranges from pruritus to anaphylactic shock.

Two immunologic mechanisms are responsible for the reaction to latex.

The most common type of latex-induced allergic reaction is contact dermatitis, which is caused by a type IV (delayed hypersensitivity) reaction. This reaction does not require antibodies but is mediated by T lymphocytes.

The second, more threatening type of reaction is latex-induced anaphylaxis. This reaction eventually leads to the development of shock and is based on a type I (immediate hypersensitivity) reaction involving IgE-antibodies [58].

Several groups of patients have been identified to be at and increased risk for latex-associated complications.

Besides medical stuff and rubber product workers, children with congenital malformations such as spina bifida, myelomeningocele, and urogenital abnormalities are considered to have a high susceptibility to develop latex hypersensitivity. It is believed that recurrent exposition to latex containing materials due to frequent operations and catheterizations cause sensitization in these children [58, 59].

Indeed, Theissen et al. found that the number of operations undergone in the past, was the most important discriminator between sensitized and non-sensitized children. However, it has to be mentioned that the predictive value of IgE-antibodies against latex for the development of anaphylaxis during anaesthesia was low in this study [60].

Patients with certain food allergies constitute a second risk group. In these patients cross-reacting IgE-antibodies recognizing both latex and fruit allergens can be detected with RAST-inhibition test. Cross reactivity has been demonstrated for allergens found in a variety of tropical fruits like avocado, banana, pineapple, mango, kiwi, peach and tomato. This condition is termed the "latex-fruit syndrome" [61].

Finally, atopic individuals appear to have an increased likelihood to develop hypersensitivity reactions to latex [61].

Latex allergy is detected by a thorough history, skin test, and IgE-assays [62]. Once the diagnosis "latex allergy" is established, all potential sources of latex (catheters, gloves, anaesthesia equipment) should be replaced by synthetic substitutes.

Severe latex-induced anaphylactic reactions are treated by removing the antigen and application of an antihistamine, epinephrine and steroids [58].

Conclusions

Alterations of physiologic processes are inevitable during the perioperative period and may be regarded as side effects of the surgical procedure. It is the anaesthesiologist's duty to anticipate, diagnose and manage these hazards.

Clinical studies performed during the past decade have brought about an increased understanding of the mechanisms involved, and provide a rational basis for the anaesthesiologist to develop specific therapeutic strategies, that will hopefully lead to a further increase in the patient's safety and convenience.

References

1. Mangano DT (1990) Perioperative cardiac morbidity. Anesthesiology 72:153-184
2. Ouchterlony J, Arvidsson S, Sjostedt L et al (1995) Perioperative and immediate postoperative adverse events in patients undergoing elective general and orthopaedic surgery. The Gothenburg study of perioperative risk (PROPER). Part II. Acta Anaesthesiol Scand 39: 643-652
3. Dripps RD (1963) New classification of physical status. Anesthesiology 24:111
4. Goldman L, Caldera DL, Nussbaum SR et al (1977) Multifactorial index of cardiac risk in noncardiac surgical procedures. N Engl J Med 297:845-850
5. Detsky AS, Abrams HB, McLaughlin JR et al (1986) Predicting cardiac complications in patients undergoing non cardiac surgery. Gen Intern Med 1:211-219
6. Prause G, Ratzenhofer-Comenda B, Pierer G et al (1997) Can ASA grade or Goldman's cardiac risk index predict perioperative mortality? A study of 16,227 patients. Anaesthesia 52: 203-206
7. Eagle KA, Brundage BH, Chaitman BR et al (1996) Guidelines for perioperative cardiovascular evaluation for noncardiac surgery. Report of the American College of Cardiology/American Heart Association Task Force on Practice Guidelines (Committee on Perioperative Cardiovascular Evaluation for Noncardiac Surgery). J Am Coll Cardiol 27:910-948
8. Guidelines for assessing and managing the perioperative risk from coronary artery disease associated with major noncardiac surgery (1997) American College of Physicians. Ann Intern Med 127:309-312
9. Palda VA, Detsky AS (1997) Perioperative assessment and management of risk from coronary artery disease. Ann Intern Med 127:313-328
10. Berlauk JF, Abrams JH, Gilmour IJ et al (1991) Preoperative optimization of cardiovascular hemodynamics improves outcome in peripheral vascular surgery. A prospective, randomized clinical trial. Ann Surg 14:289-297
11. Sinclair S, James S, Singer M (1997) Intraoperative intravascular volume optimisation and length of hospital stay after repair of proximal femoral fracture: randomised controlled trial. BMJ 315:909-912
12. Boyd O, Grounds RM, Bennett ED (1993) A randomized clinical trial of the effect of deliberate perioperative increase of oxygen delivery on mortality in high risk surgical patients. JAMA 270:2699-2707
13. Guest JF, Boyd O, Hart WM et al (1997) A cost analysis of a treatment policy of a deliberate perioperative increase in oxygen delivery in high risk surgical patients. Intensive Care Med 23:85-90
14. Roizen MF (1988) Should we all have a sympathectomy at birth? Or at least preoperatively? Anesthesiology 68:482-484

15. Nicolaou G, Chen AA, Johnston CE et al (1997) Clonidine decreases vasoconstriction and shivering thresholds, without affecting the sweating threshold. Can J Anaesth 44:636-642
16. Vanderstappen I, Vandermeersch E, Vanacker B et al (1996) The effect of prophylactic clonidine on postoperative shivering. A large prospective double blind study. Anaesthesia 51:351-355
17. Horn EP, Werner C, Sessler DI et al (1997) Late intraoperative clonidine administration prevents postanesthetic shivering after total intravenous or volatile anesthesia. Anesth Analg 84:613-617
18. Quintin L, Bonnet F, Macquin I et al (1990) Aortic surgery: effect of clonidine on intraoperative catecholaminergic and circulatory stability. Acta Anaesthesiol Scand 34:132-137
19. Ellis JE, Drijvers G, Pedlow S et al (1994) Premedication with oral and transdermal clonidine provides safe and efficacious postoperative sympatholysis. Anesth Analg 79:1133-1140
20. Quintin L, Bouilloc X, Butin E et al (1996) Clonidine for major vascular surgery in hypertensive patients: a double blind, controlled, randomized study. Anesth Analg 83:687-695
21. Zhang X, Wulfert E, Hanin I (1997) Mivazerol, a new alpha 2 adrenergic agonist, blunts cardiovascular effects following surgical stress in pentobarbital anesthetized rats. Acta Anaesthesiol Scand 41:694-700
22. Guyaux M, Gobert J, Noyer M et al (1998) Mivazerol prevents the tachycardia caused by emergence from halothane anesthesia partly through activation of spinal alpha 2 adrenoceptors. Acta Anaesthesiol Scand 42:238-245
23. Bruandet N, Rentero N, Debeer L et al (1998) Catecholamine activation in the vasomotor center on emergence from anesthesia: the effects of alpha 2 agonists. Anesth Analg 86:240-245
24. Richer C, Gobert J, Noyer M et al (1996) Peripheral alpha 2 adrenoceptor mediated sympathoinhibitory effects of mivazerol. Fundam Clin Pharmacol 10:529-537
25. McSPI Europe Research Group (1997) Perioperative sympatholysis. Beneficial effects of the alpha 2 adrenoceptor agonist mivazerol on hemodynamic stability and myocardial ischemia. Anesthesiology 86:346-363
26. Stone JG, Foex P, Sear JW et al (1988) Myocardial ischemia in untreated hypertensive patients: effect of a single small oral dose of a beta adrenergic blocking agent. Anesthesiology 68:495-500
27. Mangano DT, Layug EL, Wallace A et al (1996) Effect of atenolol on mortality and cardiovascular morbidity after noncardiac surgery. Multicenter Study of Perioperative Ischemia Research Group. N Engl J Med 335:1713-1720
28. Wallace A, Layug B, Tateo I et al (1998) Prophylactic atenolol reduces postoperative myocardial ischemia. McSPI Research Group. Anesthesiology 88:7-17
29. Hannes W, Seitelberger R, Christoph M et al (1995) Effect of perioperative diltiazem on myocardial ischaemia and function in patients receiving mammary artery grafts. Eur Heart J 16:87-93
30. Malhotra R, Mishra M, Kler TS et al (1997) Cardioprotective effects of diltiazem infusion in the perioperative period. Eur J Cardiothorac Surg 12:420-427
31. Podesser BK, Schwarzacher S, Zwoelfer W et al (1995) Comparison of perioperative myocardial protection with nifedipine versus nifedipine and metoprolol in patients undergoing elective coronary artery bypass grafting. J Thorac Cardiovasc Surg 110:1461-1469
32. Boldt J, Rothe G, Schindler E et al (1996) Can clonidine, enoximone, and enalaprilat help to protect the myocardium against ischaemia in cardiac surgery? Heart 76:207-213
33. Frank SM, Higgins MS, Breslow MJ et al (1995) The catecholamine, cortisol, and hemodynamic responses to mild perioperative hypothermia. A randomized clinical trial. Anesthesiology 82:83-93
34. Frank SM, Fleisher LA, Breslow MJ et al (1997) Perioperative maintenance of normothermia reduces the incidence of morbid cardiac events. A randomized clinical trial. JAMA 277:1127-1134

35. Murry CE, Jennings RB, Reimer KA (1986) Preconditioning with ischemia: a delay of lethal cell injury in ischemic myocardium. Circulation 74:1124-1136
36. Kuzuya T, Hoshida S, Yamashita N et al (1993) Delayed effects of sublethal ischemia on the acquisition of tolerance to ischemia. Circ Res 72:1293-1299
37. Okazaki Y, Kodama K, Sato H et al (1993) Attenuation of increased regional myocardial oxygen consumption during exercise as a major cause of warm up phenomenon. J Am Coll Cardiol 21:1597-1604
38. Deutsch E, Berger M, Kussmaul WG et al (1990) Adaptation to ischemia during percutaneous transluminal coronary angioplasty. Clinical, hemodynamic, and metabolic features. Circulation 82:2044-2051
39. Kloner RA, Shook T, Przyklenk K et al (1995) Previous angina alters in hospital outcome in TIMI 4. A clinical correlate to preconditioning? Circulation 91:37-45
40. Lu EX, Chen SX, Hu TH et al (1998) Preconditioning enhances myocardial protection in patients undergoing open heart surgery. Thorac Cardiovasc Surg 46:28-32
41. Illes RW, Swoyer KD (1998) Prospective, randomized clinical study of ischemic preconditioning as an adjunct to intermittent cold blood cardioplegia. Ann Thorac Surg 65:748-752
42. Liu GS, Thornton J, Van Winkle DM et al (1991) Protection against infarction afforded by preconditioning is mediated by A1 adenosine receptors in rabbit heart. Circulation 84:350-356
43. Auchampach JA, Grover GJ, Gross GJ (1992) Blockade of ischaemic preconditioning in dogs by the novel ATP dependent potassium channel antagonist sodium 5-hydroxydecanoate. Cardiovasc Res 26:1054-1062
44. Mentzer RM Jr, Rahko PS, Molina-Viamonte V et al (1997) Safety, tolerance, and efficacy of adenosine as an additive to blood cardioplegia in humans during coronary artery bypass surgery. Am J Cardiol 79:38-43
45. Brooks-Brunn JA (1997) Predictors of postoperative pulmonary complications following abdominal surgery. Chest 111:564-571
46. Nunn JF, Milledge JS, Chen D et al (1988) Respiratory criteria of fitness for surgery and anaesthesiology. Anaesthesia 43:543-551
47. Kheradmand F, Wiener-Kronish JP, Corry DB (1997) Assessment of operative risk for patients with advanced lung disease. Clin Chest Med 18:483-494
48. Warner DO, Warner MA, Barnes RD et al (1996) Perioperative respiratory complications in patients with asthma. Anesthesiology 85:460-467
49. May HA, Smyth RL, Romer HC et al (1996) Effects of anaesthesia on lung function in children with asthma. Br J Anaesth 77:200-202
50. Cheney FW, Posner KL, Caplan RA (1991) Adverse respiratory events infrequently leading to malpractice suits. A closed claims analysis. Anesthesiology 75:932-939
51. Pizov R, Brown RH, Weiss YS et al (1995) Wheezing during induction of general anesthesia in patients with and without asthma. A randomized, blinded trial. Anesthesiology 82:1111-1116
52. Hirota K, Hashimoto Y, Sakai T et al (1998) In vivo spasmolytic effect of ketamine and adrenaline on histamine-induced airway constriction. Direct visualization method with a superfine bronchoscope. Acta Anaesthesiol Scand 42:184-188
53. Jahangir SM, Islam F, Aziz L (1993) Ketamine infusion for postoperative analgesia in asthmatics: a comparison with intermittent meperidine. Anesth Analg 76:45-49
54. Erskine RJ, Murphy PJ, Langton JA (1994) Sensitivity of upper airway reflexes in cigarette smokers: effect of abstinence. Br J Anaesth 73:298-302
55. Schwilk B, Bothner U, Schraag S et al (1997) Perioperative respiratory events in smokers and nonsmokers undergoing general anaesthesia. Acta Anaesthesiol Scand 41:348-355
56. Rezaiguia S, Jayr C (1996) Prevention of respiratory complications after abdominal surgery. Ann Fr Anesth Reanim 15:623-646

57. Laxenaire MC (1993) Drugs and other agents involved in anaphylactic shock occurring during anaesthesia. A French multicenter epidemiological inquiry. Ann Fr Anesth Reanim 12: 91-96
58. Vasallo SA (1998) Perioperative care of latex-allergic patients. In: Lake CL, Rice LJ, Sperry JS (eds) Advances in anesthesia vol. 15. Mosby, St. Louis, pp 107-131
59. Meeropol E, Kelleher R, Bell S et al (1990) Allergic reactions to rubber in patients with myelodysplasia. N Eng J Med 323:1072
60. Theissen U, Theissen JL, Mertes N et al (1997) IgE-mediated hypersensitivity to latex in childhood. Allergy 52:665-669
61. Brehler R, Theissen U, Mohr C et al (1997) "Latex-fruit syndrome": frequency of cross-reacting IgE antibodies. Allergy 52:404-410
62. Turjanmaa K, Palosuo T, Alenius H et al (1997) Latex allergy diagnosis: in vivo and in vitro standardization of a natural rubber latex extract. Allergy 52:41-50

CLINICAL ANAESTHESIA

Standards in Anaesthetic Practice

A.R. AITKENHEAD

A "standard" is defined in the Oxford Dictionary as "a quality or measure serving as a basis or example or principle to which others conform or should conform or by which the quality of others is judged", or "the degree of excellence required for a particular purpose". Many national and international bodies have published recommendations for standards of care in a wide variety of areas of anaesthetic practice, with the intention of improving safety for patients, and eliminating the unacceptable practices of the worst anaesthetists. Not all of the published standards are evidence-based, some are illogical, and others become outdated. However, in many instances, the published "standards" come to be regarded both by the "authorities" within anaesthesia, and by lawyers, as mandatory instructions. This has led to situations in which anaesthetists have been threatened with removal of their licence to practise medicine, even though their practice conformed to that which would be regarded as acceptable by the majority of their peers.

Standards relating to anaesthetic techniques may result in uniformity of practice. This eliminates the worst extremes of practice, and the exercise of "clinical judgement", which is prone to abuse and error. However, it also saps the morale of competent anaesthetists, who may become disillusioned by the inability to use their skills to adapt techniques for individual patients. In addition, in those countries with physician-based anaesthesia services, it increases the pressure to delegate the administration of anaesthesia to nurses.

There are some areas in which standards are clearly appropriate, and obviously reduce the risk of accidents. Medical equipment design is regulated by a set of standards [1]. In addition, standards can be described for the administrative and educational activities of departments of Anaesthesia, which are designed to ensure that adequate provision of anaesthetic services, training requirements, continuing medical education and audit processes exists [2, 3].

How do doctors set standards?

Ideally, individual anaesthetists set personal standards, and assess their performance relative to these standards. These standards may include clinical standards as well as standards of education and professional development. However, individuals may not set appropriate standards, may not set standards at all, and may use inappropriate methods of assessing performance. While this system works well for the caring and conscientious anaesthetist, it leaves much scope for failure on the part of the poorly performing or lazy doctor.

Clinical teams may set local collective standards. These teams may be based on an anaesthetic department or subspecialty within a department, or may comprise anaesthetists, surgeons and other members of the operating team. Standards are set as a group, and local audit is conducted to establish outcome. This system has the advantages that the standards can take account of local factors and that poor performance by an individual or group of individuals should be detected, the cause identified, and appropriate strategies put in place to improve performance. However, it has the disadvantage that a poorly performing department may set inappropriate standards, may use ineffective methods of audit, and may fail to take remedial steps when inadequate performance is detected.

Consequently, the task of setting standards has, for the most part, been adopted by national and international bodies. National professional standards are set by committees of "experts". In theory, this should ensure that the highest standard is achieved. However, there is a risk that the national committee may comprise a significant proportion of individuals who are out of touch with current practice (because of age or because political activities have removed them from the operating room), or that it may set standards which are so rigorous that they are not achievable. In addition, it is extremely difficult for a national or international body to audit compliance with, or outcome associated with, a set of standards.

Examples of standards applicable to anaesthesia

Management, organisation and planning

These are essential components in the attempt to minimise risk. There are four recognised stages of risk management:

– Identification
– Analysis
– Control
– Funding

Risk can be divided into non-clinical risks, which are those arising from the environment, and clinical risks, which are linked directly to patient care. The head of an anaesthetic department needs to formulate specific advice on anaesthetic risk, and may wish to identify individual anaesthetists to take responsibility for various aspects, e.g. staffing, equipment, training, etc. Risk identification and analysis lead logically to policies for risk reduction. Risk control involves the investigation of accidents and incidents, the formulation of plans to minimise the financial consequences of these events, and the development of plans to prevent recurrence.

Every department should be aware of the numbers and grades of staff required to meet its clinical, professional and contractual obligations. These include service provision, training, continuing medical education, research, audit and management. Allowance must be made for vacations and for absences related to educational and external professional activities. Clearly defined arrangements must be in place to provide continuous on-call cover.

An area of risk which is often ignored relates to familiarisation of new staff with the geography of the hospital, the procedures of the department, and the use of the anaesthetic equipment which is provided. There is often an assumption that new staff will be able to adapt to the local working environment on the basis of their previous experience, but such an assumption is inherently flawed. All new members of staff should undergo an induction procedure, such as that shown in Table 1.

Table 1. An example of information which is required by new members of staff

The clinical director is responsible for ensuring that all new members of the department (including locum appointments) are:

1. familiarised with the general layout of the hospital and specifically the operating theatres, Accident and Emergency Department, wards, on-call rooms and catering facilities;
2. shown how to gain access to the hospital at night, and to pertinent areas of the hospital protected by security locks;
3. instructed in the use of the telephone and paging systems;
4. familiarised with the checking and operation of anaesthetic and monitoring equipment provided for use in all locations in which the new member of staff may be expected to work;
5. familiarised with the procedures and protocols for recovery from anaesthesia and for discharge to surgical wards;
6. shown the locations of emergency equipment (e.g. defibrillator, difficult intubation kit) and drugs (e.g. dantrolene);
7. told about the expectations of the department with regard to preoperative assessment, postoperative follow-up and reporting and recording of complications;
8. shown the anaesthetic record, and told the expectations of the department regarding its completion;
9. told about the procedures for ordering urgent investigations and for obtaining blood or blood products in an emergency;
10. informed about local protocols for clinical management, e.g. protocols used in the obstetric and intensive care units, criteria for notifying a more senior anesthetist including the on-call consultant;
11. informed about local protocols for specific emergency situations, e.g. malignant hyperthermia, difficult intubation, or anaphylaxis;
12. told about the role of the department of anaesthesia in the hospital's Major Incident Plan;
13. informed about local educational and audit activities, including critical incident reporting.

It may be appropriate for items 7-13 to be presented in written form as an "Information Pack" together with a list of useful paging system and telephone numbers.

(Modified from [2])

New trainees should also take part in an induction procedure, which should include clear instructions on the following matters:
- trainees should know the identity and location of the responsible consultant;
- trainees should communicate any problems to a consultant;
- trainees must be discouraged from undertaking any activity which is not comfortably within their competence and experience in the absence of senior assistance (other than in life-threatening situations);
- trainees should notify the responsible consultant of any clinical incident which either resulted in, or which might have resulted in, material sequelae.

Standards for training are usually set by national bodies, and assessed by examinations or by local arrangements prescribed by the national body.

The employment of locums should be kept to a minimum. Locums must be appropriately qualified and experienced for the work expected of them. References from previous employers must be taken up, candidates must undergo formal interview, and successful candidates must be supervised on arrival and undergo an induction procedure.

Staff should be registered with the Occupational Health Department and immunised against hepatitis B as necessary. Needle-stick injuries are common, and local procedures for dealing with them should be in place. Staff should adhere to the regulations for the Control of Substances Hazardous to Health, to the lifting and handling procedures, and to the waste disposal procedures. Staff should be aware of the risks associated with the use of electrical equipment during anaesthesia and surgery. Protective clothing must be available for patients and staff when ionising radiation, lasers, ultraviolet light and other non-ionising radiations are to be used.

There must be an agreed system of record-keeping. Comprehensive anaesthetic records not only provide guidance for future anaesthetic management, but are also very powerful in the successful defence of a claim for negligence. The ideal anaesthetic record has yet to be devised, but a suggested anaesthesia record data set is shown in Table 2. Automated printouts from anaesthetic machines may form part of the record, and provide an objective summary of intraoperative events.

It is widely accepted that the practice of individual anaesthetists may vary where evidence supports a range of different techniques. However, there are circumstances in which standards of care are more likely to be maintained if there are agreed guidelines within a department or within the hospital. Guidelines for clinical practice are particularly appropriate if:
- *a problem is life-threatening*

   for example: management of the difficult airway
                  cardiopulmonary resuscitation
                  anaphylaxis
                  management of massive haemorrhage

Table 2. Sample anaesthetic data set for anaesthesia record

Preoperative information

Patient identity
    Name/ID no./gender
    Date of birth

Assessment & risk factors
    Date of assessment
    Assessor, where assessed
    Weight (kg), [height (m) optional]
    Basic vital signs (BP, HR)
    Medication, incl. contraceptive drugs
    Allergies
    Addiction (alcohol, tobacco, drugs)
    Previous GAs, family history
    Potential airway problems
    Prostheses, teeth, crowns
    Investigations
    Cardiorespiratory fitness
    Other problems
    ASA grade ± comment

Urgency
    Scheduled – listed on a routine list
    Urgent – resuscitated, not on a routine list
    Emergency – not fully resuscitated

Peroperative information

Checks
    Nil by mouth
    Consent
    Premedication, type and effect

Place & time
    Place
    Date, start and end times

Personnel
    All anaesthetists involved
    Operating surgeon
    Qualified assistant present
    Duty consultant informed

Operation planned/performed

Apparatus
    Check performed, anaesthetic room, theatre

Vital signs recording/charting
    Monitors used and vital signs (specify)

Drugs & fluids
    Dose, concentration, volume
    Cannulation
    Injection site(s), time & route
    Warmer used
    Blood loss, urine output

(Modified from [2])

    – a problem is unusual

       for example: abnormal haemoglobins
                        malignant hyperthermia

    – a problem is routine but is managed by different people in various wards and departments

       for example: blood ordering schedule
                        postoperative pain relief
                        day case anaesthesia
                        perioperative management of diabetes
                        endocarditis prophylaxis
                        preoperative investigation
                        preoperative fasting

Clinical management

Preoperative assessment

Unless there are overriding circumstances, every patient should be assessed by their anaesthetist before transfer to the operating theatre suite. Departments of anaesthesia should design protocols for pre-operative investigations; this minimises the risk of operations being postponed, and avoids unnecessary investigations being ordered. The anaesthetist should ensure that an adequate volume of blood has been cross-matched and is available.

Patients should receive appropriate information regarding anaesthesia. They should be warned of material risks, and consent should be obtained for the proposed anaesthetic technique before premedication is administered. If special risk factors exist for an individual patient, then these should be explained, and a summary of the explanation should be recorded.

Perioperative management

Appropriate procedures must be in place to ensure the correct identification of the patient and the proposed surgical procedure. The operating theatre list should be published in good time, and should not be altered. If alterations are necessary, it is the responsibility of the person making the changes to ensure that all appropriate members of staff are notified of the changes.

It is the duty of the surgeon and the anaesthetist to confirm that the correct patient has been brought to the anaesthetic room, together with the correct records.

The anaesthetist should have the appropriate experience and grade for the intended procedure and the condition of the patient. The anaesthetist should have skilled, dedicated assistance throughout the procedure.

It is the joint responsibility of the surgeon and the anaesthetist to ensure that the patient is positioned appropriately and safely to minimise the risk of physical damage.

Monitoring equipment which conforms to national and international recommendations must be available in every anaesthetising location. Individual anaesthetists should be made aware of the consequences of failing to use appropriate monitoring throughout anaesthesia.

An equipment standard should be agreed by the Department of Anaesthesia. This should be able to cope safely with the diversity of the workload. It is the duty of the head of department to ensure that staff are trained in the use of the equipment available. This includes not only the equipment in the operating theatre, but also equipment which may be employed in the postoperative period on instructions from the anaesthetist (e.g. patient-controlled analgesia systems).

Before every operating theatre list starts, the anaesthetic and monitoring equipment must be checked by the anaesthetist. Recommended methods of checking anaesthetic equipment have been published [4]. Further checks should be undertaken if equipment is changed during an operating list.

All equipment associated with anaesthesia and patient monitoring should be subject to regular maintenance and servicing. Instruction manuals for equipment should be readily available to users. Alarms should be set appropriately, and should not be disabled. It is the responsibility of the head of department to ensure that hazard warning and safety action bulletins issued by central sources should be scrutinised, and appropriate action taken.

The anaesthetist is responsible for the drugs given during anaesthesia, even when other members of staff draw the drugs up into syringes or administer them. Syringes and drug infusions should be clearly labelled.

The recovery area (post-anaesthesia care unit [PACU])

The PACU should be appropriately staffed and equipped. Patients should be transferred to the PACU from the operating theatre by, or under the direct supervision of, the anaesthetist. A full and formal hand-over should take place on arrival. The completed anaesthetic record must be made available to the PACU staff, and specific verbal and written instructions should be given for postoperative care. The anaesthetist should ensure that the patient's condition is stable, and that the PACU staff are happy to take over responsibility, before leaving the patient.

One-to-one staffing is required at least until the patient is conscious and able to maintain a clear airway. Each patient must be kept under continuous clinical observation. Physiological variables should be measured and recorded at regular intervals. Administration of opioid analgesics by PACU staff should be subject to local protocols. A formal checklist or scoring system should be established for staff to satisfy themselves that a patient is fit to be discharged.

Patients to be discharged home directly from a PACU require special arrangements to ensure an adequate level of after-care.

The department of anaesthesia should be aware of its responsibilities for acute pain management in the postoperative period. Protocols and policies should be disseminated widely and ward staff provided with appropriate training.

Professional competence and ethical framework

A doctor's principal duty is to benefit patients. This requires detailed, up-to-date knowledge together with proficiency in practical skills. Every anaesthetist needs to be involved in a programme of continuing education and training at a local and national level.

The degree of trust and confidence which patients have in their anaesthetist is crucially dependent on the relationship which the anaesthetist establishes. A clear explanation should be provided in language which the patient can understand. The patient's anxieties and concerns should be listened to, and questions should be answered fully and honestly. Written information about anaesthesia may be helpful, particularly for day-stay patients, but should not be used as a substitute for personal explanation.

Anaesthetists work as part of a team with other doctors and health professionals. Anaesthetists will often take the lead in decision-making. However, there is no place for individuals who pursue a predetermined course of action irrespective of the views and wishes of their colleagues. Professional independence is important, but the limits of acceptable behaviour must be recognised.

How do doctors maintain standards?

Audit which is properly conducted plays an important part in improving patient care, in improving the provision of anaesthetic services, and in providing continuing medical education. Audit may include individual case reports of mortality and morbidity, reviews of critical incidents, perceptions of patients and other healthcare workers about the anaesthetic service, complaints about the anaesthetic service, and formal reviews of areas of clinical practice and service provision. Audit may extend to investigation of cost:benefit ratios of new drugs. The audit cycle (collect data; analyse and review; agree change and set standards; implement change; collect data, etc.) is well known, but departments must ensure that the cycle is repeated.

A recommended pattern for audit programmes is shown in Table 3.

National reporting systems also exist (e.g. National Confidential Enquiry into Perioperative Deaths; Australian Incident Monitoring Study). These schemes have the advantages that they collect much larger quantities of information than local schemes, and that they usually have the resources to ensure objective

Table 3. A recommended pattern of local audit activities for an anaesthetic department

Monthly	Review of deaths, complications, unexpected outcomes, critical incidents
2-3 times per year	Joint audits with other departments, e.g. surgery, obstetrics, paediatrics, orthopaedics
Annually	Review of anaesthetic record-keeping
Every 2-3 years	Review of local guidelines

(Modified from [3])

scrutiny and analysis of the data. However, it is more difficult to complete the audit "cycle" when data have been gathered from large numbers of institutions.

In many countries, standards of training are assessed regularly either by national bodies, or by international bodies such as the European Academy of Anaesthesiology. By encouraging scrutiny of individual training schemes by those with wide experience of training schemes in other centres, recommendations can be made regarding improvements in training, or in respect of provision of resources to facilitate improvements in training.

Reference has already been made to national recommendations for continuing medical education. Continuing professional development includes the facility to acquire and practise new skills, to change patterns of clinical work cyclically, and to undergo regular appraisal to identify objectives and aims as well as to judge the degree to which previous objectives have been achieved successfully.

How are these standards revised when necessary?

The medical profession has a poor track record in terms of implementation and revision of standards. "Good" departments of anaesthesia revise their guidelines at regular intervals; however, not all departments are "good". Consequently, in a number of countries, systems have been introduced centrally to impose revision.

– National societies of anaesthetists usually review standards on a regular basis, although their efficiency in doing so varies widely. In addition, there is no compulsion on individual anaesthetists to heed the revised standards.

– Insurers are increasingly encouraging the setting and regular revision of standards in order to reduce their liability. Although their primary motive is financial, it is generally true that safety and financial liability for injury are linked. Thus, factors which reduce financial liability for insurers also increase safety for patients.

– Government bodies, keen to avoid adverse publicity associated with criticisms of the healthcare system, are beginning to impose concepts such as "clinical governance", which places a requirement on the managers of a hospital to ensure quality of care. Hospital managers, in attempting to fulfil their statutory duty, will increasingly require departments of anaesthesia to put in place, and to review regularly, standards covering managerial, educational and clinical activities, and to present evidence that the standards are effective.

How does the profession ensure compliance with these standards?

The risks of failing to ensure compliance with standards vary among countries, but are becoming increasingly more serious.

– Failure to comply with standards increases the risk of successful litigation. The possibility of defending local failure to comply with nationally agreed "standards" is becoming progressively more difficult, even when these standards are not evidence-based.

– Failure of a department of anaesthesia, or the head of department, to comply with agreed standards may result in sanctions imposed by the hospital administration.

– Failure to comply with nationally agreed standards results, in some countries, in the possibility that training recognition will be withdrawn. This has many adverse implications both for the department and the hospital.

– Failure of an individual to perform his clinical duties satisfactorily is associated increasingly with the likelihood that the individual will be subjected to local disciplinary action, or referred to a national body for assessment; that assessment may result in the conclusion that the doctor requires retraining, or, in extreme circumstances, that the individual is incapable of continuing clinical practice safely. Poor performance may be related to personal misconduct, professional misconduct or impaired health.

– Serious failure to perform satisfactorily results in referral to national bodies which assess whether a doctor is guilty of serious professional misconduct. Until recent years, serious professional misconduct was a charge associated either with personal misconduct with a patient, or with evidence of inappropriate clinical management on multiple occasions. More recently, national registration bodies have been considering whether shortcomings in the clinical management of a single patient, and particularly failure to conform to national "standards", represents serious professional misconduct and should result in the withdrawal of the doctor's licence to practice medicine.

– In a number of countries, it has become an obligation on doctors to report under-performance by other doctors: "You must protect patients when you believe that a doctor's or other colleague's health, conduct or performance is a threat to them" [5].

Conclusion

At present, standards in medicine are set primarily by the profession. Changes in recent years have extended beyond scientific and technological developments, and have engulfed the social context in which doctors work. Medical practice takes place within a political and economic framework over which doctors have little control, but both politicians and patients expect them to make the system work. Self-regulation will be tolerated by patients and politicians only if it is seen to be effective, and if the profession deals promptly and effectively with doctors who fall below the accepted standard. Failure of the medical profession to set, maintain and audit adherence to standards is likely to result in the imposition of standards by hospital managers or by government.

References

1. Greenbaum R, Paterson IG (1996) Safety of equipment. Baillière's Clinical Anaesthesiology: International Practice and Research 10:317-331
2. Association of Anaesthetists of Great Britain and Ireland (1998) Risk management. London
3. Royal College of Anaesthetists and Association of Anaesthetists of Great Britain and Ireland (1998) Good practice: a guide for departments of anaesthesia. London
4. Association of Anaesthetists of Great Britain and Ireland (1997) Checklist for anaesthetic apparatus 2. London
5. General Medical Council (1998) Good medical practice; Guidance from the general medical council. London

Hypnotics

P. Mastronardi, T. Cafiero, A.E. Rossi

A hypnotic drug has to be able to achieve and maintain the suppression of consciousness (sleep) as its main activity. The pharmacological induced sleep is defined as hypnosis but it has not to be confused with that particular condition of consciousness susceptible to be influenced (hypnotic suggestion). The modern hypnotics available in the Italian anaesthesiological pharmacopoeia (propofol and midazolam) are able to work, in proportionally reduced doses, as sedative agents too; therefore, they can reduce or abolish the excitatory states or psychomotor agitation making patients calm and quiet. On the basis of a modulated and progressive central nervous system (CNS) depression, propofol and midazolam can produce either sedation or hypnosis. Therefore they can be injected intravenously to induce general anaesthesia and to maintain unconsciousness as the hypnotic component of a balanced anaesthetic technique just founding on the triad: hypnosis, analgesia and muscle relaxation. Without the suppression of consciousness (hypnosis) the last two components could not be able to attenuate the stress response during surgical procedures.

Mechanism of action

Although undoubted concepts do not exist about the mechanism of action of hypnotics, a theory has been widely accepted on the interaction with the principal inhibitory neurotransmitter in the CNS: γ-aminobutyric acid [1]. The γ-aminobutyric acid receptor complex is divided in two subtypes GABAa and GABAb, structurally consisting of up to five glycoprotein subunits. Activation of the GABA increases chloride conductance through the membrane hyperpolarizing and reducing the excitability of the post-synaptic neuron. It has been suggested that propofol has the same mechanism of action on the GABA receptor in comparison with barbiturates: increase the duration of GABA activated chloride ion channel opening. The binding of benzodiazepines to a specific receptor on the GABA-receptor complex enhances the interaction between GABA and chloride channels. The discovery of the specific benzodiazepines binding sites allowed to identify endogenous benzodiazepine-like substances. It also seems that the clinical effect is a function of benzodiazepine receptor occupancy: occupancy below 20 per cent is sufficient to produce the anxiolytic effect, sedation requires 30-50 per cent and unconsciousness requires 60 per cent or higher receptor occupancy. Although increasing the dose of benzodiazepines it is not possible to produce more than certain clinical effects: the so-called "ceiling effect"; for example, midazolam cannot produce "burst suppression". Midazolam given as epidural injection can exert an analgesic effect; it could be explained by enhancing the GABA activity on spinally GABAa receptors [2, 3] for which muscymol and isoguvacine are agonists.

Propofol

It is a derivative of phenol, insoluble in water, available as a 1 or 2 per cent solution in a lipid emulsion widely used for parenteral nutrition and consisting of soybean oil, glycerol and purified egg phosphatide. Pain on propofol injection can be reduced by using a large vein or adding lidocaine 1 per cent or administering a premedication with opiates. Pain on injection could be related to the amount of propofol in aqueous phase; in fact an experimental reformulation with long-chains triglycerides increasing the amount of propofol in lipid phase minimizes pain without influencing the characteristics of the induction [4]. Propofol is rapidly metabolized in the liver by conjugation to glucuronide and sulfate to produce inactive water-soluble metabolites which are excreted by the kidneys. The rapid metabolism of propofol is also evidenced by the blood radioactivity that becomes less than 40 per cent at 10 minutes after radio labelled propofol injection while it passes from 14 per cent after 1 hour to 5 per cent after 6 hours from injection [5]. Extrahepatic metabolism (lungs) has been confirmed because of the high clearance of propofol (1.7-2.2 L/min^{-1}) exceeding hepatic blood flow. Propofol has a protein binding of 98 per cent and a very rapid clearance from the central compartment with a value of $t1/2\alpha$ ranging from 2.5 to 5 minutes. The pharmacokinetics of propofol are not affected by sex and age, in fact in children (age > 4 years) no significant differences were recorded in comparison with adults and only the elderly have decreased clearance rates. In adults the induction dose of propofol is 2-2.5 mg/kg^{-1}, being highest in children (> 30-50%) because of the larger volume of distribution and the more rapid clearance [6]. In the elderly the induction dose of propofol has to be reduced of 1/3 because of the smaller volume of distribution and the slower clearance. After an induction dose of propofol a transitory increase in respiratory frequency and tidal volume reduction occur and then in a similar percentage as compared with thiopental apnea occurs. The duration of apnea is greater with propofol than with other intravenous hypnotics. Propofol induces bronchodilation in patients with chronic obstructive pulmonary disease without affecting the ventilatory response to hypoxaemia. Propofol decreases the cerebral metabolism of oxygen (CMRO$_2$), the intracranial pressure (ICP), the cerebral blood flow (CBF) and the cerebral perfusion pressure (CPP) without affecting autoregulation and cerebral reactivity to carbon dioxide. The neuroprotective effect could be likely due to the antioxidant properties of the structure of propofol with an alkylphenol ring. With high infusion rates propofol produces burst suppression rapidly reversed reducing the speed of injection. Propofol administration is associated sometimes with excitatory side effects also defined as non-epileptogenic myoclonia, being not associated with epileptogenic EEG activity [7]. It has been shown in several reports a direct anticonvulsant activity of propofol [8]. Propofol possesses a direct myocardial depressant effect and produces decreases in systemic vascular resistance. Both myocardial depression and vasodilation appear to be dose dependent and the vasodilatory effect of propofol appears to be due to the intracellular calcium mobilization and to the increased production of nitric oxide. Recently it has been suggested that propofol affects the baroreflex mechanism inducing a de-coupling between systemic arterial hypotension and heart rate thus decreasing the tachycardic response to hypotension. Therefore bradycardia occurring during propofol administration could be detrimental to the patient especially when a concomitant administration of other vagomimetic drugs is necessary; premedication with atropine attenuates bradycardia. Although the mechanism of action is not completely understood, propofol also exerts significant antiemetic effect at low doses (10-20 mg). Propofol has been used to treat nausea and wry-neck and also to relieve pruritus induced by spinal opiates [9]. Finally, propofol is reported to be safe in the anaesthetic management of patients with malignant hyperthermia and porphyria.

Midazolam

The first water-soluble benzodiazepine in aqueous solution in a buffered acidic medium (pH 3.5) which becomes the most lipid-soluble in vivo because of its pH-dependent solubility. The local tolerance to midazolam is higher in comparison with other benzodiazepines given parenterally; as such it causes minimal, if any, local irritation after intravenous or intramuscular injection [10]. Midazolam undergoes oxidation-reduction by the cytochrome P450 in the liver producing water-soluble hydroxylated compounds excreted via the kidney. Among these metabolites only the α-hydroxymidazolams possess little intrinsic CNS depressant activity, nevertheless the clearance of α-hydroxymidazolams is more rapid than that of midazolam thus their activity is clinically insignificant as compared with diazepam which forms two active metabolites. Cytochrome P450 3A4 is involved in the metabolism of other substances given for therapeutic use (erythromycin, cyclosporine) or in anaesthesia (alfentanil) which can interfere with their metabolisms [11]. The volume of distribution of benzodiazepines is relatively similar and ranges for midazolam, lorazepam and diazepam from 0.7 to 1.7 L/kg^{-1}; consequently the elimination half-life differs depending on the clearance which ranges from 6.4 to 11 ml/g^{-1}/min^{-1} for midazolam and from 0.2 to 0.5 for diazepam. Therefore the t1/2β ranges from 1.7 to 2.6 hours for midazolam while it is greater for diazepam ranging from 20 to 50 hours. Midazolam has anxiolytic, sedative, hypnotic, amnestic, anticonvulsant, centrally produced muscle relaxant and analgesic properties in a dose-related manner. Midazolam exerts the same effects as compared with propofol and thiopental regarding $CMRO_2$, CBF and ICP [12]. Owing to the "ceiling effect" midazolam cannot produce burst suppression. The mean time for exerting its maximum effect on CNS is about 3 minutes, thus, ignoring this parameter it could be possible to administer additional amount of drug with a potential risk for the patient. Midazolam produces dose-related central respiratory system depression; this depression is clinically insignificant in healthy patients but becomes significant in patients with chronic obstructive pulmonary disease especially with concomitantly administered opioids [13]. The benzodiazepines receptors are located in several tissues; they can interact with calcium channels producing, together with the sympathetic central activity, the cardiocirculatory effects [14] which are very modest in healthy patients but haemodynamically prominent in hypovolaemic patients. Midazolam as well as other benzodiazepines can produce a paradoxical effect likely due to the lack of inhibitory control revealing with excitement, confusion and disorientation; such a situation can be treated with further doses of midazolam up to induce hypnosis, if necessary; it also can be antagonized by flumazenil administration. Alternatively when particular conditions restrain the previous techniques it is possible to administer boluses of haloperidol, 5 mg, repeated up to abolish symptoms [15]. Midazolam can be administered intravenously, intramuscularly and also via the oral and nasal routes in children for sedation, using the drug without dilution. Transmucosal drug delivery through the nasopharynx in dose of 0.2-0.3 mg/kg^{-1} reaches the maximum effect after 10 minutes. Midazolam acidic solution (pH 3.5) is irritating for the nasal mucosal membranes; conversely midazolam in dose of 0.5-1.0 mg/kg^{-1} mixed with a tasty drink improves patient comfort. It has been suggested that midazolam in association with clonidine could play a positive role in treating chronic not malignant pain [16] and it is a suitable drug in the anaesthetic management of patients with porphyria. Finally midazolam can be antagonized by flumazenil with high affinity to specific receptors in CNS.

Table 1 summarized the prescribed induction doses of midazolam in relation to age, physical status and concomitant administration of other drugs affecting CNS.

Table 1. Prescribed induction doses of midazolam

Age	ASA	Route	Initial dose (ID)	Interval	Further dose
		Not premedicated adult patients			
≤ 60 yrs	I or II	i.v.	0.3-0.35 mg/kg^{-1}	3 min	25% of ID
> 60 yrs	III or IV	i.v.	0.2-0.25 mg/kg^{-1}	4 min	25% of ID
		Premedicated adult patients			
≤ 60 yrs	I or II	i.v.	0.2-0.25 mg/kg^{-1}	3 min	25% of ID
> 60 yrs	III or IV	i.v.	0.1-0.15 mg/kg^{-1}	4 min	25% of ID
		Pediatric patients			
		i.m.	0.15-0.2 mg/kg^{-1}	Ketamine association	

Context-sensitive half-time

The context-sensitive half time is the time it takes for the plasma concentration in the central compartment to decrease by 50 per cent. This parameter is calculated in a three-compartment model. The context-sensitive half-time for propofol increases in a slow and progressive manner for prolonged infusions ranging from a few minutes after 2 hours to 20-30 minutes after 8 hours. The context-sensitive half-time for midazolam is the most favourable as compared with other benzodiazepines; in fact, with diazepam this parameter increases to 150 minutes after 30 minutes of infusion while with midazolam ranges from 20 minutes after 1 hour to about 65 minutes after 8 hours of infusion [17].

Continuous infusion

Now it is widely accepted the concept that the technique of intermittent boluses for drugs administration is inadequate to give stability both to plasma concentrations and to biophase. Continuous infusion technique can provide much more stability to the above mentioned parameters with minor side effects and more predictable recovery times. Nevertheless the infusion dosing scheme could be based on the anaesthetic dose requirements, especially when the plasma concentrations can be easily evaluated (Table 2).

Table 2. Correlation between plasma concentrations and surgical stimulus

	Major surgery	Minor surgery	Sedation
Propofol	4-6 μg/ml^{-1}	2-4 μg/ml^{-1}	1.5-2 μg/ml^{-1}
Midazolam	100-200 ng/ml^{-1}	50-150 ng/ml^{-1}	40-100 ng/ml^{-1}

Fortunately computerized infusion systems are available and by means of software based on pharmacological parameters automatically they regulate the infusion speed to achieve and maintain pre-selected plasma concentrations. These concentrations are the infusion target; the relative technology is just called "Target controlled infusion".

Co-induction

It is the sequential administration of two or more drugs to induce anaesthesia. This anesthetic technique is based on the synergism between hypnotics and opioids. Table 3 shows the advantages related to the dose requirements for co-induction.

Table 3. Dose requirements for co-induction (mg/kg^{-1})

		Midazolam
Thiopental	1.57	0.02
Propofol	0.7	0.02
Fentanyl	0.002	0.02-0.1
Alfentanil	0.027	0.02
Alfentanil	0.003	0.14
Alfentanil	0.018	0.036 + propofol 0.181

Co-induction makes the induction of anaesthesia much more predictable and controlled because it reduces the inter-individual variability; furthermore, it reduces the side effects which each drug could cause when given alone.

References

1. Franks NP, Lieb WR (1994) Molecular and cellular mechanisms of general anaesthesia. Nature 367:607
2. Goodchild CS, Serrao IM (1987) Intrathecal midazolam in the rat: Evidence for spinally mediated analgesia. Br J Anaesth 59:1563
3. Niv D, Whitwam JG, Loh L (1983) Depression of nociceptive sympathetic reflexes by intratechal administration of midazolam. Br J Anaesth 55:541
4. Doenicke A, Roizen MF, Rau J et al (1996) Reducing pain during propofol injection: The role of the solvent. Anesth Analg 82:472
5. Simons PJ, Cockshott ID, Douglas EJ et al (1985) Blood concentrations, metabolism and elimination after a subanaesthetic intravenous dose of C-propofol to male volunteers. Postgrad Med J 61[Suppl 3]:64
6. Saint-Maurice C, Landais A, Cockshott ID et al (1987) Le propofol comme agent d'induction en anesthésie pédiatrique. Etude clinique préliminaire. Ann Fr Anesth Réeanim 6:269
7. Reddy RV, Moorthy SS, Dierdorf SF et al (1993) Excitatory effects and electroencephalographic correlation of etomidate, thiopental, methohexital and propofol. Anest Analg 77:1008
8. Ebrahm ZY, Schubert A, van Ness P et al (1994) The effect of propofol and the electroencephalogram of patient with epilepsy. Anesth Analg 78:275
9. Borgeat A, Wilder-Smith OHG, Suter PM (1994) The non-hypnotic therapeutic application of propofol. Anesthesiology 80:642
10. Reves JG, Fragen RJ, Vinik HR et al (1985) Midazolam - Pharmacology and uses. Anesthesiology 62:310
11. Kronbach T, Mathys D, Umeno M et al (1989) Oxidation of midazolam and triazolam by human liver cytocrome P450 3A4. Mal Pharmacol 36:89
12. Strebel S, Kaufmann M, Guardiola PM et al (1994) Cerebral vasomotor responsiveness to carbon dioxide is preserved during propofol and midazolam anesthesia in humans. Anesth Analg 78:884
13. Bailey PL, Pace NL, Ashburn MA et al (1990) Frequent hypoxemia and apnea after midazolam and fentanyl. Anesthesiology 73:826
14. Laurent J (1989) Mècanismes d'action centraux et péripherique des benzodiasepines. In: Les benzodiazepines en anestésie-réanimation. Arnette, Paris, p 1-12
15. Khan LC, Lustik SJ (1997) Treatment of paradoxical reaction to midazolam with haloperidol. Anesth Analg 85:213
16. Borg PAJ, Krijnen HJ (1996) Long-term intrathecal administration of midazolam and clonidine. Clin J Pain 12:63
17. Hughes MA, Jacobs JR, Glass PSA (1992) Context-sensitive half-time in multicompartment pharmacokinetic models for intravenous anesthesia. Anesthesiology 76:334

Analgesics

C. MELLONI

This review will proceed in a scholarly manner, starting from basic pharmacokinetic-pharmacodynamic principles, partly corrected by the arrival of new concept and new information, and arriving later at the clinical application of the new drugs.

Pharmacokinetic-pharmacodynamic principles governing the fentanyl derivatives

We will assume that for all fentanyl derivatives the most suitable model is represented by the three exponential model; the terminal half life for drugs with three exponential terms is not useful in predicting the decrease in concentration after a bolus or an infusion [1]. As a matter of fact, the terminal half life is always greater than the time it takes for drug concentration to decrease by 50% following administration of a drug, particularly after a prolonged infusion.

In clinical practice, the most interesting moments are two; the speed with which a therapeutic concentration is reached and the rate at which the plasma concentration decreases, this latter being particularly important because it determines the recovery time; its kinetics will be described in a greater detail introducing the concept of context sensitive plasma half time, defined as the length of time required for the central compartment concentration to fall by 50% following cessation of an infusion designed to maintain a constant C_p for a specific period of time (the context). Determining the half time with respect to a specific context is important because for most drugs the half time increases markedly as the infusion duration varies from few minutes to many hours; also in clinical practice rate of infusion and therefore dosage might vary. It is to underline that this context sensitive plasma half time is not related with distribution or elimination halflives, which are virtually useless in the clinical context, since they derive from simple 1 compartment model, the hybrid rate constant β used to compute $t \frac{1}{2} \beta$ is a consequence of both distribution and elimination processes, as are α and γ; moreover, the relative roles of distribution and elimination at any time is a function of the degree at which the drug concentrations in the central and peripheral compartments are equilibrated, which is a function of the nature and duration of the dosing regimen. The context sensitive half time indicates only the time to 50% decrease of the plasma concentration at the end of the infusion; other half times could be described, as 80%, 25%, 10%, but 50% was chosen because the half time context sensitive establishes a superior limit for the time necessary for a drug concentration to fall below the threshold levels needed for recovery, always assuming that the patients did not require a plasma concentration 2 fold greater of the concentration needed for recovery. From the conceptual point of view, continuous vigilance paid by the anaesthesiologist on infusion rate should indicate that at the end of the operation (or even before) there should be no need to wait for the 50% fall in plasma concentration in order to obtain the functional recovery of the patient.

The importance of context sensitive half times resides in the fact that it provides a quantitative description of the distribution and elimination phenomena much more practical than other descriptors, since, for instance, drugs classified as having long elimination half lives can present short context sensitive plasma half times; moreover, even drugs with clearances (Cl) and volumes of distribution (V_d) values very different can exhibit very similar context sensitive plasma half times (CSHT).

In a specific model, a small V_1/Cl_1 or small Cl leads to short CSHTs even following long infusions, since $V_1/Cl_1 = V_1/V_1 k_{10}$, $V_1/Cl_1 = 1/k_{10}$, indicating that small V_1/Cl_1 possess a large k_{10}, indicating that drug is removed rapidly from the central compartment; therefore a model with a small V_1/Cl_1 ratio can have relatively short half times; this is true for alfentanil and remifentanil.

Context sensitive half times could be short even in cases where clearances ratios are small; this happens because small Cl_i/Cl_1 ratios suggest sluggish peripheral compartments. The explanation is as follows: when infusion ends and unless it has been running long enough to reach equilibrium between central and peripheral compartments, concentrations in the peripheral compartments will be lower than that in the central one, so that peripheral compartments will continue to take up drug until each peripheral compartment will reach equilibrium with that of central compartment, when net transfer of drug between the two compartments will cease, but elimination processes will continue removing drug from the body and the central compartment drug concentration will drop below that in the peripheral compartment. At this point the peripheral compartment will begin returning drug in the plasma, but this transfer is limited by the slugginess of the peripheral compartment, i.e. the return of drug from the peripheral compartment will be slow relative to the ability of central clearance processes to remove drug from the body, the end result being that plasma drug concentration will not be elevated by a rapid influx of drug from the peripheral compartment.

Designing the dosages upon pharmacokinetic-pharmacodynamic principles

For a 1 compartment model, the desired plasma concentration could be simply achieved by a bolus loading dose of V_1C_{pd}, C_{pd} being the desired plasma concentration; and maintenance of a desired concentration is attained by the immediate initiation, following the loading, of an infusion characterized by $V_1k_{10}C_{pd}$, called maintenance infusion. If at any time during a continuous infusion one desires to increase plasma concentrations by 50%, it would be required to administer another loading dose of $V_1C_{pd}/2$ and to increase immediately thereafter the maintenance infusion rate by 50%. After the drug administration has ceased, plasma drug concentration in the 1 compartment model will decrease 50% every t½ β minutes, being the only half life in the 1 compartment model, defined as t½ β = ln2/β or 0.693/β.

Because distribution infusion schemes for drugs exhibiting multicompartment kinetics are more complex than those for a 1 compartment model, administering a loading dose of V_1C_{pd} + immediate start of a continuous infusion $V_1k_{10}C_{pd}$ will achieve C_{pd} initially and later at steady state, but there will be a subtherapeutic period due to the transfer of drug into the peripheral compartments, during which the plasma drug concentration will fall below C_{pd}. Therefore the loading dose should be modified as V_TC_{pd}, in order to obtain initially a substantially higher concentration than C_{pd}, that will fall later below C_{pd} because an appreciable amount of the loading dose will be cleared from the central compartment.

The most satisfying way to achieve and maintain C_{pd} consist in the administration of a loading dose of V_1C_{pd}, + a constant rate infusion of $V_1k_{10}C_{pd}$ plus an exponentially declining infusion of $k_{13}e^{-k_{31}}$ consisting in the 3 compartment variant of the BET infusion scheme [2], whereby the loading bolus dose (B) brings the plasma drug concentration up to C_{pd} immediately, the constant infusion replaces drug lost through elimination (E) processes and the exponentially declining infusion accounts for drug distribution or transfer (T) into the peripheral compartments. In order to follow this scheme a computer controlled infusion pump is required; however, therapeutic plasma drug concentrations do not need to be maintained with rigid precision, so that many algorithms have been devised to assist in the development of dosing schemes and some examples will be later offered. However, we should recognize that it is not plasma the predominant site of action of drugs, as has been demonstrated with some of the measures of drug effects mentioned before; using EEG for instance, a delay has been noted between changes in plasma drug concentration and effect on the EEG and this phenomenon of kinetic-dynamic dissociation is characterized by hysteresis in a graph of effect versus plasma drug concentration. This apparent discrepancy has been solved with the addition of an effect compartment to the classic pharmacokinetic modeling. It has been assumed that this effect compartment is so small as to not contribute anything in terms of volumes, but having its own rate constant k_{eo}, drug considered irreversibly cleared from the plasma. A numerical value for k_{eo} is determined according to nonlinear regression modeling of simultaneous measurements of plasma drug concentration and the specified drug effect. Given a value for k_{eo}, its half life, according to 1 compartment kinetics, is $t_{1/2}k_{eo}$ and can be computed as $0.693/k_{eo}$; from the practical point of view large k_{eo} predict relatively large equilibration between plasma and effect compartment drug concentration and thus between plasma drug concentration and effect. Following a bolus dose, the time to achieve a peak site effect concentration is a function of both pharmacokinetics and k_{eo}; if a drug has an extremely rapid decline in plasma concentration following a bolus, the effect site concentration peaks in several seconds regardless of the k_{eo}; but for drugs with a rapid keo and a slow decrease in concentration after a bolus, the time of peak effect site concentration is determined more by k_{eo} than by plasma pharmacokinetics; remifentanil and alfentanil will be more dependent on k_{eo}, while sufentanil and fentanyl less. Time to peak effect for the various opioid is (min) in decreasing order sufentanil (5,6) > fentanyl (3,6) > remifentanil (1.4) = alfentanil (1.4).

Again, in order to control the effect compartment drug concentration, many algorithms have been implemented and the basic controversy resides in the proponents of adhering to effect compartment modeling or not, since following a BET scheme a specified plasma concentration can be reached and maintained very quickly, but the effect compartment drug concentration approaches equilibrium with the plasma drug concentration at an exponential rate, determined by k_{eo}, while instead using the effect compartment dosing computation, the desired effect compartment drug concentration is obtained much more quickly, but at the cost of transiently high plasma concentration. The controversy between different dosing schemes has clinical importance, since high plasma concentrations could result in adverse effects, while concentrations below C_{pd} are subtherapeutic and may be ineffective. Moreover, if we assume that effect compartment concentrations are clinically more relevant than plasma drug concentrations, because they reflect concentrations at the site of effect, computation of context sensitive effect compartment half times would be more useful than context sensitive plasma half times as means of indicating anticipated duration of action. Effect context sensitive effect compartment half times is defined as the number in minutes that elapse from the time an infusion targeting the effect is terminated until the effect drug concentration decreases to half the maximum effect compartment drug concentration achieved with an infusion of a a given duration. The clinical implications of this novel approach indicate that a drug with effect compartment half time significantly longer than the plasma half time for a given infusion duration should be discontinued a little bit earlier than on pharmacokinetic grounds alone if a rapid recovery is desired: moreover k_{eo} could be used as a measure of onset of effect; as a matter of fact, alfentanil and remifentanil possess short k_{eo}, of the order of 1.2-1.3 min and this knowledge has even pushed further, suggesting that, in the case of remifentanil at least, being his k_{eo} short and its potency high, linked to the potential for severe respiratory depression and rigidity, a bolus dose should be avoided, provided that at least some minutes are available for its onset of action. A simple method for calculating the bolus dose to achieve a desired peak concentration at the effect site is as follows: $V_{peak\ effect} = V_1 * C_{plasma,\ initial}/C_{plasma\ at\ peak\ effect}$, where $C_{plasma,\ initial}$ is the initial concentration following a bolus and $C_{plasma\ at\ peak\ effect}$ is the concentration at time of peak effect. Since V peak effects are as follows (lt): for fentanyl 75, alfentanil 6, sufentanil 89, dose can be calculated as $= Ct*V_{peak\ effect}$: Ct is the target effect site concentration; for instance, in order to achieve 100 µg/ml with alfentanil, 600 µg will suffice and this effect will be reached within 1.4 min. The knowledge of k_{eo}, times to peak effect, V peak effect is important for the clinician; for rapid sequence induction, drugs like thiopental, remifentanil or alfentanil peak at the same time and therefore ablate the response during laryngoscopy and intubation, 80-90 sec. following their bolus injection; while using fentanyl, with a 216 sec time to peak effect, it is obvious that its administration should precede thiopental and succinylcholine of at least 2 minutes, otherwise its effect will not be maximal at the time of the greatest stimulation and this would likely result in hypertension and tachycardia during and following laryngoscopy, followed a few seconds later by hypotension as soon as fentanyl reaches its peak effect during a phase of minimal stimulation.

Dose-response relationships

Following the quantitative approach initiated, most drug effects could be described with the so called Emax model: $E = E_{max}C/EC_{50} + C$, where E is effect, C drug concentration, E_{max} the maximun effect and EC_{50} the concentration producing 50% of the maximum effect. This results in a sigmoidal curve, where it could be noted that above a certain concentration there is no further increase in effect; similarly, below a certain concentration there is no effect and when the concentration is $= EC_{50}$ the effect is half that of E_{max}. EC_{50} is equivalent to C_{p50} or IC_{50} and is a measure of efficacy, i.e. the relationship between concentration and effect: it is not a sinonym of potency, since drugs with lower potency but equal efficacy need only a higher concentration to achieve a given effect.

This sigmoidal curve has been used to characterize the probability of reaching a quantal effect, i.e. response-no response, in a population of patients: for example Ausems et al. [3] studied the relationship between the opioid alfentanil effect and its concentration in patients undergoing general anaesthesia; using logistic regression they were able to define the probability of no response to three usual surgical stimuli, namely skin incision or closure and intubation, at a given concentration, where patients could be categorized as responders or non responders. The steepness of the sigmoidal curve is related to the amount of variability in the study group; drugs with little variability between concentration and effect have steep curves and drugs with more variability have gently sloping curves. These graphs could be used to define the concept of therapeutic window; relating concentrations to desired effect and toxic or excessive effect, so that knowing the relationship between concentration and theraputic effect the therapeutic window could be identified at which most subjects will present the desired effect and while few will exhibit the toxic effect. The therapeutic windows for alfentanil, fentanyl and sufentanil are presented in Table 1.

Table 1. Therapeutic windows for opioids

Clinical anaesthesia	Fentanyl (µg/ml)	Alfentanil (µg/ml)	Sufentanil (µg/ml)
Induction and intubation:			
with pentothal	3-5	250-400	0,4-0,6
with N_2O	8-10	400-750	0,8-1,2
maintenance:			
with N_2O/volatile agent	1,5-3	100-300	0,25-0,5
with N_2O only	1,5-10	100-750	0,25-1
with O_2 only	15-60	1000-4000	2-8
ventilation adequate at emergence:	1.5	125	0,25

Applying some of the described concepts into clinical practice the terminal half lives of alfentanil and sufentanil are 2 and 9 hours respectively and it could therefore be deducted that sufentanil is not amenable to continuous infusion; but for infusion duration < 10 hours, sufentanil concentrations fall much faster than those of alfentanil, so that the drug is not only useful, but even better suited than alfentanil, which is however more handly for infusion lasting < 2 hours.

From the pharmacokinetic parameters and the CSHT fentanyl is the less useful drug for continuous infusion, while remifentanil is by far the more useful.

Clinical implications of physico-chemical parameters and pharmacokinetics-pharmacodynamics

A closer look at Table 2 will reveal other interesting insights into the more useful opioids.

Table 2. Chemical-physical parameters of important drugs

Drug	Pka	% nonionized	Part. coefficient.	Penetration half time	Onset time
Thiopentone	7.6	0,61	3	3.3	1.4
Morphine	7.9	0.24	1.4	0.336	15-30
Meperidine	8.5	0.05	39	1.95	10-15
Fentanyl	8.4	0.09	860	4-6	4.5
Alfentanil	.6.5	0.89	130	0,9	1.2
Sufentanil	8.0	0.20	1778	4-6	5
Remifentanil	7.1	0,68	18	1.6	1.4

We have already quoted the pharmacokinetic-pharmacodynamic paradox, where the clinical emergence following sufentanil infusion is more rapid than fentanyl: but sufentanil accumulates more than fentanyl; moreover, remifentanil is the less lypophilic of the group, but its onset is very fast, almos equal to alfentanil... These data associated with the fact that half lives do not correlate with emergence times induced the editorial "(Almost) everything you learned about pks was (somewhat) wrong!" [4].

However, large Vd_{ss} (fentanyl: 358; sufentanil: 541) indicate the potential for a great reservoir, while Vd_{ss} small indicate a lesser propensity for the drugs (alfentanil: 24; remifentanil: 20,5) to move elsewhere. This could be significant in clinical practice; having to reanaesthetize a patient briefly following the emergence from a previous anaesthesia, if the patient was maintained under a continuous infusion of sufentanil, you may assume that a large quantity of the drug is still in the body and therefore a very small quantity of the same drug will most probably suffice for analgesia, while in the case of a previous alfentanil infusion, this will be of lesser concern.

Speed of onset of the central nervous system effect of an opioid can be approximated or ranked in relation to other opioids calculating its "effective partition coefficient", determined by multiplying the fraction of the drug that is nonionized at the pH value of interest (7.4 in terms of the plasma-csf interphase) by the partition coefficient of the drug in some suitable system (n octanol/water). This approach proved reliable in predicting the rank of order of penetration of barbiturates and other agents into the csf and could be important, perhaps, even in the termination of effects, corrected by the effect of the CSHT. Where speed of recovery from the sedative and respiratory depressant effects of opioids are priorities, remifentanil may represent the optimal agent, as it is also ideal from the CSHT point of view, since it is practically devoid of a CSHT, being so rapidly hydrolized that even following very prolonged infusion, its CSHT is of the order of a few minutes.

Since analgesics are titrated during surgery in response to evidence of inadequate analgesia, speed of onset would be an area open for future drug development, alfentanil and remifentanil approaching the ideal, while the others, with effect site equilibration times of several minutes, are less than optimal in terms of patient comfort and protection.

Since the introduction of the concept of MAC for the inhalation anaesthetics, the use of drugs became less qualitative and a new series of studies appeared, relating concentration to effects, in order to maximize efficacy and minimize toxicity. Anaesthesia is a threshold event; there cannot be degrees or depths of anaesthesia and the most obvious and reliably measured effect of an anaesthetic is lack of movement in a group of animal or patients exposed to a standardized noxious stimulus. Other responses produced by anaesthetic drugs have been measured in the attempt to relate drug concentration and effect, but there is no other accepted definition of anaesthesia. The motor response to a noxious stimulus consists normally in the withdrawal of the stimulated part or simply in a movement of the body; suppression of this involuntary movement by a certain dose of a drug is used as one of the main indicators of anaesthetic potency for inhaled drugs [5]. The concept of MAC is the minimum alveolar concentration of an inhaled anaesthetic at one athmosphere which results in immobility in 50% of patients exposed to a noxious stimulus. It is assumed that alveolar partial pressure is transmitted without change to the arterial blood and that, given time for equilibration, the partial pressure of gas at the site of drug action equals that of arterial blood. Under normal circumstances, these are reasonable assumptions, but neither the inspired gas concentration nor the drug concentration in blood bears such a constant relationship to the concentration or partial pressure at the anaesthetic site of action.

One of the most surprising properties of MAC is its constancy within and between different species. Also, its value is not dependent on the intensity of stimulus, duration of drug administration, sex, acid-base status, carbon dioxide or oxygen tensions in arterial blood (within certain limitations). Values are altered by circadian rhythms, body temperature, diseases such as thyrotoxicosis and other drugs, like benzodiazepines. Age has a marked effect, since it has been shown that the MAC for halothane falls from 1 per cent in the neonate to 0.63 per cent in the 70-year-old patient.

For intravenous anaesthetic drugs the concept of minimum infusion rate (MIR) was proposed as an attempt to compare potencies; this was defined as the infusion rate of an intravenous anaesthetic drug necessary to prevent movement in response to surgical incision in 50 per cent of patients; however, the relationship between infusion rate and plasma concentrations is governed by many factors, even after the 25-minute period allowed in the calculation of MIR. There is not always a linear relationship between infusion rate and blood concentrations using this method. Ausems [6] analysed alfentanil plasma concentration data from patients in the presence of 66 per cent nitrous oxide and calculated dose-response curves for different surgical stimuli; response was defined as any movement or arterial pressure or pulse rate variation or an increase in sweating. Plasma concentrations associated with a 50% probability of no response (IC_{50}) are shown in Table 3.

Table 3. IC_{50} for alfentanil

Event	Mean conc	(95% confidence limits) (ng/ml)
Intubation	475	418-532
Skin incision	279	238-320
Skin closure	150	103-196
Ventilation	223	197-249

From the aforementioned numbers it can clearly be seen that the concentration required for skin closure is less than skin incision: therefore, the opioid could be slowly titrated downward towards the end of the procedure, allowing an even faster recovery.

In studies on MAC and MIR patients moving in response to surgical stimulation did not recall surgery or anaesthesia; thus it appears that plasma concentrations of drugs necessary to suppress somatic motor response is higher than that required for amnesia and unconsciousness.

In paralyzed patients lack of response to a stimulus is not a good indicator of anaesthesia depth; Tunstall used a sphygmomanometer cuff to isolate one forearm from the effects of neuromuscular blocking agents administered to the other arm; he showed that all patients moved the arm at the time of skin incision, patients breathing only low concentrations of nitrous oxide responding to command but no patient had postoperative recall. It is clear that, in paralyzed patients, other indicators than movement must be used as indicator of response to anaesthetic drugs.

Noxious stimuli may result in involuntary responses of the autonomic nervous system; observations of pulse rate, arterial pressure, sweating or tears have been the mainstay of the clinical assessment of adequacy for years since neuromuscular blocking agents were used commonly.

In 1981, the concept or MAC-BAR was added; it is the alveolar concentration of an inhaled agent which suppresses haemodynamic and adrenergic responses to a noxious stimulus in 50 per cent of patients; the ratio of MAC-BAR to MAC is 1.45 for halothane, 1.6 for enflurane: in general, autonomic signs bear no relationship to conscious awareness or semi-purposeful movements seen with the isolated arm technique; no constant or close relationship has been demonstrated between autonomic signs and cortical activity and autonomic signs may be modified by drugs independently of their anaesthetic effects.

The electroencephalogram and in particular the processed EEG (pEEG) has been increasingly used as a measure of anaesthetic depth of anaesthesia; the particular type of EEG processing applied has been decided empirically and pharmacodynamic modeling has been applied to remove the lag between change in plasma concentration and change in EEG. Spectral Edge Frequency (SEF) is an attempt to circumvent the problems of different EEG frequencies at similar anaesthetic concentrations; the SEF is the frequency below which 95 per cent of the EEG power is present; in the awake man it is 25-30 Hz and it falls rapidly in response to increases in concentration of enflurane, halothane or thiopental. Enflurane anaesthesia reduces the SEF by 20 Hz/MAC, while halothane decreases by 8 Hz/MAC. Thiopental administration shifts the SEF down to 4 to 8 Hz. There is a classic sigmoid relationship between the venous serum concentrations and the SEF; a value for IC_{50} (the serum concentration needed to cause one half of the maximal slowing) can be calculated. From these data it is possible to determine brain responsiveness to thiopentone and to demonstrate that repeated administration, a history of alcohol intake or old age have no effect on brain sensitivity. In addition, if the SEF is reduced below 5 Hz during induction of anaesthesia, a marked rise in arterial pressure in response to laryngoscopy and tracheal intubation is unlikely. Although the change in SEF mirrors increasing anaesthetic concentrations during induction anaesthesia, there is a considerable lag in recovery of SEF when anaesthetic concentrations fall. The median frequency (MF) of the EEG power spectrum may be a better index of anaesthetic drug activity. It is 9 Hz in fully conscious subjects and must fall to below 5 Hz for subjects to become unresponsive to verbal commands. It shows dose related changes with anaesthetic drugs and, compared with SEF, there is less lag during recovery. However, there is some lag and MF is not ideal to monitor anaesthesia itself.

All these studies and others gave the plasma concentrations required to suppress responses and to maintain a reasonable stable depth of anaesthesia; for alfentanil the range was between 140-44 nanogr/ml and for fentanyl a comparable plasma concentration was between 3-5 nanogr/ml; for semplification, a target plasma concentration of 250 microgr/ml of alfentanil could be obtained with a bolus dose of 50 µg/kg and maintained by an infusion of 50 µg/kg/h; for fentanyl the loading dose could be obtained by a loading dose of 5 µg/kg, aiming at a concentration of 4 nanogr/ml, followed by a continuous infusion of 3 µg/kg/h. The advantage of using a continuous infusion is that to achieve stable blood concentrations so that concentrations at the site of effect (biophase) are likey to be in equilibrium with it within 10 min or so after the start of the infusion.

Having so far approached the problem from a quantitative point of view, it is necessary to invoke mathematical modeling to describe pharmacokinetic and pharmacodynamic modeling, in order to continue to provide a quantitative basis for the understanding of a drug dose-response relationship, which in turn may provide a formal rationale for dosage regimens design. Numerous assumptions are necessary; first of all since the effect site concentrations is largely unknown, the effect site concentration of a drug is constantly in the process of equilibrating with the concentration of drug in the plasma, which can be sampled easily and therefore serve as our window into the biophase. A second assumption is that drug acting at the biophase should be free drug, not bound to plasma proteins or other binding sites; however, there are insufficient data to date to speculate about the potential significance of free drug concentrations alone.

Therefore we remain obligated to characterize the temporal relationship between intravenous dosages administered and concentration of total drug in the blood (or plasma or serum) and its relationship with a measure of effect, more or less specific, like anaesthesia, or, more precisely, IC_{50}, IC_{95}, etc.

EEG derived effect compartment models indicate that k_{eo} is a reasonable indicator of the time required for plasma and brain (effect site?) drug concentations to equilibrate and has been used to investigate effect compartment kinetic-dynamic behavior.

Dose response relationships have been approached determining C_{p50} values for various drugs and different surgical stimuli and since plasma and effect compartment concentrations are supposedly equal, or at least in equilibrium, at steady state, pharmacodynamics could be discussed in terms of k_{eo} and C_{p50}; unfortunately there is a marked inter- and intrasubject variability, at least as much as in pharmacokinetics and the study of population dynamics and kinetics coupling is just beginning. However, empirical dosing regimens for continuous infusion of i.v. drugs are more and more based on the application of kinetic and dynamic principles and it would appear very soon that the implementation of these studies be incorporated into syringe pumps, controlling the theoretical plasma or/and effect compartment drug concentrations. In the meantime we'll like to present at the end of this paper some examples of dosing schemes aimed at a total intravenous anaesthesia with continuous infusion.

The C_{p50} & C_{p50} BAR for fentanyl are reported in Table 4 from various sources (in association with N_2O 70%).

Table 4. C_{p50} & C_{p50} BAR for fentanyl

Author	C_{p50}	C_{p50} BAR
Glass 1997	3,26	4,17
Glass 1990	3	
Glass 1997	6	
White 1983	1	
White 1983	4	

A different approach tries to identify the 50% MAC reduction by opiates (Table 5) [7-9]

Table 5. Opiate concentration reducing MAC by 50%

	Plasma concentration
Fentanyl	1
Alfentanil	38
Sufentanil	15

or, more clinically, trying to find a 50% suppression of EEG spectral edge by opiates fentanyl/alfentanil/sufentanil (Table 6) [10, 11].

Table 6. Plasma opiate concentration reducing EEG by 50%

	Plasma concentration
Fentanyl	6,9
Alfentanil	520
Sufentanil	0,68

Please, keep always in mind that opiates are not complete anaesthetics and since they cannot abolish the MAC completely, a minimum amount (MAC AWAKE) of the inhalatory agent will be always necessary to obtain a status of general anaesthesia, whereby it is demonstrated that anaesthesia requires both the inhibition of noxious stimuli by analgesics and provision of loss of consciousness by hypnotics.

Isoflurane MAC is decreased by 50% with a concentration of 1.7 ng/ml of fentanyl and this is in turn reached by a bolus dose of 4 µg/ml followed by a continuous infusion of 1.75 µg/kg/min, since the minimum effective analgesic concentration of fentanyl is around 0.6 ng/ml and a good analgesic effect lies somewhere between 1 and 2 ng/ml, with the steepest reduction in isoflurane MAC, and because clinical significant respiratory depression occurs at fentanyl concentration > 2 ng/ml, it is a nonsense trying to reach a very high level of fentanyl, because there is a ceiling effect at a MAC 80% reduction at 5 ng/ml of fentanyl in plasma. The most intelligent course of action is therefore to establish a therapeutic window with the opiate, playing the fine tuning with the volatile agent.

The practice of continuous infusion

The postulates upon which infusion is claimed to be superior to intermittent boluses have been demonstrated over the last years in many papers [12-15]; from these papers and many others it has emerged that infusion is generally better than intermittent injections, allowing better control, especially since a proper infusion regimen avoids peaks and valleys, i.e. circumvent the transient high plasma levels resulting from the administration of relatively large bolus and the relatively low plasma concentrations typically occurring before the administration of the next bolus. Continuous infusion helps to maintain the plasma (or effect site) concentrations within relatively narrow limits, eliminating overshoots and subtherapeutic valleys. Kinetic and dynamic coupling should be complemented by a continuous titration from the anaesthesiologist, in order to continuously monitor and anticipate the patients responses, the ultimate goal being to maintain the plasma (or effect site) drug concentrations only slightly above those required for the desired effect; unless there has been a sudden and dramatic increase in surgical stimulation, the appearance of signs of inadequate anaesthesia (increase in heart rate, blood pressure, tears, sweat, movements) suggest that the effect site drug concentration has fallen just below the therapeutic threshold and therefore small increases in the effect site drug concentration are necessary to prevent or ablate a response.

That means that the anaesthesiologist should be always vigilant to titrate up and down as required, as has been always practiced with the most potent gases and vapors.

Similarities between inhalation and i.v. drugs are many and fundamentally the same type of reasoning could be applied for both; the differences being only in the different equipment used: syringe pumps instead of vaporizers, i.v. lines instead of tubes and breathing circuit. In both cases preoperative and intraoperative checks are continuously needed, as is the need for careful titration. Loading i.v. dose could be equated with the concept of "overpressure" and in either case a continuous background administration of a drug could reduce the requirement of a second one, as happens with the continuous inhalation of N_2O, that contributes heavily to the MAC.

The most important practical points during administration is to try to maintain the plasma or effect site drug concentration at a concentration that is only slightly above that required for recovery, so that recovery from the drug effects could be fast at the end of the infusion; as a matter of fact, the percentage decrease in plasma drug concentration required for recovery depends on the manner in which the infusion was titrated, the slope of the concentration-response drug for the given drug, the clinical end point being monitored and the presence of other anaesthetic drugs. The theoretical knowledge of context sensitive half times should be again emphasized, as is continuous vigilance.

Continuous infusion should be constantly inspected as happen with the vaporizers and gases delivered in the context of inhalational anaesthesia; a few recommendations are to often chart boluses, rate changes and cumulative totals, i.e. every 10-15 minutes, provided that vital signs are to be charted at least every 5 min. Titration should be applied aggressively and continuously, at least every 5 min, based on anticipated and observed responses; titration up is better attained with a small bolus followed by increase in rate, while titration down is better attained with a slowly downward titration. Inserting needles through a capped y site is not recommended, because of the ease of disconnection, the danger of needle sticks and of easier line occlusion in case of very low infusion rates.

Microbore extension tubings are to be recommended to reduce waste, albeit excessively high pressures are to be avoided. The carrier fluid should be chemically compatible with all drugs; in case of uncertainty, it is better to use a second dedicated i.v. line and this is to be recommended in case of need of large volumes of fluids or plasma expansion with colloids and/or blood.

As far as practical suggestions concerning titration, it is obvious that there could be no uniformity, being too different the goals to be investigated depending on patients, type of surgery, drugs and so on; however, apart from the loading dose and choice of a certain level of a maintenance infusion, it is our practice to titrate downward continuously by 5-10% every 10-15 min if the patient has not responded to surgical stimulation within the last 10-15 minutes and if no increase in the level of surgical stress is anticipated. If the patient begins responding, the infusion rate should be titrated upward by 20-25% and a small bolus dose rapidly injected, the amount of the bolus being calculated as the amount of drug given in the last 5 min and that of infusion evaluated halfway between the present and the previous rate. If the surgical stress could be anticipated as being very short or otherwise occurring near the end of the anaesthetic, the bolus dose could be administered alone, without any adjustment in the infusion rate.

Dosages of muscle relaxants should be kept at the minimum compatible with the presence of only the first or second twitch in the train of four modality of stimulation; unfortunately, balanced i.v. anaesthesia does not potentiate muscle relaxation and therefore dosages of neuromuscular blocking agents are often relatively high; therefore neuromuscular monitoring is highly recommended.

In general, hypnotics precede the administration of analgesics, so that patients are unconscious from the very start and will remain so; if hypnotics are also amnesics, then amnesia would be assured and this very useful combination is, in my opinion, better obtained with small titrated doses of midazolam, hypnosis induced and maintained with propofol. As a matter of fact, it is probably more important to maintain sleep relatively constant, with analgesics titrated up and down according to the varying changes in surgical stimulation required by the procedure. Because pain intensity varies throughout the procedure, with intubation, skin incision, visceral manipulation and traction, etc., the anaesthesiologist should be able to efficiently raise or lower the blood levels of analgesics and this can be better obtained with computer assisted infusion pumps, since the plasma concentrations of many anaesthetic drugs required for the suppression of the autonomic signs associated with surgical stimulation have been determined and are presented in Table 7.

Table 7. Plasma drug concentration ranges for the most useful anaesthetic drugs (ng or μg/ml)

Drug	Skin incision	DEEP surgery	Surface surgery	Awake	Analgesia (sedation)
Alfentanil	200-300	300-450	100-250	–	25-75
Fentanyl	3-6	14-8	2-5		1-2
Sufentanil	0.3-1.5	0.5-2	0.3-1.5		0.02-0.2
Propofol	3-5	4-7	3-5	1	1-2
Midazolam	50-250	50-250	100-200		40-100

Knowing the desired plasma level to be reached (and maintained) for a given stimulus, the implementation of the BET scheme or other algorithms is simply made introducing some data on a microcomputer; age, weight would be required, since these data modify the calculations; other questions could be sex, some information on kidney or liver function, and so on. The computer connected to the infusion pump will then start calculating the infusion rate theoretically required to obtain the desired plasma concentration; therefore, stable levels could be attained, in plasma or at the effect site and varied according to the surgical needs, continuously guided by the information inputted by the clinician.

This problem has been approached, and solved, by many authors; the ultimate goal being to establish the IC_{50} and IC_{95}, i.e. the blood concentrations, and hence the amount of drug to be given in a given period of time in order to achieve that concentration, inhibiting an undesired response or producing a certain effect. However, data in the literature confirm that different stimuli require different concentration of drugs: for instance, propofol and fentanyl infusion rates should be varied according to the patient responsiveness to stimulation in order to maintain a satisfactory anaesthetic and surgical conditions and to provide a satisfactory and prompt return of consciousness with minimal side effects and "hangover". Particularly useful are the following end points:

– C_{p50} (plasma concentration that results in a 50% probability of no response)
– C_{p95} (plasma concentration that results in a 95% probability of no response)

For noxious stimulations, the most important of which could be graded:

– no response to verbal commands
– no response to skin incision
– no response to tetanic stimulation
– no response to laryngoscopy
– no response to endotracheal intubation.

Since drug concentration at the site of effect governs the drug effect and stability of response over a period of time implies stability in the biophase concentration, but it is not currently feasible to measure such concentration directly, equilibration should be assumed and this can be achieved maintaining a constant site effect concentration; this could be obtained with continuous infusion stable for some minutes, at least 10 for propofol and 20 for fentanyl, as done in the studies by Kazama et al. [16]. Since considerable interpatient variability has been reported and the relationship between infusion rates and measured blood concentrations varies greatly between studies, the direct approach chosen by Kazama, relating patient response to predicted and measured blood concentration, is particularly promising.

Smith et al. [17] reported that for propofol alone the C_{p50} loss of consciousness was 3.3 µg/ml and the C_{p95} loss of consciousness 5.4 µg/ml; on the other hand, a propofol blood concentration of 2.5 µg/ml was required for satisfactory hypnosis during surgery [18]. In the Kazama study C_{p50} loss of consciousness was 4.4 µg/ml when propofol was administered alone, but this difference could arise from the different form of stimulation used by the authors, comprising both vocal and tactile (shoulder rubbing) stimulation. The reduction by fentanyl of the propofol C_{p50} loss of consciousness was minimal and this is in agreement with Smith. Davidson [19] reported following temazepam premedication a C_{p50} skin incision of propofol of 8.1 µg/ml, while Kazama et al. reported 10 µg/ml and Smith et al. 15.2 µg/ml. Reduction of C_{p50} skin incision by fentanyl was higher in the studies of Smith: 63% with 1 ng/ml and 89% with 3 ng/ml of fentanyl, while Kazama et al. reported 32% and 55% respectively. Differences are unclear, but may be related to the site of incision.

Response to tetanic stimulation, while appealing because of its reproducibility, could not bear a clinical significance, because MAC tetanus where consistently lower than MAC skin incision in the studies by Saidman and Eger [20]: anaesthetic depth defined using various noxious stimuli during isoflurane/oxygen anaesthesia was studied using tetanic stimulation also [21-23]; so Kazama demonstrated that there was no significant difference in somatic response between C_{p50} skin incision and C_{p50} tetanus; but differences existed in haemodynamic responses.

The somatic response to surgical incision has shown C_{p50} and C_{p95} values of 1.7 and 3.4 microgr/ml respectively, in patients given a constant infusion of propofol after morphine premedication and a standardized induction with propofol [24]; the study by Kazama gave higher values, C_{p50} 10 µg/ml and C_{p95} 17.7 µg/ml, less than the values reported by Smith et al. (15.2 µg/ml) for C_{p50} and 27.4 for C_{p95}.

Skin incision has been used as a standard stimulus in most concentration versus response relationship studies for anaesthetics [25], but it has the disadvantage of allowing only one measurement for patient and of possibly not being representative of all noxious stimuli encountered in surgery; skin incision also elicits a response that depends from site and size of incision (see Zbinden); moreover, determination of whether a reaction is positive may be subjective because not all reactions may be classified into "gross purposeful movements" as established originally in the MAC concept [26].

Moreover, skin incision does not represent the most intense stimulation, since the inception of MACei (endotracheal intubation), i.e. the end tidal concentration of an agent needed by 50% of the population to prevent all movements during and immediately after endotracheal intubation, is more useful, because there are many situations during an operation where not only adequate conditions for laryngoscopy are requested, but also are required to prevent coughing or bucking. In effect laryngoscopy followed by intubation was the strongest stimulus confirming the previous studies [27]. The ratio C_{p50} intubation/C_{p50} skin incision was 1.7-1.9 for propofol alone or in propofol + fentanyl, higher than 1.5 for isoflurane and lower than 2.17 for alfentanil + nitrous oxide.

However, each stimulation has to be applied in the non paralyzed patient if a motor response has to be evaluated; sufficient anaesthetic depth is a prerequisite without muscle relaxation and certain anaesthetics do depress the laryngeal reflexes more than others, i.e., propofol depresses the larynx more than ketamine does [28].

Doses needed to blunt haemodynamic responses to intubation were greatly influenced by fentanyl, the association between 6.4 µg/ml of propofol and 2.6 µg/ml of fentanyl being more protective than 7.8 µg/ml of propofol alone; the lack of motor response was not an accurate predictor of the ability of an agent to depress haemodynamic reaction, so that the correlation between somatic response and haemodynamic response to noxious stimuli was poor.

The same type of work needs to be done with alfentanil, remifentanil and propofol, between midazolam and fentanyl/alfentanil/remifentanil and the interactions between all these drugs.

But the graphs presented by Kazama et al. should be used in the programming of CACI (Computer Assisted Continuous Infusion) and adopted according to the different degrees of surgical stimulation; for instance, assuming as a target a fentanyl 2.6 µg/ml concentration and a 4 µg/ml concentration of propofol, at skin incision BP increase should be between 6.8-10.2, according to the figures presented.

The next step could be to link the delivery sistems to some measure of drug effect, like the EEG previously discussed; in this case, a closed loop will be established and the system could run by itself. More recently, the bispectral index has been used as a monitor for the titration of the hypnotic component of a balanced anaesthesia; this bispectral index is a dimensionless number varying between 0 and 100, empirically derived from a large data base of cases. The EEG is analyzed through Fourier and bispectral analysis and broken into frequencies and amplitudes and coherence of waveforms; features associated with increasing sedation and loss of consciousness were identified and served to accumulate the database upon which the BIS number was obtained and validated [29]. Knowing the drug interaction, it should be possible to provide adequate anaesthesia by any combination of sedative-hypnotics and analgesics opioids; providing not only adequate intraoperative analgesia and anaesthesia, but even assuring a rapid recovery, that implies return of consciousness and adequate spontaneous respiration; from the quantitative point of view we have been considering since the beginning, that the aim should be to obtain an ED_{95} for adequate anaesthesia during surgery, returning to a combination associated with an ED_{95} for consciousness and adequate ventilation. Time of recovery is therefore dependent both on CSHT required for both drugs used intraoperatively to decrease to that required for recovery. The lower the opioid dose, the more the time depends from the hypnotic and vice versa.

Vuyk et al. performed a brilliant analysis determining the interaction between alfentanil and propofol [30] and observing at the same time the time of awakening at each of these combinations; therefore, data were collected on prevention of response to skin incision and concentration at recovery. The shortest recovery time occurs at an alfentanil concentration of 80 ng/ml and propofol concentration of 3 µg/ml; when the concentration of propofol is increased, the dosage of alfentanil can be decreased, but overall recovery time is increased, and it similarly happens with increased alfentanil concentration, allowing a lower propofol concentration, but a longer recovery. For all drug combinations, including volatile agents like isoflurane, the infusion regimen should provide an analgesic concentration equivalent to 1-2 ng/ml of fentanyl. Propofol or the inhalatory anaesthetic should provide a minimal C_{p50} awake concentration or a MAC awake end tidal concentration (03-0.4%). If the patient demonstrates signs of inadequate anaesthesia, it is preferable to increase the volatile agent or the hypnotic as these drugs will have less effects on prolonging the wake up times than increasing the opioid, with less probability of awareness. All the suggestions so far advanced could not be relevant for remifentanil, since it has the shortest CSHT of 3-5 min, with a 80% CSHT of 10-15 min, irrespective of the infusion duration and even fastest than most volatile anaesthetics; therefore, the most rapid recovery will be obtained with the combination of a high dose remifentanil and a minimum amount of hypnotic, independ of the duration of anaesthesia. High remifentanil concentration of 4-8 ng/ml could be maintained with a continuous infusion of 0.15-0.30 µg/kg/min (900 µg/h in the average adult), adding just enough hypnotic as to ensure unconsciousness. If the patient responds, it could be more advantageous, in terms of recovery times, to increase the remifentanil infusion instead of the hypnotic. As a matter of fact, the unique metabolism of remifentanil could change our way to approach the analgesics; an overdose of remifentanil could not represent a real problem, since it will disappear incredibly faster, in comparison with the fear of residual depression following fentanyl; from this point of view, remifentanil could be considered a "forgiving" anaesthetic.

General pharmacology

We cannot conclude this review on analgesics without recalling at least the basic about them; therefore a brief discussion on general pharmacology of this class of drugs will follow, with special attention to points of clinical interest.

The peculiar large V_d (3-6 lt/kg) of fentanyl as been already alluded to; it may derive from its lipophilicity and may cause a rapid and prolonged peripheral tissue uptake, limiting its hepatic metabolism and causing a slow and variable decline in the blood plasma levels, where a secondary peak has often be noted in the postoperative phase, attributed to the rise in muscle blood flow typical of the early postoperative period and pain. Because fentanyl is metabolized primarily in the liver, decreases in hepatic blood flow decrease its elimination and hence patients with hepatic insufficiency should be treated cautiously with the drug.

CSHT for fentanyl is such that following a 60 min infusion, it will take the same time for a 50% fall in the effect site (and plasma) concentration; therefore, unless cautiously and continuously titrated up to the effects, this drug is the least suitable for continuous infusion analgesia.

Sufentanyl is approximately 10 times as potent as fentanyl; since its V_d is smaller (2.9 lt/kg), its receptor binding tighter and also higher is its degree of plasma protein binding, t½ β and duration of action are shorter than fentanyl and the drug is much more suitable for continuous infusion; its CSHT is 30 min following a 2-hour infusion and increases slower than the other opioids, so that its clinical recovery may be even faster than alfentanil.

Alfentanil is characterized by a small V_d and this is the main reason for its short t½ β; however, after one-hour infusion, its CSHT starts to increase faster, reaching one hour following a two-hour infusion, but remaining around 60 min even for prolonged infusion of 3-6 hrs. Unfortunately, P_{450} 3A is involved in the drug disposition and patients deficient in this enzyme may, unpredictably, present very prolonged recoveries and CSHTs.

Remifentanil is a unique derivative metabolized by non specific tissue esterases and hence characterized by very high clearance (3 lt/min), small Vd_{ss} (32 lt) and short mean residence time (11 min); its CSHT is little affected by impressive variations in dosage and from this point of view clinical recovery is incredibly faster than the other opioids, being of the order of a few minutes even following very prolonged infusion. However, this appealing characteristics imply the need to provide postoperative analgesia far in advance of the end of the infusion of the drug, assuring a smooth transition from remifentanil to another analgesic. Following major abdominal surgery, morphine 10-12 mg injected 30 min before the last suture has been found adequate, without prolonging clinical emergence.

The ED_{50} has been found 0.020 µg/kg/min for the incision at one hospital and 0.087 µg/kg/min in another [31] for all surgical manoeuvers: 0.52 µg/kg/min (Dershwitz), 4.25 µg/kg/min (Jooshi) for loss of consciousness. The ED_{50} for delta EEG activity is: 0.97 ng/ml vs 7.7 for alfentanil (data in the dog) [32], and for the technique of monitored anaesthesia care: 0.014-0.17 µg/kg/min [33], i.e. 5.6-714 µg per hour for 70 kg, with an incredible variability between 0,3-36 ml/h, at a concentration of 20 µg/ml.

Simple mathematical calculations demonstrate that 0.4 µg/kg/min means 84 ml/h:
– 0.02 µg * 60 min * 70 kg = 84 µg in one hour in a man of 70 kg;
– 0.09 µg * 60 min * 70 kg = 378 µg in one hour in a man of 70 kg;
– 0.52 µg * 60 min * 70 kg = 2184 µg in one hour in a man of 70 kg;
– due to this inherent variability, for an average patient of 70 kg body weight and diluting the drug to 20 µg/ml, the suitable dosages are of the order of ⇒: 4.2, ⇒ 18.9⇒ 109 ml/h!

At dosages > 0,3 µg/kg/min = 1260 µg/h/70 kg, i.e. 63 ml/h of a dilution of 20 µg/ml, only 14% of patients react to a surgical manipulation, and 0.1 µg/kg/min are adequate.

Spontaneous respiration is possible at dosages < 0.1 µg/kg/min or 0.05 µg/kg/min with isoflurane 1.1%: in another study 0.05 µg/kg/min + propofol 133 µg/kg/min allowed the maintenance of spontaneous ventilation. Sebel et al. have shown that remifentanil 2-5-15-30 µg/kg in 1 min does not release histamine, but reduces significantly PAS, PAD, FC (20%), independent from the dose [34].

From these unique characteristics, remifentanil appears the opiate of choice in every situation where a potent opiate with a rapid recovery is required, especially in patients with major organ dysfunction.

Recommended injectate concentrations and pharmaceutical forms available in Italy today are presented in Table 8.

Table 8.

Drug	Supply	Recommended concentration for infusion
Alfentanil	500 µg/ml	50 or 100 µg/ml
Fentanyl	50 µg/ml	5 µg/ml
Ketamine	50 mg/ml	10 mg/ml
Midazolam	5 mg/ml	500 µg/ml
Propofol	10 mg/ml	10 mg/ml
Sufentanil	50 µg/ml	5 µg/ml

In Table 9 guidelines relative to infusion schemes are shown ("end" means end of surgical procedure including termination of any dressings).

Table 9. Opioids infusion as analgesics in supplement to other primary anaesthetics in the presence of 60-65% nitrous oxide (+ eventually 0.3-0.4 MAC of alogenated anaesthetics)

Drug	Loading dose	Infusion	Stop before end
Alfentanil	10-30 µg/kg	0.5-1 µg/kg/min	10-20'
Fentanyl	2-4 µg/kg	0.010-0.025 µg/kg/m	30'
Sufentanil	0-5-1 µg/kg	0.05-0.008 µg/kg/min	10-20'
Ketamine	0.5-1 mg/kg	20-25 µg/kg/min	10-20'
Remifentanil	1 µg/kg	0.1-0.2 µg/kg/min	at end

N_2O should be continued until the very end of procedure, dressing included.

In case of simultaneous administration of hypnotic, better to titrate the hypnotic and leave the analgesic constant.

Table 10. Continuous infusion of sedatives/hypnotics in the presence of N_2O, following analgesic premedication

Drug	Induction	Maintenance
Propofol	1-2 mg/kg	150 µg/kg/min
until skin incision; then decrease 10-20 µg/kg min every 10-15 min; minimum 6 mg/kg/h (lower in geriatrics): stop 10-15 min before end		
Midazolam	0-1-0.2 mg/kg	1 µg/kg/min
until skin incision; decrease 0.2 µg/kg/min every 10-15 min; stop 30 min before end		

Continuous infusion of analgesics, with N_2O, but without hypnotics or sedatives (patients premedicated with full dosage of benzodiazepines or other major tranquilizers) as reported in the following table:

Table 11.

Drug	Induction	Maintenance
Alfentanil	50-150 µg/kg	0.5-3 µg/kg/min stop 10-20 min before end
Fentanyl	5-15 µg/kg	0.02-0.1 µg/kg/min stop 30 min before end
Sufentanil	1-3 µg/kg	0.01-0.03 µg/kg/min stop 20-30 min before end
Remifentanil	1-2 µgr/kg	0.1-0.4 µg/kg/min stop at the end of procedure

Table 12. Total intravenous anaesthesia (TIVA) without N_2O

Drug	Induction	Maintenance
Propofol	1-2 mg/kg	0.5-3 µg/kg stop 10-15 min before end
Midazolam	0-1-0.2 mg/kg	0.5-2 µg/kg/min stop 30 min before end
Alfentanil	10-30 µg/kg	0.5-2 µg/kg/min stop 10-20 min before end
Fentanyl	2-4 µg/kg	0.02-0.08 µg/kg/min stop 30 min before end
Sufentanil	0.5-1 µg/kg	0.005-0.02 µg/kg/min stop 20-30 min before end
Ketamine	0.5-1 mg/kg	20-100 µg/kg/min
Remifentanil	1-2 µg/kg	stop at the end of procedure

The dosages suggested are merely indicative and a continuous titration is advised; the best approach is not to be dogmatic and be ready to supplement a TIVA with N_2O or isoflurane; in selected cases, clonidine (0.5-1 µg/kg) could be a useful alternative in cases of hypertension not controlled with the usual doses of opioids.

It is personal opinion of the author that continuous infusion of midazolam is less practical, especially if a fast recovery is desired; in my practice midazolam is very helpful in coinduction and/or premedication, but has not been used as a continuous infusion. A last point to be carefully considered is the knowledge of the hypnotic interactions between the drugs; these effects can be graphically plotted on the so called isobolograms and inspected to see the additive or synergistic effects. For most drugs these effects have been already calculated [35].

In general, the commonest drug combination (thiopental or propofol or midazolam and fentanyl or alfentanil or sufentanil or remifentanil) demonstrate synergistic effects allowing the clinician to markedly reduce the amount of each drug to be used.

In terms of potency, the scale of magnitude is alfentanil < fentanyl 5 < remifentanil 25 < sufentanil 50, but comparing opiates by dose alone is no longer adequate, since doses do not correspond to plasma levels having comparable clinical effects; using EEG sufentanil is 12 times more potent than fentanyl, fentanyl 12 times more potent than alfentanil and remifentanil 75 times more potent than alfentanil [36].

References

1. Hughes MA, Glass PSA, Jacobs JR (1992) Context sensitive halftime in multicompartment pharmacokinetic models for intravenous anesthetic drugs. Anesthesiology 76:334-341
2. Schwilden H, Schuttler J, Stoekel H (1983) Pharmacokinetics as applied to total intravenous anesthesia: theoretical considerations. Anesthesia 38[Suppl]:51-51
3. Ausems ME, Hug C, Stanski DR et al (1986) Plasma concentrations of alfentanil required to supplement nitrous oxide anesthesia for general surgery. Anesthesiology 65:362-373
4. Fisher DM (1996) (Almost) everything you learned about pks was (somewhat) wrong! Editorial. Anesth Analg 83:901-903
5. Eger EI (1974) Anesthetic uptake and action. Williams & Wilkins, Baltimore 1-25
6. Ausems ME, Vuyp J, Hug CC et al (1988) Comparison of a computer assisted infusion versus intermittent bolus administration of alfentanil as a supplement to nitrous oxide for lower abdominal surgery. Anesthesiology 68:851-861
7. McEwan AI, Smith C, Dyar O et al (1993) Isoflurane Mac reduction by fentanyl. Anesthesiology 78:864-869
8. Brunner MD, Braithwaite P, Jihaveri R et al (1994) The Mac reduction of isoflurane by sufentanil. Br J Anesth 72:42-46
9. Lang E, Kapila E, Shlugman D et al (1996) The reduction of isoflurane MAC by remifentanil. Anesthesiology 85:71-78
10. Scott JC, Ponganis KV, Stanski DR (1985) EEG quantitation of narcotic effect: the comparative pharmacodynamics of fentanyl and alfentanil. Anesthesiology 62:234-241
11. Scott JC, Cooke JE, Stanski JR (1991) Electroencephalographic quantitation of opioid effect: comparative pharmacodynamics of fentanyl and sufentanil. Anesthesiology 74:34-42
12. White PF (1989) Clinical uses of intravenous anesthetic and analgesic infusions. Anesth Analg 68: 61-171
13. White PF, Dworsky W, Trevor AJ (1983) Comparison of continuous infusion fentanyl or ketamine versus thiopental-determining the mean effective serum concentrations for outpatient surgery. Anesthesiology 59:564-569
14. White PF (1983) Use of continuous infusion versus intermittent bolus administration of fentanyl or ketamine during outpatient anesthesia. Anesthesiology 59:294-300

15. Pathak KS, Brown RH, Nash CL et al (1983) Continuous opioid infusion for scoliosis fusion surgery. Anesth Analg 62:841-845
16. Kazama T, Ikeda K, Morita K (1997) Reduction by fentanyl of the C_{p50} values of propofol and haemodynamic responses to various noxious stimuli. Anesthesiology 87:213-227
17. Smith C, McEwan AI, Jhaveri R et al (1994) The interaction of fentanyl on the C_{p50} of propofol for loss of consciousness and skin incision. Anesthesiology 81:820-828
18. Wessen A, Persson PM, Nisson A et al (1993) Concentration effect relationships of propofol after total intravenous anesthesia. Acta Anaesth Scand 37:458-464
19. Davidson JAH, Macleod AD, Howie JC et al (1993) Effective concentration 50 for propofol with and without 67% nitrous oxide. Acta Anesth Scand 37:458-464
20. Saidman LJ, Eger EI (1964) Effect of nitrous oxide and of narcotic premedication on the alveolar concentration of halothane required for anesthesia. Anesthesiology 25:302-306
21. Zbinden AM, Maggiorini M, Petersen-Felix S et al (1994) I. Motor reactions. Anesthesiology 80:253-260
22. Hornbein TF, Eger EI, Winter PM et al (1982) The minimum alveolar concentration of nitrous oxide in man. Anesth Analg 61:553-556
23. Kopman AR, Lawson (1984) Milliampere requirements for supramaximal stimulation of the ulnar nerve with surface electrodes. Anesthesiology 61:83-85
24. Spelina KR, Coates D, Monk CR et al (1986) Dose requirements of propofol by infusion during nitrous oxide anaesthesia in man. I: Patients premedicated with morphine sulfate. Br J Anaesth 58:1080-1084
25. Quasha AL, Eger FI, Tinker JH (1980) Determination and applications of MAC. Anesthesiology 53:315-334
26. Eger EI, Saidman LJ, Brandstrater B (1965) Minimum alveolar anesthetic concentration: A standard of anesthetic potency. Anesthesiology 26:56-63
27. Ausems ME, Vuyk J, Hug CC et al (1988) Comparison of a computer-assisted infusion versus intermittent bolus administration of alfentanil as a supplement of nitrous oxide for lower abdominal surgery. Anesthesiology 68:851-861
28. Pedersen CM, Thirstrups Nielsen-Kudsk JE (1993) Smooth muscle relaxant effects of propofol and ketamine in isolated guinea pig trachea. Eur J Pharmacol 238:75-80
29. Glass PSA, Bloom M, Kearse L et al (1997) Bispectral analysis measures sedation and memory effects of propofol, midazolam, isoflurane and alfentanil in healthy volunteers. Anesthesiology 86:836-847
30. Vuyk J, Lim T, Engbers FHM et al (1995) The pharmacodynamic interaction of propofol and alfentanil in lower abdominal surgery in female patients. Anesthesiology 83:8-22
31. Dershwitz M, Randell GI, Rosow CE et al (1995) Initial clinical experience with remifentanil, a new opioid metabolized by esterases. Anesth Analg 81:619-623
32. Cunningham FE, Koke JF, Muir KT et al (1995) Pharmacokinetic/pharmacodynamic evaluation of remifentanil GR90291 and alfentanil (abstract). Anesthesiology 83:A376
33. Schnider TH, Minto C, Camu F (1997) Model based calculation of safe remifentanil infusion rates for conscious sedation from non steady state data. Anesthesiology A355
34. Sebel et al (1995) Histamine concentrations and hemodynamic responses after remifentanil. Anesth Analg 80:990-993
35. Vinik HR, Bradley EL, Kissin I (1994) Triple anesthetic combination: propofol, midazolam, alfentanil. Anesth Analg 78:354-358
36. Egan TD, Minto C, Hermann DJ (1996) Remifentanil versus alfentanil: comparative pharmacokinetics and pharmacodynamics in healthy adult male volunteers. Anesthesiology 84:821-833

Muscle Relaxants in Clinical Anaesthesia: An Update

V. Vilardi, M. Sanfilippo, M.K. Verdi

Most of the drugs actually used in general anaesthesia resemble high stereospecifity, receptors affinity, short duration of action, short recovery time, rapid distribution and redistribution in high degradation tissues. A short sleeping time and muscle relaxation is needed to ensure a rapid recovery and early deambulation. Since 60% of the total surgical procedures are nowadays performed in outpatient regimen, it is necessary to satisfy such requirements. The question is, whether this need has really improved the quality of the drugs currently available. In the case of non-depolarizing muscle relaxants (NMBAs), the short onset time, action and recovery are combined with low potency [1]. None of the muscle relaxants can substitute succinylcholine in terms of onset, duration, quality of muscle relaxation and recovery despite its well known side effects [2]. The other muscle relaxants have a different behaviour. The rate of maximal block reached at laryngeal muscles by rocuronium and mivacurium is 77% and 90% respectively [3], which is lower than thumb adductor muscle. In the case of mivacurium, the time of permanence on neuromuscular laryngeal endplates [4] is so short that it is impossible to perform any procedure on vocal chords even if a complete block is registered on the adductor pollicis muscle. Another problem concerns the method of measurement of the onset time. It is defined as the time interval from the beginning of the injection to the maximal action (peak effect) of a drug [5]. The measurement of the onset time should be performed without either any additive or synergistic drugs (propofol, etomidate, halotane, isoflurane, enflurane, etc.) [6, 7], or priming and timing principle [8] which often cause patient discomfort [9]. All the other parameters, recently suggested by many researchers, including the lag time [10], misunderstand the definition of the onset time. A long lasting electric stimulation or clinical criteria are not suitable to define the quality of intubation [5].

Tracheal intubation can be considered excellent when mechanomiography or accelerometry show maximal block on orbicular muscle or on vocal chords [11]. TOF ratio value has been increased to 0,9 and new recovery indexes and clinical tests [12] have been suggested in order to a safe discharge of patients. A decrease of mortality due to PORC (postoperative residual curarisation) has been registered by the use of vecuronium and atracurium, but the use of pancuronium is correlated with a deeper residual block and a higher incidence of

PORC [13]. In the case of microdoses of mivacurium, healthy volunteers one hour after administration showed dyplopia, caused by sensibility of extraocular muscles, and facial weakness even if the recovery index was 0,9-1 [14, 15]. A possible obstruction of the high respiratory airways in the immediate postoperative period [16] is due to the use of analgesics and halogenated anaesthetics alone or associated with residual block [2, 17-23]. In the early experimental and clinical studies muscle relaxants were not given in the right dose for intubation in adults or pediatric patients. In the case of mivacurium, good intubating conditions in adults and children can be obtained with doses higher than 0,15 mg/kg (0,25 mg/kg and 0,3 mg/kg) respectively [24, 25], but with such doses, clinical signs of histamine release are evident [26]. The intubation dose of cisatracurium is 0,2 mg/kg [27] and not 0,15 mg/kg as suggested by Glaxo Wellcome. Rocuronium [25] allows good intubating conditions in adults and children with doses higher than 0,6 mg/kg (0,9-1,1 mg/kg to 1,2 mg/kg). The detritment is represented by an increased clinical duration, higher MRT (mean residence time) and higher rate of vagolytic effects [28, 29].

Steroidal compounds

Rocuronium

Rocuronium bromide has a steroidal molecular structure similar to that of vecuronium bromide. It has an ED_{95} of 0,3 mg/kg and only 20% of vecuronium potency [30]. This low potency allows very short onset times with good and excellent intubating conditions especially with doses of 3-4 x ED_{95} [1, 31]. With such doses, the onset time is 60-90 seconds but the DUR 25 and DUR 75 are increased (40-50 minutes) [31]. Women [32] are 30% more sensitive to rocuronium than men. During pediatric anaesthesia [33] excellent intubating conditions are performed with 0,9 mg/kg (3x ED_{95}) despite occurrence of tachycardia within the third minute after its administration. The haemodynamic profile of a 0,6 mg/kg bolus of rocuronium is stable [34]. In patients undergoing acute normovolaemic haemodilution [35], the neuromuscular block is decreased.

End-stage renal failure patients show a decreased clearance and increased MRT, in spite of 30% of injected dose is eliminated via kidney [36, 37]. Patients with hepatic failure show increased onset time and recovery index, high volume of distribution at steady state (V_{dss}) low clearance, and high individual variability [38-40]. It is suggested in these patients to titrate doses and monitorize neuromuscular function (first dose 0,12 mg/kg, maintainance doses 0,07-0,2 mg/kg) [41].

Neuromuscular block is also prolonged after reperfusion of a liver allograft transplantation [42] compared with the native diseased liver. In myasthenic patients [43, 44], rocuronium should be administered in a bolus dose of 0,15 mg/kg, that is 1/4 of the standard intubating dose. In obese and asthenic patients, the bolus dose or infusion rate of rocuronium [45] should be reduced. It has been proposed an intramuscular use of rocuronium in doses of 1-1,8 mg/kg in children, but only in 50% of these small patients onset times of 3-4 minutes had been obtained and intubating conditions were not satisfactory [46]. Poor intubating conditions were obtained in patients undergoing caesarean section who received a bolus of 0,6 mg/kg [47]. A dose of 0,05 mg/kg of rocuronium is recommended [48, 49] to avoid succinylcholine fasciculations. Some authors reported residual paralysis after cardiac [50], carotid and breast surgery [51] with rocuronium. Epinephrine [52] and ephedrine [53] seem to reduce the onset time of rocuronium. Patients receiving chronic anticonvulsant treatment with sodium valproate and primidone [54] showed accelerated recovery and unchanged half time elimination and clearance of rocuronium. Chronic treatment with beta blockers or calcium entry blocking drugs [55] reduce the duration of action of rocuronium probably because of a mechanism of receptors up regulation.

Rocuronium mixed with mivacurium did not show any particular advantage in addition to synergic and additive effects which were already noticed in mixtures of other muscle relaxants [56, 57].

ORG 9487

This compound first appeared in 1992 in clinical studies [58]. It has low potency, high lipophilia and inhibits voltage activated calcium channels. All these properties cause short lag time (18 sec) and vasodilation by inhibiting receptors and voltage activated calcium channels [59]. This ability enables a rapid onset.

In vitro [60] on rat phrenic nerve/hemidiaphragm preparation, ORG 9487 showed a significant anticholinesterasic activity. This negative aspect was emphasized by the inability of antiacetylcholinesterases (AchES) to reverse the effects of the experimentally induced block.

Haemodynamic properties of this blocking agent reported by Wierda et al. [61], Lictor et al. [62] and Bikhazi et al. [63] seem to be dose-dependent and probably mediated by histamine. The available data are controversial and the methods used arouse some perplexities. Van den Broeck et al. [64] and Schiere et al. [65] suggested that this drug is a short acting compound good for intubation. Although proceedings take longer and maintenance doses are requested, ORG 9487 becomes a muscle relaxant with an intermediate-long duration of action.

The most interesting aspect suggested by Wierda et al. [66] is the possibility of an early recovery from a deep block already two minutes after ORG 9487 administration.

Histamine release is evident for doses of 2,5-3 mg/kg [66]. Tachycardia [67] is dose-related and it may occur in 7% of hearth failure patients, 13% of neonates and 17% of adults for doses of 1,5 mg/kg. In women undergoing caesarean section, bolus doses of 2,5 mg/kg enable good intubating conditions and fetal outcome [68, 69].

In cirrhotic patients after administration of 1,5 mg/kg bolus dose, pharmaco-dynamic and pharmacokinetic changes have been observed [70]. Org 9487 does not interfere with ocular tone and can be also administered in ophtalmic surgery [71]. In pediatric anaesthesia with bolus doses of 0,3-2,5 mg/kg, the onset time was 67-150 seconds without significant changes in cardiocirculatory parameters [72-74]. The response of vocal chords does not differ from that observed with other muscle relaxants [75].

New steroidal compounds

ORG 9488, desacetil-metabolite of ORG 9487, is actually on experimental trial. Its recovery index is 25-75 times lower than its precursor, while the ED_{90} and DUR 25 are longer [76]. It has been administered in short infusion times and it showed kinetic and dynamic characteristics similar to those of ORG 9487 [76].

Benzylisoquinolinic compounds

Mivacurium

Mivacurium is a member of the benzylisoquinolinium family. It has a half-life of 5 minutes [77], the lowest actually available for a non depolarizing neuro-muscular blocking agent. A bolus dose of 0,25 mg/kg in adults [4] and of 0,3 mg/kg in children [78] permits good intubating conditions. Histamine release is more frequent with these doses (53%) respect to 0,2 mg/kg (15-20%) [78].

Since it is metabolized by plasma cholinesterases, all physiological and pathological conditions which can interfere with these enzymes should be care-fully considered. In homozygotes patients, mivacurium is 4-5 times more potent with a duration of action 30-50% longer, even with doses of 0,12 mg/kg [79]. The interferences with other drugs which decrease plasma cholinesterase activi-ty, like esmolol, should be also considered [80]. Mivacurium should not be used in the myasthenic patients treated with anticholinesterasic drugs and with a re-duced cholinesterasic activity [81]. Pretreatment with 0,02 mg/kg [82] is effec-tive in preventing the increase of intraocular pressure after suxamethonium ad-ministration.

Mixtures of non depolarizing drugs have a competitive action on Ach recep-tors of mivacurium [83]. Halogenated anaesthetics potentiate its action [6, 7]. A low dose (0,04-0,08 mg/kg) of mivacurium facilitate the insertion of the laryn-geal mask [84]. In the case of long lasting infusion [85], the cis-cis isomer plas-ma concentration is increased and especially in patients with low cholinesteras-es activity, the rate and dose should be reduced (from 4-6 µg/kg/min to 2,4 µg/kg/min) in order to achieve a satisfactory recovery. In patients with liver or renal failure, the bolus dose and infusion rate should be also reduced [86-89].

Cisatracurium

Cisatracurium is a stereoisomeric compound (1 R cis – 1 R^I cis Atracurium) which represents 15% of the isomeric mixture of atracurium. It is more potent than atracurium and rapidly eliminated via Hofmann reaction [90]. The resultant metabolite laudanosine is 4-times lower than atracurium [91] and its histamine releasing property is 8-times lower than atracurium [92]. The relationship between Vd_{ss} and total body clearance [93] means organ independent elimination. The half life is independent either from total body clearance or from Vd_{ss} [93]. Infusion rates should be reduced with inhalation anaesthetics [94], especially with desflurane and sevoflurane [95]. The haemodynamic profile [96] is stable at 2-3 and $4xED_{95}$ indicating a high degree of cardiovascular safety. It can be used also in patients with renal or liver disorders [97]. Bronchospasm and other side-effects have been scarcely reported during long lasting infusions [98].

New benzylisoquinolinic compounds

Savarese [99] hypothesized the synthesis of ultra short-acting benzylisoquinolinic compounds as BW785U. This old compound has an onset time of 60-90 seconds, a duration of action of 10-15 minutes and a recovery index of 2-3 minutes. It has been abandoned because of the high incidence of adverse reactions due to histamine release. Actually a new compound with similar pharmacokinetics (GW2804XX) is going to be tested in experimental setting by Glaxo Wellcome laboratories.

Conclusions

A goal of a compound with a very low recovery index and a short onset time has not been still reached.

The mortality due to difficult or impossible intubation conditions is not related to the onset time but to the long recovery of a non depolarizing muscle relaxant. The use of a short-acting neuromuscular blocking agent does not reduce the intensive care unit or hospital stay [100].

Mivacurium is the only compound with a short duration of action and a recovery index of 5-7 minutes, a period which is considered too long to avoid any complication.

References

1. Donati F (1993) Effect of dose and potency on onset. Anaesth Pharmacol Rev 1:34-43
2. Meistelman C, Mc Loughlin C (1993) Suxamethonium. Curr Anaesth Crit Care 4:53-58
3. Belmont MR, Rubin LA, Lien CA et al (1995) Mivacurium. Anaesth Pharmacol Rev 3: 156-167
4. Plaud B, Debaene B, Lequeau F et al (1996) Mivacurium neuromuscular block at the adductor muscles of the larynx and adductor pollicis in humans. Anesthesiology 85:77-81
5. Viby-Mogensen, Engbaeck J, Eriksson LI et al (1996) Good clinical research practice (GCRP) in pharmacodynamic studies of neuromuscular blocking agents. Acta Anaesth Scand 40:59-74
6. Meretoja OA, Wirtavuori K, Taivainen T et al (1996) Time course of potentiation of mivacurium by halothane and isoflurane in children. Br J Anaesth 76:235-238
7. Kansanaho M, Olkkola K (1996) Quantifying the effect of isoflurane on mivacurium infusion requirements. Anaesthesia 51:133-136
8. Sieber TJ, Zbinden AM, Curatolo M et al (1998) Tracheal intubation with rocuronium using the "timing principle". Anesth Analg 86:1137-1140
9. Aziz L, Jahangir SM, Choudhury SNS et al (1997) The effect of priming with vecuronium and rocuronium on young and elderly patients. Anesth Analg 85:663-666
10. Puehringer FK, Khuenl-Brady KS, Koller J (1992) Evaluation of the endotracheal intubating conditions of Rocuronium (ORG 9426) and succinylcholine in outpatient surgery. Anesth Analg 75:37-40
11. Werner MU, Nielsen HK, May O et al (1988) Assessment of neuromuscular transmission by the evoked acceleration response. An evaluation of the accuracy of the acceleration transducer in comparison with a force displacement transducer. Acta Anaesth Scand 32:395-400
12. Brull SJ (1997) Indicators of recovery of neuromuscular function: time for change? Anesthesiology 86:755-757
13. Berg H, Viby-Mogensen J, Roed J et al (1997) Residual neuromuscular block is a risk factor for postoperative pulmonary complications. Acta Anaesthesiol Scand 41:1095-1103
14. Kopman AF, Ng J, Zank LM et al (1996) Residual postoperative paralysis. Anesthesiology 85: 1253-1259
15. Kopmann AF, Yee PS, Neuman GG et al (1997) Relationship of the Train-of-four fade ratio to clinical signs and symptoms of residual paralysis in awake volunteers. Anesthesiology 86: 765-771
16. D' Honneur G, Lofaso F, Drumond GB et al (1998) Susceptibility to upper airway obstruction during partial neuromuscular block. Anesthesiology 88:371-378
17. Jan GSK, Tong WN, Chan AMH et al (1996) Recovery from mivacurium block with or without anticholinesterase following continuous infusion in obstetric patients. Anaesth Intens Care 24:585-589
18. Abdulatif M, Al-Ghamdi A, Al-Sanabary M et al (1996) Edrophonium antagonism of intense mivacurium-induced neuromuscular block in children. Br J Anaesth 76:239-244
19. Hunter JM (1996) Is it always necessary to antagonize residual neuromuscular block? Do children differ from adults? Br J Anaesth 77:707-709
20. Abdulatif M, Mowafi H, Al-Ghamdi A et al (1996) Dose-response relationships for neostigmine antagonism of rocuronium-induced neuromuscular block in children and adults. Br J Anaesth 77:710-715
21. Okum GS, Keikhah MM, Horrow JC et al (1997) Is reversal of mivacurium detrimental? Anesthesiology 87:A845
22. Erkola O, Rautoma P, Meretoja O (1996) Mivacurium when preceded by pancuronium becomes a long acting muscle relaxant. Anesthesiology 84:562-565
23. Olkkola KT, Tammisto T (1994) Quantifying the interaction of rocuronium (ORG 9426) with etomidate, fentanyl, midazolam, propofol, thiopental and isoflurane, using closed-loop feedback control of rocuronium infusion. Anesth Analg 78:691-696

24. Shorten GD, Crawford MW, St Louis P (1996) The neuromuscular effects of mivacurium chloride during propofol anesthesia in children. Anesth Analg 82:1170-1175
25. Pino MR, Ali HH, Denman WT et al (1998) A comparison of the intubation conditions between mivacurium and rocuronium during balanced anesthesia. Anesthesiology 88:673-678
26. Hunter JM (1993) Histamine release and neuromuscular blocking drugs. Anaesthesia 48: 561-563
27. Rimaniol JR (1997) Intubating conditions using cis-atracurium after induction of anaesthesia with tiopenthone. Anaesthesia 52:998-1000
28. Booth MG, Marsh B, Bryden FMM et al (1992) A comparison of the pharmacodynamics of rocuronium and vecuronium during halothane anaesthesia. Anaesthesia 47:832-834
29. Wierda JMKH, Schuringa M, Van den Broek L (1997) Cardiovascular effects of an intubating dose of rocuronium 0,6 mg/kg⁻¹ in anaesthetized patients, paralysed with vecuronium. Br J Anaesth 78:586-587
30. Durant NN, Marshall IG, Savage DS et al (1979) The neuromuscular and autonomic blocking activities of pancuronium, ORG NC45 and other pancuronium analogues, in the cat. J Pharm Pharmac 31:831-836
31. Agoston S (1995) Onset time and evaluation of intubating conditions-rocuronium in perspective: A review. Eur J Anaesth 12(11):31-37
32. Xue FS, Tong SY, Liao X et al (1997) Dose-Response and Time course of effect of Rocuronium in male and female anesthetized patients. Anesth Analg 85:667-671
33. Fuchs Buder T, Tassonyi E (1996) Intubating conditions and time course of rocuronium induced neuromuscular block in children. Br J Anaesth 77:335-338
34. Hudson ME, Rothfield KP, Tullock WC et al (1998) Haemodynamic effects of rocuronium bromide in adult cardiac surgical patients. Can J Anaesth 45:139-143
35. Xue FS, Liao X, Tong SY et al (1998) Influence of acute normovolaemic haemodilution on the relation between the dose and response of rocuronium bromide. Eur J Anaesthesiol 15:21-26
36. Cooper RA, Wierda JMKH, Mirakhur R et al (1994) Pharmacodynamics and pharmacokinetics of rocuronium bromide in patients with and without renal failure. Eur J Anaesth 11[Suppl] 9:82-86
37. Cooper RA, Maddineni VR, Mirakhur MK et al (1993) Time course of neuromuscular effects and pharmacokinetics of rocuronium bromide (ORG 9426) during isoflurane anaesthesia in patients with or without renal failure. Br J Anaesth 71:222-229
38. Bevan DR (1994) Rocuronium bromide and organ function. Eur J Anaesth 11[Suppl]9:87-91
39. Khalil M, D'Honneur G, Duvaldenstin P (1994) Pharmacokinetics and pharmacodynamics of rocuronium in patients with cirrhosis. Eur J Anaesthesiol 11[Suppl]9:85-86
40. Magorian T, Wood P, Caldwell J et al (1995) Pharmacokinetics and neuromuscular effects of rocuronium bromide in patients with liver disease. Anesth Analg 80:754
41. Servin F, Lavaut E, Desmonts JM (1993) Pharmacokinetics of repeated doses of rocuronium in cirrhotic and control patients. Anesthesiology 79:A962
42. Marcel RJ, Ramsay MAE, Tillmann Hein HA et al (1997) Duration of rocuronium-induced neuromuscular block during liver transplantation: A predictor of primary allograft function. Anesth Analg 84:870-874
43. Proost JH (1997) A pharmacokinetic/pharmacodynamic model explaining the altered potency and time course of action of neuromuscular blocking agents in myasthenic patients. Eur J Anesthesiol 14[Suppl]16:32
44. Sanfilippo M, Fierro G, Cavalletti MV et al (1997) Rocuronium in two myasthenic patients undergoing thymectomy. Acta Anaesthesiol Scand 41:1365-1366
45. Puehringer FK, Khuenl-Brody KS, Mitterschiffthaler G (1995) Rocuronium bromide: Time course of action in underweight, normal weight, overweight and obese patients. Eur J Anaesth 12(11):107-110
46. Reynolds LM, Lau M, Brown R et al (1997) Bioavailability of intramuscular rocuronium in infants and children. Anesthesiology 87:1096-1105
47. Kelly MC, Mirakhur RK, Carabine UA et al (1996) Rocuronium: Placental transfer and neonatal effects. Anesthesiology 85:A883

48. Motamed C, Choquette R, Donati F (1997) Rocuronium prevents succinylcholine fasciculations. Can J Anaesth 44:1262-1268
49. Demers-Pelletier J, Drolet P, Girard M et al (1997) Comparison of rocuronium and d-tubocurarine for prevention of succinylcholine-induced fasciculations and myalgia. Can J Anaesth 44:1144-1147
50. McEwin L, Merrick PM, Bevan DR (1997) Residual neuromuscular blockade after cardiac surgery: Pancuronium vs rocuronium. Can J Anaesth 44:891-895
51. Coveler LA, Gallacher BP (1997) Postoperative rocuronium reparalysis. Can J Anaesth 44:1127
52. Arndt GA, Gerry T, White P (1997) Postoperative reparalysis after rocuronium following nebulized epinephrine. Can J Anaesth 44:321-324
53. Munoz HR, Gonzàlez JA, Dagnino JA et al (1997) The effect of ephedrine on the onset time of rocuronium. Anesth Analg 85:437-440
54. Driessen JJ, Robertson EN, Booij LHD et al (1998) Accelerated recovery and disposition from rocuronium in an end-stage renal failure patient on chronic anticonvulsant therapy with sodium valproate and primidone. Br J Anaesth 80:386-388
55. Loan PB, Connolly FM, Mirakhur RK et al (1997) Neuromuscular effects of rocuronium in patients receiving beta-adrenoreceptor blocking, calcium entry blocking and anticonvulsant drugs. Br J Anaesth 78:90-91
56. Kim DW, Joshi G, White P et al (1996) Interactions between mivacurium, rocuronium and vecuronium during general anaesthesia. Anesth Analg 83:818-822
57. Stevens J, Shepherd J,Vories P et al (1996) A mixture of mivacurium and rocuronium is comparable in clinical onset to succinylcholine. J Clinical Anaesth 8:486-489
58. Wierda JMKH, Van den Broeck L, Smeulers NJ et al (1992) Early reversibility of Org 9487, a new steroidal muscle relaxant. Anesthesiology 77:A970
59. Yamaguchi K, Huraux C, Szlam F et al (1998) Vascular effects of ORG 9487 in human mammary arteries, a new short acting muscle relaxant. Anesth Analg 86:SCA109
60. Prior C, Tian L, El Mallah AI et al (1995) Neuromuscular blocking profile of the vecuronium analogue, Org 9487, in the rat isolated hemidiaphragm preparation. Br J Pharmacol 116: 3049-3055
61. Wierda JMKH, Beaufort AM, Kleef UW et al (1994) Preliminary investigations of the clinical pharmacology of three short acting non depolarizing neuromuscular blocking agents: Org 9453, Org 9489, Org 9487. Can J Anaesth 41:213-220
62. Lictor JL, Korttila K, Lane B et al (1996) Onset time, peak effect and cardiovascular effects in adult patients after three different doses of ORG 9487. Anesthesiology 85:A805
63. Bikhazi GB, Deepika KD, Fonseca J et al (1996) Cardiovascular effects of ORG 9487 under nitrous oxide, barbiturate, fentanyl anaesthesia. Anesth Analg 82:S29
64. Van den Broeck L, Wierda JMKH, Smeulers NJ et al (1994) Pharmacodynamics and pharmacokinetics of an infusion of ORG 9487, a new short acting steroidal neuromuscular blocking agent. Br J Anaesth 73:331-335
65. Schiere S, Van den Broeck L, Proost JH (1997) Comparison of Vecuronium with ORG 9487 and their interaction. Can J Anaesth 44:1138-1143
66. Wierda JMKH, Proost JH, Muir AW et al (1993) Design of drug for rapid onset. Anaesth Pharmacol Rev 77:579-584
67. Witkowski TA, Bartkowsky RR, Huffnage S et al (1997) Haemodynamic effects of bolus injection of ORG 9487: A comparison with mivacurium and succinylcholine. Anesthesiology 87:A865
68. Abboud TK, Bikhazi G, Mroz L et al (1997) ORG 9487 vs succinylcholine in rapid sequence induction for cesarean section patients: maternal and neonatal effects. Anesthesiology 87:A906
69. Fragen RJ, Shanks CA (1997) Time course of onset and recovery of ORG 9487: A comparison with mivacurium and succinylcholine. Anesthesiology 87:A867
70. Duvaldestin P, Slavov V, Rimaniol JR (1997) Pharmacodynamique de l'ORG 9487 chez les patients ayant une cirrhose. 39° Congrès de la SFAR. Ann Fr Anesth Reanim R380

71. Whitford AM, Godschalkx A, Robertson EN (1997) A clinical comparison of some cardiovascular and intraocular effects of ORG 9487, vecuronium and succinylcholine. Anesthesiology 87:A848
72. Meretoja OA, Taivainen T, Jalkanen L et al (1996) A fast-onset short-acting non-depolarizing neuromuscular blocker, ORG 9487 in infants and children. Br J Anaesth 76[Suppl]2:A304
73. Kaplan RF, Fletcher JE, Hannallah R et al (1996) The ED_{50} of ORG 9487 in infants and in children. Anesthesiology 85:A1059
74. Motsch J, Meakin G, Meretoja OA et al (1996) A dose ranging study of ORG 9487 on endotracheal intubating conditions in infants and children. Anesthesiology 85:A1084
75. Debaene B, Billard V, Lieutaud T et al (1995) Org 9487 induced neuromuscular block at the adductor pollicis muscle and laryngeal adductor muscles in humans. Anesthesiology 83:A919
76. Schiere S (1997) Pharmacokinetics and pharmacodynamic relationship of the Org 9488, the 3-desacetyl metabolite of ORG 9487. Anesthesiology 87:A377
77. Basta SJ (1992) Clinical pharmacology of mivacurium chloride. A review. J Clin Anaesth 4:153-163
78. Brandom BW, Simhi E, Lloyd ME et al (1997) Intubation in children after 0,3 mg/kg of mivacurium. J Clin Anesth 9:576-581
79. Østergaard D, Jensen FS, Skovgaard T (1995) Dose-response relationship for mivacurium in patients with phenotypically abnormal plasma cholinesterase activity. Acta Anaesth Scand 39:1016-1018
80. Kim KS, Kim KH, Shin WJ et al (1998) Neuromuscular interaction between mivacurium and esmolol in rabbits. Anaesthesia 53:140-145
81. Paterson IG, Hood JR, Russell SH et al (1994) Mivacurium in the myasthenic patient. Br J Anaesth 73:494-498
82. Chui CL, Lang CC, Wong PK et al (1998) The effect of mivacurium pretreatment on intraocular pressure changes induced by suxamethonium. Anaesthesia 53:486-510
83. Stevens J, Shepherd J, Vories P et al (1996) A mixture of mivacurium and rocuronium is comparable in clinical onset to succinylcholine. J Clinical Anaesth 8:486
84. Chui PT, Cheam EWS (1998) The use of low-dose mivacurium to facilitate insertion of the laryngeal mask airway. Anaesthesia 53:486-495
85. Goudsouzian N, Chakravorti S, Denman W et al (1997) Prolonged mivacurium infusion in young and elderly adults. Can J Anaesth 44:955-962
86. Cook RA, Freeman JA, Lai AA (1992) Pharmacokinetics of mivacurium in normal patients and in those with hepatic or renal failure. Br J Anaesth 69:580B
87. Devlin JC, Head-Rapson AG, Parker CJR (1993) Pharmacodynamics of mivacurium chloride in patients with hepatic cirrhosis. Br J Anaesth 71:227-231
88. Philips BJ, Hunter JM (1992) Use of mivacurium chloride by constant infusion in anephric patient. Br J Anaesth 68:492-495
89. Mangar D, Kirchoff GT, Rose PL (1993) Prolonged neuromuscular block after mivacurium in a patient with end-stage renal disease. Anesth Analg 76:866-870
90. Wastila WB, Maehr RB, La Munion GL et al (1996) Preclinical pharmacology of cisatracurium besylate. Curr Op Anesthesiol 9[Suppl 1]:S2-S8
91. Boyd AH, Eastwood NB, Parker CJR et al (1996) Comparison of pharmacodynamics and pharmacokinetics of an infusion of cis-atracurium (51W89) or atracurium in critically ill patients undergoing mechanical ventilation in an Intensive Therapy Unit. Br J Anaesth 76:382
92. Lien CA, Belmont MR, Abalos A et al (1995) The cardiovascular effects and histamine-releasing properties of 51W89 in patients undergoing nitrous oxid/opioid/barbiturate anaesthesia. Anesthesiology 82:1131-1138
93. Kisor DF, Schmith VD, Wargin WA et al (1996) Importance of the organ independent elimination of cisatracurium. Anesth Analg 83:1065-1071
94. Hemmerling T (1997) Determination of the therapeutic infusions (ETI) of cis-atracurium during isoflurane or propofol/alfentanyl anaesthesia by closed-loop feedback control. Anesthesiology 87:A843

95. Wulf H, Kahl M, Ledowski T (1998) Augmentation of the neuromuscular blocking effects of cisatracurium during desflurane, sevoflurane, isoflurane or total i.v. anaesthesia. Br J Anaesth 80:308-312
96. Savarese JJ, Viby-Mogensen J, Reich D et al (1996) The haemodynamic profile of cisatracurium. Curr Opin Anesthesiol 9[Suppl 1]:S36-S41
97. Hunter JM, De Wolf A (1996) The pharmacodynamics and pharmacokinetics of cisatracurium in patients with renal or hepatic failure. Curr Op Anesthesiol 9[Suppl 1]:S42-S46
98. Newman PJ (1997) A comparison of cis-atracurium (51W89) and atracurium by infusion in critically ill patients. Crit Care Med 25:1139-1142
99. Savarese JJ, Wastila WB (1995) The future of the benzylisoquinolinium relaxants. Acta Anaesth Scand 39[Suppl]106:91
100. Butterworth J, James R, Prielipp RC et al (1998) Do shorter acting neuromuscular blocking drugs or opioids associate with reduce intensive care unit or hospital lengths of stay after coronary artery bypass grafting? Anesthesiology 88:1437-1446

Total Intravenous Anaesthesia

L. Barvais, B. Ickx, P. Pandin

A pharmacokinetic relation between the dose the anaesthesiologist injects and the generated blood concentration and a pharmacodynamic relation between measured or calculated blood concentrations and the hypnotic or analgesic effects are described for most of the intravenous agents.

In the past, intravenous (IV) agents were given as large single bolus doses or multiple smaller intermittent doses for induction and maintenance of anaesthesia. Different studies indicate that IV anaesthetics given by variable infusion rates have several advantages over intermittent boluses [1, 2]. These include greater haemodynamic stability, fewer haemodynamic breakthroughs and other signs of patient's responsiveness and reduced requirements for supplemental anaesthetics or vasoactive drugs.

Recently, new IV hypnotic and opioid drugs with a short duration of action have become available. These drugs enhance the interest of a total IV anaesthetic (TIVA) technique for general anaesthesia but their administration by continuous infusion is particularly recommended and their independent titration by separate infusion devices must be preferred.

Up to now, no study demonstrates any major advantage of any TIVA technique using these new drugs compared with a conventional volatile anaesthetic technique. However, after ambulatory surgery, Green et al. show that the length of stay in hospital was longer when isoflurane was used for maintenance of anaesthesia compared to propofol infusion simply due to a greater percentage of postoperative nausea (44% versus 19%) [3]. In a retrospective analysis of 27 investigations on N_2O and the incidence of nausea and vomiting, Hartung et al. show that 24 of the 27 studies demonstrate a greater percentage of emesis when N_2O is associated [4].

One of the major drawbacks of a TIVA technique was the lack of a convenient delivery system comparable to the commonly used easy volatile anaesthetic vaporizer. Recently, the Diprifusor system based on pharmacokinetic modeling and using a conventional three compartment pharmacokinetic set [5] has been commercialised thanks to the collaboration of the infusion system manufacturers and the Zeneca pharmaceutical company. This target controlled infusion (TCI) system controls the amount of propofol delivered to achieve and maintain calculated plasma target propofol concentrations for adult patients.

The purpose of this review will not debate between TIVA and inhalational techniques for general anaesthesia but if a TIVA technique is indicated or selected, it will focus on the way to improve the titration of a TIVA technique when using the Diprifusor system for the hypnotic component and remifentanil given by continuous infusion for the analgesic component.

Use of the Diprifusor system for the titration of the hypnotic component

The Diprifusor TCI system has been developed as a standardised infusion system for the administration of propofol by target controlled infusion. It consists in a software module in which infusion control algorithms are linked to a pharmacokinetic simulation program which includes a three compartment pharmacokinetic set. This module can be incorporated in any conventional infusion pump. The Diprifusor TCI system will operate only on recognition of an electronically tagged prefilled syringe containing "Diprivan" 1% or 2% injection.

The specific set of parameters for propofol [5] has been selected by Zeneca Pharmaceuticals on the basis of the predictive performance of different studies [6-8]. The pharmacokinetic set published by Gepts et al. [9] and modified as described by Marsh et al. [5] has been demonstrated to be associated with a low bias (+ 5.7%) and an acceptable precision (25.5%) in healthy adult patients [6]. Swinhoe et al. have evaluated the predictive performance of the pharmacokinetic set of Marsh et al. in three different age groups (18-40 years, 41-55 years and 56-80 years) and have found no significant difference between these age groups in bias and precision [8]. In patients undergoing CABG surgery the same set of Marsh et al. has underestimated the measured propofol concentrations in blood during the prebypass period with a low positive bias of + 21%, but the precision was acceptable (23%) [7]. In children, the set of Marsh has shown a negative bias and up to now, the Diprifusor is not recommended for children. Other factors can influence the predictive performance of the Diprifusor system over time within the same subject such as acute blood loss, haemodilution, episodes of low cardiac output states or hypothermia.

The field of the Diprifusor system application is the same as which is generally recommended for propofol given by infusion. Successful use of the Diprifusor in an adult patient requires the knowledge of the therapeutic blood concentrations appropriate for the different anaesthetic and surgical events.

Clinical studies have provided guidance for target propofol concentrations settings required for induction and maintenance of anaesthesia. Table 1 shows a proposed range of target propofol concentrations using the Diprifusor system when low or high doses of opioids are coadministered.

Figure 1 shows the profile of the propofol target concentrations required in adult and elderly patients according to the events of a minor surgical procedure when associated with low doses of opioids.

Table 1. Proposed range of the target propofol concentrations for the use of the Diprifusor system according to the coadministered opioid doses and the noxious stimulus in healthy adult patients

	Low doses of opioids	Large doses of opioids
Loss of consciousness	4-6 µg/ml	2-4 µg/ml
Minor surgery	3-8 µg/ml	2-6 µg/ml
Major surgery	3-10 µg/ml	2-8 µg/ml
Recovery	1-3 µg/ml	0.5-2 µg/ml

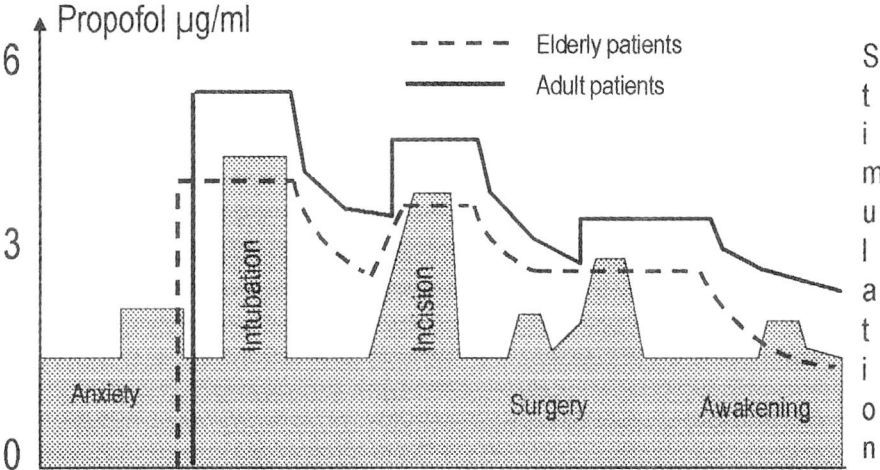

Fig. 1. Profile of the propofol target concentrations required in adult and elderly patients according to the events of a minor surgery when associated with low doses of opioids

Due to large interindividual pharmacokinetic variability target concentrations should always be titrated against clinical effect. If the target concentration must be titrated up and down, increments or decrements of 1-2 µg/ml in adult healthy patients or of 0.5-1 µg/ml in elderly or high risk patients are generally adequate. An increase of the target concentration is associated with a bolus and an increase of the maintenance infusion whereas a decrease of the target concentration is accompanied by the cessation of the propofol delivery for a short period followed by its automatic rerun at a lower infusion rate. If the target concentration is titrated according to the haemodynamic parameters without the use of a monitoring of the depth of anaesthesia such as EEG or evoked potentials, a lower safety limit of minimum 3 µg/ml is recommended in young adult patients without any premedication and minimum 2 µg/ml if benzodiazepines are given as premedication.

The Diprifusor system gives also information on the theoretical effect site concentration of propofol. During the recovery period, it also gives on-line information on the time required to reach a predefined awakening concentration. Finally, anaesthetists without any previous experience of propofol infusion express a clear preference for the Diprifusor system compared with a manual control and find it easier to use [2, 10].

Use of the opioids especially remifentanil for titration of the analgesic component

Fentanyl, sufentanil and alfentanil are generally administered by multiple repeated titrated boluses associated or not with a continuous infusion. However, Glass et al. have demonstrated that a TCI of fentanyl provides an acceptable accuracy within a homogeneous patient population of ASA 1-2 adult patients [11]. Other studies have demonstrated a good predictive accuracy for remifentanil, alfentanil, fentanyl and sufentanil [12-15]. Figures 2 and 3 show the plasma concentrations of these opioids required according to the level of surgery and the concomitant hypnotic level. Unfortunately, up to now, there is no commercialised TCI systems for the opioids except those developed by some university centers [11, 12, 15]. Consequently, opioid infusion schemes are generally titrated according to the surgical stimulation, the patient's requirements, the concomitant other anaesthetic drugs and the clinician experience. In the clinical practice, continuous infusions of sufentanil or alfentanil are preferred to fentanyl infusion due to their shortest context sensitive half lives [16].

Remifentanil is a new ultra-short acting pure μ opioid analgesic for use in anaesthesia. An ester linkage renders it susceptible to rapid metabolism by blood and tissue esterases that are nonsaturable and its context sensitive half life is very short (3-10 minutes). Remifentanil metabolism is not affected by a defi-

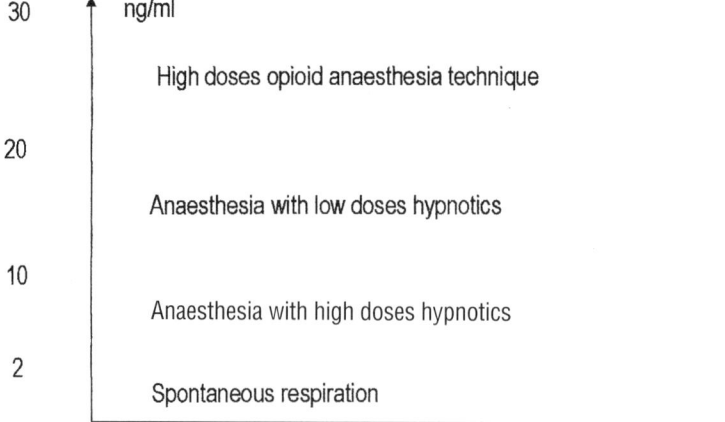

Fig. 2. Range of the target remifentanil and fentanyl concentrations

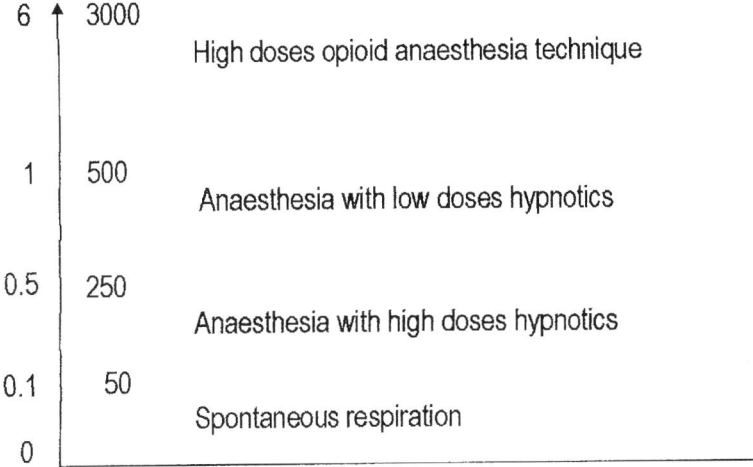

Fig. 3. Range of the target sufentanil and alfentanil concentrations

ciency of the plasma cholinesterase enzymes and by anticholinesterases such as neostigmine. Due to his particular pharmacokinetic profile, there is a good relation between his administration by constant infusion rate and measured plasma concentrations with a 1/30 ratio. A 1 µg/kg/min continuous infusion rate generates a plasma concentration of 30 ng/ml.

The pharmacokinetics and pharmacodynamics of remifentanil were not altered in patients with hepatic or renal diseases but the elimination of its principal metabolite is markedly reduced. This metabolite has a potency ratio in animals of 1/330 and is not associated with significant opioid effects in human after a 12 hour-infusion of 1µg/kg/min [17].

The pharmacodynamics of remifentanil is modified with increasing age. To reach the same peak effect EEG, the bolus dose required in a 80-yr-old person is approximately one half the bolus dose of a 20-yr-old person of similar lean body mass [12]. Moreover, the peak effect site concentration occurs later in elderly patients. The infusion rate required to maintain 50% EEG effect in a 80-yr-old is approximately one third of that required in a 20-yr-old person [12].

In unpremedicated healthy patients, the median effective dose and concentration for loss of consciousness with remifentanil were 12 µg/kg and 53.8 ng/ml, respectively [18]. In this study, minimal haemodynamic changes were observed but remifentanil was not considered as an adequate induction agent when administered alone.

The MAC reduction of isoflurane by remifentanil is similar to that produced by other opioids. A 50% isoflurane MAC reduction is produced by 1.37 ng/ml remifentanil whole blood concentration compared with fentanyl (1.67 ng/ml) or sufentanil (0.14 ng/ml) [19]. Remifentanil alone at extremely high concentrations (32 ng/ml) did not provide adequate anaesthesia [19]. Use of remifentanil alone also did not provide optimal sedation during local anaesthesia [20]. The combination of minimum 2 mg midazolam with 0.05 to 0.1 µg/kg/min remifentanil provides effective sedation and analgesia in ASA 1-2 women scheduled for elective breast biopsy procedures. However, midazolam produces a dose dependent potentiation of remifentanil depressant effect on respiratory rate [20].

In a multicenter evaluation studying 161 patients undergoing elective general surgery and anaesthetised using a TIVA technique combining propofol (0.5-1 mg/kg loading dose followed by a constant rate infusion of 4.5 mg/kg/hour) and remifentanil (0.5-1 µg/kg loading dose followed by a variable infusion rate from 0.25 to 4 µg/kg/min), the authors have observed an effective haemodynamic control of the responses to tracheal intubation and to the intraoperative stimuli and a rapid emergence from anaesthesia [22].

For tracheal intubation, a combination of 3 µg/kg remifentanil infused over 90 seconds and propofol 2 mg/kg infused over 5 seconds co-administered intravenously were demonstrated to provide adequate conditions for tracheal intubation in healthy patients without neuromuscular relaxants. This combination of drugs allows the rapid return of spontaneous ventilation [21].

The transition from remifentanil intraoperative anaesthesia to postoperative analgesia must be planned carefully due to its short context sensitive half life. After major abdominal surgery, Schüttler et al. have compared the efficacy and safety of remifentanil and alfentanil [23]. Fewer patients who received remifentanil responded to tracheal intubation, skin incision and surgery. In the postoperative period, time to extubation was shorter in the remifentanil group but an unacceptable high incidence of muscle rigidity, respiratory depression and apnoea was observed and attributed to rapid administration of bolus doses and infusion rate increments [23]. A multicenter evaluation of remifentanil for early postoperative analgesia was also associated with a too large incidence of respiratory adverse events (29%) and apnoea episodes (7%) [24]. In the immediate extubation period, 0.05 to 0.23 µg/kg/min remifentanil was associated with greater successful analgesia (58% of patients) than an intraoperative pretreatment using a standard bolus of 0.15 mg/kg morphine given 20 minutes before the anticipated end of surgery (33% of patients) [25]. In this study, the effects of remifentanil dissipated rapidly after ending the remifentanil infusion and alternate analgesia was required.

Vinik and Kissin have observed that tolerance to analgesia during a 3-hour remifentanil infusion administered to healthy volunteers is profound [26]. However, in this study, the acute remifentanil tolerance was not described in all the volunteers. In the clinical practice of TIVA, acute opioid tolerance is not frequently observed but can be evoked if one patient requires increasing opioid plasma concentrations over time for a stable and constant noxious stimulus.

Rational TIVA management

Only two abstracts have tried to evaluate the effectiveness of additional sedative or analgesic medication to treat haemodynamic responses during TIVA. In 62 patients presenting for lower limb or lower abdominal surgery, Glass et al. found that during a fentanyl-propofol TCI technique, it is preferable to maintain fentanyl constant at a low plasma concentration of 1.5 ng/ml and to titrate propofol to maintain adequate anaesthesia than to maintain TCI propofol stable at 2.5 µg/ml and to vary the TCI of fentanyl [27]. On the contrary, in 22 patients undergoing radical prostatectomy and anaesthetised by a propofol-alfentanil TIVA technique, Monk et al. showed that the recovery was more rapid when alfentanil was titrated to treat the acute haemodynamic responses than propofol [28].

These controversial results can be partially explained by the opioid selection and their respective therapeutic level. Recently, Vuyk et al. have determined by pharmacokinetic simulations the optimal effect site propofol opioid concentration window that assures adequate anaesthesia in 50% and 95% of healthy young patients for combinations of propofol with alfentanil, fentanyl, sufentanil and remifentanil for duration of infusion lasting 15-600 minutes [29].

They also demonstrate that the target concentrations or the infusion rates of propofol and of the opioid with which propofol is combined should be adjusted in relation to the selected opioid and the duration of the infusion to allow an optimal rapid return of consciousness [29].

A remifentanil-propofol TCI combination allows a more rapid return of consciousness than the other propofol-opioid combinations whatever the duration of infusion (15 to 600 minutes). It allows a recovery in less than 8 minutes if the target propofol concentration is around 2.5 µg/ml even for long-lasting procedures.

After a one hour TCI of propofol combined with either alfentanil, fentanyl or sufentanil, the shortest time to awakening is minimum 10 minutes. To optimise the time to awakening at the end of such a TIVA technique, the required propofol concentration must be around 3.5 µg/ml and to avoid any respiratory depression the target concentrations of alfentanil, fentanyl or sufentanil must be around 100, 1.5 and 0.1 ng/ml, respectively.

Figures 4 and 5 propose a TIVA technique combining either a variable TCI profile of propofol and sufentanil or a stable TCI of propofol with a variable TCI of remifentanil, respectively.

Prolonged time to awakening may be observed if the sufentanil administration is not correctly adapted or stopped at the end of the procedure (Fig. 4). In such a TIVA combination, surgical stimuli at the end of the anaesthesia procedure must be treated preferably by propofol titration rather than by sufentanil titration (Fig. 4). Due to the shortest context sensitive half life of remifentanil compared with propofol, target concentrations of propofol can be maintained at a stable 2.5 µg/ml level and associated with up and down titration of the remifentanil concentration according to the patient's responses (Fig. 5).

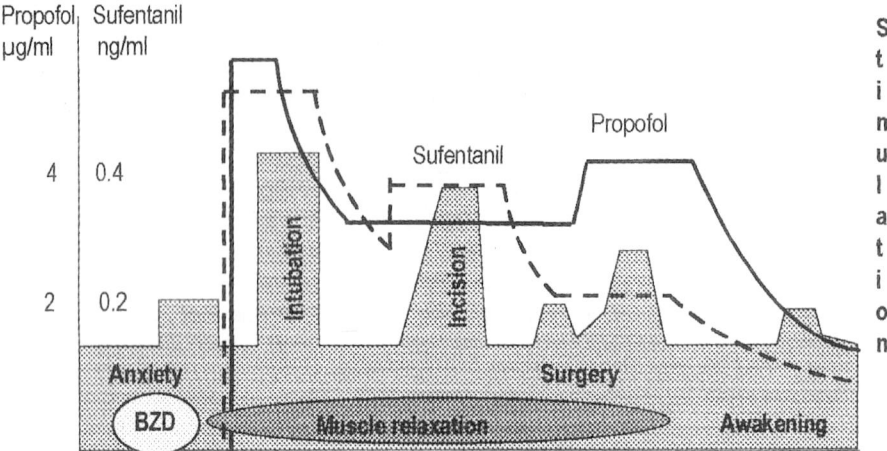

Fig. 4. TIVA technique combining propofol and sufentanil administered by TCI systems

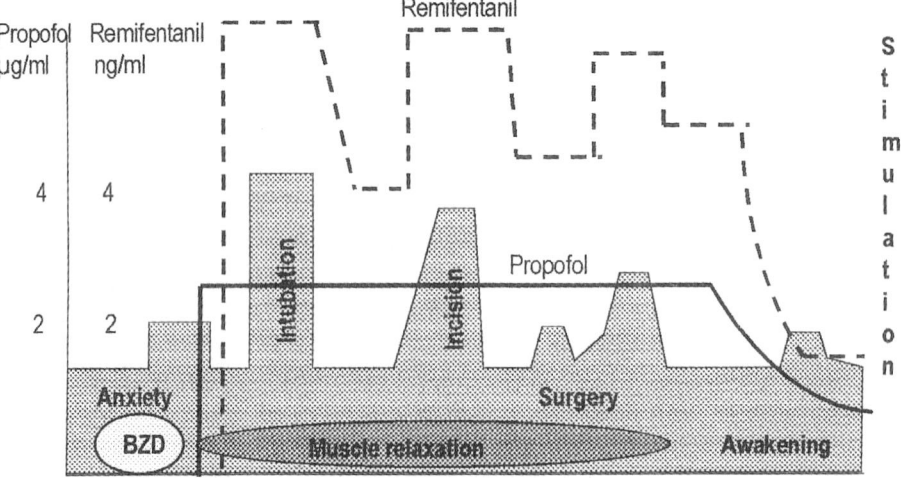

Fig. 5. TIVA technique combining propofol and remifentanil administered by TCI systems

Conclusions

General anaesthesia is a dynamic balance between hypnosis, amnesia and analgesia. This anaesthetic balance must be adapted to the clinical profile of the patient, the effects of the noxious stimulation (anaesthesia instrumentation and surgical stimulation) and the drug interaction.

A total IV anaesthetic technique allows the independent titration of the hypnotic and analgesic drugs.

The Diprifusor represents what may be the first of a new generation of infusion systems for hypnosis titration. It enables the anaesthetist to reach as rapidly as possible a steady plasma target concentration of propofol, to assess the adequacy of hypnosis and to modify this target concentration in a simple and intuitive manner.

The unique pharmacokinetic properties of remifentanil make it suitable for use in an analgesia-based anaesthesia balanced technique. It gives the anaesthetist a greater easiness of up and down analgesia titration without the disadvantages normally associated with high dose classical opioid regimens.

The combination of Diprifusor and a variable remifentanil infusion regimen reduces the consumption of each drug but such a TIVA anaesthetic technique remains more expensive than a standard technique using fentanyl as the analgesic component. However, the awakening with such a remifentanil technique is more predictable especially for the very long surgical procedures and the elderly patients [12, 29]. Finally, the postoperative analgesia regimen must be adapted and anticipated before the cessation of the remifentanil infusion. Remifentanil infusion (0.05-0.1 µg/kg/min) can only be administered as a postoperative analgesic agent on a separate and independent line in the presence of adequate supervision and monitoring of the patient. Administration of bolus doses of remifentanil is not recommended in this setting [23].

References

1. Alvis M, Reves JG, Govier AV et al (1985) Computer-assisted continuous infusions of Fentanyl during cardiac anesthesia: comparison with a manual method. Anesthesiology 63:41-49
2. Servin FS (1998) TCI compared with manually controlled infusion of Propofol: a multicentre study. Anaesthesia 53:82-86
3. Green J, Jonsson L (1993) Nausea: the most important factor determining length of stay after ambulatory anesthesia. A comparative study of Isoflurane and/or Profopol technics. Acta Anaesthesiol Scand 37:742-746
4. Hartung J (1996) Twenty-four of twenty-seven studies show greater incidence of emesis associated with nitrous oxide than with alternative anesthetics. Anesth Analg 83:114-116
5. Marsh P, White M, Morton N et al (1991) Pharmacokinetic model - driven infusion of Propofol in children. Br J Anaesth 67:41-48
6. Coetzee JF, Glen JB, Wium CA et al (1995) Pharmacokinetic model selection for target controlled infusions of Propofol. Anesthesiology 82:1328-1345
7. Barvais L, Rausin I, Glenn JB et al (1996) Administration of Propofol by target-controlled infusion in patients undergoing coronary artery surgery. J Cardiothorac Vasc Anesth 10:877-883
8. Swinhoe CF, Peacock JE, Glen JB et al (1998) Evaluation of the predictive performance of a Diprifusor TCI system. Anaesthesia 53:61-67
9. Gepts E, Camu F, Cockshott ID et al (1987) Disposition of Propofol administered as constant rate intravenous infusions in human. Anesth Analg 66:1256-1263
10. Russel D, Wilkes MP, Hunter SC et al (1995) Manual compared with target controlled infusion of Propofol. Br J Anaesth 75:562-566
11. Glass PA, Jacobs JR, Smith LR et al (1990) Pharmacokinetic model-driven infusion of Fentanyl: assessment of accuracy. Anesthesiology 73:1082-1090

12. Minto CF, Schnider TW, Shafer SL (1997) Pharmacokinetics and pharmacodynamics of Remifentanil - Model application. Anesthesiology 86:24-33
13. Raemer DB, Buschman A, Varvel JR et al (1990) The prospective use of population pharmacokinetics in a computer-driven infusion system for alfentanil. Anesthesiology 73:66-72
14. Shafer SL, Varvel JR, Aziz N et al (1990) Pharmacokinetics of Fentanyl administered by computer-controlled infusion pump. Anesthesiology 73:1091-1102
15. Pandin P, Ewalenko P, D'Hollander A et al (1997) Long-term predictive accuracy of target controlled infusion of Propofol and Sufentanil. Anesthesiology 87:A319
16. Hughes MA, Glass PA, Jacobs JR (1992) Context-sensitive half time in multicompartment pharmacokinetic models for intravenous anesthetic drugs. Anesthesiology 76:334-341
17. Hoke JF, Shlugman D, Dershwitz M et al (1997) Pharmacokinetics and pharmacodynamics of Remifentanil in persons with renal failure compared with healthy volunteers. Anesthesiology 87:533-541
18. Jhaveri R, Joshi P, Batenhorst R et al (1997) Dose comparison of Remifentanil and Alfentanil for loss of consciousness. Anesthesiology 87:253-259
19. Lang E, Kapila A, Shlugman D et al (1996) Reduction of Isoflurane minimal alveolar concentration by Remifentanil. Anesthesiology 85:721-728
20. Avramov MN, Smith I, White PF (1996) Interactions between Midazolam and Remifentanil during monitored anesthesia care. Anesthesiology 85:1283-1289
21. Hogue CW, Bowdle TA, O'Leary C et al (1996) A multicenter evaluation of total intravenous anesthesia with Remifentanil and Propofol for elective inpatient surgery. Anesth Analg 83: 279-285
22. Stevens JP, Wheatley L (1997) Tracheal intubation in an ambulatory surgery patients: using Remifentanil and Propofol without muscle relaxants. Anesth Analg 86:45-49
23. Schüttler J, Albrecht S, Breivikh et al (1997) A comparison of Remifentanil and Alfentanil in patients undergoing major abdominal surgery. Anaesthesia 52:307-317
24. Bowdle TA, Camporesi EM, Maysick L et al (1996) A multicenter evaluation of Remifentanil for early postoperative analgesia. Anesth Analg 83:1292-1297
25. Yarmush J, D'Angelo R, Kirkhart P et al (1997) A comparison of Remifentanil and Morphine sulfate for acute postoperative analgesia after total intravenous anesthesia with Remifentanil and Propofol. Anesthesiology 87:235-243
26. Vinik HR, Kissin I (1998) Rapid development of tolerance to analgesia during Remifentanil infusion in humans. Anesth Analg 86:1307-1311
27. Glass P, Dyar O, Jhaveri R et al TIVA (1998) Propofol and combinations of Propofol with Fentanyl. Anesthesiology 75:A44
28. Monk TG, Ding Y, Smith I et al (1991) Modifying the stress response during total intravenous anesthesia. Anesthesiology 75:A42
29. Vuyk J, Mertens MJ, Olofsen E et al (1997) Propofol anesthesia and rational opioid selection. Anesthesiology 87:1549-1562

PERIOPERATIVE CARE
OF CARDIAC RISK PATIENTS

Perioperative Care of Cardiac Risk Patients: New Pharmacological Strategies

P. Coriat

Taking into account the nature of perioperative cardiac complications and the moment when they occur during the operating period, it has become possible to define perioperative managements, which may improve the cardiac risk in patients suffering from coronary artery disease (CAD) undergoing non-cardiac surgery. The main goal of the perioperative management of patients with coronary artery disease is to control increased sympathetic tone or its circulatory effects. Two types of cardiovascular drugs have been recommended to achieve this goal: β adrenergic blocking drugs and α-2 adrenoreceptor agonists.

Physiopathology of perioperative cardiac complications

The most serious postoperative coronary complication is myocardial infarction which compromises short and medium term life expectancy in surgical patients [1]. The most frequent coronary event is the occurrence of episodes of myocardial ischaemia which, on the one hand play an important role in the etiopathology of acute postoperative myocardial infarction and, on the other hand, through their deleterious effects on left ventricular function may lead to postoperative congestive heart failure [2]. In vascular surgery patients or general surgery patients with coronary risk factors the degree of incidence of intraoperative myocardial ischaemia, is identical or even lower to that from which the patient suffers when not submitted the surgery (provided that the circulatory status be controlled throughout surgery) and that the anaesthetic technique does not influence the risk of perioperative ischaemia. By contrast, the incidence of ischaemic episodes is very significantly increased postoperatively. Studies by MacCann [3], Raby [4] and Landesberg [5] confirm the relationship between perioperative myocardial ischaemia and postoperative myocardial damage which is further illustrated by the fact that the occurrence of a postoperative episode of myocardial ischaemia doubles the risk of mortality in the years following surgery.

The incidence of perioperative myocardial infarction varies from 1.3 to 6% according to the different studies and the deleterious effect of a perioperative myocardial damage on short and long term survival of the surgical patients is now firmly established [1, 2]. Along with immediate postoperative mortality should be added the repercussions of myocardial infarction on the life expectancy of the operated patients. They are of particular importance since the occurrence of perioperative myocardial infarction even located to the subendocardium multiplies the mortality rate by 7 in the first two postoperative years [6].

The dosage of cardiac troponin in the plasma which can be determined routinely in numerous laboratories, now provides a highly specific marker for acute myocardial necrosis, the result of which is not affected by surgery [7]. This biological marker, which should be dosed at any moment during the operating period whenever myocardial infarction is suspected, enables a very reliable diagnosis of this complication in clinical practice. The plasmatic troponin level observed after surgery shows the extent of myocardial cellular necrosis which influences morbidity and mortality of this complication in the short and medium term [8].

Two essential mechanisms, hypercoagulability and circulatory problems are involved in the constitution of acute postoperative myocardial necrosis. These two mechanisms are favoured by intra and postoperative haemodynamic and metabolic constraints [9, 10]. They appear individually or more often in association. In fact, each mechanism favours and/or potentializes the deleterious effects of the other on myocardial oxygenation. Indeed, coagulation disorders restrict perfusion of the sub-endocardic layers (those most threatened by ischaemia) by encouraging the formation of micro-thrombi in the coronary arteries or in the intra-myocardial arterioles.

Studies undertaken in the 1980s when postoperative myocardial infarction was detected by means of electrocardiogram recordings every 12 hours following operation [11, 12] suggested that this complication occurred on the second or third postoperative day. More recent studies where postoperative myocardial necrosis has been detected by means of continuous electrocardiogram in the operative period on by repeated troponin dosages have revealed that, in fact, postoperative myocardial infarction appears much earlier between 12 and 32 hours after the end of surgery [5, 7, 8]. In all these studies, myocardial infarction is preceded by episodes of myocardial ischaemia. Therefore, acute postoperative myocardial necrosis appears not as a fatality on the third day, but rather as the consequence of episodes of myocardial ischaemia occurring during surgery or in the first postoperative day.

Better knowledge of the physiopathological mechanisms involved in postoperative coronary complications now enables to define perioperative managements for CAD patients undergoing non cardiac surgery and thus limit the coronary risk of anaesthesia. Since ischaemic episodes have not been raised during anaesthesia, one can consider that the problems posed by perioperative management have been solved. This is not the case postoperatively. After surgery, humoral mechanical inflammatory and hypercoagulability phenomena add up their deleterious effects on myocardial oxygen balance.

Pharmacological management: when should we use what medication?

The main goal of the perioperative management of CAD patients undergoing non cardiac surgery is to limit postoperative stress and to control increased sympathetic tone or its circulatory effects [13].

β blockers

Since the use of postoperative epidural analgesia may be limited, numerous authors have envisaged the administration of cardiovascular medication to effectively limit the sympathetic stimulation which persists several days after surgery. Two types of cardiovascular drugs have been recommended: β adrenergic blocking drugs and α-2 adrenoreceptor agonists.

Administered prior to anaesthesia, β blockers very significantly limit the haemodynamic response to noxious stimuli related to surgery and to postoperative metabolic stress [14]. Furthermore, these agents do not increase the hypotensive effects of general anaesthesia [14-16]. In vascular surgery patients, suffering from poorly-controlled hypertension, the preoperative administration of β blockers was effective to blunt the increased blood pressure and tachycardia and to prevent myocardial ischaemia associated with intubation and the recovery period (16). β blockers administered by intravenous route and then orally as soon as abdominal transit has resumed also have a beneficial effect in the days following surgery. In a recent study, prophylactic β-blocking therapy was installed throughout the operative period, to patients with coronary risk factors [17]. Continuous electrocardiogram recordings with the holter method used in this study, confirmed that the administration of atenolol decreased by half the incidence of episodes of post-operative myocardial ischaemia [15]. Whereas the incidence of postoperative complications observed on leaving hospital did not differ in the group receiving β blockers vs the placebo group of patients, the occurrence of coronary complications in the year following surgery was significantly decreased in the patients receiving β blockers during the week of surgery. The follow-up of patients two years after the operation showed that survival rate was improved in those receiving atenolol (90% compared to 79% in the placebo group) and that a smaller percentage of patients was free from any cardiovascular incident in the treated group (83% vs 68%) [17]. Therefore, interactions between the β blockers and circulatory response to anaesthesia and surgery are much more beneficial than deleterious. The patients operated upon fully benefit from the beneficial effects of this medication on myocardial oxygen balance without any threat to their circulatory system. These beneficial effects appear to improve the cardiac risk of anaesthesia in the medium and long term.

α-2 adrenoceptors agonists

The α-2 adrenoceptors agonists have been used as anti-hypertensive medication for a long time now. In fact, they possess many other properties which result from a large distribution of the α-2 adrenergic receptors in the body and their contributions to different physiologial regulations [18]. Apart from their haemo-dynamic properties, which limit the acceleration of heart rate and the increase in the loading condition of the heart which characterizes the postoperative period, another major property of the α-2 adrenoceptors agonists is that of inducing se-dation and providing analgesia, thus decreasing the overall metabolic postopera-tive stress [19, 20].

In the perioperative period the α-2 adrenoceptors agonists have a particularly marked beneficial effect, as they directly oppose step by step all the physiologi-cal mechanisms which may lead to the occurrence of heart failure or acute coro-nary complications. In fact, they very successfully limit the increase in plasma catecholamines, control the rise in global oxygen consumption and spectacular-ly anticipate postoperative shivering [19-22]. As a result, the incidence of episodes of postoperative ischaemia is significantly diminished with the admin-istration of preventive α-2 adrenoceptors agonists [23].

α-2 adrenoceptors agonists can be safety administered several days after sur-gery as they "modulate" but not totally block the sympathetic system and inter-feres little with the chronotropic, inotropic and vasopressor effects of its agonists [8]. Today, one of the limitations of their prophylactic administration is related to the duration of effect of clonidine characterized by a long half life elimina-tion. This is why the two α-2 adrenoreceptors agonists which are being devel-oped (mivazerol [23] and dexmedetomidine [24]) and which have a much short-er half-life, appear in practice to be much better adapted to perioperative admin-istration (in continuous perfusion) in high risk cardiac patients undergoing sur-gery [23]. Mivazerol is a drug with α-2 agonist properties which reduces sympa-thetic outflow (spinal and/or post-ganglionic) and effectively controls the in-crease in plasma catecholamines, heart rate and blood pressure which occur in the postoperative period. As a result, the incidence of postoperative ischaemia is significantly diminished. It has been shown that mivazerol can be safely admin-istered several days after surgery. Because of its much shorter half-life (com-pared with clonidine), it appears in practice to be well adapted to perioperative administration (in continuous perfusion: 1.5 mcg/kg/hour) in high risk cardiac patients undergoing surgery. This rationale led to carry out a final outcome study: to determine whether a continuous (double blind) infusion of mivazerol given during non cardiac surgery and during 3 postoperative days will reduce perioperative incidence of myocardial infarction and death. Initially, patients with or at risk for CAD were included, but early experience showed that the overall event rate was so low (4%) in those at risk that no significant benefit could be expected. Assessments of the primary end point were restricted, there-fore the results of this final outcome study reinforce those of an intermediate outcome study which showed that mivazerol reduced perioperative tachycardia and ischaemia. They lead to envisage more extended administration of mivazerol in patients with documented history of CAD undergoing vascular surgery to the cardiac risk of surgery in this high risk population: to 1897 patients with previous documented CAD. Overall, there was a 12% decrease in myocardial infarction and/or death and a 37% reduction in all cause deaths in the mivazerol group, but neither decline was statistically significant. However, a pre-planned test of heterogeneity revealed that the vascular surgery group was the only stratum with reasonable power (about 60%) to detect the 33% risk reduction. In the subgroup the beneficial effects of mivazerol were readily apparent since this α-2 agonists reduced the incidence of 1) MI death (primary objective) by 32% ($p < 0.04$), 2) death from all causes by 59% ($p < 0.03$), 3) cardiac death by 68% ($p < 0.02$).

In conclusion, interactions between the β blockers and circulatory response to anaesthesia and surgery are much more beneficial than deleterious. Administered pre, intra and postoperatively, β blockers very significantly limit the haemodynamic response to noxious stimuli, decrease the incidence of myocardial ischaemia and the occurrence of coronary complications in the year following surgery. The α-2 adrenoceptors agonists have a particularly marked beneficial effect, as they directly oppose step by step all the physiological mechanisms which lead to perioperative heart failure or acute coronary complications. As a result, the incidence of episodes of postoperative ischaemia is significantly diminished. They can be safety administered several days after surgery as they "modulate" but not totally block the sympathetic system. The α-2 adrenoreceptors agonists which are being developed (mivazerol and dexmedetomidine) and which have a quite short half-life, appear in practice to be well adapted to perioperative administration. On the grounds of the results of the multicenter study which demonstrated that mivazerol significantly limit postoperative cardiac complications and improve survival rate in CAD patients, we can envisage more extended prophylactic administration of this agent to improve cardiac risk of surgery.

References

1. Mangano DT (1990) Perioperative cardiac morbidity (review). Anesthesiology 72:153-184
2. Mangano DT, Browner WS, Hollenberg M et al (1990) Associations of perioperative myocardial ischemia with cardiac morbidity and mortality in men undergoing non cardiac surgery. N Engl J Med 323:1781-1788
3. McCann RL, Clements FM (1989) Silent myocardial ischemia in patients undergoing peripheral vascular surgery: Incidence and association with perioperative cardiac morbidity and mortality. J Vasc Surg 9:583-587
4. Raby KE, Barry J, Creager MA et al (1992) Detection and significance of intraoperative and postoperative myocardial ischemia in peripheral vascular surgery. JAMA 268:222-227
5. Landesberg G, Luria MH, Cotev S et al (1993) Importance of long-duration postoperative ST-segment depression in cardiac morbidity after vascular surgery. Lancet 341:715-719
6. Mangano DT, Browner WS, Hollenberg M, Tateo IM (1992) Long term cardiac prognosis following non cardiac surgery. JAMA 268:233-239
7. Adams J, Sicard A, Allen T et al (1994) Diagnosis of perioperative myocardial infarction with measurement of cardiac troponin I. N Engl J Med 330:670-674
8. Metzler H, Gries M, Rehak P et al (1997) Perioperative myocardial cell injury: the role of troponins. Br J Anaesth 78:386-390
9. Collins GJ, Barber JA, Zajtchuk R et al (1977) The effects of postoperative stress on the coagulation profile. Am J Surg 133:612-616
10. Rosenfeld B, Beattie C, Christopherson R et al (1993) The effects of different anesthetic regimen on fibrinolysis and the development of postoperative arterial thrombosis. Anesthesiology 79:435-443
11. Tarhan, Moffitt EA, Taylor WF, Giuliani ER (1972) Myocardial infarction after general anesthesia. JAMA 220:1451-1454
12. Rao, Jacobs KH, Al-Etr AA (1983) Reinfarction following anesthesia in patients with myocardial infarction. Anesthesiology 59:499-505
13. Goldman L (1992) Perioperative myocardial ischemia. To every thing there is a season. Anesthesiology 76:331-333
14. Warltier DC (1998) Beta-adrenergic-blocking drugs: Incredibly useful, incredibly underutilized. Anesthesiology 88:2-5
15. Mangano DT, Layug EL, Wallace A et al (1996) Effect of atenolol on mortality and cardiovascular morbidity after noncardiac surgery. N Engl J Med 335:1713-1720
16. Stone JG, Foex P, Sear JW et al (1988) Myocardial ischemia in untreated hypertensive patients: effect of a single small oral dose of a beta-adrenergic blocking agent. Anesthesiology 68:495
17. Wallace A, Layug B, Tateo I et al (1998) Prophylactic atenolol reduces postoperative myocardial ischemia. Anesthesiology 88:7-17
18. Longnecker DE (1987) Alpine Anesthesia. Can pretreatment with clonidine decrease the peaks and valleys? Anesthesiology 67:1-2
19. Ellis JE, Drijvers G, Pedlow S et al (1994) Premedication with oral and transdermal clonidine provides safe and efficacious postoperative sympatholysis. Anesth Analg 79:1133-1140
20. Quintin L, Viale JP, Annat G et al (1991) Oxygen uptake after major abdominal surgery: effect of clonidine. Anesthesiology 74:236-241
21. Quintin L, Bouilloc X, Butin E et al (1996) Clonidine for major vascular surgery in hypertensive patients: a double-blind, controlled, randomized study. Anesth Analg 83:687-695
22. Delaunay L, Bonnet F, Liu N et al (1993) Clonidine comparably decreases the thermoregulatory thresholds for vasoconstriction and shivering in humans. Anesthesiology 79:470-474
23. McSpi, European Research Group (1997) Perioperative sympatholysis. Anesthesiology 86:346-363
24. Jalonen J, Hynynen M, Kuitunen A et al (1997) Dexmedetomidine as an anesthetic adjunct in coronary artery bypass grafting. Anesthesiology 86:331-345

Biochemical Markers of Myocardial Cell Injury

H. Metzler, M. Gries, S. Fruhwald, W. Toller

Clinical symptoms, ECG, biochemical markers

The assessment of myocardial cell injury and infarction is usually based on the combination of clinical symptoms, electrocardiographic changes and a particular pattern of biochemical markers.

For nonsurgical patients WHO criteria for the diagnosis of acute myocardial infarction (AMI) requires that at least two of the following three elements be present [1]:

1. History of ischaemic type - chest discomfort
2. Evolutionary changes on serially obtained ECG tracings
3. Rise and fall in biochemical cardiac markers.

In surgical patients undergoing noncardiac surgery the assessment of injury and infarction is more difficult. Definition problems arise from the low incidence of typical chest discomfort (only about 15%) because of anaesthesia, analgesia, sedation and surgery-related pain [2-4]. Perioperative ECG changes indicating myocardial ischaemia or infarction are also of limited sensitivity and specificity. ST-segment changes may not be ischaemia-related, but may result from electrolyte abnormalities, controlled ventilation, etc. Uncodeable ECGs (left bundle branch block, pacemaker ECG, etc.) may not allow interpretation. In contrast to nonsurgical patients with predominant Q-wave infarction this type of AMI occurs not so frequently in the perioperative period (only about 20%) [2, 4, 5].

The limited information of perioperative ECG findings and the low incidence of typical chest pain emphazise the need to look for biochemical markers allowing early and definite assessment of myocardial cell injury and infarction.

Biochemical markers: benefits and problems

An ideal marker of myocardial cell injury should:

– be found in high concentrations in myocardium
– not be found in other tissues

– be released rapidly and completely after injury
– be released in direct proportion to the extent of myocardial injury
– persist in plasma for several hours to provide a convenient diagnostic time window [6].

For more than three decades creatine kinase (CK) and the MB-isoenzyme (CK-MB) have been the test of choice for the detection and confirmation of AMI. CK is abundant in most tissues. Results with sensitive assays have shown that most skeletal muscles contain small amounts of CK-MB (1-3%) [6]. Therefore, increases of CK-MB in plasma are only attributable to release from myocardium in the absence of conditions known to increase CK-MB in muscle [6]. Especially in the perioperative and intensive care setting CK-MB increases are often not-specific for myocardial cell injury. Because of these limitations alternative markers have been investigated. Kinetics of and potential indications for new molecular markers are listed in Table 1 and 2 [7].

According to their origin, the available cardiac markers can be subdivided into three different groups.

Table 1. Kinetics of new molecular markers for acute myocardial infarction

Marker	Molecular weight D	First rise h	Peak (occlusion) h	Peak (reperfusion) h	Return to normal
CK-MB (mass)	86,000	4	24	16	48-72 h
CK-MB subforms	86,000	2	10	?	?
Myoglobin	17,800	2	6-7	4	24 h
Troponin T	33,000	2-4	38	14	10-20 d
Troponin I	22,500	2-4	16	12	6-8 d

CK, creatine kinase
(Reproduced with permission of Lippincott Williams & Wilkins)

Table 2. Potential indications for new molecular markers

	CK-MB (mass)	CK-MB subforms	Myoglobin	Troponin T	Troponin I
Early infarction	Potential use	Useful	Useful	Potential use	Potential use
Late infarction	No use	No use	No use	Useful	
Reperfusion	Useful		Useful	Useful	
Unstable angina	No use	Potential use		Useful	
Infarct size	Useful		No use	Useful	
Myocarditis	No use		No use	Potential use	
Perioperative infarction	No use		No use	Useful	Useful
AMI with skeletal muscle injury	No use	No use	No use	Useful	Useful

AMI, acute myocardial infarction; CK, creatine kinase
(Reproduced with permission of Lippincott Williams & Wilkins)

Free cytosolic proteins

– Myoglobin

– Fatty acid binding proteins (FABP)

– Glycogen phosphorylase BB isoforms

– CK, CK-MB

They are rapidly washed out from a damaged myocardium into the circulation, are particularly useful for the early detection of AMI and for monitoring of the perfusion of the infarcted zone. Because of its low molecular weight (17 800) and rapid kinetics, myoglobin is currently the earliest marker in clinical use. It is elevated within two hours after the onset of AMI. The presence in both cardiac and skeletal muscle limits its usefulness in the perioperative period.

Structural bound proteins

– Myosin light and heavy chains (MLC, MHC)

They are released after degradation of contractile proteins, which is a time consuming process, independent from perfusion. These markers are useful to test the size of AMI.

Combined markers

– Troponin-T, Troponin-I

– Tropomyosin (?)

Some proteins, especially Troponin-T and I, are both structural proteins of striated muscle fibers and are found in small concentrations in the cytosolic pool. The contractile apparatus consists of two different filaments, the thick and thin ones. The thick filament consists of myosin molecules with two heavy chains (MHC) and four light chains (MLC). The thin filament comprises actin, tropomyosin and troponin-complexes (Fig. 1) [8].

Now, commercial immuno-assays with high specificity are available for cardiac troponin-T (cTNT) and cardiac troponin-I (cTNI).

TNT and TNI have been shown to be equally effective as markers for diagnosis of AMI and injury in patients with unstable angina. There are, however, some differences between these two proteins [9]. The molecular weight of TNT and TNI are 37 000 and 24 000 dalton resp. Despite the larger size, TNT is released earlier than TNI, possibly because of a 6 to 8% free cytosolic pool compared to 2.8 to 4.1% free TNI. In addition, TNT exists as a relatively stable complex, whereas TNI appears predominantly as a binary complex and nearly no free TNI. Free TNI is bound to other proteins and surfaces because of its hydrophobic nature.

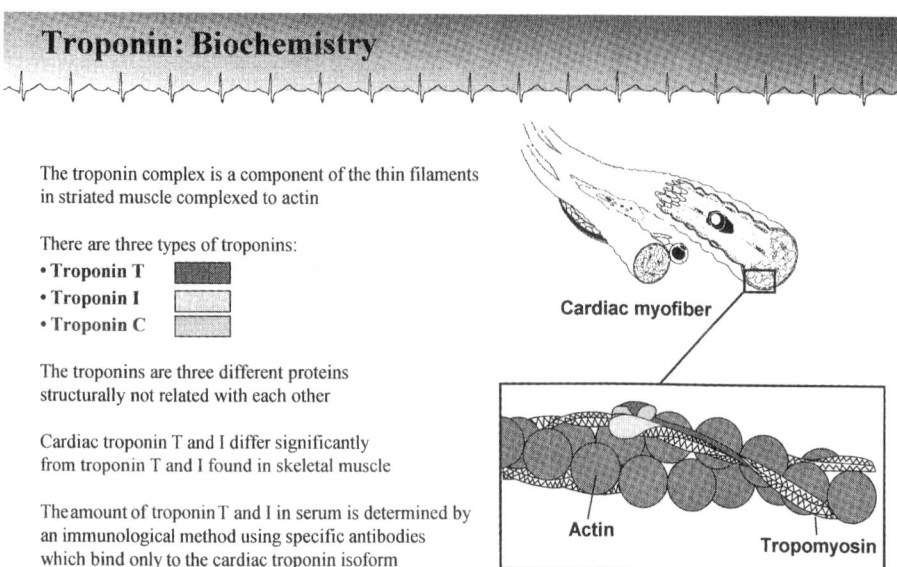

Fig. 1.

The role of troponins to assess perioperative myocardial cell injury

In 1994 Adams et al. published the first study using the new marker troponin [10]. They demonstrated the high sensitivity and specificity of troponin for the diagnosis of perioperative AMI avoiding the high incidence of false diagnosis associated with the use of CK-MB. Lee et al. investigated 1175 patients undergoing major noncardiac surgery [11]. Analysis indicated that troponin-T had a performance for the diagnosis of AMI similar to CK-MB, but a significantly better correlation with other major cardiac complications in patients without definite infarction. They also evaluated the prognostic significance of TNT and found that values > 0.1 ng/ml were an independent correlate of cardiac events [12]. Recently, Metzler et al. studied 67 cardiac risk patients undergoing noncardiac surgery [13]. All patients with normal TNT had a good outcome. Patients with only slightly elevated TNT concentrations (0.32 to 0.99 ng/ml) also had a good outcome indicating some degree of minor myocardial cell injury, whereas patients with cardiac complications had higher TNT concentrations (0.47 to 9.8 ng/ml) (Fig. 2). Because of the excellent results, troponin-T will probably be included into the definition criteria of AMI in large scale trials [2, 4].

In the future there is an increasing interest, not only to properly assess perioperative AMI, but also to detect "minor myocardial cell injury" which may have an impact on outcome. Lee et al. and Metzler et al. demonstrated in their studies that increases of TNT – without an AMI by traditional definition – may result in cardiac complications, like LV-dysfunction, congestive heart failure and

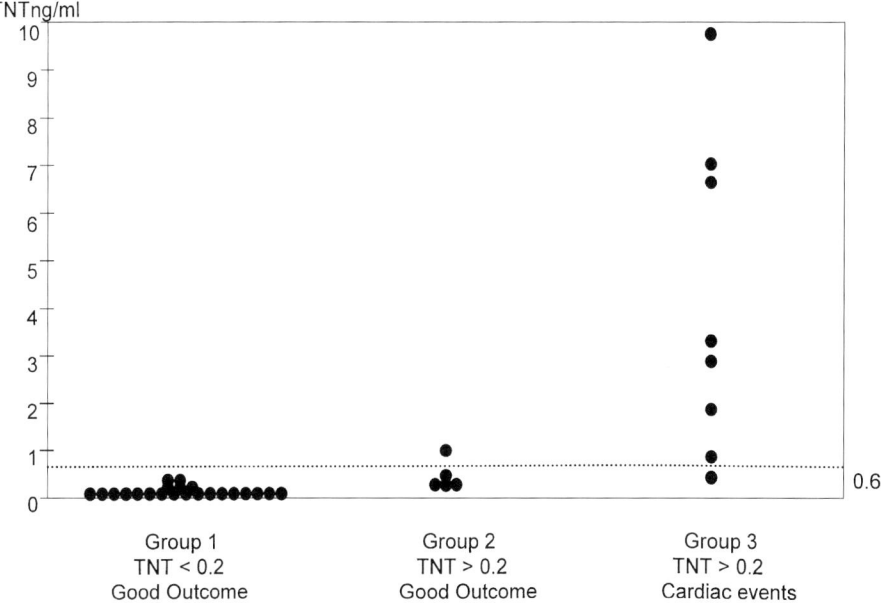

Fig. 2. TNT-concentrations in relation to outcome (Reproduced with permission of BMJ Publishing Group)

severe arrhythmias. In the cardiologic literature large scale trials confirmed, that troponins are superior compared to routine CK and CK-MB laboratory tests in patients with unstable angina [14-17]. Cardiac troponins are also used more frequently in critically ill patients to assess other myocardial cell injury. Guest et al. determined the incidence of myocardial cell injury in 209 critically ill patients [18]. Defined by elevated levels of troponin, myocardial injury was relatively high (15%) and associated with increased morbidity and mortality.

Conclusions

1. A low incidence of typical, ischaemia-related chest pain and a decreased sensitivity and specificity of ECG are typical for the perioperative period and aggravate the proper detection of myocardial cell injury and infarction.

2. Although the traditional biochemical markers, like myoglobin, CK and CK-MB are still the standard biochemical tests for the diagnosis of AMI in non-surgical patients, the applicability of these tests is limited in surgical patients because of decreased specificity.

3. New biochemical markers, especially the troponins T and I, offer a new dimension. Because of their characteristics, their high sensitivity and speci-

ficity, they seem to have substantial advantages if they are used in the perioperative scenario.

4. In addition to the proper assessment of perioperative AMI, the new markers
   give the clinician the opportunity also to detect minor myocardial cell injury
   and to quantify myocardial damage.

5. Similar to findings in cardiologic studies, these new markers may help to
   improve risk stratification and to predict perioperative short and long-term
   outcome in surgical patients.

References

1. Antman EM, E Braunwald (1997) Acute myocardial infarction, 5th edn. In: Braunwald E (ed)
   Heart Disease. WB Saunders, Philadelphia, pp 1184-1202
2. Oliver M, Goldman L, Desmond J et al (1998) Effect of mivazerol on peri-operative cardiac
   complications during non-cardiac surgery in patients with coronary heart disease: The European Mivazerol Trial (EMIT). Lancet (in press)
3. Ashton CM, Petersen NJ, Wray NP et al (1993) The incidence of perioperative myocardial infarction in men undergoing noncardiac surgery. Ann Intern Med 118:504-510
4. Badner NH, Knill RL, Brown JE et al (1998) Myocardial infarction after noncardiac surgery.
   Anesthesiology 88:572-578
5. Landesberg G, Luria MH, Cotev S et al (1993) Importance of long-duration postoperative ST-
   segment depression in cardiac morbidity after vascular surgery. Lancet 341:715-719
6. Adams JE, Abendschein DR, Jaffe AS (1993) Biochemical markers of myocardial injury: Is
   MB creatine kinase the choice for the 1990s? Circulation 88:750-763
7. Hamm CW, Katus HA (1995) New biochemical markers for myocardial cell injury. Curr
   Opin Cardiol 10:355-360
8. Mair J, Dienstl F, Puschendorf B (1992) Cardiac troponin T in the diagnosis of myocardial injury. Crit Rev Clin Lab Sci 29:31-57
9. Wu AHB (1998) Biochemical differences betwen cTnT and cTnI and its significance for diagnosis of acute coronary syndromes. European Expert Panel Meeting Cardiac Markers, Sor-
   rento, Italy
10. Adams JE, Sigard GA, Allen BT et al (1994) Diagnosis of perioperative myocardial infarc-
    tion with measurement of cardiac troponin I. N Engl J Med 330:670-674
11. Lee TH, Thomas EJ, Ludwig LE et al (1996) Troponin T as a marker for myocardial ischemia
    in patients undergoing major noncardiac surgery. Am J Cardiol 77:1031-1036
12. Lopez-Jimenez F, Goldman L, Sacks DB et al (1997) Prognostic value of cardiac troponin T
    after noncardiac surgery: 6-month follow up data. J Am Coll Cardiol 29:1241-1245
13. Metzler H, Gries M, Rehak P et al (1997) Perioperative myocardial cell injury: the role of tro-
    ponins. Br J Anaesth 78:386-390
14. Hamm CW, Ravkilde J, Gerhard W et al (1992) The prognostic value of serum troponin T in
    unstable angina. N Engl J Med 327:146-150
15. Seino Y, Tomita Y, Takano T et al (1993) Early identification of cardiac events with serum tro-
    ponin T in patients with unstable angina. Lancet 342:1236-1237
16. Lindah B (1997) Troponin T identifies patients with unstable coronary artery disease who
    benefit from long-term antithrombotic protection. J Am Coll Cardiol 29:43-48
17. Ohman EM, Armstrong PW, Christenson RH et al (1996) Cardiac troponin T levels for risk
    stratification in acute myocardial ischemia. N Engl J Med 335:1333-1341
18. Guest TM, Ramanathan AV, Tuteur PG et al (1995) Myocardial injury in critically ill patients.
    JAMA 273:1945-1949

Postoperative Intensive Care Therapy - In Which Patients and for How Long?

T. MÖLLHOFF

Cardiovascular disease is the leading cause of death in developed and undeveloped countries. It is estimated that in the beginning of the next millenium 33% of all patients undergoing surgery will be older than 65 years of age or having two or more cardiovascular risk factors. 10% of these patients at risk for cardiovascular complications in the perioperative period will suffer a myocardial infarction [1]. In a recently published study in patients at risk for perioperative myocardial infarction (PMI) by Badner et al., the incidence of PMI was 5.6% of which 17% were fatal [2]. Two major findings of this study are of great importance for postoperative surveillance of patients at risk:

1. only 17% of all patients experiencing PMI had chest pain whereas 56% of the patients had other clinical signs;
2. the majority of PMI occurred on the day of surgery.

PMI in these high risk patients will result in a decreased 2 year survival rate by at least 50%, thereby increasing aggregate world health care costs by an additional 50 billion dollars [3].

Identifying preoperative risk factors

Two recent guidelines have been published on perioperative evaluation and management of cardiac risk patients undergoing noncardiac surgery [4, 5]. Whereas the American College of Physicians provides an evidence-based approach to preoperative risk stratification, the American College of Cardiology and the American Heart Association (ACC/AHA) define the optimal perioperative management for the high risk patient based on the evidence as well as expert opinion.

The original publication by Goldman et al. [6] describing a cardiac risk index to predict perioperative cardiac complications has been modified by a lot of investigators who implemented risk factors for cardiac complications like angina and major vascular surgery in their risk index [7]. In all studies the highest perioperative risk resulted from the presence of congestive heart failure. However, it is clinically important to distinguish heart failure from a non-ischaemic origin from patients with ischaemic cardiomyopathy at high risk for ventricular dysfunction and perioperative myocardial infarction.

Major clinical predictors of increased perioperative risk according to the guidelines of the ACC/AHA include [5]:

1. recent myocardial infarction
2. unstable or severe angina (Canadian Class III or IV)
3. decompensated congestive heart failure
4. significant arrhythmias
5. severe valvular diseases

Traditionally, recent myocardial infarction has been an important risk, particularly within 3-6 months after the event. However, recent advances in the management of MI has led the ACC/AHA to the definition that the acute period only includes the first thirty days. However, high risk can continue up to six weeks after MI and it seems reasonable to await this time period before proceeding with elective surgery [5].

Intermediate risk factors include:

1. angina (Canadian Class I or II)
2. prior MI by history or pathological Q-waves
3. compensated or prior congestive heart failure
4. Diabetes mellitus

Minor risk factors include advanced age, abnormal ECG, rhythm other than sinus, low functional capacity, history of stroke, and uncontrolled hypertension.

It also has to be stressed that the surgical procedure itself has been stratified to cardiac risk and is related to several important factors.

1. The type of surgery itself may identify a patient with greater likelihood of underlying heart disease. Major vascular surgery for example is associated with among the highest incidence of cardiac complications [8] because underlying coronary artery disease is present in a substantial portion of patients.

2. The degree of haemodynamic cardiac stress associated with surgery-specific techniques. Certain operations may be associated with profound alterations in heart rate, blood pressure, vascular volume, pain, bleeding, clotting tendencies, oxygenation, neurohumoral activation, and others.

3. The quality of anaesthesia during surgery. For example, one study did not find any difference in patients' outcome in vascular surgery regardless of the anaesthetic technique. However, in a group of patients that had inadequate spinal anaesthesia so that the anaesthetic regimen had to be switched to general anaesthesia, mortality was significantly higher [9]. In another study comparing morphine/halothane anaesthesia to sufentanil anaesthesia in congenital heart surgery, intraoperative determination of stress hormones re-

vealed significantly higher epinephrine and norepinephrine levels in the halothane/morphine group resulting in higher postoperative morbidity [10].

The ACC/AHA has published cardiac risk stratification for noncardiac surgical procedures [5].

Surgical procedures accompanied by a high incidence of perioperative cardiac complications (> 5%) include emergent major operations (particularly in the elderly), aortic-, peripheral-, and major vascular surgery, and prolonged surgical procedures that are associated with large fluid shifts and/or blood loss.

Intermediate cardiac risk (< 5%) results from carotid endarterectomy, head and neck surgery, intraperitoneal, intrathoracic, orthopaedic and prostate surgery.

At low risk (< 1%) are patients undergoing endoscopic or superficial procedures, cataract and breast surgery.

Monitoring the cardiac risk patient in the postoperative period

Perioperative myocardial ischaemia can be documented by serial electrocardiography analyses. Perioperative myocardial infarction can be documented by ECG, cardiac-specific enzyme analyses, echocardiography and radioisotopic studies specific for myocardial necrosis. However, nonspecific ST and T wave changes that are not associated with impaired outcome have been described in the postoperative period. Cardiac enzyme analyses usually check CK-MB and/or cardiac troponin-I or troponin-T, the latter have also been linked to short and long-term prognosis [11]. There are only few studies that have examined the optimal protocol for diagnosing a perioperative myocardial infarction. In patients without evidence of CAD, surveillance should be restricted to patients who develop signs of cardiovascular dysfunction. In patients with known or suspected heart disease undergoing procedures with a high incidence of cardiovascular morbidity, it is recommended that ECGs at baseline, immediately after the surgical procedure (in the recovery room), and daily on the first two days postoperatively have to be performed. Measurements of cardiac enzymes are best reserved for patients at high risk or those who demonstrate ECG or haemodynamic evidence of cardiovascular dysfunction [5].

Invasive monitoring (i.e. arterial and central venous line) might be necessary in selected patients.

The use of pulmonary artery catheterization has recently been questioned [12]. However, the ACC/AHA recommends use of the PAC in patients at risk for major haemodynamic disturbances who are undergoing a procedure that is likely to cause these haemodynamic changes (i.e. aortic aneurysm repair in a patient with angina). These patients have to be observed on an intermediate or critical care unit.

Therapeutic strategies in the postoperative period

Overall it is important to stress that the patient with heart disease is not necessarily at risk during anaesthesia, however, the problem starts during emergence and the immediate postoperative phase. This is also the time period of the occurrence of most ischaemic events and perioperative myocardial infarctions. Multiple promising approaches for the best intra- and postoperative management have been published. While there is no evidence that there is a best intraoperative technique (i.e. regional versus general anaesthesia) different perioperative strategies have aimed at improving patients short and long-term outcome. Overall, perioperative administration of atenolol has improved short and long-term outcome of cardiac risk patients undergoing noncardiac procedures [13]. Thus, the perioperative use of atenolol in patients with known coronary artery disease (CAD) or risk factors for CAD has been recommended by the American College of Physicians [4]. Other promising strategies include the use of α-2-agonists like mivazerol [14] or the use of thoracic epidural anaesthesia [15, 16]. The patients having epidural anaesthesia/analgesia have demonstrated lower opiate dosages, better ablation of the catecholamine response, and a less hypercoagulable state [17]. Most important, an effective analgesic regimen has to be included in the perioperative plan, which should be supervised by an acute pain service. Most studies that did not find a difference in outcome between general and regional anaesthesia have implemented the following postoperative strategies:

1. effective postoperative analgesia (i.e. by epidural [18, 19], or intravenous analgesia [19]). Last year, Bois and co-workers published their results of TEA in vascular surgery. Postoperative analgesia using the epidural catheter was continued for 24 hours. In this study pain (VAS) was significantly reduced in the epidural group. However, there was a clear trend that in patients treated with TEA there was an improvement regarding the occurrence of myocardial ischaemia [19];

2. postoperative surveillance either on an intermediate care or a post anaesthetic care unit [9, 18, 20].

General ward – intermediate care unit – critical care unit – which patient where?

In order to determine which patient has to be transferred to a specialized unit, a description of the different standards of care between general ward, intermediate care unit, and critical care is given.

General ward

Under normal circumstances the general ward is not able to give the same safety standards as the recovery room in patients after surgery because the number of nursing personal is not comparable. Additionally, continuous monitoring of vital parameters (ECG, invasive blood pressure measurement, breathing, pulse oximetry) is usually not applicable in the general ward.

Intermediate care unit

In most hospitals so called "intermediate care units" have been established. They are usually operated by the surgeon. However, a surgeon may not be continuously on the ward. The nursing ratio is usually based on acuity. The minimum nurse/patient ratio is 1:3 with ability to increase 1:2 if acuity demands. A continuous postoperative surveillance even with invasive monitoring is performed on these wards. Noninvasive ventilation can be performed on these wards as well as differentiated drug therapy of heart failure. In some intermediate wards, especially those run by cardiac surgeons or cardiologists, mechanical support of the heart (intra-aortic-balloon pumping) is performed. However, for more invasive procedures like mechanical ventilation, continuous veno-venous haemofiltration and others patients have to be transferred to the critical care unit.

Critical care unit

The following principles categorize the critical care unit as described by the Society of Critical Care Medicine [21]:

1. Critical care units appropriately concentrate critically ill patients within specified areas of the hospital.
2. Within these units, there is concentrated not only the equipment and supplies necessary to support these patients, but also the personnel with special training and expertise in the care of the critically ill.
3. Patients in critical care units must be cared for by specially trained nurses.
4. The management of critically ill patients must involve the participation of specially trained physicians that shall be readily available throughout the 24-hr day.
5. Efficient delivery of care to the critically ill patient depends on "state-of-the-art" support services and equipment.
6. The nurse/patient ratio is minimum 1:2 with ability to increase to 1:1, or 2:1 if acuity demands.

To determine which patient needs postoperative surveillance on the intermediate care or the critical care unit several principals have to be stated:

1. preoperative risk stratification is mandatory, and patients preoperative status might warrant postoperative surveillance on the intermediate ward or on the critical care unit;
2. the surgical procedure itself demands postoperative care on the intermediate ward or critical care unit;

3. perioperative complications in the cardiac risk patient undergoing noncardiac surgery warrant postoperative surveillance and therapy on the intermediate ward or critical care unit, regardless of preoperative risk factors and surgery specific risks.

It is not feasible and necessary (and also financially not applicable) to demand continuous surveillance for every cardiac risk patient undergoing noncardiac surgery. For example, a patient with intermediate or minor risk factors with moderate or excellent functional capacity undergoing noncardiac procedure could be transferred to the general ward after uneventful stay in the recovery room.

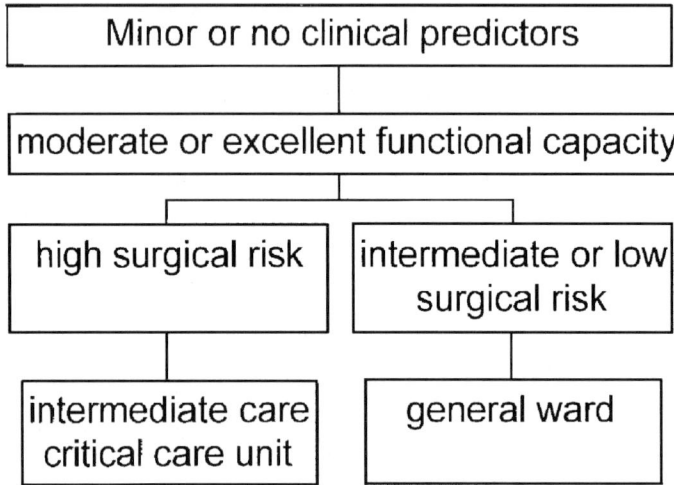

Fig. 1. Postoperative transferral of patients with minor or no clinical predictors of cardiac risk and moderate or excellent functional capacity

However, in patients with major cardiac risk factors as described above elective surgery is usually cancelled. When surgery is performed of whatsoever reason the patient has to be transferred to an intermediate care ward or even to the critical care unit. Here, medical management and risk factor modification is performed, and the subsequent care is dictated by the findings and treatment results [5].

If intermediate clinical predictors have been identified, the patients functional capacity is poor, and the patient is subjected to elective surgery of whatsoever reason, the patient has to be transferred to an intermediate ward postoperatively for postoperative surveillance, risk stratification, and risk reduction. Preoperative identification of cardiac risk factors is mandatory for perioperative management of these patients at increased risk.

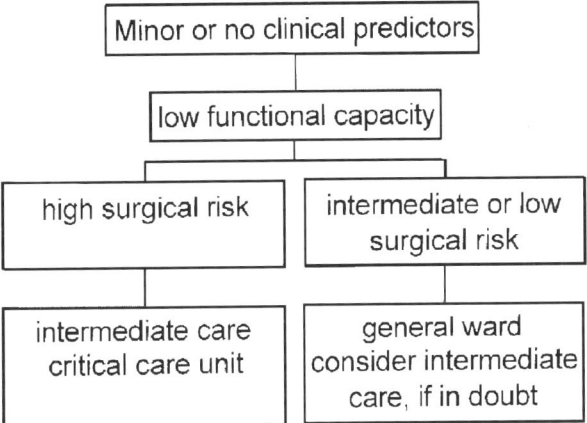

Fig. 2. Postoperative transferral of patients with minor or no clinical predictors of cardiac risk and low functional capacity

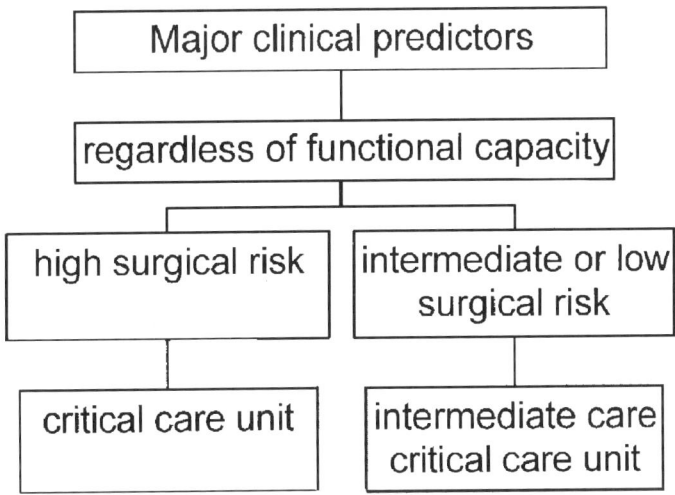

Fig. 3. Postoperative transferral of patients with major clinical predictors of cardiac risk

In conclusion four important observations are highlighted:

1. In case of perioperative cardiac deterioration (congestive heart failure, myocardial ischaemia, myocardial infarction and others) postoperative transferral to an intermediate or critical unit might be necessary.

2. Preoperative low functional capacity or poor ASA physical status might warrant postoperative transferral to the intermediate care or even critical care unit.

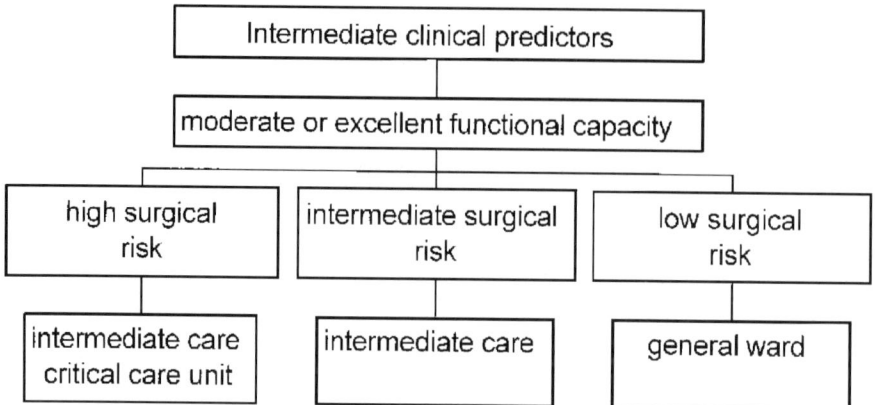

Fig. 4. Postoperative transferral of patients with intermediate clinical predictors of cardiac risk and moderate or excellent functional capacity

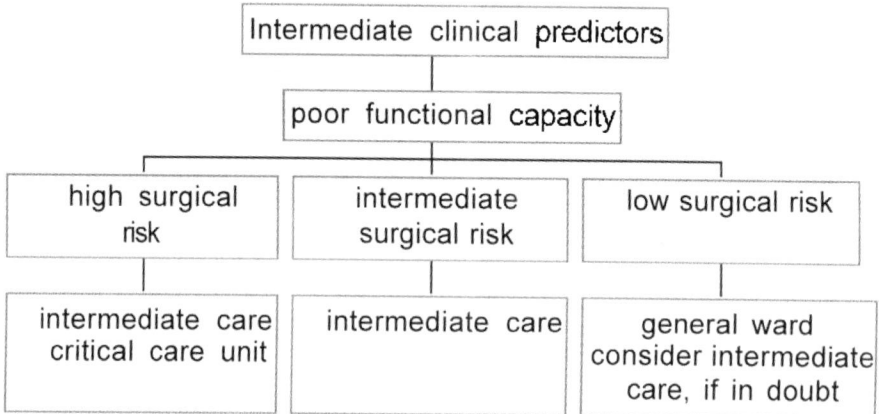

Fig. 5. Postoperative transferral of patients with intermediate clinical predictors of cardiac risk and poor functional capacity

3. It also has to be stressed that most studies dealing with patients at cardiac risk undergoing noncardiac surgery have been performed in patients undergoing vascular surgery.

4. In most of the studies postoperative care of these patients was performed on an intermediate or critical care unit.

References

1. Mangano DT (1998) Adverse outcomes after surgery in the year 2001 – a continuing odyssey. Anesthesiology 88:561-564
2. Badner NH, Knill RL, Brown JE et al (1998) Myocardial infarction after noncardiac surgery. Anesthesiology 88:572-578
3. Mangano DT, Browner WS, Hollenberg M et al (1992) Long-term cardiac prognosis following noncardiac surgery. The Study of Perioperative Ischemia Research Group. JAMA 268: 233-239
4. American College of Physicians (1997) Guidelines for assessing and managing the perioperative risk from coronary artery disease associated with major noncardiac surgery. Ann Intern Med 127:309-312
5. Eagle KA, Brundage BH, Chaitman BR et al (1996) Guidelines for perioperative cardiovascular evaluation for noncardiac surgery. Report of the American College of Cardiology/American Heart Association Task Force on Practice Guidelines. Committee on Perioperative Cardiovascular Evaluation for Noncardiac Surgery. Circulation 93:1278-1317
6. Goldman L, Caldera DL, Nussbaum SR et al (1977) Multifactorial index of cardiac risk in noncardiac surgical procedures. N Engl J Med 297:845-850
7. Detsky AS, Abrams HB, Forbath N et al (1986) Cardiac assessment for patients undergoing noncardiac surgery. A multifactorial clinical risk index. Arch Intern Med 146:2131-2134
8. Krupski WC, Layug EL, Reilly LM et al (1993) Comparison of cardiac morbidity rates between aortic and infrainguinal operations: two-year follow-up. Study of Perioperative Ischemia Research Group. J Vasc Surg 18:609-615
9. Bode RH, Lewis KP, Zarich SW et al (1996) Cardiac outcome after peripheral vascular surgery: comparison of general and regional anesthesia. Anesthesiology 84:3-13
10. Anand KJ, Hickey PR (1992) Halothane-morphine compared with high-dose sufentanil for anesthesia and postoperative analgesia in neonatal cardiac surgery. N Engl J Med 326:1-9
11. Galvani M, Ottani F, Ferrini D et al (1997) Prognostic influence of elevated values of cardiac troponin I in patients with unstable angina. Circulation 95:2053-2059
12. Connors Jr AF, Speroff T, Dawson NV et al (1996) The effectiveness of right heart catheterization in the initial care of critically ill patients. SUPPORT Investigators. JAMA 276:889-897
13. Mangano DT, Layug EL, Wallace A et al (1996) Effect of atenolol on mortality and cardiovascular morbidity after noncardiac surgery. Multicenter Study of Perioperative Ischemia Research Group. N Engl J Med 335:1713-1720
14. McSPI – Europe Research Group (1997) Perioperative sympatholysis. Beneficial effects of the alpha 2-adrenoceptor agonist mivazerol on hemodynamic stability and myocardial ischemia. Anesthesiology 86:346-363
15. Rolf N, Meissner A, Van Aken H et al (1997) The effects of thoracic epidural anesthesia on functional recovery from myocardial stunning in propofol-anesthetized dogs. Anesth Analg 84:723-729
16. Meissner A, Rolf N, Van Aken H (1997) Thoracic epidural anesthesia and the patient with heart disease: benefits, risks, and controversies. Anesth Analg 85:517-528
17. Liu S, Carpenter RL, Neal JM (1995) Epidural anesthesia and analgesia. Their role in postoperative outcome. Anesthesiology 82:1474-1506
18. Baron JF, Bertrand M, Barre E et al (1991) Combined epidural and general anesthesia versus general anesthesia for abdominal aortic surgery. Anesthesiology 75:611-618
19. Bois S, Couture P, Boudreault D et al (1997) Epidural analgesia and intravenous patient-controlled analgesia result in similar rates of postoperative myocardial ischemia after aortic surgery. Anesth Analg 85:1233-1239
20. Christopherson R (1993) Perioperative morbidity in patients randomized to epidural or general anesthesia for lower extremity vascular surgery. Anesthesiology 79:422-434
21. Society of Critical Care Medicine (1991) Guidelines for categorization of services for the critically ill patient. Task Force on Guidelines. Crit Care Med 19:279-285

Diagnosis in the Early Phase of Aortic Dissection

S. Klugmann, A. Alberti, F. Faletra, A. Rampoldi

Aortic dissection is an emergency with an extremely high early mortality, time dependent (1-2% per hour) if not treated [1]. Survival however can be significantly improved by an appropriate therapy, medical or surgical. A prompt diagnosis therefore is mandatory in the treatment of this disease [2].

The diagnostic flow chart of a patient with a suspected aortic dissection can vary significantly according to the clinical presentation and the admitting hospital facilities. There are different options for example if we consider:

– a well-founded clinical suspicion or an incidental observation (for example a chest X ray with an ascending aorta dilatation in a patient with a different illness);
– the presence or absence of an invasive cardiology and of a cardiac surgery department and easy access to contrast enhanced CT or MRI facilities.

The first diagnostic step is mainly clinical and if one of the imaging techniques confirms an aortic dissection the patient must be rapidly transferred, in case of the absence of a cardiac surgery department to a referring hospital.

The optimal care of the patients requires also a rapid identification of the site of origin and the extension of the disease.

The Stanford classification system divides aortic dissection depending on the location [3]. In type A dissection there is an involvement of the ascending aorta (this includes De Bakey types I and II) [4]. All the aortic dissections without an ascending aorta involvement are considered of type B (De Bakey type III).

The patients with type A dissection require in the vast majority of cases an urgent surgical repair whereas those with an uncomplicated type B dissection can be successfully treated medically.

Symptoms

The most common presenting symptom of aortic dissection is severe pain that is present in more than 70% of patients [5, 6]. The pain is of abrupt onset, often migrating (generally following the direction of the dissection) and its location is correlated with the site of the dissection; when it is located only in the anterior chest there are high probabilities that the disease involves the ascending aorta while an interscapular pain suggest a descending thoracic aorta disease [5, 6].

The other symptoms are less frequent and involve the aortic branches, the aortic valve or the pericardium: cerebrovascular accidents, paraplegia, cardiac arrest, syncope, congestive heart failure.

Physical findings

The physical findings are related to the extension of the disease and to the cardiovascular involvement [6].

Hypertension is a common finding, particularly in the descending aorta dissection. The exploration of peripheral pulses often demonstrates a deficit of one or more pulses, sometimes transient or migrating with the dissection. The presence of a murmur of aortic regurgitation is frequent in the ascending aorta location. The extension of the dissection into the carotid or innominate artery may cause severe neurologic deficit, while the involvement of the coronary ostium, of the renal or mesenteric arteries is related to ischaemic signs in the interested district.

Diagnostic techniques

Echocardiography

Nowadays it is well documented that, in experienced hands, combined echocardiography (transthoracic, transoesophageal, color doppler) is a powerful diagnostic tool in acute aortic dissection [7-11].

Echocardiography is a noninvasive imaging technique that is widely available, does not require the use of intravenous contrast agents or ionizing radiation and can be performed rapidly in the Cardiac Care Unit by one well trained operator and during the study the patient remains accessible to the medical and nursing staff.

Echocardiography, used in connection with doppler and color doppler flow imaging, as it can give simultaneous anatomic and flow imaging, provides the unique opportunity to study the distribution of intracavitary flow patterns while observing cardiac dynamics in real time.

Transthoracic echocardiography (TTE) has lower sensitivity and specificity (59-85% and 63-96% respectively) but a high positive predictive accuracy (90-96%) [7, 10, 12, 13]. TTE study includes evaluation of ascending aorta from the standard and high parasternal windows, the aortic arch from the suprasternal noch window, the descending aorta from parasternal and apical windows. When a left pleural effusion is present, the descending aorta can be imaged through the effusion with the transducer positioned on the left posterior chest wall.

When a definite, undulating intimal flap is seen within a dilated aortic lumen, the specificity of transthoracic ecocardiography for diagnosis of dissection is high [14]. Its sensitivity is highest for dissections involving the ascending aorta, ranging from 78% to 100% [10, 13, 15], whereas for dissections of the descending aorta its sensitivity is as low as 31-55% [10, 13].

Furthermore, the presence of pericardial and/or left pleural effusion, the estimation of aortic regurgitation and ventricular regional motion and global function are easily detected in the majority of patients.

The major limitations of TTE include its inability to visualize the thoracic aorta in its entirety, poor quality of images in approximately 10-30% of patients, especially those with chronic lung disease, obesity, abnormal chest wall configuration and previous thoracic surgery.

Transoesophageal echocardiography (TEE) overcomes most of these limitations. TEE images of the aorta are far superior to TTE images due to: 1) shorter distance between the transducer and the aorta, without the interference from the chest wall or the overlying lung, 2) the use of a higher frequency transducer and 3) better ultrasound penetration (higher signal-to-noise ratio).

Despite the need for oesophageal intubation, TEE may take only 5 to 10 minutes to complete [8]. It is well tolerated in the majority of patients, and is contraindicated only in patients with known oesophageal diseases including varices, strictures and tumors.

A number of studies examining the use of TEE in a large number of patients have demonstrated a sensitivity of 94% to 100% in identifying an intimal flap and 77% to 87% in identifying the site of entry [8, 16, 17]. Its specificity ranges from 68% to 98%, the highest values being related to the operator's skill and the use of biplane or multiplane probes [8, 18].

The aortic root is seen on TEE imaging in the transverse plane at the aortic level. Evaluation of the ascending aorta depends on the use of longitudinal plane; this aortic segment cannot be adequately assessed with a single-plane transoesophageal probe.

The descending thoracic aorta can be examined in its entirety from the diaphragm to the arch in both long and short-axis planes. Biplane and multiplane TEE probes allow better visualization of the arch, ascending and thoracic descending aorta. Recently Keren A. et al. [18], using biplane or multiplane probes, reported high sensitivities for intimal fenestration in the ascending aorta, arch and descending aorta (89%, 83%,100% respectively). In this setting color flow imaging associated with TEE is very useful, as it can show the slower swirling flow pattern in the false lumen and the rapid color doppler flow signals moving during systole in the true lumen.

A dissection flap appears as a linear, bright echogenic structure in the aortic lumen with undulating motion [8]. Some authors state that the intimal flap should be seen in more than one view, should have a defined motion that is not parallel to the motion of any other cardiac or aortic root structure [8, 19, 20], and should not be confused with an extension or reverberation of any other cardiac structure. Often the false lumen is filled with a spontaneous echo contrast phenomenon because of low blood velocity. In cases in which the false lumen is thrombosed, it has been proposed that central displacement of intimal calcification, separation of the intimal layers from the thrombus and shearing of the different wall layers from the thrombus are criteria for diagnosing a dissection [8, 18]. The sensitivity and specificity for identifying the presence of a thrombus range from 64% to 78% and from 91% to 100% respectively [8, 18]. In some cases it is impossible to distinguish between a thrombosed false lumen and an intramural haematoma. However in a recent paper from Keren and coworkers [18] a high sensitivity and specificity for intramural haematoma were reported (90% and 99% respectively).

Color flow imaging, in conjunction with TEE, allows one to identify not only the entry and reentry sites, but also the flow dynamics in the true and in the false lumen. This is of paramount importance because it has been demonstrated that the presence of an open false lumen with persistent communication between it and the true lumen, as well as the extravasation of fluid in the pleural cavity or the mediastinum have a significant negative impact on the long-term outcome of these patients [21].

The complications of aortic dissection are well recognized by TEE associated to color doppler.

In the diagnosis of aortic insufficiency TEE has a sensitivity of 100% and allows the definition of its origin: 1) aortic root dilatation, 2) leaflet fail due to inadequate leaflet support for the retrograde extension of the dissection. This information is very useful in order to perform the more appropriate surgical correction.

In the diagnosis of pericardial effusion both the sensitivity and specificity are 100% [7-9, 13].

Some studies moreover have reported a good sensitivity (90%) in the visualization of the dissection extending into the coronary vessels (ostia and proximal segment) [8, 22]. The coronary artery ostial occlusion may also occur as the result of the compression of the vessel and the resultant wall motion abnormalities are easily detected.

The principal limitations of echocardiography in aortic dissection are:
– small dissected sections of the ascending aorta can be missed because TEE has a "blind spot" in the distal part of the ascending aorta which is hidden behind the trachea;

– false positive findings have been reported because of the misinterpretation of ultrasound artifacts, such as riverberations (especially in calcific aortic disease), beam width artifacts and oblique imaging planes;
– the branch vessel involvement is rarely recognized.

In conclusion this technology, in presence of a trained echocardiographic team, provides the information required to plan the appropriate management of patients with a (suspected) aortic dissection. Its easy availability, moreover, safety and low costs make echocardiography a first choice tool, especially in clinically unstable patients.

Aortography

Aortography has been considered mandatory in the past for the diagnosis of aortic dissection [8] and was the only accurate imaging method in vivo. The introduction, however, of other, non invasive, tests has gradually reduced its use.

The diagnosis of aortic dissection with the retrograde aortography is based on direct and indirect findings. The characteristic signs are the presence of the intimal flap and a double lumen; the longitudinal extension of these alterations can be easily detected with this technique [23]. The indirect signs are the compression of the aorta or other arteries by the false lumen, the presence of an aortic insufficiency, abnormalities of the branch vessels [23, 24].

The advantages of retrograde aortography are the possibility to identify the longitudinal extension (determining the presence of a type A or a type B dissection) and the sites of entry and reentry together with the extent of branch-vessel involvement (especially coronary arteries) [8].

The sensitivity of this method is limited in comparison with the other imaging techniques and varies between 80% and 90% [25]. False negative angiograms are due to the presence of a thrombosis of the false lumen, a faint opacification of the false lumen or the difficulty of the visualization of the intimal flap [26]. Other limitations of aortography are the increased risk due to the necessity of the use of contrast agents (potentially nephrotoxic, particularly in patients with an acute renal insufficiency) and the high cost of the procedure. There may be also a substantial delay in the diagnosis because of the time required to assemble the angiographic team and to trasport the patient to the catheterization laboratory [8].

CT scanning

In the investigation of acute cases of aortic dissection, a combined use of echocardiography and CT is most appropriate, because of its speed, accuracy and low complication rate.

The diagnosis of aortic dissection by CT requires consistent aortic opacification using rapid-sequence contrast-enhanced scans and has been shown to be accurate in detecting dissection flaps with reported sensitivities of 88% to 100% and a specificity of 92%.

CT images para-aortic structures but has the disadvantage of not assessing aortic regurgitation or ventricular function, and may not detect all dissection flaps, particularly rapidly moving flaps in the ascending aorta.

CT should therefore not be used as the unique method for excluding aortic dissection.

The benefits of spiral CT compared with standard CT have been well established and include considerably shorter examination times and the potential for better evaluation of vascular structures, as more images will be obtained during peak levels of enhancement due to better tracking of the contrast material bolus [27, 28].

Spiral CT can be used to create two-dimensional reconstructions of excellent quality, and these reconstructions proved useful invisualising the course of the dissection membrane in the aortic arch relative to the origin of the left subclavian artery in type B dissection.

This information is especially important for the exclusion of retrograde dissection into the arch, which was recently shown to occur in 30% of type B dissections and is associated with a high mortality rate [29].

Spiral CT, including thin sections, proved to be highly accurate in the detection of arch vessel involvement.

Spiral CT requires intravenous administration of contrast medium, which may be a limiting factor in patients with severe cardiac failure, impaired renal function, or intolerance to contrast medium.

Conclusions

Which is the preferred imaging method for the evaluation of a patient with a suspected aortic dissection? Probably transoesophageal echocardiography today, when available, should be considered first, especially in cases with a low likelihood of coronary artery disease and without an involvement of the major artery trunks. Expert and skilled readers are however necessary with this technique. Aortography is often preferred by some cardiac surgeons, mainly because it excludes an involvement of coronary arteries. This imaging technique is expensive, confined to few centers and has a definite risk particularly in patients with cadiac failure and/or renal insufficiency. CT scanning is acceptable for the rapid screening of the cases.

Every institution has to determine its preferred diagnostic method on the basis of the local human and material resources available.

References

1. Hirst AE Jr, Johns VJ Jr, Kime SW Jr (1958) Dissecting aneurysm of aorta: a review of 505 cases. Medicine 37:217
2. Daily PO, Trueblood HW, Stinson EB et al (1970) Management of acute aortic dissection. Ann Thorac Surg 10:237
3. DeBakey ME, Mc Cullum CH, Crawford ES et al (1982) Dissection and dissecting aneurysms of the aorta: twenty year follow-up of five hundred twenty-seven patients treated surgically. Surgery 92:1118
4. Spittel PC, Spittel JA Jr, Joyce JW et al (1993) Clinical features and differential diagnosis of aortic dissection: experience with 236 cases (1980 through 1990). Mayo Clin Proc 68:642
5. Isselbacher EM, Eagle KA, Desanctis RW (1997) Diseases of the aorta. In: Braunwald E (ed) Heart disease. A textbook of cardiovascular medicine. WB Saunders, Philadelphia, pp 1546-1581
6. Harris PD, Malm JR (1969) The management of acute aortic dissection of the thoracic aorta. Am Heart J 78:419-422
7. Erbel R, Daniel W, Visser C et al and the European Cooperative Study Group for Echocardiography (1989) Echocardiography in diagnosis of aortic dissection. Lancet 1:457-461
8. Cigarroa JE, Iselbacher EM, DeSanctis RW, Eagle KA (1993) Diagnostic imaging in the evaluation of suspected aortic dissection. N Engl J Med 328:35-43
9. Nienaber CA, von Kodolitsch Y, Nicholas V et al (1993) The diagnosis of thoracic aortic dissection by non invasive imaging procedures. N Engl J Med 328:1-9
10. Khanderia BK (1993) Aortic dissection, the last frontier. Circulation 87:1765-1768
11. Erbel R, Mohr-Kahalay S, Rennollet H et al (1987) Diagnosis of aortic dissection: the value of transesophageal echocardiography. Thorac Cardiov Surg 2:126-133
12. DeSanctis RW, Doroghazi RM, Austen WG, Buckley MJ (1987) Aortic dissection. N Engl J Med 317:1060-1067
13. Nienaber CA, Spielman RP, von Kodolitsch Y et al (1992) Diagnosis of thoracic aortic dissection: Magnetic resonance imaging versus transesophageal echocardiography. Circulation 85:434-447
14. Otto S, Pearlman AS (1995) Textbook of clinical echocardiography. WB Saunders, Philadelphia
15. Illiceto S, Nanda NC, Rizzon P et al (1987) Color Doppler evaluation of aortic dissection. Circulation 75:748-755
16. Adachi H, Omoto R, Kyo S et al (1991) Emergency surgical intervention of acute aortic dissection with the rapid diagnosis by transesophageal echocardiography. Circulation 84;III: 14-19
17. Hashimoto S, Kumada T, Osakada G et al (1989) Assessment of transesophageal doppler echocardiography in dissecting aortic aneurysm. JACC 14:1253-1262
18. Keren A, Kim CB, Hu BS et al (1996) Accuracy of biplane and multiplane transesophageal echocardiography in diagnosis of typical acute aortic dissection and intramural hematoma. JACC 28:627-636
19. Goldman AP, Kotler MN, Scanlon MH et al (1986) The complementary role of magnetic resonance imaging, doppler echocardiography and computed tomography in the diagnosis of dissecting thoracic aneurysm. Am Heart J 111:970-981
20. Victor MF, Mintz GS, Kotler MN et al (1981) Two dimensional echocardiography diagnosis of aortic aneurysm. Am J Cardiol 48:1155-1159
21. Erbel R, Oelert H, Meyer J and The Cooperative Study Group on Echocardiography (1993) Effect of medical and surgical therapy on aortic dissection evaluated by transesophageal echocardiography: implications for prognosis and therapy. Circulation 87:1604-1615
22. Ballal RS, Nanda NC, Gatewood R et al (1991) Usefulness of transesophageal echocardiography in assessment of aortic dissection. Circulation 84:1903-1914

23. Hayashi K, Maney TF, Zelch JV et al (1974) Aortographic analysis of aortic dissection. AJR Am J Roentgenol 122:769-782
24. Petasnik JR (1991) Radiologic evaluation of aortic dissection. Radiology 180:297-305
25. Pretre R, Segesser LK (1997) Aortic dissection. Lancet 343:1461-1464
26. Earnest F IV, Muhm JR, Sheedy PF II (1979) Roentgenographic findings in thoracic aortic dissection. Mayo Clin Proc 54:43-50
27. Costello P, Damian E, Dupuy Dem Ecker CP, Tello RJ (1992) Spiral CT of thorax with reduced volume of contrast material: a comparative study. Radiology 183:663-666
28. Ney DR, Fishman EK, Niederhuber JE (1991) Threedimensional vascular imaging of the liver with spiral CT (abstract). Radiology 181:293
29. Erbel R, Oelert H, Meyer J et al (1991) Effect of medical and surgical therapy on aortic dissection evaluated by transesophageal echocardiography. Circulation 894[Suppl iii]:14-19

Surgical Strategies in the Management of Acute Aortic Dissection

B. ZINGONE

Aortic dissection is an acute, catastrophic disease leading the majority of patients to death due to aortic rupture, aortic valve insufficiency or end-organ malperfusion. In the absence of surgical treatment 50% of patients die within 48 hours and an additional 30% are lost within the following two weeks since the onset of symptoms [1]. The mortality rate is substantially higher when the ascending aorta is involved, and of course lower when it is not, irrespective of the site of the entry tear [1]. A useful classification for analysing therapeutic strategies and results is reported in Fig. 1. It retains the basic simplicity of the popular Stanford scheme and also includes the notion of where the entry tear is located [2].

involvement of the ascending aorta	entry tear site
yes: <u>TYPE A</u>	*ascending*
	arch
	descending
	other
no: <u>TYPE B</u>	*arch*
	descending
	other

Fig. 1. Stanford classification of aortic dissections. (Modified from [2])

Stanford type A acute aortic dissection

About two thirds of aortic dissections belong to this group. As previously mentioned, the majority of patients die early due to the propensity for rupture of the dissected intrapericardial aorta. End-organ malperfusion and heart failure from aortic valve insufficiency account for the remaining fatalities. Any delay to surgery not only increases the risk of preoperative death but also, by allowing more time for the appearance or the progression of malperfusion, aortic regurgitation and cardiac tamponade, significantly curtails the chances of a successful operation [3, 4]. Thus, it is of paramount importance that acute type A dissection be identified as early as possible and, to this end, that the diagnostic work-up be kept simple and expeditious. Transoesophageal Echocardiography (TEE), Computed Axial Tomography and Nuclear Resonance Imaging all share a higher diagnostic accuracy compared to angiography and are therefore preferred except for selected cases with regional malperfusion [5-7].

Most surgeons would currently accept whichever test can be first available, given that the incremental accuracy yelded by integrated testing may not outweigh the delay imposed to the operation [7]. TEE can be quickly performed at the bedside, with the additional advantage of not requiring the administration of contrast media, and probably is the most popular diagnostic tool in the field at this point in time.

Surgical access for the treatment of acute type A dissection is gained through a median sternotomy incision. It is always worth emphasizing that the primary goal of the operation is to replace the ascending aorta in order to neutralise the risk of rupture. At the same time care should be taken of the aortic valve if it is incompetent.

It has long been debated whether the resection of the entry tear should be an obligatory step of the procedure. Of course the tear is removed with the vessel whenever it is located within the ascending aorta. When the dissection propagates retrogradely from a more distal tear, as it happens in nearly one out of every four patients, it may be questionable whether the resection should be extended into the aortic arch or even farther, potentially increasing the magnitude and the risks of the operation [4, 8, 9]. Things to be weighted are operator experience, coexistence of additional risk factors and the understanding that an unattended tear may be associated with a significant incidence of delayed fatal and non-fatal failures. The latter argument has favored the current trend towards extending the resection to most arch tears, also based on the appreciation that they are generally quite proximal and readily managed when an "open distal anastomosis" (see below) strategy is selected, while individualising the decision for more distal tears [10-13].

This brings also into focus some strategic details that have been credited for the improved outcome reported in the more recent literature. For the sake of discussion they may be separated into "distal" and "proximal" details. The "open distal anastomosis" [14] is that option by which a properly sized vascular graft is connected to the wide open mouth of the arch without an intervening vascular clamp during a period of deep hypothermic circulatory arrest (DHCA). This approach carries a number of important advantages, the first being the opportunity to resect more of the ascending aorta and, if needed, of the proximal arch. Since most arch tears are quite proximal it follows that radicality is enhanced by this approach. Suturing also is far more accurate while the chances of producing secondary tears at the suture line are lessened. Finally, the clamp-crushed aorta is no longer left in site with its attending risk of secondary intimal tears [15-17].

Actually, some surgeons avoid altogether crossclamping the ascending aorta in order to prevent the compartmentalization of the vessel, and simply wait for the desired level of hypothermia before arresting the pump and perform the aortotomy [18]. In fact, as cardiopulmonary bypass is carried out by retrograde arterial perfusion from a femoral artery, preferential perfusion of the false lumen may take place through a distal intimal tear. That may be unconsequential as long as the false lumen is vented through the proximal entry tear. At the time of cross-clamping the ascending aorta, and in the absence of any additional intervening tears, the pressure may indeed increase within the false lumen to the point of compressing both the true lumen and the origin of important aortic side-branches. Intraoperative TEE is quite useful for diagnosing true lumen obstruction by observing the intimal flap and recording any shift of it following the application of the aortic clamp though, if intraoperative TEE is not available, it may be safer to adhere to a no-clamp strategy [19].

Similar arguments also support a strategic choice at the time of reinstitution of cardiopulmonary bypass following DHCA. At this stage preferential perfusion of the false lumen may, in addition to favoring malperfusion, exhert excessive tension against the distal aortic anastomosis and increase the likelihood of secondary intimal tears or bleeding. The arterial return from the heart-lung machine is therefore best moved to a newly-placed cannula through the vascular graft so that antegrade perfusion may take place while the femoral arterial limb of the circuit is kept shut [17]. Combined with the radicality allowed by the "open distal anastomosis", switching to antegrade perfusion at resumption of cardiopulmonary bypass may contribute to lower false lumen patency at follow-up [17].

Aortic root involvement varies among patients, and so does its anatomic substrate. It may look grossly normal in Marfan's patients, yet it is now aknowledged that radical root replacement is warranted to prevent the late development of aneurysms or severe aortic insufficiency [20]. The same is in order when the root is dilated, whether in a Marfan's circumstance or not, and one should certainly not be reluctant in adopting this option [21, 22]. Whether a bicuspid aortic valve should be replaced is arguable, though most surgeons would. In that case, as well as for any other intrinsic valvular deformity, separate replacement of both the aortic valve and the supra-coronary ascending aorta can be performed. Finally, a basically normal valve in a basically normal root, by far the most common occurrence, may prolapse due to dissection of the commissures and produce significant regurgitation, yet can be easily made competent by properly resuspending the commissures [23, 24]. A selective "proximal" strategy is therefore adopted by carefully matching the procedure to the particular circumstances encountered (Fig. 2). A further option deserves consideration when the walls of the aortic sinuses are ectatic or badly dissected while the leaflets are intrinsecally normal. Rather than resorting to implant a valved con-

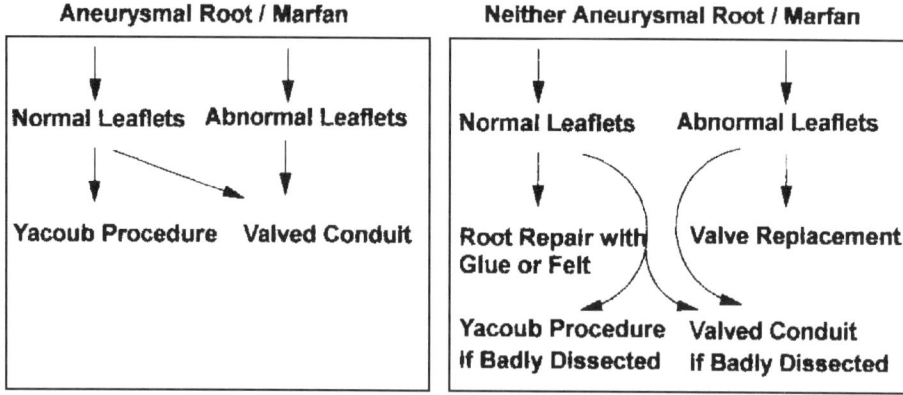

Fig. 2. Aortic root management options with acute type A aortic dissection

duit, with the attendant inconvenience of a prosthetic valve, the aortic sinuses can be resected leaving the leaflets in place with their commissures attached to a small rim of aortic wall. A properly sized vascular graft is then tailored at one extremity so as to reproduce the aortic sinuses and sutured to the aortic remnants along the leaflet hinges. Reimplantation of the coronary ostia completes the procedure [25].

As discussed above, DHCA has become a common step in surgery for aortic dissection involving the ascending aorta. Though initially reserved to arch operations, its use has gradually expanded to almost all ascending operations for the reasons previously mentioned. More recently it has been combined with retrograde cerebral perfusion (RCP) through the superior vena cava in order to minimise the risk of perioperative brain damage.

The time allowed for DHCA depends on the temperature of the brain. At 22°C nasopharyngeal up to 20′ of circulatory arrest is safe and is therefore accepted for straightforward open distal anastomosis [14, 24]. Lower temperatures (i.e. below 20°C rectal or 15°C nasopharyngeal) are necessary for longer procedures involving the arch though, if the time required is longer than 45 minutes, one should probably consider antegrade perfusion of arch vessels and certainly do so when it is longer than 60 minutes [26, 27]. In addition, packing the head with ice is a useful and cost-effective adjunct.

The relationship of DHCA to perioperative brain damage is made more complex by other mechanisms affecting cerebral perfusion. It has been previously discussed how aortic cross-clamping and retrograde arterial perfusion may jeopardise carotid flow and how that can be prevented. Furthermore, working within an empty arch also introduces the likelihood of debris and air embolism entering the carotid arteries. To this regard it remains controversial whether retrograde cerebral perfusion may contribute – and how – in decreasing the risk of brain damage [28]. Most surgeons would agree that RCP greatly facilitates getting rid of air and debris emboli at the end of the arrest period. Most also feel that it may help enhancing and maintaining brain hypothermia during the arrest interval. Despite some evidence that RCP also contributes to the metabolic needs of the brain, the extent to which it may surrogate for proper antegrade perfusion remains unsettled. There are also concerns that currently prescribed pressure and flow limits will not prevent some degree of cerebral oedema and microvascular damage from prolonged RCP. It may be therefore confidently stated that incorporating RCP in any DHCA strategy should be done within the previously established time constraints, with the expectation that it will probably decrease the risk of brain damage and may provide a safety net should the anticipated arrest time be exceeded [27].

In conclusion, the most popular strategy for dealing with acute type A dissection currently is to start hypothermic cardiopulmonary bypass between the right atrium and one femoral artery, reserving femoro-femoral perfusion prior to sternotomy to patients with cardiac tamponade. Once the appropriate temperature is reached, the circulation is arrested and the superior vena cava is perfused retrogradely through a cannula branched to the arterial limb of the circuit. The aorta is opened and appropriately resected, and the distal anastomosis to a vascular graft is performed. Next, air is evacuated by retrogradely filling the arch. The arterial cannula is then removed from the vena cava and introduced into the prosthesis, which is now cross-clamped proximally, so that antegrade systemic perfusion can be reinstituted. The proximal reconstruction is finally performed while systemic rewarming proceeds and the operation is completed in a routine manner (Fig. 3). The heart is adequately protected by hypothermia alone, though some form of cardioplegia is to be preferred for ischaemic times longer than 30-45 minutes.

Stanford type B acute aortic dissection

Compared to acute type A, Stanford type B aortic dissection has a less ominous prognosis because of the much lower propensity for the descending aorta to freely rupture while on medical treatment [29]. Coupled with unsatisfactory historical surgical outcomes, this has long prompted a selective approach by which surgery was more often contemplated for the complicated cases [4, 30]. As a matter of fact, direct aortic surgery is currently undertaken either in the presence of symptoms or signs suggesting rapid aortic expansion (> 5 cm) and impending rupture, or because of persisting pain and uncontrolled hypertension [31]. The appearance of visceral or limb malperfusion is also a strong indications for surgery though not necessarily on the thoracic aorta itself, as will be discussed below.

When surgery is focused on the descending aorta for threatened rupture the goal is that of resecting roughly the proximal one third of the vessel, which is

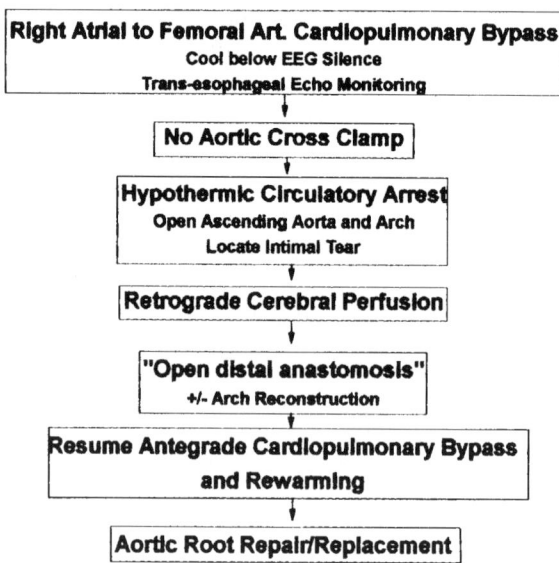

Fig. 3. Intraoperative flow chart for acute type A aortic dissection

likely to contain the entry tear and is also the most dilated and rupture-prone segment. The access is obtained through a left lateral thoracotomy. Out of the several options available to support the distal circulation and protect the spinal cord while operating on the descending aorta, when it comes to acute dissection most surgeons would favor a left heart bypass with low-dose heparinization [31]. A simplified circuit is employed which includes a centrifugal pump and two short lengths of tubing for left atrial and femoral connection to the respective pump ports. The procedure is performed at normothermia, and the sacrifice of the first few pairs of intercostal is unconsequential [31]. Once the graft has been connected proximally, an "open distal anastomosis" may be performed in order to resect the distal clamp-bearing aorta. The femoral perfusion is therefore reduced to trickle flow for the lower body while the upper body is perfused by heart action. In selected occasions, such as when the arch has to be resected or a proximal clamp cannot be safely placed, DHCA may be induced through femoro-femoral cardiopulmonary bypass and allow a completely no-clamp technique [32].

As an alternative the descending aorta may be managed with an "elephant trunk" procedure, which consists in opening the arch under DHCA and inserting a vascular graft into the distal true lumen past the entry tear site [33]. Once the proximal end of the graft is sutured to the arch and the circulation is reinstituted, the prosthesis will be floating within the descending aorta. A cul-de-sac will form around the prosthesis promoting thrombotic obliteration at the entry tear site and lessening the chances of aortic rupture. This is by no means an intriguing approach whose role has yet to be established.

Malperfusion

Angiographic evidence of obstructed flow either to limbs or internal organs is very common in acute aortic dissections and results in symptoms in nearly 1/3 of the patients. The obstruction may be severe enough to jeopardise organ or limb function and viability, as manifested by either neurologic deficits, myocardial infarction, renal failure, ileus or limb weakness and paresis, and constitute a risk factor for an adverse outcome despite a seemingly successful aortic repair [34].

The surgical strategy is based on the understanding that malperfusion is generally the consequence of collapse of the true lumen involving the take-off of aortic side-branches due to a pressurised false channel lacking a distal re-entry tear. Prioritization of treatment may vary according to circumstances.

With acute type A dissection the previously described ascending aortic procedure deserves full priority due to the impending risk of fatal rupture and to the expectation that by resecting the proximal entry tear the aortic layers will coapt and so restore perfusion to jeopardised regions [34, 35]. Classically, this would be immediately followed by a secondary procedure, perhaps before leaving the operating room, if the suspicion of unrelieved ischaemia persisted [34]. While this holds true in the majority of cases, an inverse sequence can be considered when organ failure is already established such as may occur in cases presenting for surgery after a significant diagnostic delay [36]. What might have been an early ischaemia several hours previously then becomes an incipient gangrene deserving immediate treatment coupled with intensive monitoring and anti-hypertensive medication. A further consideration is that the hazard function for aortic rupture, peaking sometimes within the first 48 hours, may be largely over at the time these decisions must be taken.

It follows that under these circumstances the timing of the aortic repair can be individualised.

With acute type B dissection the malperfusion syndromes constitute the most frequent indication for surgery. Some surgeons may opt for thoracic aortic replacement in some selected circumstances, and perhaps the "elephant trunk" may be an option here, but most would settle now for the time-honored – and transiently disreputed – abdominal fenestration procedure, completed with some vascular grafting when the former fails [34, 37]. Flap fenestration within the abdominal aorta is meant to decompress the false channel and relieve the obstruction to flow through side-branches. It should be noted, however, that a growing proportion of malperfusions is being successfully treated by percutaneous catheter interventions, the so-called "fen/sten" approach [38]. When the appropriate technology and skills are available the patient can have the flap fenestrated at the time of the diagnostic study. Expandable stents and endovascular prostheses are also being employed to expand the true aortic lumen or the orifice of a compromised side-branch.

Conclusions

The ingredients of successful management of acute aortic dissections include timeliness, appropriate strategy and adequate surgical skill. The latter was enphasised first and further supported by the adoption of impervious vascular grafts and hardening glues. Next came the appreciation that end-organ malperfusion plays a significant role in favoring postoperative sepsis and multiple organ failure unless it is timely relieved. Awareness of the need for cutting down the preoperative time interval and for improving upon intraoperative perfusion management has evolved into diagnostic and surgical strategies which have been associated with improved surgical outcomes.

References

1. Anagnostopoulos CE, Prabhakar MJS, Kittle CF (1962) Aortic dissections and dissecting aneurysms. Amer J Cardiol 30:263-273
2. Lansman SL, Galla JD, Schor JS et al (1994) Subtypes of acute aortic dissection. J Card Surg 9:729-733
3. Butler J, Ormerod OJ, Giannopoulos N et al (1991) Diagnostic delay and outcome in surgery for type A aortic dissection. Q J Med 79:391-396
4. Fann JI, Smith JA, Miller DC et al (1995) Surgical management of aortic dissection during a 30-year period. Circulation 92[Suppl II]:II-113-II-121
5. Nienaber CA, von Kodolitsch Y, Nicolas V et al (1993) The diagnosis of thoracic aortic dissection by noninvasive imaging procedures. N Engl J Med 328:1-9
6. Cigarroa JE, Isselbacher EM, DeSanctis RW et al (1993) Diagnostic imaging in the evaluation of suspected aortic dissection. Old standards and new directions. N Engl J Med 328: 35-43
7. Sarasin FP, Louis Simonet M, Gaspoz JM et al (1996) Detecting acute thoracic aortic dissection in the emergency department: time constraints and choice of the optimal diagnostic test. Ann Emerg Med 28:278-288
8. Yun KL, Glower DD, Miller DC et al (1991) Aortic dissection resulting from tear of transverse arch: is concomitant arch repair warranted? J Thorac Car diovasc Surg 102:355-368
9. Crawford ES, Kirklin JW, Naftel DC et al (1992) Surgery for acute dissection of ascending aorta: should the arch be included? J Thorac Cardiovasc Surg 104:46-59
10. Kazui T, Kimura N, Yamada O et al (1994) Total arch graft replacement in patients with acute type A aortic dissection. Ann Thorac Surg 58:1462-1468
11. Okita Y, Takamoto S, Ando M et al (1996) Surgery for aortic dissection with intimal tear in the transverse aortic arch. Eur J Cardiothorac Surg 10:784-790
12. Bachet J, Goudot B, Dreyfus G et al (1997) The proper use of glue: a 20-year experience with the GRF glue in acute aortic dissection. J Card Surg 12[Suppl]:243-253
13. Kazui T, Tamiya Y, Tanaka T et al (1996) Extended aortic replacement for acute type A dissection with the tear in the descending aorta. J Thorac Cardiovasc Surg 112:973-978

14. Livesay JJ, Cooley DA, Duncan JM et al (1982) Open aortic anastomosis: improved results in the treatment of aneurysms of the aortic arch. Circulation 66[Suppl I]:I-122-I-127
15. Miller DC (1992) Invited letter concerning: concomitant arch repair in acute type A aortic dissection. J Thorac Cardiovasc Surg 104:206-208
16. Kipfer B, Striffeler H, Gersbach P et al (1995) Surgery for acute ascending aortic dissection: closed versus open distal aortic repair. Eur J Cardiothorac Surg 9:248-252
17. Yamashita C, Okada M, Ataka K et al (1997) Open distal anastomosis in retrograde cerebral perfusion for repair of ascending aortic dissection. Ann Thorac Surg 64:665-669
18. Bavaria JE, Woo YJ, Hall RA et al (1996) Circulatory management with retrograde cerebral perfusion for acute type A aortic dissection. Circulation [Suppl II]:II-173-II-176
19. Yamada E, Matsumura M, Kimura S et al (1997) Usefulness of transesophageal echocardiography in detecting changes in flow dynamics responsible for malperfusion phenomena observed during surgery of aortic dissection. Am J Cardiol 79:1149-1152
20. Smith JA, Fann JI, Miller DC et al (1994) Surgical management of aortic dissection in patients with the Marfan syndrome. Circulation 90[Suppl II]: II- 235-II-242
21. Ergin MA, McCullough J, Galla JD et al (1997) Radical replacement of the aortic root in acute type A dissection: indications and outcome. Eur J Cardiothorac Surg 10:840-845
22. Niederhauser U, Rudiger H, Vogt P et al (1998) Composite graft replacement of the aortic root in acute dissection. Eur J Cardiothorac Surg 13:144-150
23. Fann JI, Glower DD, Miller DC et al (1991) Preservation of aortic valve in type A aortic dissection complicated by aortic regurgitation. J Thorac Cardiovasc Surg 102:62-73
24. Westaby S, Katsumata T, Freitas E (1997) Aortic valve conservation in acute type A dissection. Ann Thorac Surg 64:1108-1112
25. Pepper J, Yacoub M (1997) Valve conserving operation for aortic regurgitation. J Card Surg 12:151-156
26. Svensson LG, Crawford ES, Hess KR et al (1993) Deep hypothermia with circulatory arrest. Determinants of stroke and early mortality in 656 patients. J Thorac Cardiovasc Surg 106: 19-31
27. Griepp RB, Ergin MA, McCullough JN et al (1997) Use of hypothermic circulatory arrest for cerebral protection during aortic surgery. J Card Surg 12:312-321
28. Usui A, Abe T, Murase M (1996) Early clinical results of retrograde cerebral perfusion for aortic arch operations in Japan. Ann Thorac Surg 62:94-104
29. Masuda Y, Yamada Z, Morooka N et al (1991) prognosis of patients with medically treated aortic dissections. Circulation 84[Suppl III]:III-7-III-13
30. Glower DD, Fann JI, Speier RH et al (1990) Comparison of medical and surgical therapy for uncomplicated descending aortic dissection. Circulation [Suppl IV]:IV-39-IV-46
31. Schor JS, Yerlioglu ME, Galla JD et al (1996) Selective management of acute type B aortic dissection: long-term follow-up. Ann Thorac Surg 61:1339-1341
32. Kouchoukos NT, Daily BB, Rokkas CK et al (1995) Hypothermic bypass and circulatory arrest for operations on the descending thoracic and thoracoabdominal aorta. Ann Thorac Surg 60:67-77
33. Palma JH, Almeida DR, Carvalho AC et al (1997) Surgical treatment of acute type B aortic dissection using an endoprosthesis (elephant trunk). Ann Thorac Surg 63:1081-1084
34. Borst HG, Heinemann MK, Stone CD (1996) Surgical treatment of aortic dissection. Churchill Livingstone, New York
35. Okita Y, Takamoto S, Ando M et al (1995) Surgical strategies in managing organ malperfusion as a complication of aortic dissection. Eur J Cardiothorac Surg 9:242-246
36. Deeb GM, Williams DM, Bolling SF et al (1997) Surgical delay for acute type A dissection with malperfusion. Ann Thorac Surg 64:1669-1677
37. Elefteriades JA, Hartleroad J, Gusberg RJ et al (1992) Long-term experience with descending aortic dissection: the complication-specific approach. Ann Thorac Surg 53:11-20
38. Slonim SM, Nyman U, Semba CP et al (1996) Aortic dissection: percutaneous management of ischemic complications with endovascular stents and balloon fenestration. J Vasc Surg 23:241-251

Early Complications and Management After Bypass Circulation

J.O.C. Auler Jr, M.J.C. Carmona

Aortic dissection could be defined as a splitting of the aortic tunica media with extraluminal blood in the aortic wall. This blood penetrates the diseased medial layer and cleaves the laminar plane of the media in two, thus dissecting the aortic wall. The association of some medial degeneration, recurring flexion of the aorta and tensions applied to the aortic intima by hydrodynamic forces operating within the aorta may lead to an intimal tear and installation of a dissection. The majority of tears occur at the ascending aorta (60-65%). Subsequent propagation of the dissecting haematoma is related to hydrodynamic forces in the aorta, the pulse wave in the aorta being most important. Acute aortic regurgitation, cardiac tamponade, myocardial ischemia and heart block are the principal causes of death following aortic dissection. The peak incidence of aortic dissection is in the sixth and seventh decades of life, being twice more common in men [1]. In nontraumatic aortic dissection the pathogenesis is a degeneration of the medial collagen and elastin of the medial layer of the aortic wall [2, 3]. Although the mechanisms of such medial deterioration remain to be totally elucidated, aging process and coexisting history of hypertension are present in the majority of the cases of aortic dissection [1]. Due to its catastrophic evolution, acute aortic dissection requires prompt clinical diagnosis and treatment. Acute or chronic dissection is based on the time of onset of the dissection. Arbitrarily, acute dissection is defined when the onset is less than 2 weeks in duration. This classification is based on clinical data that reported 70% of untreated patients dying within 1 week and 90% dying within 3 months. In one fourth of the patients suffering acute aortic dissection, an aneurysm develops in the following 5 years. Chronic dissecting aneurysm may rupture or dissect again with symptoms and signs similar to acute dissection. Evidently the mortality rate, problems in postoperative management and complications, that we intend to discuss in advance, are related to the clinical conditions that the patients present at the moment of surgical treatment [4]. After aortic dissection onset, classification has also been proposed to define the location of initial tear and extent of aortic involvement. Debakey types I, II and III; Stanford types A and B as well as anatomical classification of proximal or distal, all share the same principle of distinguishing the site of the tear and the involvement or not of the ascending aorta [5, 6]. Simplistically, aortic involvement before the proximal to the left subclavian artery origin or ascending aorta, requires immediate surgical treatment; distal involvement or descending aorta, beyond the left subclavian artery origin could be treated initially by medical management. When this fails, surgical approach could be considered [4]. It is important to consider that aortic dissection may also occur in aortic aneurysm. Aneurysm has been defined as when the aortic transverse diameter exceeds twice the normal aortic diameter. The pathogenesis of true aortic aneurysm is related to a medial degenerative disease. According to its localisation in the aorta, the aneurysms are classified as thoracic, thoracoabdominal or abdominal. Although most aneurysms are asymptomatic, controversy exists when their surgical correction is indicated. Due to the high risk of rupture most of the surgeons indicated surgical repair of the aorta when the aneurysm exceeds 5 cm in diameter for thoracic, and 4 cm for abdominal [7, 8].

Early complications and management after bypass circulation

A large proportion of patients with aortic disease are elderly and present coexisting diseases. Emergency surgery, cardiogenic shock due to cardiac tamponade, myocardial ischemia or aortic valvar regurgitation, obstruction of other arteries arising from the aorta causing strokes in addition to renal and bowel ischemia all carry high incidence of postoperative complications.

Surgery on the thoracic aorta presents some serious problems that require specific management. It is important to divide the aorta in regions based on the site of aneurysm or dissection since these will determine the degree of cardiovascular stress, risk of organ or tissue ischemia and the necessity for special procedures such as cardiopulmonary bypass, intra-arterial shunts, hypothermia, circulatory arrest, and special spinal cord protection. Cardiopulmonary bypass in general is necessary for interventions to treat dissections or aneurysms in the ascending aorta including the aortic root, aortic arch and eventually the descending aorta. This is best achieved utilising cardioplegia for cardiac arrest and protection, and, if necessary, deep hypothermia with circulatory arrest and retrograde brain perfusion for cerebral protection. Surgery on the descending thoracic aorta presents some important clinical problems. First, cross clamping of the aorta creates major haemodynamic alterations, proximal and distal to the clamp. Second, there is a significant risk of haemorrhage from surgical bleeding and or coagulopathy. Third, there is elevated risk of paraparesis or paraplegia due to spinal cord injury, during aortic cross clamping and surgical correction. Several clinical and pharmacological strategies have been proposed to minimise or to prevent acute spinal cord lesions during aortic cross clamping [9]. Atriofemoral bypass is increasingly used to support haemodynamics in patients who need descending or thoracoabdominal aortic repairs. Clinical data from this procedure are consistent to significantly decrease spinal cord injury. Oxygenated blood is drained from the atrium and pumped into the femoral artery with a centrifugal pump. This method also seems to protect the kidneys, and reduces the need for vasodilators during aortic cross clamping and decreases the risk of hypotension with aortic unclamping [10]. In 1997, 1,926 cardiac or vascular surgeries that required cardiopulmonary bypass were performed at the Heart Institute in São Paulo, Brazil. Among them, 42 patients were submitted to some type of surgery in the ascending aorta or aortic arch and 12 patients with interventions in the descending aorta (Table 1).

Table 1.

	Patients
Cardiovascular operations with CPB	1926
Ascending aorta or aortic arch surgeries with CPB	42
Descending aortic surgeries with CPB	12

Year 1997
CPB, cardiopulmonary bypass

Harmful effects of cardiopulmonary bypass

Aneurysms or acute dissection in ascending or aortic arch, need cardiopulmonary bypass (CPB). This method activates a generalised inflammatory response characterised by postoperative alterations, mainly in cardiovascular and pulmonary function. The degree of this response and subsequent organ dysfunction may be quite different among patients considering its magnitude and morbidity. In its most severe form, this adverse response to CPB has been termed the post perfusion syndrome and may include, to a greater or lesser extent, clinical signs of pulmonary and renal dysfunction, systemic vasodilation with hypotension, abnormal bleeding diathesis, fever, increased susceptibility to infection, interstitial oedema and leukocitosis. When severe lung injury occurs, mortality is elevated (50 to 60%) [11]. The initiation of systemic inflammatory response during CPB includes: blood exposure to nonendothelial surfaces, shear stress, development of ischemia and reperfusion injury as well as the presence of endotoxaemia. Release of endotoxin during CPB is associated with reductions in mesenteric blood flow. Endotoxin is a powerful potential producer of the inflammatory reaction that causes the production of cytokines, complement and neutrophil activation [12]. An integral part of this whole body inflammatory response process involves the so-called humoral and cellular amplification system. Once installed, the systemic inflammatory response is continued by several factors including cytokine production (TNF, interleukins, interferons) [13], endothelial activation expressed by neutrophil activation [14], increased production and release of nitric oxide, under the influence of endotoxin and cytokines [15]. Activation of Hageman factor (XII) and other substances, leads to the activation of other kallikrein system and production of bradykinin. Activation of the fibrinolytic system is also initiated at the onset of CPB and plasmin may also activate prekallikrein, the complement system and Hageman factor (XII) [16]. High circulating levels of bradykinin have been documented during CPB. Bradykinin is related to vascular permeability increase and hypotension [17]. Complement is activated by means of the alternative pathway, due to exposition of blood to foreign surfaces, which has been described as part of inflammatory amplification [18]. Although the systemic inflammatory response is self-limiting in the majority of the patients, the magnitude of the response and clinical symptoms is influenced by many endogenous and exogenous factors. Several specific antagonists that exert antinflammatory effects have been identified, including anti TNF and anti interleukin receptors. Once triggered, the inflammatory response to CPB may be self limited by an internal reaction against proinflammatory substances. Pulmonary dysfunction is one of the worst adverse effects caused by the inflammatory reaction in operations, including aortic surgery that requires CPB. Otherwise, several strategies can be proposed to minimise the inflammatory response or limit its effects during CPB and consequently in the cardio-respiratory system.

Extracorporeal devices

Type of oxygenator, priming composition, the use of mechanical filtration during bypass, type of flow during perfusion, and temperature degree during CPB could influence the results of the surgery [19-22]. Specific therapeutic strategies related to CPB can be useful to minimise early complications due to inflammatory reaction after extracorporeal circulation. Use of haemoconcentration filters to remove proinflammatory cytokines, membrane oxygenators instead of bubble oxygenators in bypass circuits, heparin bonded CPB circuits, pulsatile perfusion and hypothermic bypass are being proposed to achieve these targets. The question of the neuroprotective benefits of a hypothermic versus normothermic bypass temperature management strategy appears to remain open. The biological rationale for hypothermic cerebral protection is based on the decrease of metabolic rate and excitotoxic cascade inhibition [23]. To reduce the incidence of postoperative brain injury, deep hypothermic bypass with circulatory arrest, is an invaluable and relatively safe adjunct for proximal aortic operations. To avoid undesirable "hyperthermic cerebral temperatures" during the cooling or rewarming process, three or more monitors of cerebral temperature should reflect the desired magnitude of hypothermia, and an additional 5-10 minutes of supplementary cooling after achieving the preferred core temperature, should be used before starting the circulatory arrest. Hypothermic CPB and prolonged rewarming increases the risk of cerebral microembolism and is associated with cerebral hyperperfusion. Retrograde perfusion of the brain via veins during circulatory arrest may provide some controversial benefits; flushing out of microemboli in the brain capillary network, aside from providing substrates, oxygen, keeping the brain cold and avoiding undesirable over temperature during core rewarming [24, 25]. The major issues with deep hypothermia during circulatory arrest are: temperature and rewarming, acid base management and the safety period of circulatory arrest. Comparing the alpha stat versus pH stat, more recent studies have shown less decline in cognitive performance when alpha stat management is used, especially in cases with prolonged bypass [26, 27].

Pharmacological agents

Pharmacological neuroprotection is a very exciting field because many procedures involving aortic surgery need CPB with deep hypothermia and at times circulatory arrest. With intracellular calcium being a central and final pathway; nitric oxide, oxygen free radicals, excitatory amino acids, arachidonic acid metabolites, endothelin, cytokines and complement all play a role in the pathophysiological process of ischemia. Despite methods to protect the brain like hypothermia and retrograde cerebral perfusion, a significant number of patients may present temporary or permanent neurologic deficits. However, there are a lot of discrepancies among clinical and experimental data in the attempts to block the inflammatory cascade responsible for brain injury. There is substantial evidence that free radicals and excitatory amino acids (e.g., glutamate and aspartate) play an important role in ischaemic reperfusion cerebral lesions. Several insults including ischaemia, hypoxia and trauma have been demonstrated to cause accumulation of excitatory amino acids. The mechanisms for release of excitatory amino acids probably involves depolarization of presynaptic neurons by increased extracellular potassium concentration resulting from failure of ATP-dependent pumps. Although therapeutic antioxidant has produced conflicting results, substances designed to block glutamate neurotoxicity show substantially positive effects in animal models submitted to both focal and global cerebral ischaemia and reperfusion [28].

Corticosteroids seem to be associated with the improvement of some aspects of inflammatory response. There are controversies among different reports, however it has been related that reduced levels of proinflammatory cytokines and complement activation reduced integrin receptor up-regulation with corticosteroids use [29].

Protease inhibitors, agents like aprotinin and ulinastatin, have been shown to exert antinflammatory activity including inhibition of complement activation and subsequent reduction in cytokine release and serum protease activation [30].

Conclusions

The successful outcome of aortic operations is dependent on the upright comments, and careful monitoring of cardiovascular haemodynamics and other or-

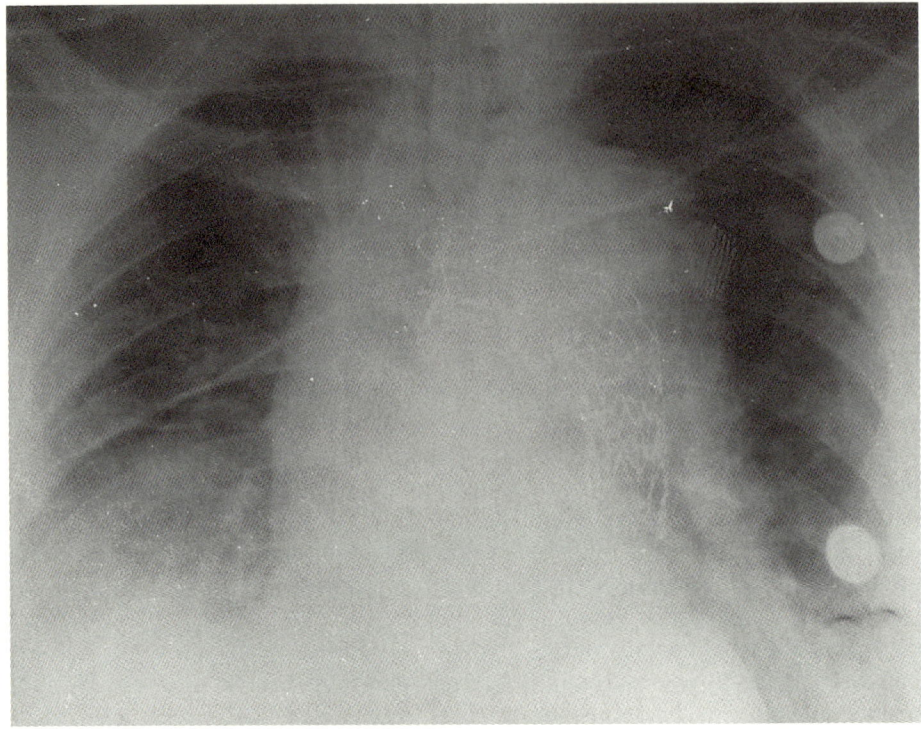

Fig. 1.

gan functions. Specifically discussing strategies in the management of aortic dissection, the incidence of early complications and successful management after bypass circulation, directly depends on pre-establishment and rigorous protocol. Thus invasive monitoring of cardiac function, exhaled CO_2, peripheral oxygen saturation, coagulation, electrocardiography and alfa stat acid base gas interpretation are all very important. During hypothermic bypass, the controversy over temperature correction of blood gases remains open to discussion. This discussion is fixed on myocardial and on cerebral outcome resulting from the two greatly different types of acid-base management, alpha or pH stat. There are three ways to measure blood gases: 1) measuring apparatus itself at body temperature. This is quite a new method utilising optical fluorescence, but the clinical validity has not been fully established yet, 2) blood sample is warmed anaerobically and measured in an analyzer at 37 degrees Celsius, and then corrected back to body temperature utilising calculations or nomograms (pH stat). The practical consequence of the pH stat method is the necessity of flushing carbon dioxide into oxygenator to keep the CO_2 at normal values. This may cause intracellular acidosis 3-alpha stat; uncorrected values for hypothermia, obtained

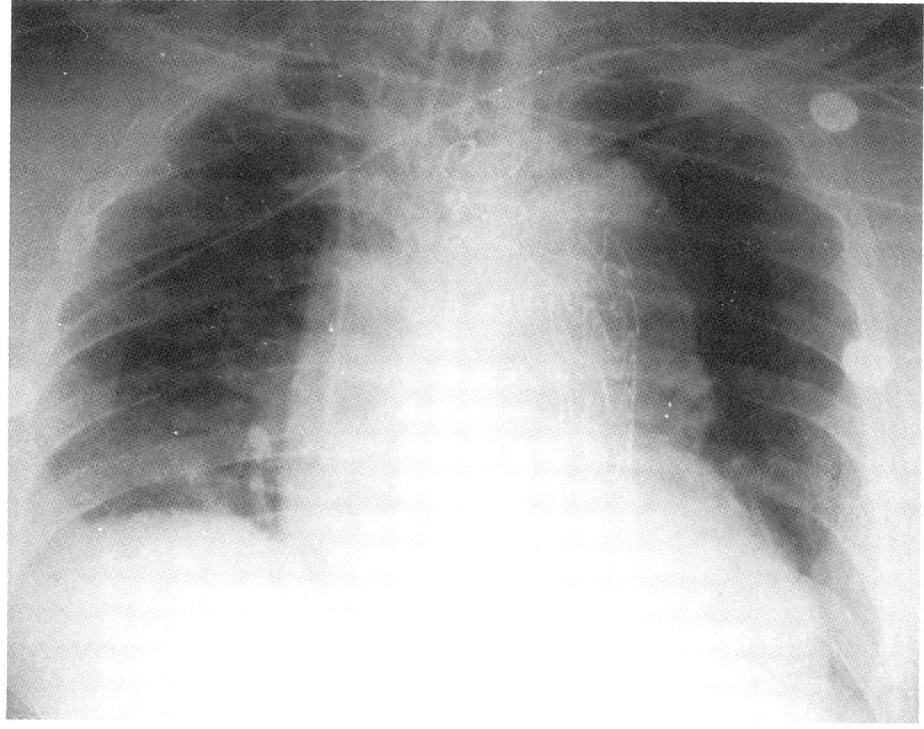

Fig. 2.

from anaerobically warmed blood, are kept at a pH of approximately 7.4 and $paCO_2$ 30 to 40 mmHg by relative hyperventilation. Because of the risks associated with intracellular metabolism, some authors, including our Department, have favoured the alpha stat method of pH control on the belief that this may reduce the risk of intracellular acidosis [24]. However, recent research in this field suggests that the pH stat method may be better than the pH alpha stat for infants under hypothermic circulatory arrest [31]. In operations to treat acute or chronic dissection on the ascending aorta, aortic arch or both, bilateral radial catheters are inserted and temperature should be monitored from the oesophagus (aortic temperature), nasopharynx (brain temperature), tympanic membrane (brain temperature), rectum (core temperature) and pulmonary catheter (blood temperature) [32]. To help the interpretation of cardiac contractility, transoesophageal echocardiography has increasingly been advocated in aortic surgeries. Before or after bypass, cardiac index should be maintained higher than 2.5 L/min². Epinephrine and or dobutamine are the preferable drugs. Pulmonary hypertension and systemic hypertension should be controlled with intravenous vasodilators, nitroglycerine and nitroprusside, respectively. Hypoxaemia, bronchospasm and

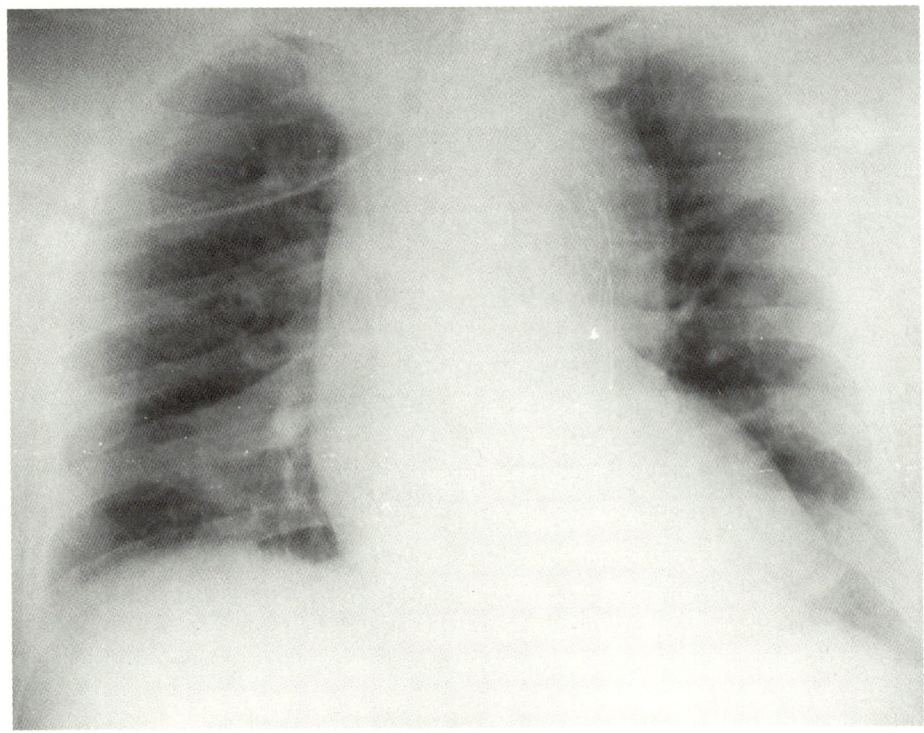

Fig. 3.

pulmonary hypertension during bypass weaning suggest vasoactive mediators in the lungs. Inhalational anaesthetics and specific therapy with adrenergic agonists may revert the process. Uncontrolled bleeding due to clotting defects and massive transfusion were the marks in the pioneer years of aortic surgeries. Uncontrolled bleeding further exacerbated by disseminated intravascular coagulation and fibrinolysis, may be responsible to up to one third of postoperative deaths [33]. Careful strategies should be directed during aortic operations to minimise bleeding and homologous transfused blood. An attempt should be made by the surgeon to guarantee adequate haemostasis as much as possible with the use of pledgeted sutures before aorta unclamping. Together with intra-operative use of plasmapheresis, at the bypass weaning, haematocrit, platelet count, prothrombin (PT) and partial thromboplastin time (PTT), fibrinogen and fibrin split products should be monitored. Fresh frozen plasma is administered if PT is enlarged as well as further protamine, if PTT is abnormal. All blood and blood products should be filtered with 40 μm filter, and stored bank packed red cells units should also be filtered utilising a white cell 5 μm filter. Platelet count should remain higher than 150,000/mm^3 and 5 to 10 units of cryoprecipitate are

given if fibrinogen is lower than 100 ug/ml. Evidence of fibrinolysis characterised by abnormal and fragile clots, the presence of increased levels of fibrin
split or degradation products, require the administration of antifibrinolytic
agents. There are three known agents, epsilon aminocaproic acid, tranexanic
acid and aprotinin. Some protocols suggest the prophylactic use of antifibrinolytic drugs to minimise the possibility of fibrinolysis and abnormal bleeding.
Although widely accepted in Europe, aprotinin is still being debated. Two studies from the US showed complications related to the use of aprotinin, one of
them related higher incidence of myocardial infarction and vein graft occlusion
after coronary bypass graft reoperations [34]. Following hypothermic circulatory arrest, other reports have related death and renal failure due to microvasculature thrombosis [35]. Postoperative mental status of the patients remains a central role of care in aortic surgery with CPB. Ancillary measures such as barbiturates and membrane stabilizers (e.g., lidocaine, methylprednisolone sodium suc-
cinate) has been used in the last years as protection for the brain. Recent findings that thiopental may be harmful to the brain during deep hypothermia, possible increase in the incidence of sepsis with steroids have declined their routine
utilization [36]. It can be foreseen, however, that further thought of the pathophysiological processes of ischemia and the associated uses of therapeutic
agents would result in a practical and effectual approach in the prevention of ischemia induced injury. Postoperative management plays a fundamental role in
successful surgery of aortic dissections. General surgical or postoperative cardiac wards represent the ideal place for this kind of patient. Our protocol for
these patients is centered in careful haemodynamic monitoring, X-rays every 12
hours, transoesophageal echocardiography, immediately after and the day following surgery as well as whenever necessary. Systemic arterial hypertension is
very common in the first hours after surgical correction. We manage this utilizing sodium nitroprusside and β-blockers according to cardiac function. We utilize pressure controlled ventilation, PEEP according to compliance curve and
pressure support preceding extubation. After acute aortic dissection that requires
CPB and emergency surgery it is common to observe radiological and functional signals of lung hydric infiltrations. This can be observed in the following X-
ray sequence: one patient in the postop after surgical correction of acute aortic
dissection (Figs. 1, 2, 3). Fluid restriction, 24 hours of ventilation after circulatory arrest and extubation are conditioned according to mental status, cardiovascular stability and absence of bleeding.

Finally, the results of managing patients with aortic dissection undergoing
cardiopulmonary bypass have improved considerably in the last years, due to
earlier diagnosis and improvement in intra and postoperative care.

References

1. Spittell PC, Spittell JA, Jr Joyce JW et al (1993) Clinical features and differential diagnosis of aortic dissection: Experience with 236 cases (1980 through 1990). Mayo Clin Proc 68: 642-651

2. Marsales DL, Moodie DS, Lytl BW et al (1990) Cystic medial necrosis of the aorta in patients without Marfan's syndrome: Surgical outcome and long term follow up. J Am Coll Cardiol 16:68-73

3. Coselli JS, Büket S, Djukanovic B (1995) Aortic arch operation: current treatment and results. Ann Thorac Surg 59:19-27

4. Svensson LG & Crawford ES (1992) Aortic dissection and aortic aneurysm surgery: clinical observations, experimental investigations and statistical analyses. Part II. Curr Probl Surg 29: 913-1057

5. Debakey ME, Cooley DA, Creech O Jr (1955) Surgical considerations of dissecting aneurysms of the aorta. Ann Surg 142:586-592

6. Daily PO, Trueblood W, Stinson EB et al (1970) Management of acute aortic dissections. Ann Thorac Surg 10:237-247

7. Crawford ES, Hess KR, Cohen ES et al (1991) Ruptured aneurysm of descending thoracic and thoracoabdominal aorta: analysis according to size and treatment. Ann Surg 213:417-425

8. Crawford ES, Hess KR (1989) Abdominal aortic aneurysm. N Engl J Med 321:1040-1042

9. Urban M (1997) Spinal cord ischemia: recognition and prevention. In: TJJ Blanck (ed) Neuroprotection vol. 6. Williams & Wilkins, Baltimore, pp 135-162

10. Verdant A, Cossette R, Page A et al (1995) Aneurysms of the descending thoracic aorta: three hundred sixty six consecutive cases resected without paraplegia. J Vasc Surg 21:385-390

11. Messent M, Sullivan K, Keogh BF et al (1992) Adult respiratory distress syndrome following cardiopulmonary bypass: incidence and prediction. Anaesthesia 47:267-268

12. Kharazmi A, Andersen LW, Baek L et al (1989) Endotoxemia and enhanced generation of oxygen radicals by neutrophils from patients undergoing cardiopulmonary bypass. J Thorac Cardiovasc Surg 98:381-385

13. Hennein HA, Ebba H, Rodriguez JL et al (1994) Relationship of the proinflammatory cytokines to myocardial ischemia and dysfunction after uncomplicated coronary revascularization. J Thorac Cardiovasc Surg 108:62-35

14. Tönz M, Mihaljevic T, von Segesser LK et al (1995) Acute lung during cardiopulmonary bypass: are the neutrophils responsible? Chest 108:1515-1556

15. Delgado R, Rojas A, Gloria LA et al (1995) Calcium independent nitric oxide synthase activity in human lung after cardiopulmonary bypass. Thorax 50:403-404

16. Backmann F, McKenna R, Cole ER, Najafi H (1975) The hemostatic mechanisms after open heart surgery. I. Studies on plasma coagulation factors and fibrinolysis in 512 patients after extracorporeal circulation. J Thorac Cardiovasc Surg 70:76-85

17. Ellison N, Behar M, MacVaugh H III, Marschall BE (1980) Bradykinin, plasma protein fraction and hypotension. Ann Thorac Surg 29:15-19

18. Boyle EM Jr, Pohlman TH, Johnson MC, Verrier ED (1997) Endothelial cell injury in cardiovascular surgery: the systemic inflammatory response. Ann Thorac Surg 63:277-294

19. Jansen PG, Te Velthuis H, Wildevuur WR et al (1996) Cardiopulmonary bypass with modified gelatin and heparin-coated circuits. Br J Anaesth 76:13-19

20. Johnson D, Thomson D, MycykT et al (1995) Depletion of neutrophils by filter during aorto-coronary bypass surgery transiently improves postoperative cardiorespiratory status. Chest 107:1253-1259

21. Driessen JJ, DhaeseH, Fransen G et al (1995) Pulsatile compared with nonpulsatile perfusion using a centrifugal pump for cardiopulmonary bypass during coronary bypass grafting: effects on systemic hemodynamics, oxygenation and inflammatory response parameters. Perfusion 10:3-12

22. Nilsson L, Tydén H, Johansson O et al (1990) Bubble and membrane oxygenators: comparison of postoperative organ dysfunction with special reference to inflammatory activity. Scand J Thorac Cardiovasc Surg 24:59-64

23. McLean RF, Wong BI, Naylor CD et al (1994) Cardiopulmonary bypass, temperature and central nervous system dysfunction. Circulation 90(2):250-255

24. Svensson LG, Crawford ES, Hess KR et al (1992) Deep hypothermia with circulatory arrest: determinants of stroke and early mortality in 656 patients. J Thorac Cardiovasc Surg 106: 19-31

25. Mora MC (1997) Cardiac surgery and central nervous injury: the importance of hypothermia during cardiopulmonary bypass. In: TJJ Lanck (ed) Neuroprotection. Williams & Wilkins, Baltimore, 89:197-237

26. Murkin JM, Martzke JS, Buchan AM et al (1995) A randomized study of the influence of perfusion technique and pH management strategy in 316 patients undergoing coronary artery bypass surgery. II. Neurological and cognitive outcomes. J Thorac Cardiovasc Surg 110:349-362

27. Hall RI, Smith SM, Graeme R (1997) The systemic inflammatory response to cardiopulmonary bypass: pathophysiological, therapeutic and pharmacological considerations. Anesth Analg 85:766-782

28. Park CK, Hall ED (1994) Dose response of the 21-aminosteroid tirilazad mesylate, upon neurological outcome and ischemic brain damage in permanent focal cerebral ischemia. Brain Res 645:157-163

29. Engelman RM, Rousou JÁ, Flack JE III et al (1995) Influence of steroids on complement and cytokine generation after cardiopulmonary bypass. Ann Thoracic Surg 60:801-804

30. Boldt J, Osmer C, Schindler E et al (1995) Circulating adhesion molecules in cardiac operations: influence of high dose aprotinin. Ann Thoracic Surg 59:801-804

31. Newburger JW, Jonas RA, Wernovsky G et al (1993) A comparison of the perioperative neurological effects of hypothermic circulatory arrest versus low-flow cardiopulmonary bypass in infant heart surgery. New Engl J Med 329:1057-1064

32. Svensson LG & Crawford ES (1992) Aortic dissection and aortic aneurysm surgery: clinical observations, experimental investigations and statistical analyses. Part I. Curr Probl Surg 29: 817-911

33. Jex RK, Schaff HV, Piehler JM et al (1986) Early and late results following repair dissections of the descending thoracic aorta. J Vasc Surg 3:226-237

34. Cosgrove DMI, Heric B, Lytle BW et al (1992) Aprotinin therapy for reoperative myocardial revascularization: a placebo controlled study. Ann Thoracic Surg 54:1031-1038

35. Sundt TMI, Kouchoukos NT, Saffitz JE et al (1993) Renal dysfunction and intravascular coagulation with aprotinin and hypothermic circulatory arrest study. Ann Thoracic Surg 55: 1418-1424

36. Sigman MG, Anderson RV, Balaban RS et al (1992) Barbiturates impair cerebral metabolism during hypothermic circulatory arrest. Ann Thorac Surg 54:1126-1130

New Concepts of Antiarrhythmic Strategies

J.L. ATLEE

Concept of substrates and imbalance

Cardiac arrhythmias are an important cause of morbidity and mortality in hospital settings. They are more likely to occur in patients with heart disease, which provides the substrate for genesis of arrhythmias. However, arrhythmias often will not occur without some destabilizing factor (imbalance). For example, patients with *chronic* ischemic heart disease may have zones of fibrous scar tissue intermingled with surviving, normal fibers. The latter provide potential pathways (the substrate) for anatomical reentry. However, arrhythmias do not occur without some trigger, which could be premature beats from an automatic focus in response to digitalis excess, catecholamines, acute electrolyte or other imbalance. The latter might even be produced by an antiarrhythmic drug administered to suppress ventricular extrasystoles [1, 2]. If so, the premature beat encounters refractory tissue (due either to prematurity of the beat or increased refractoriness secondary to acute imbalance) and blocks in one direction. However, it conducts slowly in another part of the anatomical circuit and returns to re-excite no longer refractory tissues of the circuit. Thus, a reentry ventricular tachycardia could be initiated and sustained. With *acute* ischemic heart disease, we envision a different substrate, one not defined by anatomical boundaries. Rather, the substrate is defined by nonuniform electrophysiologic properties, produced by compromised coronary flow to some tissues. Consequently, depolarization and repolarization of myocardial fibers is inhomogeneous due to variable activation and inactivation of Na and K channels. Conduction and refractoriness may be normal in some fibers, but prolonged in others. The stage is set, but still some trigger is required. The inciting imbalance might be coronary spasm or thrombosis, hypoxia, a surge in catecholamines, or drug toxicity. This could stimulate a focus of abnormal automaticity or triggered automaticity (from early or delayed afterpotentials) to generate premature beats required to initiate reentry [3]. Thus, the concept of substrates and imbalance, key to understanding contemporary antiarrhythmic strategies.

Proarrhythmia

If transient imbalance does alter normal or abnormal myocardium to cause or aggravate arrhythmias, then prevention and management should include treatment for structural heart disease and corrective intervention for obvious imbalance. This idea is especially important in the post-CAST (Cardiac Arrhythmia Suppression Trials) era, where we learned that chronic administration of class 1C antiarrhythmics to suppress chronic ventricular arrhythmias (encainide, flecainide, moricizine) increased expected mortality two- to three-fold, presumably by aggravation of arrhythmias or provocation of new ones [1, 2]. The latter phenomenon, aggravation or provocation of arrhythmias by antiarrhythmic drug, is termed proarrhythmia [4, 5]. Thus, when undertaking treatment of arrhythmias, one must be aware of the proarrhythmic potential of antiarrhythmic drugs, as well as of devices, used to treat arrhythmias. Examples of device proarrhythmia include 1) provocation of ventricular fibrillation during attempted cardioversion of tachyarrhythmias in patients with digitalis toxicity, and 2) programming an atrial-tracking temporary pacing mode in a patient with bradycardia and paroxysmal atrial tachycardia.

Pathophysiologic approach to management

Recognition of proarrhythmia (i.e., CAST I and II [1, 2]) and limitations of the Vaughan Williams drug classification system (below) led a group of the world's leading cardiologists, meeting first in Taormina, Sicily (1990) and later (1993) in Harriman, New York, to rethink strategies for pharmacologic management of arrhythmias [6, 7].

Class 1 - Na channel blockers, with variable potency as blockers of open or inactivated Na channels and recovery from blockade (1A, 1B, 1C)

Class 2 - β-adrenergic receptor antagonists

Class 3 - Drugs that prolong repolarization, primarily by block of K-channel repolarization currents

Class 4 - Ca-channel blockers (delay recovery from inactivation of the L-type cardiac Ca-channel)

Some antiarrhythmic drugs, especially the class 3 drugs amiodarone and sotolol, have more than one class action and/or different actions in different tissues. For example, amiodarone has all four class actions, with class II and IV effects more prominent following acute (parenteral) administration, and class I and III effects more prominent after prolonged administration. Sotolol, a class III drug is also a β-blocker. Lidocaine, a class 1B drug with a rapid onset of action and short time-constant for recovery, exerts greater effects in depolarized (ischemic, hypoxic) myocardium and at fast heart rates than in normal myocardium at slower heart rate.

So, instead of selecting a drug based on its electrophysiologic classification in normal cardiac tissue, the Sicilian Gambit suggested a more pathophysiologic approach, one based on recognition that drugs may act on one or several "targets" (e.g., ion channels, receptors, ion pumps, and other cardiac or extracardiac loci). Such targets are important not only to the genesis and perpetuation of arrhythmias, but also to normal sinus rhythm and conduction.

To illustrate the Gambit approach, let us consider AV nodal reentry tachycardia, one type of paroxysmal supraventricular tachycardia. The older empiric approach would have us make the diagnosis, then select an intervention (e.g., adenosine, verapamil) based on that diagnosis. The Gambit's pathophysiologic approach would have us consider: 1) known or suspected mechanisms (AV node with or without accessory AV pathway); 2) critical components (anatomical atrial pathway - fast or slow conduction; AV node - slow conduction); 3) vulnerable parameters (AV node or accessory pathway or atrial - action potential); and 4) targets for therapy (L-type Ca-channel; Na-channel). Thus, the Gambit approach represents an expansion of the older empiric approach to management. It offers us far more options for intervention and in planning strategies for prevention, much as does the Queen's gambit, a classic move in the game of chess.

Magnesium and perioperative ventricular arrhythmias

Magnesium (Mg^{2+}) and potassium (K^+) contribute importantly to the regulation of ion channel transport processes and generation of the action potential in myocardium. Both cations are essential for normal cellular excitability, uniform impulse propagation, and regular ventricular recovery. Experimental and clinical studies have shown that low K^+ and Mg^{2+} plasma concentrations increase the risk of ventricular tachyarrhythmias [8-10]. Administration of both Mg^{2+} and K^+ appears effective in reducing tachyarrhythmias with chronic heart failure [11, 12], and Mg^{2+} for perioperative ischemic tachyarrhythmias in patients undergoing coronary artery bypass surgery [13-15].

The concept that cardiac electrical stability might be increased by preservation of positive K^+ and Mg^{2+} balance is attractive due to its simplicity, safety and possible cost-effectiveness compared to chronic antiarrhythmic drug therapy, with the attendant risk of proarrhythmia and other adverse drug effects. The MAGICA (Magnesium in Cardiac Arrhythmias) multicenter trial assessed potential antiarrhythmic effects of oral Mg^{2+} and K^+ repletion in 307 patients with frequent but stable ventricular arrhythmias (> 720 VPB/24 hr, mean frequency > 300 VPB/h) [16]. Patients with "malignant" ventricular arrhythmias (> 6 consecutive VPB > 120 beats/min or history of sustained ventricular tachycardia - VT or fibrillation - VF) were excluded from study. Patients were assigned to two, randomized, three week periods of treatment with Mg^{2+} and K^+ (dietary intake increased by 50%) or placebo after a one-week placebo run-in period. Primary data analysis was based on 232 patients who presented low spontaneous arrhythmia variability both before (baseline) and after the placebo run-in (> 720 VPB/24 hr, both times). Secondary analysis included all patients with > 720 VPB/24 hr at baseline. Compared to three weeks of placebo, patients who received Mg^{2+} and K^+ had 2.4-fold increased suppression of VPB. Also, two response criteria for suppression of VPB were tested: 1) Primary analysis - predefined as a ≥ 60% reduction in the frequency of VPB; 2) Secondary analysis - a ≥ 70% reduction in VPB based on observed spontaneous arrhythmia variability in the 232 patients with low spontaneous arrhythmia variability. The likelihood of ≥ 60% or 70% reductions, respectively, were 1.5 and 1.7 times greater in patients receiving Mg^{2+} and K^+ compared to placebo. Finally, there was no effect of Mg^{2+} or K^+ repletion on the incidence of repetitive ventricular (paired VPB or salvos - ≥ 3 VPB) or supraventricular arrhythmias.

These findings are of interest, because new-onset tachyarrhythmias, particularly atrial tachyarrhythmias, often complicate the perioperative course of patients having cardiothoracic and major vascular surgery [17]. Many of these patients are elderly, and have chronic, stable atrial and/or ventricular arrhythmias. New-onset tachyarrhythmias are a destabilizing factor, have an adverse impact on outcomes, and increase the cost of hospitalization. It would be worthwhile if we could find a safe, low cost and effective means to prevent complications from tachyarrhythmias. Drugs are not necessarily the answer, for – in addition to proarrhythmia – they often compound haemodynamic imbalance with arrhythmias or have adverse interactions with anaesthetics and other drugs during the perioperative period. It should be noted here that proarrhythmia are completely undefined for antiarrhythmic drugs in perioperative settings.

There are no data that point to an association between new-onset atrial or ventricular tachyarrhythmias and preexisting "lesser" atrial or ventricular arrhythmias (premature beats, couplets, salvos, or non-sustained tachycardia < 15 sec) or chronic Mg^{2+} and K^+ depletion. Assuming there are such associations, should we empirically replete Mg^{2+} and K^+ in all patients undergoing cardiothoracic and vascular surgery? The Magica do not support such preemptive Mg^{2+} and K^+ repletion in all patients. However, in patients with "lesser" arrhythmias and established associations with Mg^{2+} and/or K^+ deficiency (e.g., chronic diuretic therapy, alcoholism, cirrhosis, diabetes, etc.), consideration should probably be given to preemptive repletion, at least until contrary data appear.

Prophylaxis for postoperative atrial fibrillation

Acute onset atrial flutter or fibrillation frequently complicate the postoperative course following cardiothoracic anaesthesia and surgery. The reported incidence ranges from 10 to 40 per cent with coronary artery bypass grafting (CABG), to 50 per cent or more with valvular or combined valvular and CABG surgery [17]. There is interest in new strategies for prophylaxis. Evidence is equivocal for efficacy of the Ca-channel blockers diltiazem and verapamil [18]. Possibly, they suppress Ca-mediated triggered action potentials that might initiate atrial flutter or fibrillation. However, Ca-channel blockers have no effect on atrial conduction and may reduce refractoriness, which could increase the atrial rate of atrial flutter or fibrillation. This is especially dangerous in a patient with ventricular preexcitation (Wolff-Parkinson-White syndrome) and a short antegrade refractory period of the accessory pathway. Digoxin is not effective for prevention of atrial flutter and fibrillation after cardiac surgery [18]. While class IA (procainamide) and IC drugs (flecainide, propafenone) can prevent recurrences of atrial flutter or fibrillation, a 5-10 per cent incidence of ventricular proarrhythmia complicates their use for prophylaxis in patients with ischemic or other cardiomyopathies.

Daoud et al. performed a double-blind, randomized comparison of placebo (N = 60) and oral amiodarone (N = 64) as prophylaxis for atrial fibrillation in patients having elective cardiac surgery (CABG = 52; valvular = 41; combined CABG and valvular = 22; other = 9 patients) [17]. The cumulative preoperative dose of amiodarone (600 mg x 7 days, then 200 mg/day until discharge) was 4.8 ± 1.0 gm over a period of 13 ± 7 days. The prevalence of atrial fibrillation during hospitalization was 16 of 64 patients (32 per cent) receiving amiodarone compared to 32 of 60 patients (53 per cent) with placebo. The duration of atrial fibrillation was similar in both groups, but the maximum ventricular rate was greater in the group receiving placebo (135 ± 31 vs. 112 ± 21 beats/min). DC cardioversion was performed on two patients receiving placebo, but none who received amiodarone (NS). Both length of stay and hospital costs were significantly reduced in the amiodarone compared to placebo treatment groups. Finally, while major morbidity and mortality were similar for both groups, patients who received amiodarone were more likely to remain free of atrial fibrillation 40-50 days after surgery. An earlier study of prophylactic IV amiodarone administered following completion of cardiac surgery also reported a reduced incidence of atrial fibrillation, but only for the first 48 hours postoperatively [19]. Thus, the actual incidence of post-operative atrial fibrillation may be underreported compared to the study with oral amiodarone [17]. Furthermore, amiodarone infusions were stopped in 18 per cent of patients due to adverse effects.

Amiodarone has a number of electrophysiologic actions by virtue of its diverse effects on specialized and nonspecialized atrial and ventricular tissue: 1) it slows atrial and ventricular conduction by virtue of use-dependent Na channel blockade (Class 1 action); 2) it slows sinus rate and AV node conduction time by β-adrenergic and Ca-channel blockade (class II and IV actions); 3) atrial and ventricular repolarization are prolonged due to block of K-repolarization currents (class III action); 4) amiodarone also produces noncompetitive α-adrenergic blockade [19, 20]. However, the time course for development of these actions differs [20]. Antiadrenergic effects and Ca-channel blockade develop soon after IV dosing. These could explain early suppression of atrial fibrillation, if triggered activity was required for initiation of atrial microreentry. Na- and especially K-channel blockade do not develop until later, but may render atrial myocardium incapable of sustaining microreentry. That β-blockade may be important to the effectiveness of amiodarone as prophylaxis for atrial fibrillation is suggested by studies demonstrating efficacy of β-blockers for prophylaxis of postoperative atrial fibrillation [21-28]. As noted earlier, evidence is equivocal for efficacy of Ca-channel blockade in prevention of postoperative atrial fibrillation [18].

Clearly, the early experience with oral amiodarone is quite promising [17], but confirmatory data from a larger, multicenter study will be required before amiodarone can be recommended as universal prophylaxis. Certainly, prophylactic oral amiodarone circumvents limitations of IV amiodarone and β-blockers, especially haemodynamic intolerance. Also, amiodarone is not as likely as β-blockers to aggravate preexisting medical conditions. Nonetheless, heart block, sinus arrest, and haemodynamic instability have been reported in patients receiving amiodarone and volatile anaesthetics [29, 30].

References

1. The Cardiac Arrhythmia Suppression Trial (CAST) Investigators (1989) Preliminary report: effect of encainide and flecainide on mortality in a randomized trial of arrhythmia suppression after myocardial infarction. N Engl J Med 321:406-412
2. The Cardiac Arrhythmia Suppression Trial (CAST) Investigators (1992) Effect of the antiarrhythmic agent moricizine on survival after myocardial infarction. N Engl J Med 327:227-233
3. Janse M, Wit A (1989) Electrophysiological mechanisms of ventricular arrhythmias resulting from myocardial ischemia and infarction. Physiol Rev 69:1049-1169
4. Morganroth J (1992) Proarrhythmic effects of antiarrhythmic drugs: evolving concepts. Am Heart J 123:1137-1139
5. Kerin N, Somberg J (1994) Proarrhythmia: Definition, risk factors, causes, treatment, and controversies. Am Heart J 128:575-586
6. The Sicilian Gambit (1991) A new approach to the classification of antiarrhythmic drugs based on arrhythmogenic mechanisms. Task force of the working group on arrhythmias of the European Society of Cardiology. Circulation 84:1831-1851
7. The Sicilian Gambit (1994) Antiarrhythmic therapy: A pathophysiologic approach. Futura Publishing, Armonk, pp 3-337
8. Tsuij H, Venditti FJ, Evans JC et al (1994) The association of levels of serum potassium and magnesium with ventricular premature complexes (the Framingham Heart Study). Am J Cardiol 74:232-235
9. Gettes L (1994) Electrolyte abnormalities as triggers for lethal ventricular arrhythmias. In: Akhtar M, Myerburg RJ, Ruskin JN (eds) Sudden cardiac death. Williams and Wilkins, Philadelphia, pp 327-340
10. Arsenian MA (1993) Magnesium and cardiovascular disease. Progr Cardiovasc Dis 4: 271-310
11. Gottlieb SS, Fisher ML, Pressel MD et al (1993) Effects of intravenous magnesium sulfate on arrhythmias in patients with cogestive heart failure. Am Heart J 125:1645-1650
12. Leir CV, Dei Cas L, Metra M (1994) Clinical relevance and management of the major electrolyte abnormalities in congestive heart failure: hyponatremia, hypokalemia, and hypomagnesemia. Am Heart J 128:564-574
13. Yusuf S, Teo K, Woods K (1993) Intravenous magnesium in acute myocardial infarction. Circulation 87:2043-2046

14. Woods KL, Fletcher S, Roffe C, Haider Y (1992) A randomized trial of intravenous magnesium in suspected acute myocardial infarction: results of the second Leicester Intravenous Magnesium Intervention Trial (Limit-2). Lancet 339:1553-1558

15. Schechter M, Hod H, Chouraqui P et al (1995) Magnesium therapy in acute myocardial infarction when patients are not candidates for thrombolytic therapy. Am J Cardiol 75:321-323

16. Zehender M, Meinertz T, Faber T et al for the MAGICA Investigators (1997) Antiarrhythmic effects of increasing the daily intake of magnesium and potassium in patients with frequent ventricular arrhythmias. J Am Coll Cardiol 29:1028-1034

17. Daoud EG, Strickberger SA, Man K et al (1997) Preoperative amiodarone as prophylaxis against atrial fibrillation after heart surgery. N Engl J Med 337:1785-1791

18. Hohnloser SH, Meinertz T, Dammbacher T et al (1991) Electrocardiographic and antiarrhythmic effects of intravenous amiodarone: results of a prospective, placebo-controlled study. Am Heart J 121:89-95

19. Kowey PR, Marinchak RA, Rials SJ, Filart RA (1997) Intravenous amiodarone. J Am Coll Cardiol 29:1190-1198

20. Mitchell LB, Wyse G, Gillis AM, Duff HJ (1989) Electropharmacology of amiodarone therapy initiation: time courses of onset of electrophysiologic and antiarrhythmic effects. Circulation 80:34-42

21. Rubin DA, Nieminski KE, Reed GE, Herman MV (1987) Predictors, prevention, and long-term prognosis of atrial fibrillation after coronary bypass graft operations. J Thorac Cardiovasc Surg 94:331-335

22. White HD, Antman EM, Glynn MA et al (1984) Efficacy and safety of timolol for prevention of supraventricular tachyarrhythmias after coronary artery bypass surgery. Circulation 70:479-484

23. Daudon P, Corcos T, Gandjbakhch I et al (1986) Prevention of atrial fibrillation or flutter by acebutolol after coronary bypass grafting. Am J Cardiol 58:933-936

24. Lamb RK, Prabhakar G, Thorpe JAC et al (1988) The use of atenolol in the prevention of supraventricular arrhythmias following coronary artery surgery. Eur Heart J 9:32-36

25. Janssen J, Looomans L, Harink J et al (1986) Prevention and treatment of supraventricular tachycardia shortly after coronary bypass grafting: a randomized open trial. Angiology 37:601-609

26. Suttorp MJ, Kingma JH, Tjon Joe Gin JG et al (1990) Efficacy and safety of low- and high-dose sotalol versus propranolol in the prevention of supraventricular tachyarrhythmias early after coronary bypass operations. J Thorac Cardiovasc Surg 100:921-926

27. Aranki SF, Shaw DP, Adams DH et al (1996) Predictors of atrial fibrillation after coronary artery surgery: current trends and impact on hospital resources. Circulation 94:390-397

28. Nystrom U, Edvardsson N, Berggren H et al (1993) Oral sotalol reduces the incidence of atrial fibrillation after coronary artery bypass surgery. Thorac Cardiovasc Surg 41:34-37

29. Navalgund AA, Alifimoff JK, Jakymec AJ, Bleyaert AL (1986) Amiodarone-induced sinus arrest successfully treated with ephedrine and isoproterenol. Anesth Analg 65:414-416

30. Gallagher JD, Lieberman RW, Meranze J et al (1981) Amiodarone-induced complications during coronary artery surgery. Anesthesiology 55:186-188

Emergency Treatment of Bradycardic and Tachycardic Arrhythmias

A.S. MONTENERO

Cardiac arrhythmic disorders are defined as bradycardia or tachycardia on the basis of ventricular response that is less than 60 b/m for bradyarrhythmias and more than 100 b/m for tachyarrhythmias. Arrhythmias are a common cause of syncope and must be considered in all patients in whom syncope occurs, particularly when cardiac disease is present. Either extreme of ventricular rate, bradycardia or tachycardia, can depress cardiac output to the point of critical hypotension and syncope. Cerebral blood flow is well maintained in supine, healthy individuals over a wide range of heart rates, from approximately 35 to 190 beats for minute. Pulse rates outside this range may reduce cerebral circulation and function. The most common arrhythmias producing syncope or presyncope are profound sinus bradycardia, high-grade atrioventricular (AV) block, supraventricular tachycardia, ventricular tachycardia, pacemaker malfunction, pacemaker induced arrhythmias, and pacemaker syndrome. Arrhythmias can occur as an isolated phenomenon (e.g. Wolff-Parkinson-White syndrome), but are commonly secondary to such disorders as ischaemic heart disease, cardiomyopathy, and valvular hearth disease.

Bradyarrhythmias

Bradyarrhythmic disorders depend on sinus node and AV node dysfunction or a combination of both [1].

Sinus node dysfunction

Bradycardia in the sinus node syndrome may result from a failure of sinus node impulse formation or failure of conduction of the impulse through the specialized atrial conduction system. Primary degenerative or fibrotic lesions in the sinus node and the specialized conduction tissue is the most frequent cause of the sick sinus syndrome, it may also occur as a secondary phenomenon in a variety of cardiac disorders. The most important electrocardiographic features of this disease are episodes of sinus arrest and sino-atrial block alternating with

episodes of atrial tachyarrhythmias (mainly atrial fibrillation) or intense bradycardia. The appearance of alternating sinus bradycardia with atrial fibrillation or
atrial flutter is quite common and is referred to as the *bradycardia-tachycardia
syndrome.* Syncope often occurs after abrupt termination of tachycardia, when
there is overdrive suppression of the sinoatrial or junctional pacemakers or of
AV conduction [2].

Atrial pause or sino-atrial block rarely require an emergency treatment, unless they determine a haemodynamic compromise, whereas episodes of prolonged sinus arrest or atrial fibrillation, with a very rapid ventricular response,
should be promptly treated to avoid syncope, dizziness or haemodynamic deterioration.

AV node block

High grade of AV block may be due to disease of AV node or of the His-Purkinje system. It may be caused by a primary degenerative disease of the AV node or
may be secondary to an acute episode of ischaemia or a combination of these
factors. Disease of AV node is associated with an intact junctional pacemaker
and a normal QRS complex that can be easily identified on the basis of the standard electrocardiogram as a first or second degree (Mobitz 1 or Mobitz 2).

Advanced second (Mobitz 2) and third degree AV block is due to disease
of the His-Purkinje system and usually associated with a wide idioventricular
escape rhythm that often require an emergency treatment to avoid syncope
(Morgagni-Adams-Stokes syndrome), dizziness or haemodynamic deterioration. The syncopal episodes are caused by either cardiac arrest or ventricular
arrhythmia [1].

Emergency therapy for patients with bradyarrhythmias

An intravenous infusion of saline drip should be provided as a first step, then
the acute treatment of bradyarrhythmic events depends on the recognition of the
arrhythmia. Symptoms like syncope or dizziness may be related to several factors other than prolonged bradycardia or complete acute AV block, therefore to
make interventions more appropriate is mandatory to differentiate between sinus
or junctional bradycardia and second or third degree AV block and to establish
the presence of a haemodynamic compromise.

Sick sinus syndrome is often asymptomatic or the symptoms are mild or
nonspecific. An intravenous infusion of isoproterenol might be considered as a
first step of the therapy in presence of prolonged asystole or intense bradycardia
and temporary pacing may be delayed until the patient is more clearly symptomatic.

In all patients, symptoms must be carefully correlated to arrhythmia manifestations. In the clearly symptomatic patient, treatment may include a combination of antiarrhythmic agents and temporary pacing. Ironically, eventual development of atrial fibrillation in patients with sick sinus syndrome may alleviate symptoms. Pacing is usually ventricular, but may be atrial when atrioventricular conduction and atrial stability can be reasonably assured.

First degree AV block is never symptomatic and is not an indication for temporary pacing.

Mobitz type 1 AV block, or the Wenckebach phenomenon is usually associated with an adequate ventricular rate and is rarely symptomatic. Rarely, the effective ventricular rate is slow and patients are symptomatic requiring temporary prophylactic pacing.

It may be common in the acute phase of inferior wall myocardial infarction; however it rarely requires temporary pacing in this setting and reversion is usually prompt.

Mobitz type 2 is less common but implies more significant conduction system disease. The site of block is almost always below the AV node, and usually below the His bundle, therefore, slower escape rhythms and risk of progression to complete heart block are of concern. Temporary pacing is indicated and the purpose of pacing is primarily to protect against symptomatic events, e.g. syncope, and thus protect the patient from injury to himself or herself or others.

Complete heart block may be acute in onset and produce significant symptoms, or may be chronic and discovered incidentally [3]. When acute and symptomatic, evaluation and rate support are urgently needed. Pharmacological intervention with atropine or isoproterenol are most readily available. The latter should be avoided in the ischaemic setting and external pacing instituted if needed until temporary ventricular pacing is provided. In any case, reliable rate control is achieved by ventricular temporary cardiac pacing.

Tachyarrhythmias

Management of cardiac tachyarrhythmias has become far more comprehensive in recent years, compared to the simple pharmacological approaches of the past. There is better understanding of the underlying systemic and cardiac factors which can be modified to influence outcome of the arrhythmias, and the range of pharmacological and nonpharmacological interventions has been expanded.

A complete management for any tachyarrhythmia must distinguish between: the specific underlying etiology, the contributing factors which interact with the underlying etiology. Contributing factors may be systemic or cardiac. The major metabolic abnormalities include hypoxia, acidosis, electrolyte disturbance, toxic or proarrhythmic drug effect and endocrine abnormalities. Central nervous system abnormalities may cause or aggravate specific arrhythmias; systemic haemodynamic disturbances may be involved in the genesis of the arrhythmias.

An arrhythmia which results from an electrophysiologic disturbance is defined as a *primary arrhythmia*; an arrhythmia which results from an electrical disturbance initiated by haemodynamic deterioration or metabolic abnormalities is a *secondary arrhythmia*.

Supraventricular arrhythmias

This category includes all tachycardias which originate above the His bundle, or incorporate tissues proximal to the bifurcation of the bundle of His in a reentrant circuit. The diagnosis requires an atrial chamber rate of 100 or more b/m; the ventricular rate may be less when AV conduction is incomplete. Supraventricular arrhythmias usually show narrow QRS complexes, but they may be wide because of aberrant conduction due to the presence of bundle branch block or by pass tract.

Supraventricular arrhythmias may be categorized into three subgroups based on duration: paroxysmal, persistent or chronic, therefore the management is dictated not only by its mechanism but also by its duration.

Emergency therapy for patients with supraventricular tachyarrhythmias

The reentrant paroxysmal supraventricular tachycardia

Paroxysmal supraventricular tachycardia (PSVT) may be due to AV nodal reentry, to Wolff-Parkinson-White syndrome (WPW), or interatrial or sinus node reentry. PSVT due to AV nodal reentry is the most common form of PSVT. It is a benign disturbance, requiring intervention solely for the patient's confort and sense of well-being, except when it coexists with other cardiac or non cardiac abnormalities that lead to a haemodynamic deterioration.

Rest, sedation and vagotonic maneuvers are simple means for reverting acute episodes. Pharmacological interventions, when required, include Ca+ entry blockers or β-adrenergic blockers. A 5 mg bolus of verapamil, followed by one or two additional 5 mg boluses 10 minutes apart if the initial doses does not convert the arrhythmia, is an effective regimen in up to 90% of patients [4].

The class Ic antiarrhythmic agents such as propafenone or flecainide (1 mg/kg of body weight in 10 min) may be tried if verapamil fails. It is worth of noting that when the QRS is wide class Ic agents should be avoided.

In patients with coexisting haemodynamically significant underlying heart disease, either i.v. verapamil or propranolol should be used with caution; when the clinical setting demands an immediate return to sinus rhythm either a transoesophageal catheter overdrive or a low-energy DC shock (10 to 50 joules) may be the right option.

Paroxysmal supraventricular tachycardia (PSVT) due to Wolff-Parkinson-White syndrome (WPW) is also common and amenable to a broad range of interventions. Careful attention to the details of therapy is required because a sub group is at risk for potentially lethal arrhythmias due to very rapid conduction across the accessory pathway during atrial flutter or fibrillation. This concern may influence the pharmacological approaches to PSVT in the WPW syndrome, since drugs have different effects on by pass tract and AV node. The class Ic antiarrhythmic agents such as propafenone or flecainide (1 mg/kg of body weight in 10 min) should be used as the first choice [5], whereas verapamil and digoxin should be avoid because they may accelerate the ventricular rate during atrial flutter or atrial fibrillation and evolve to a life-threatening tachyarrhythmia due to delay of conduction into the AV node and rapid accessory pathway conduction. In patients with coexisting haemodynamically significant underlying heart disease, or very rapid atrial fibrillation, even if they do not suffer other than WPW, an immediate return to sinus rhythm by using a low-energy DC shock (10 to 50 joules) should be achieved.

Atrial flutter

Atrial flutter may be paroxysmal, persistent or chronic.

Treatment of acute paroxysmal atrial flutter differs from that of PSVT due to AV nodal or reciprocating mechanisms. Carotid sinus massage slows the ventricular rate by partially blocking AV conduction, but may increase the flutter rate. The pharmacological therapy of atrial flutter should be directed to reversion to a sinus rhythm or to control of the ventricular rate. Drugs such as verapamil or β-blockers may be indicated to reduce ventricular rate; reversion may be achieved with amiodarone, flecainide or propafenone but their efficacy is unpredictable [6]. When the ventricular rate is poorly tolerated, an attempt to entrain the atrium with rapid transoesophageal or endocavitary pacing results in conversion to a more manageable atrial fibrillation or to sinus rhythm. Failing conversion or achieving an acceptable ventricular rate during atrial fibrillation may require cardioversion with DC shock.

Atrial fibrillation

Atrial fibrillation may be paroxysmal, persistent or chronic.

Short paroxysm of atrial fibrillation (AF) in the absence of underlying heart disease are usually managed conservatively. Propafenone, flecainide, amiodarone or ibutilide [7] may be used either to control the ventricular rate or to achieve restoration to sinus rhythm.

In the presence of heart disease, particularly when the haemodynamic circumstances require either atrial kick or a slow ventricular rate, immediate reversion to sinus rhythm may be mandatory. The presence of clinical signs of heart failure require immediate cardioversion to achieve this goal. Anticoagulation is not required prior to reversion when AF last from less than 48 hours.

Ventricular arrhythmias

When the algorithm of the electrocardiographic forms, clinical settings and end-points of treatment is applied to ventricular arrhythmias, they may be separated into the various patterns of triggering PVCs and of potentially lethal sustained ventricular tachycardia or fibrillation (VT or VF). However, this distinction is an oversimplification because of the lack of a uniformly accepted classification system to estimate risk.

The conventional definition of VT (three or more consecutive ventricular ectopic impulses at rate of 120 b/m or more) is too broad to apply to current evaluation and management procedure. A distinction between short runs of three to five consecutive complexes, burst of non sustained VT lasting for up to 30 seconds, and sustained VT lasting 30 seconds or more is necessary to properly evaluate bedside clinical information and target the therapy.

Emergency therapy for patients with ventricular tachyarrhythmias

The indications and methods for treating ventricular arrhythmias are complex and controversial, thus there often exist a conflict between the need to treat and the urge to treat. Despite these problems, there are many elements of arrhythmia management which are based upon scientifically developed pathophysiologic and pharmacodynamic concepts. Application of these concepts to clinical problems requires a clear analysis of the interrelationship between electrocardiographic forms of the arrhythmias, clinical setting and goals of therapy.

Sustained monomorphic ventricular tachycardia

This form of VT may occur in acute or chronic ischemic heart disease syndromes, dilated or hypertrophic cardiomyopathy, and less frequently in inflammatory or infiltrative disease or as a primary electrical disturbance. Management depends upon the clinical setting, and the clinical characteristic of the tachycardia.

In acute myocardial infarction VT may occur within 24-48 of the onset and in presence of stable haemodynamic condition 75-100 mg bolus of i.v. lidocaine, followed by a continuous infusion of 1 to 4 mg/min, may be tried. If the VT does not revert immediately, or in presence of haemodynamic compromise or hypotension, immediate DC cardioversion is required. Following cardioversion, i.v. lidocaine is continued to prevent recurrences. If VT recurs with lidocaine, amiodarone alone or in combination may be tried or even bretylium tosylate.

A form of sustained VT that occurs in late phase of myocardial infarction or complicate long-term follow up has a somewhat less ominous prognosis than acute phase VT, but is still considered lifethreatening, and requires special intervention. Management of the acute event requires intravenous antiarrhythmic drugs and/or cardioversion.

Automatic forms of VT that arise from the ventricular outflow tract of the right ventricle or from the left fascicular bundle of the left ventricle are sensitive to verapamil or β-blockers, but their diagnosis might be more difficult to be achieved. Usually they are very well tolerated, self terminating and rarely require cardioversion because of self terminating and not resulting to hypotension.

Ventricular fibrillation

Ventricular fibrillation is a terminal arrhythmia, uniformly requiring rapid initiation of emergency measures. Basic life support with standard CPR is used only until emergency defibrillation at 200 or more joules can be performed. Immediate steps to improve metabolic and electrolyte disturbances are required, paramount of which is to establish an airway, followed by technique to support ventilation.

After successful defibrillation, careful attention to total clinical status of the patient and prophylactic antiarrhythmic drugs or ventricular pacing, when in presence of bradycardia dependent VF, are required.

References

1. Montenero AS (1984) Le aritmie ipocinetiche. Autovalutazione in aritmologia. Ed Domus Cordis, p 106
2. Chung EK (1980) Sick sinus syndrome: Current views. Modern Concepts Cardiovasc Dis 49:61
3. Denes P (1987) Atrioventricular and intraventricular block. Circulation 75[Suppl 3]:19-25
4. Rinkenberger RL, Prystowsky EN, Heger JJ et al (1980) Effects of intravenous and chronic oral verapamil administration in patients with supraventricular tachyarrhythmias. Circulation 62:996
5. Montenero AS, Natale A, Di Bona G et al (1990) Opposite effects of propafenone and flecainide in a patient with reciprocating supraventricular tachycardia. Cardiologia 35(3):253
6. Buchanan LV, Kabell GG, Gibson JK (1995) Acute intravenous conversion of canine atrial flutter: Comparison of antiarrhythmic agents. J Cardiovasc Pharmacol 25:539-544
7. Stambler BS, Wood MA, Ellenbogen KA et al (1996) Efficacy and safety of repeated intravenous doses of ibutilide for rapid conversion of atrial flutter or fibrillation. Circulation 9a: 1613-1621

Perioperative Arrhythmias and Outcome

E. Mahla, H. Metzler

Based on expert opinion and observational data "symptomatic ventricular arrhythmias in the presence of underlying heart disease" have recently been defined as "a major predictor of increased perioperative cardiovascular risk (myocardial infarction, congestive heart failure or death)" and have been regarded as ominous as unstable coronary syndromes, decompensated congestive heart failure and severe valvular lesions [1].

Perioperative ventricular arrhythmias are considered to be the electrical manifestation of structural heart disease and/or transient imbalance [2-4].

Graded catecholamine surges with associated haemodynamic changes, ischaemia, fluid shifts, respiratory and metabolic alterations and perioperatively administered drugs may provoke arrhythmias particularly in a scarred, hypertrophied and dilated ventricle [2, 5-11].

Ventricular arrhythmias may compromise haemodynamics by an inappropriate heart rate with improper AV synchrony and ineffective contractions. In the setting of acute myocardial infarction or long QT syndrome premature ventricular contractions may trigger life threatening sustained ventricular tachyarrhythmias [2, 3, 12-14].

A satisfactory classification however, grading ventricular arrhythmias by frequency, appearance, haemodynamic impact and prognostic significance, currently does not exist [15].

Prevalence and frequency of perioperative ventricular arrhythmias vary with age, underlying cardiac disease, comorbidity, type of surgery, perioperative care and monitoring technique [2, 3, 16-21].

In a multicenter study Forrest et al. investigated 17,201 predominantly healthy patients (90,7% ASA physical status 1 and 2) to identify predictors of severe perioperative outcomes. Noncontinuous ECG monitoring revealed a 6,3% incidence of perioperative ventricular arrhythmias with only 0,6% needing significant treatment or cardiopulmonary resuscitation [22].

Whether or not there is an actual causative or only an associative relationship between arrhythmias and haemodynamic compromise can only be established by continuous Holter monitoring. Available anaesthesiologic literature is rare.

In men with definite or high risk for CAD scheduled for noncardiac surgery Mangano and his Mc Spi Group used continuous 3 days perioperative Holter ECG for evaluation of perioperative ischaemia and associations with in-hospital and two years adverse cardiac outcomes defined as cardiac death, nonfatal myocardial infarction, unstable angina, congestive heart failure, and ventricular tachycardia [23, 24].

They report an altogether 44% perioperative incidence of frequent or major ventricular arrhythmias (> 30 ventricular ectopic beats/min and or ventricular tachycardia) with postoperative ventricular tachycardia predominantly occurring in patients with an ejection fraction below 30% [25, 26]. Ventricular arrhythmias were asymptomatic, did not degenerate into sustained ventricular tachycardia or ventricular fibrillation and were neither associated with in-hospital nor two years adverse cardiac outcome [23-25].

Complex ventricular arrhythmias (multiform and repetitive ventricular ectopic beats) [27] have been associated with increasing hourly arrhythmia frequency [15].

Our group therefore investigated perioperative arrhythmia trend in patients already preoperatively presenting with repetitive ventricular arrhythmias in any form of cardiac disease (CAD, dilated cardiomyopathy or valvular lesions) (Fig. 1). The incidence of perioperative ventricular arrhythmias did not differ significantly between patients with good and adverse outcome (Table 1), nor was the incidence of perioperative ventricular arrhythmias predictive of progression to sustained tachyarrhythmias [28].

Table 1. Frequency of ventricular arrhythmias with respect to outcome

	Good outcome	Adverse outcome
Medians of PVB/hour		
Preoperative	92.90	39.86
Postoperative	56.33	28.59

PVB, premature ventricular beat

These data stress the fact that perioperative ventricular arrhythmias rather reflect or occur in the presence of serious underlying cardiac disease which by itself increases the risk of surgery.

The findings of Frank et al. and Lee et al. further support this concept [19, 29].

Maintenance of normothermia by forced air warming significantly reduced the incidence of early postoperative ventricular tachycardia in patients with definite CAD or at risk for CAD undergoing abdominal, thoracic or vascular procedures [19].

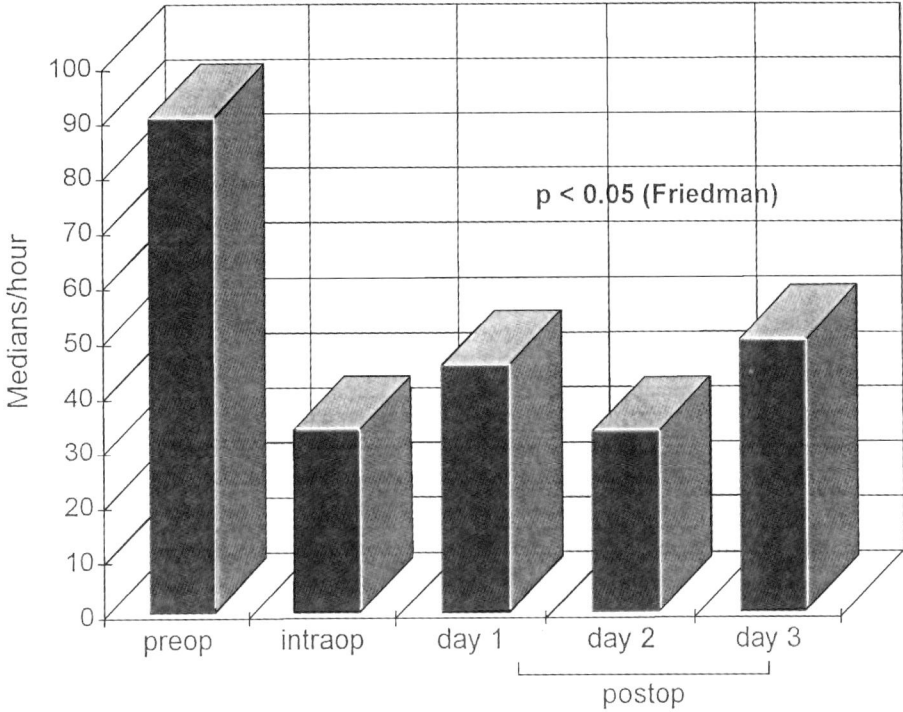

Fig. 1. Perioperative trend of premature ventricular contractions

In patients undergoing noncardiac surgery Lee et al. demonstrated a 17% incidence of perioperative Troponin T (TnT) elevation (> 0.1 ng/ml) carrying a 9.1 relative risk for major in-hospital cardiac complications (myocardial infarction, pulmonary oedema, primary cardiac arrest, ventricular fibrillation or complete heart block) which occurred in 3% of the patients. Perioperatively elevated TnT levels without major cardiac complications carried a significantly higher perioperative incidence of new sustained atrial and ventricular arrhythmias [29].

Compared to patients with perioperative TnT values less than 0.1 ng/ml, patients with elevated TnT had a 5.4% relative risk of an adverse postdischarge cardiac outcome during a 6 months follow-up period [30].

Conclusions

1. High-frequency, long-lasting ventricular arrhythmia may substantially impair an already compromised coronary perfusion or left ventricular function in the individual patient. In the setting of an acute myocardial infarction or a

long QT syndrome ventricular arrhythmias may degenerate into life-threatening sustained ventricular tachyarrhythmias.

2. Current evidence, however, suggests to regard nonsustained perioperative ventricular arrhythmias rather as concomitant marker of an underlying cardiac disease than as the actual cause of adverse cardiac outcome.

3. Recognition of the underlying cardiac disease is wanted for proper risk factor assessment and substrate oriented therapy in order to reduce in-hospital and long term morbidity and mortality.

References

1. American College of Cardiology/American Heart Association Task Force on Practice Guidelines (Committee on Peri-operative Cardiovascular Evaluation for Non-cardiac Surgery) (1996): Guidelines for peri-operative cardiovascular evaluation for non-cardiac surgery. Circulation 93:1278-1317
2. Atlee JL (1997) Perioperative cardiac dysrhythmias. Anesthesiology 86:1397-1424
3. Atlee JL (1996) Arrhythmias and pacemakers: Practical management for anesthesia and critical care medicine. WB Saunders, Philadelphia, pp 2-24
4. Task Force of the Working Group on Arrhythmias of the European Society of Cardiology. The Sicilian Gambit (1991) A new approach to the classification of anti-arrhythmic drugs based on their actions on arrhythmogenic mechanisms. Circulation 84:1831-1851
5. Naito Y, Tamai S, Shingu K et al (1992) Responses of plasma adrenocorticotropic hormone, cortisol and cytokines during and after upper abdominal surgery. Anesthesiology 77:426-431
6. Chernow B, Alexander HR, Smallridge RC et al (1987) Hormonal response to graded surgical stress. Arch Intern Med 147:1273-1278
7. Breslow MJ, Parker SD, Frank SM et al (1993) Determinants of catecholamine and cortisol responses to lower extremity revascularisation. Anesthesiology 79:1202-1209
8. Riles TS, Fisher FS, Schaefer S et al (1993) Plasma catecholamine concentrations during abdominal aortic aneurysm surgery: The link to perioperative myocardial ischemia. Ann Vasc Surg 7:213-219
9. Muller JE, Kaufmann PG, Luepker RV et al (1997) Mechanisms precipitating acute cardiac events. Circulation 96:3233-3239
10. Peters NS, Wit AL (1998) Myocardial architecture and ventricular arrhythmogenesis. Circulation 97:1746-1754
11. Kerin NZ, Somberg J (1994) Proarrhythmia: Definition, risk factors, causes, treatment, and controversies. Am Heart J 128:575-585
12. Steinbach KK, Merl O, Frohner K et al (1994) Hemodynamics during ventricular tachyarrhythmias. Am Heart J 127:1102-1106
13. Soroker D, Ezri T, Szmuk P et al (1995) Perioperative Torsades de Pointes ventricular tachycardia induced by hypocalcemia and hypokalemia. Anesth Analg 80:630-633
14. Richardson MG, Roark GL, Helfaer MA (1992) Intraoperative epinephrine-induced Torsades de Pointes in a child with long QT syndrome. Anesthesiology 76:647-649
15. Bethge KP (1991) Classification of dysrhythmias. J Cardiovasc Pharmacol 17[Suppl 6]:13-19
16. Manolio TA, Furberg CD, Rautaharju PM et al (1994) Cardiac arrhythmias on 24-h ambulatory electrocardiography in older women and men: The Cardiovascular Health Study. JACC 23:916-925
17. Bigger JT (1987) Why patients with congestive heart failure die: Dysrhythmias and sudden cardiac death. Circulation75[Suppl IV]:28-35

18. Mayet J, Shahi M, Poulter NR, Sever PS et al (1995) Ventricular arrhythmias in hypertension: In which patients do they occur? J Hypertens 13:269-276
19. Frank SM, Fleisher LA, Breslow MJ et al (1997) Perioperative maintenance of normothermia reduces the incidence of morbid cardiac events. JAMA 277:1127-1134
20. Zehender M, Meinertz T, Faber T (1997) Antiarrhythmic effects of increasing daily intake of magnesium and potassium in patients with frequent ventricular arrhythmias. J Am Coll Cardiol 29:1028-1034
21. Sueta CA, Clarke SW, Dunlap DO (1994) Effect of acute magnesium administration on the frequency of ventricular arrhythmia in patients with heart failure. Circulation 89:660-666
22. Forrest JB, Rehder K, Cahalan MK et al (1992) Multicenter study of general anesthesia. III Predictors of severe peri-operative adverse outcome. Anesthesiology 76:3-15
23. Mangano DT, Browner WS, Hollenberg M et al (1990) Association of peri-operative myocardial ischemia with cardiac morbidity and mortality in men undergoing noncardiac surgery. N Eng J Med 323:1781-1788
24. Mangano DT, Browner WS, Hollenberg M et al (1992) Long-term cardiac prognosis following noncardiac surgery. JAMA 268:233-239
25. O'Kelly B, Browner WS, Massie B et al (1992) Ventricular arrhythmias in patients undergoing non-cardiac surgery: The Study of Peri-operative Ischemia Research Group. JAMA 268:217-221
26. Halm EA, Browner WS, Tubau JF et al (1996) Echocardiography for assessing cardiac risk in patients having noncardiac surgery. Ann Intern Med 125:433-441
27. Lown B, Wolf M (1971) Approaches to sudden death from coronary heart disease. Circulation 44:130-142
28. Mahla E, Rotman B, Rehak P et al (1998) Perioperative ventricular dysrhythmias in patients with structural heart disease undergoing noncardiac surgery. Anesth Analg 86:16-21
29. Lee TH, Thomas EJ, Ludwig LE et al (1996) Troponin-T as a marker for myocardial ischemia in patients undergoing major noncardiac surgery. Am J Cardiol 77:1031-1036
30. Lopez-Jimenez F, Goldman I, Sacks DB et al (1997) Prognostic value of cardiac Troponin-T after noncardiac surgery: 6 month follow up data. J Am Call Cardiol 29:1241-1245

Therapeutic Monitoring in the Perioperative Period

O. Boyd, A. Rhodes

Monitoring in the perioperative period is traditionally performed for two reasons; firstly, to warn of life-threatening abnormalities, and secondly, to allow the maintenance of stable physiology. Although both essential, neither are themselves therapeutic. The concept of the use of the results of monitoring to guide changes in clinical treatment, which are themselves therapeutic and are greater than those required for maintaining normal physiology, is relatively new.

Most "therapeutic monitoring" is concerned with increasing tissue perfusion, at the present time two classes of monitoring have been used. The first is monitoring of cardiac output and tissue oxygen delivery by right heart catheterization, Doppler cardiac output estimation or non-invasive methods. The second is monitoring of regional tissue perfusion by gastric tonometry. What is the evidence that these forms of therapeutic monitoring improve outcome in the surgical patient?

Surgical mortality rates

Overall surgical mortality is low and is considered acceptable at about the 2% level. However, it is apparent that there are wide variations in mortality depending on the type of operation being performed and the underlying condition of the patient. It is not the purpose of this article to describe how operative factors effects surgical outcome, rather to describe factors within the patient themselves that effect outcome and to discuss how these may be modified to improve outcome. The major features which increase mortality above the average are age, co-morbidity and urgency of the surgical presentation.

Few studies are available which investigate mortality rates in these circumstances. The National Veterans Surgical Risk Study of patients with a mean age of 60 years had a mortality rate of 3.1% at 30 days, but 17% of patients had one or more major complication [1]. In a review of 900 patients aged 65 and over [2], patients with non-elective admissions (mortality rate 30% vs 5% for elective admissions), ASA grade 3+ (mortality rate 27% vs 8% for ASA < 3), age over 75 (mortality rate 20% vs 11% for patients aged 65 to 74) and major surgery (mortality rate 25% vs 10% for non-major surgery) were associated with much higher mortality at 200 days. Other studies have compared elective to more urgent surgery, and the influence of a patient's medical condition. In a population based study of colorectal surgery, the overall mortality rate was 7.6% at 30 days, but mortality rates of 21.7% were seen in patients undergoing urgent or emergency surgery [3]. Another study of urgent and emergency laparotomy showed an overall mortality of 44%, however, in patients rated as ASA 3 and over the mortality rate was 53% [4]. Considering the influence of a patients medical condition, a study of 108,878 anaesthetics between 1972 and 1977 [5], the overall mortality rate was 2.2%, but this rose considerably when there was a coexisting medical condition: 7.0% with ischaemic heart disease, 15.8% with cardiac failure and 5.7% with just diabetes. These mortality rates were increase significantly if the surgery was undertaken as an emergency.

Review of studies of treatment based on cardiac output and oxygen delivery

In 1985 Schultz and colleagues published the results of a randomized clinical trial of 70 patients undergoing operative repair of hip fracture [6]. Compared to a control group whose mortality was 29%, a monitored group treated with fluids, inotropes and vasodilators had a mortality of 2.9%. Some years later, using an approach in which cardiac index and oxygen delivery (DO_2) were increased with fluids and inotropes, Shoemaker et al. demonstrated a reduction in mortality from 33% to 4% [7]. Boyd and colleagues [8] reported the results of the largest randomized, controlled trial to date in which high risk surgical patients had a deliberate increase of DO_2 towards 600 ml/min/m^2. Results showed a significant reduction in postoperative complications, and mortality was reduced from 22.2% to 5.7%.

A number of studies have enrolled patients with lower baseline mortality rates. A randomized trial of patients undergoing limb-salvage arterial surgery showed no significant difference on mortality (9.5% in the control group and 1.5% in the protocol group), however the protocol group had fewer adverse intraoperative events, less postoperative cardiac morbidity and less early graft thrombosis than the control group [9]. Similar studies on patients undergoing aortic operations [10] and elective vascular surgery [11, 12], resulted in no significant difference in adverse postoperative events or mortality between the groups. However, in patients undergoing surgery for resection of hepatocellular carcinoma, there was a significant reduction in liver failure and hyperbilirubinemia postoperatively in patients treated to raised cardiac index and DO_2 [13].

There are three trials that have investigated the influence of increased DO_2 in trauma patients. Reduction in morbidity and mortality were seen in two of the studies [14, 15], but in a lower risk group of patients, with control group mortality of 10% no improvement in either mortality or morbidity was seen [16].

Two further studies in high-risk surgical patients have utilized pulsed Doppler to estimate cardiac output, while infusing 6% hydroxy-ethyl starch to achieve a maximum stroke volume [17, 18]. In elective cardiac surgical patients with ejection fraction > 50%, postoperative complications and hospital stay were significantly reduced, although there were no differences in the low mortality [17]. In patients undergoing repair of proximal femoral fracture the treatment group had significantly reduced hospital stay, but once again mortality was low and not significantly reduced by the intervention [18].

There have been 994 patients enrolled in the studies discussed above and the overall odds ratio for improvement in outcome is 0.35 (95% CI 0.23-0.53). As described in the text, there appears to be a difference in the likelihood of improvements in mortality related to the severity of illness of the patients studied. The six studies with mortality rates greater than 10% have a combined 451 patients and odds ratio of 0.25 (95% CI 0.15-0.43). Conversely, the seven studies with mortality rates less than 10% include 543 patients and provide an odds ratio of 0.88 (95% CI 0.39-2.00).

Gastric tonometry

Due to the special pathophysiological relationships in the gastrointestinal tract (GIT), a specific measure of regional splanchnic perfusion has become a much sought after goal in anaesthesia and critical care medicine [19]. The first modern descriptions of gastric tonometry were been in perioperative patients [20], and there are several important reasons why much attention is focused on the GIT. First, the gut of all the organs suffers the most intense vasoconstriction in response to hypovolaemia [21], leading to an increased risk of gut mucosal hypoxia in response to low flow states. Secondly, the critical DO_2 of the GIT is much higher than the rest of the body leading to pathological oxygen supply dependency states at levels of flow normally considered adequate [22]. Thirdly, it remains possible that GIT ischaemia/hypoxia may increase mucosal permeability and thus allow translocation of endotoxin and other micro-organisms setting off an inflammatory reaction [23], even if this is not the case the large mass of ischaemic tissue may itself fuel the inflammatory reaction.

Several important observations have led to the gastric tonometer being used as a marker of regional GIT perfusion. Traditionally information from the tonometer is used to calculate the gastric intramucosal pH (pH_i), although more recently the use of the directly measured pCO_2 result is being used. With a decrease in GIT blood flow there is a corresponding decrease in pH_i [24, 25]. This observation has been seen during endotoxaemia, when, if the GIT blood flow is then preserved, this reduction in pH_i is prevented [26].

The principles of tonometry have been well described [27], but some methodological problems remain. In order for the pH_i to be calculated, various assumptions have to be made. It is assumed that the arterial HCO_3^- is the same as the HCO_3^- in the gastric mucosa. However, this assumption is obviously an oversimplification [28-30]. These problems have led to recommendations that only directly measured variables from the Henderson-Hasselbalch equation be used for clinical practice i.e. the CO_2-gap ($PrCO_2$ - $PaCO_2$) [27, 31].

Further inaccuracies may result due to hydrogen ion secretion from the gastric parietal cells. These ions are able to diffuse back into the gastric mucosa which can result in an increased level of $PrCO_2$, or can react with any HCO_3^- ions that reflux back from the duodenum to create markedly raised levels of PCO_2 in the stomach. Either of these mechanisms can lead to increased levels of $PrCO_2$ (or a decreased pH_i) which are a result of buffering reactions rather than gastric mucosal ischaemia [32]. The routine use of H_2 blockers to prevent this gastric acid secretion has previously been recommended [33] but is now not thought to be of any value [34].

Clinical trials utilising tonometry

Although there have been many clinical studies in the literature utilising tonometry in critically ill or surgical patients, most have used the information as part of a predictive index for patient's outcome. There are few that have used this tool as a therapeutic monitor with the purpose of improving mortality [17, 35, 36]. Studies have described the ability of tonometry to accurately predict which patients will subsequently develop significant morbidity and mortality [37-39]. The attainment of a pH_i greater than 7.32 following 24 hours of resuscitation seems to be the best predictor of good outcome in critically ill patients [39], although some studies have suggested that in the most severely ill patients systemic acid-base variables may provide the same information [30]. The pH_i value is responsive to various forms of therapy and a variety of methods have been used including the use of colloidal fluid resuscitation [17], inotropes [40] and vasodilators [39]. Each of these has been able to demonstrate an improvement in pH_i with the protocolised treatment and thus an assumed reduction in episodes of gastric (and thus splanchnic) ischaemia. Although in none of these studies was pH_i result influencing the treatment given.

A number of studies have used the pH_i result to influence treatment. Gutierrez [36], in a multi-centre study evaluated the effect of pH_i directed therapy in 260 intensive care patients. Each patient was assigned to either maintenance of a pH_i of greater than 7.35 by manipulation of global oxygen delivery or standard intensive care therapy. Patients who were admitted with a low pH_i had no differences between protocol and control groups, however patients admitted with a normal pH_i (greater than 7.35) had a significantly improved survival (58% versus 42%, $p < 0.01$) [36]. In a study carried out on patients undergoing the above-mentioned coronary artery bypass surgery [17], the protocol group had an incidence of a pH_i less than 7.32, of 7% versus the control group who had an incidence of 56% ($p = 0.01$).

In a prospective study, Ivatury [35] randomised 57 trauma patients to either receiving pH_i directed therapy to maintain a pH_i of greater than 7.32, or therapy directed at maintaining an oxygen delivery of greater than 600 ml/min/m². They demonstrated that of the patients with a pH_i greater than 7.32 at 24 hours, 3 out of 44 died (6.8%) whereas for the other 13 patients there was 7 (53.9%) deaths ($p = 0.006$). They also found that the patients with a persistently low pH_i were frequently associated with systemic or intra-abdominal complications and the low pH_i was often the first finding in all the nonsurvivors at least 48 to 72 hours before death [35].

Conclusions

Therapeutic monitoring is a relatively new concept in care for the perioperative patient. Most trials that have been conducted have used right heart catheterization and have tended to show an improvement in outcome, especially in the trials considering the more severely ill patients [41-43]. It is important to emphasise that these trials are on perioperative patients because there are a number of trials on general critically ill patients that have not shown any advantage to this type of therapeutic monitoring [44, 45]. Although the gastric tonometer has the potential to take therapeutic monitoring into the era of organ specific, "regional" directed therapy, the widespread utilisation in the clinical setting cannot be recommended until further randomised controlled studies are performed.

References

1. Kuri SF, Daley J, Henderson W et al (1995) The national veterans surgical risk study: risk adjustment for the comparative assessment of the quality of surgical care. J Am Coll Surg 180:519-531
2. Edwards AE, Seymour DG, McCarthy JM et al (1996) A 5-year survival study of general surgical patients aged 65 and over. Anaesthesia 51:3-10
3. Mella J, Biffin A, Radcliffe AG et al (1997) Population-based audit of colorectal cancer management in two UK health regions. Colorectal Cancer Working Group, Royal College of Surgeons of England Clinical Epidemiology and Audit Unit. Br J Surg 84:1731-1736
4. Cook TM, Day CJE (1998) Hospital mortality after urgent and emergency laparotomy in patients aged 65 and over. Risk and prediction of risk using multiple logistic regression analysis. Br J Anaesth 80:776-781
5. Fowkes FGR, Lunn SC, Farrow SC et al (1982) Epidemiology in anaesthesia. III: Mortality risk in patients with coexisting physical disease. Br J Anaesth 54:819-824
6. Schultz RJ, Whitfield GF, LaMura JJ et al (1985) The role of physiologic monitoring in patients with fractures of the hip. J Trauma 25:309-316
7. Shoemaker WC, Appel PL, Kram HB et al (1988) Prospective trial of supranormal values of survivors as therapeutic goals in high-risk surgical patients. Chest 94:1176-1186

8. Boyd O, Grounds RM, Bennett ED (1993) A randomized clinical trial of the effect of deliberate perioperative increase of oxygen delivery on mortality in high-risk surgical patients. JAMA 270:2699-2707

9. Berlauk JF, Abrams JH, Gilmour IJ et al (1991) Preoperative optimisation of cardiovascular hemodynamics improves outcome in peripheral vascular surgery. Ann Surg 214:289-297

10. Valentine RJ, Duke ML, Inman MH et al (1998) Effectiveness of pulmonary artery catheters in aortic surgery: a randomized trial. J Vasc Surg 27:203-211

11. Bender JS, Smith-Meek MA, Jones CE (1997) Routine pulmonary artery catheterization does not reduce morbidity and mortality of elective vascular surgery: results of a prospective, randomized trial. Ann Surg 226:229-236

12. Ziegler DW, Wright JG, Choban PS et al (1997) A prospective randomized trial of preoperative "optimization" of cardiac function in patients undergoing elective peripheral vascular surgery. Surgery 122:584-592

13. Ueno S, Tanabe G, Yamada H et al (1998) Response of patients with cirrhosis who have undergone partial hepatectomy to treatment aimed at achieving supranormal oxygen delivery and consumption. Surgery 123:278-286

14. Fleming A, Bishop M, Shoemaker W et al (1992) Prospective trial of supranormal values as goals of resuscitation in severe trauma. Arch Surg 127:1175-1179

15. Bishop MH, Shoemaker WC, Appel PL et al (1995) Prospective, randomized trial of survivor values of cardiac index, oxygen delivery, and oxygen consumption as resuscitation endpoints in severe trauma [see comments]. J Trauma 38:780-787

16. Durham RM, Neunaber K, Mazuski JE et al (1996) The use of oxygen consumption and delivery as endpoints for resuscitation in critically ill patients. J Trauma 41:32-39

17. Mythen MG, Webb AR (1995) Perioperative plasma volume expansion reduces the incidence of gut mucosal hypoperfusion during cardiac surgery. Arch Surg 130:423-429

18. Sinclair S, James S, Singer M (1997) Intraoperative intravascular volume optimisation and length of hospital stay after repair of proximal femoral fracture: randomised controlled trial. Br Med J 315:909-912

19. Brinkmann A, Calzia E, Trager K et al (1998) Monitoring the hepato-splanchnic region in the critically ill patient. Intensive Care Med 24:542-556

20. Fiddian-Green RG, Gantz NM (1987) Transient episodes of sigmoid ischemia and their relation to infection from intestinal organisms after abdominal aortic operations. Crit Care Med 15:835-839

21. Edouard AR, Degremont AC, Duranteau J et al (1994) Heterogeneous regional vascular responses to simulated transient hypovolaemia in man. Intensive Care Med 20:414-420

22. Nelson DP, Beyer C, Samsel RW et al (1987) Pathological supply dependence of O_2 uptake during bacteremia in dogs. J Appl Physiol 63:1487-1492

23. Pastores SM, Katz DP, Kvetan V (1996) Splanchnic ischemia and gut mucosal injury in sepsis and the multiple organ dysfunction syndrome. Am J Gastroenterol 91:1697-1710

24. Grum CM, Fiddian-Green RG, Pittenger GL et al (1984) Adequacy of tissue oxygenation in intact dog intestine. J Appl Physiol 56:1065-1069

25. Elizalde JI, Hernandez C, Llach J et al (1998) Gastric intramucosal acidosis in mechanically ventilated patients: role of mucosal blood flow. Crit Care Med 26:827-832

26. Antonsson JB, Boyle III CC, Kruithoff KL et al (1990) Validation of tonometric measurement of gut intramural pH during endotoxemia and mesenteric occlusion in pigs. Am J Physiol 259:G519-G523

27. Fiddian-Green RG (1995) Gastric intramucosal pH, tissue oxygenation and acid-base balance. Br J Anaesth 74:591-606

28. Benjamin E, Polokoff E, Oropello JM et al (1992) Sodium bicarbonate administration affects the diagnostic accuracy of gastrointestinal tonometry in acute mesenteric ischemia. Crit Care Med 20:1181-1183

29. Schlichtig R, Bowles SA (1994) Distinguishing between aerobic and anaerobic appearance of dissolved CO_2 in intestine during low flow. J Appl Physiol 76:2443-2451

30. Boyd O, Mackay CJ, Lamb G et al (1993) Comparison of clinical information gained from routine blood-gas analysis and from gastric tonometry for intramural pH [see comments]. Lancet 341:142-146
31. Rhodes A, Boyd O, Bland JM et al (1997) Routine blood-gas analysis and gastric tonometry: a reappraisal [letter]. Lancet 350:413
32. Fiddian-Green RG, Pittenger G, Whitehouse Jr WM (1982) Back-diffusion of CO_2 and its influence on the intramural pH in gastric mucosa. J Surg Res 33:39-48
33. Heard SO, Helsmoortel CM, Kent JC et al (1991) Gastric tonometry in healthy volunteers: Effect of ranitidine on calculated intramural pH. Crit Care Med 19:271-274
34. Calvet X, Baigorri F, Duarte M et al (1998) Effect of ranitidine on gastric intramucosal pH in critically ill patients. Intensive Care Med 24:12-17
35. Ivatury RR, Simon RJ, Islam S et al (1996) A prospective randomized study of end points of resuscitation after major trauma: global oxygen transport indices versus organ-specific gastric mucosal pH. J Am Coll Surg 183:145-154
36. Gutierrez G, Palizas F, Doglio G et al (1992) Gastric intramucosal pH as a therapeutic index of tissue oxygenation in critically ill patients. Lancet 339:195-199
37. Marik PE (1993) A better predictor of multiorgan dysfunction syndrome and death than oxygen-derived variables in patients with sepsis. Chest 104:225-229
38. Gomershall CD, Joynt GM, Ho KM et al (1997) Gastric tonometry and prediction of outcome in the critically ill. Arterial to intramucosal pH gradient and carbon dioxide gradient. Anaesthesia 52:619-623
39. Maynard N, Bihari D, Beale R et al (1993) Assessment of splanchnic oxygenation by gastric tonometry in patients with acute circulatory failure. JAMA 270:1203-1210
40. Smithies M, Yee TH, Jackson L et al (1994) Protecting the gut and liver in the critically ill: effects of dopexamine. Crit Care Med 22:789-795
41. Boyd O, Bennett ED (1996) Enhancement of perioperative tissue perfusion as a therapeutic strategy for major surgery. New Horiz 4:453-465
42. Heyland DK, Cook DJ, King D et al (1996) Maximizing oxygen delivery in critically ill patients: a methodologic appraisal of the evidence [see comments]. Crit Care Med 24:517-524
43. Ivanov RI, Allen J, Sandham JD et al (1997) Pulmonary artery catheterization: a narrative and systematic critique of randomized controlled trials and recommendations for the future. New Horiz 5:268-276
44. Hayes MA, Timmins AC, Yau EH et al (1994) Elevation of systemic oxygen delivery in the treatment of critically ill patients. N Engl J Med 330:1717-1722
45. Gattinoni L, Brazzi L, Pelosi P et al (1995) A trial of goal-oriented hemodynamic therapy in critically ill patients. N Engl J Med 333:1025-1032

OBSTETRIC COMPLICATIONS

Uncommon Diseases in Pregnancy

G.C. Di Renzo, G. Iammarino, L. Donati

Pregnancy represents a unique alteration in physiology that usually ends without complications. The concept of "at risk pregnancy" is related to a pregnancy in which there is a risk of an adverse outcome in the mother and/or in the fetus that is greater than the incidence of that outcome in the general population. Once a risk factor known to be associated with an increased risk of a specific adverse outcome is identified, then professionals involved in pregnancy care may modify the routine antenatal care, providing to anticipate, minimise, prevent or treat that adverse outcome [1].

Sometimes, however, life-threatening complications occur, so that an intensive care with invasive monitoring and mechanical ventilation is needed. In approximately 40% of direct maternal deaths there is need for intensive care [2].

A maternal death is defined as the death of a woman while pregnant, irrespective of the duration and the site of the pregnancy, from any cause related to or aggravated by the pregnancy or its management, but not from accidental or incidental causes (Perinatal Audit, 1996) [3].

From review studies about critically ill obstetric patients admitted to intensive care units (ICUs) ranging from 0,1 to 0,9% of all deliveries, the most common causes of such admissions are hypertensive disorders with associated complications as progressive deterioration of renal function, abruptio placentae and coagulopathies. Mortality is often related to adult respiratory distress syndrome (ARDS). Haemorrhage is the second most significant cause of morbidity often due to disseminated intravascular coagulation (DIC). Morbidity results sometimes from pre-existing medical conditions, otherways well controlled, but exacerbated by the anatomical and physiological changes in pregnancy. For instance, increased cardiac output, blood volume, and heart rate increase cardiac work. This can put women with cardiovascular disorders at risk of decompensation. These effects might also be aggravated by an increase in clotting factors, because the hypercoagulable state of pregnancy predisposes to embolic events in patients with polycitemia, atrial fibrillation and cardiomyopathies. Changes in the pulmonary function also increase demands on the respiratory system and compromise patients with minimal reserve. Multiple fetuses can potentiate this effect [2].

In the present work only the less common aspects of the most frequent causes of obstetric patients' admission to ICUs will be considered.

Haemorrhagic/thromboembolic disorders

Obstetric haemorrhages are responsible for about 75% of maternal complications during pregnancy, while coagulation abnormalities, both haemorrhage and thromboembolism, are the most frequent complications of pregnancy and delivery and the first cause of maternal mortality [4].

It is critical for the obstetrician to be able to estimate rapidly the blood volume deficit in the pregnant patient that has the protective effect of the usual volume expansion of pregnancy and will show signs of blood loss only lately. An obstetric haemorrhage is traditionally defined as a blood loss of more than 500 cc after completion of the third stage of labor (ending with placental delivery) and more than 1000 cc after caesarean section [5].

Among the antepartum haemorrhage, placental pathologies are responsible for one third of excessive bleeding. In particular *abruptio placentae* (the premature separation of the normally implanted placenta from its attachment to the uterus) occurs with a frequency of 1 in 120 births, and when diagnosed, precaution should be taken to deal with the possible life-threatening consequences for both mother and fetus. At least four units of blood should be available for maternal transfusion, an intravenous line must be secured and the infusion of cristalloyd solution begun. Any attempt to arrest preterm labour and to keep the woman under close observation in case of known or suspected abruption should be weighed against the likelihood for survival and morbidity if the infant should be delivered, and the severity of the abruption. In many cases delivery is the treatment of choice. When encountering a patient with *placenta previa*, the possibility of a *placenta accreta* or one of its variations, *placenta percreta* or *placenta increta*, should be considered. In these conditions, the placenta forms an abnormally firm attachment to the uterine wall. It can be attached directly to the myometrium (accreta), invade the myometrium (increta), or penetrate the myometrium (percreta). If vaginal delivery has occurred, the patient should be in a room in which a laparotomy can be performed for possible hysterectomy.

However, the most haemorrhagic emergencies occur during and after delivery. More frequent are the *post-partum haemorrhages* that include more than 50% of maternal deaths for excessive bleeding, and that arise mainly from the following causes: uterine hypotonia/atonia, retained placenta or placental fragments, placental pathologies (placenta accreta, percreta, increta), laceration of the lower genital tract, intravasal coagulation, rupture of the uterus, inversion of the uterus [6]. Continued bleeding in the third stage of labour that is unresponsive to usual treatment should alert the clinician to consider uncommon but serious maternal coagulation disorders. Obstetric coagulopathies can be classified into: congenital and acquired or induced by pregnancy. *Congenital coagu-*

lopathies represent the smallest group in which a genetically determined defect has been identified in more steps of the coagulation process. They are usually recognised after a good clinical assessment, pertinent history and family history. Some of them (von Willebrand, factor VIII: C and IX defects) may be evident in adulthood. The most frequent pathologies are shown in Table 1.

Table 1. Congenital coagulopathies in pregnancy

Von Willebrand disease
Haemophilia A (factor VIII: C deficit)
Haemophilia B (Christmas disease, factor IX deficiency)
Deficit of α-2-antiplasmin
Glanzmann's thromboastenia (platelet glycoprotein defect)
Bernard-Soulier syndrome (platelet membrane alteration)
Hereditary thrombocytopenia
AT III deficit *

* The most common disorder of coagulation in pregnancy; from 40-70% of patients presenting this autosomic dominant trait undergo thromboembolic complications

Thromboembolic complications are not a rarity in obstetric patients since they present predisposing factors like stasis (due to the pregnant uterus obstructing venous return), damage to vascular endothelium (during vaginal delivery or caesarean section), and hypercoagulability (pregnancy has been termed a "hypercoagulability" state in that several factors involved in the coagulation cascade increase during pregnancy, i.e., fibrinogen, factors VII, VIII, IX, X, while others, i.e., AT III and protein S, decrease). Additional risks are obesity, infections, smoke, varicous veins, trauma.

The treatment of the deep venous thrombosis is based on anticoagulation by heparin, administered subcutaneously or intravenously for 10 days in order to prolong the thromboplastin time from 1,5 to 2 times the control value. If recurrent thrombosis occurs, heparin therapy must be continued until the post partum period. Coumadin derivates are not indicated in pregnancy because they cause multiple congenital fetal abnormalities during the first trimester and fetal and placental haemorrhage during the second and third trimester. Heparin is also indicated for treatment of pulmonary embolism preferably by the intravenous route. When possible a brachial catheterism is indicated in order to frame the embolus, then it is necessary to perform a systemic thrombolysis with heparin (40,000 IU/24 hours continuously for 10 days). One week after the delivery heparin can be replaced by warfarin that should be continued for three months. Heparin prophylaxis in obstetric patients at risk for thrombosis (as lacking of AT III, protein C and S and APC resistance) is performed with 2,000 IU/pro day s.c., keeping the anti Xa value at about 0,2 U/ml.

Acquired *coagulation abnormalities* are listed in Tables 2 and 3.

Table 2. Acquired coagulopathies in pregnancy

Hydiopatic thrombocitopenia (Werlhof)
Thrombotic thrombocitopenic purpura (Moskowitz)
Uremic haemolytic syndrome (Gasser)
Post-transfusional thrombocytopenia
LES anti phospholipids syndrome
Vitamine K deficiency
Hepatopathies
Acquired coagulation inhibitors *
Pharmacological thrombocytopenia

* IgG appearing in 15-20% of patients affected by deficiency of factor VIII and IX, submitted to multiple transfusion

Table 3. Pharmacological thrombocytopenia

Neurologic drugs: barbiturates, diazepam, diphenylhydantoin
Antihypertensive drugs (α-methyldopa, hydralazina, diazoxide)
Analgesics (aspirin)
Antibiotics (ampicillin, cephalosporin, isoniazid, rifampin, sulfonamides, carbenicillin)
Diuretics: tiazide, furosemide, acetozolamide
Cardiac output: digitoxin, quinine
Clorochine, indomethacin
Others: H_2 antagonists, cocaine

Patients without coagulation defects can develop haemorrhage during pregnancy or delivery in a particular situation called disseminated intravascular coagulation (DIC), which could compromise any of the mechanisms involved in the coagulation process, leading to hypofibrinogenemia, and to consumption of platelets and clotting factors V and VIII. The net result of factors' consumptions, fibrin disruption and platelets' dysfunction occurring diffusely in the vasculature is maternal bleeding. Coagulation disturbances generally resolve after correction of the initial stimulus. When it persists, it must be treated by replacing coagulation factors and red cells guided by laboratory findings. Although the overall prognosis is good, hypovolaemic shock associated with DIC may initiate other problems: acute tubular necrosis and Sheehan's syndrome (hypoperfusion and post-haemorrhagic necrosis of the anterior pituitary) [7].

Hypertensive disorders

It is a common problem of pregnancy occurring in about 12-15% of cases remaining one of the major causes of maternal mortality.

A rate of women affected by severe pre-eclampsia ranging from 4 to 12% will turn into a so called HELLP syndrome, characterised by the simultaneous occurrence of haemolysis, elevated liver enzymes and low platelets, and developing especially above the third trimester and in about 30% of cases in the post-partum period [8, 9].

Between 25 and 30 weeks' gestation a conservative management can be considered in order to provide fetal lung maturation, through an accurate monitoring of fetal and maternal conditions. Corticosteroids given to the mother have been proved to be of help in this case. In case of worst evolution of the disease and at any gestational age, delivery is mandatory (Table 4). Some alternative therapies have been proposed: plasma volume expansion, antithrombotic agents, immunosuppressive agents, plasma-exchange (post-partum), dialysis. Vaginal delivery is not contraindicated even if in the majority of cases a caesarean section is performed. In this case choice of anaesthesia should be balanced in individual situations. There is no contraindication for epidural anaesthesia, while spinal anaesthesia is associated with higher risk of hypotension and compromission of the uteroplacental circulation and there is not yet any evidence in medical literature that it is as safe as the epidural one. A major controversy is the as-

Table 4. Maternal guidelines for expedited delivery and conservative management of severe pre-eclampsia remote from term

Management	Clinical findings
Expedited delivery (within 72h)	One or more of the following: Uncontrolled severe hypertension * Eclampsia Platelet count < 100000/microl AST or ALT > 2 x upper limit of normal with epigastric pain or right upper quadrant tenderness Pulmonary oedema Compromised renal function ** Persistent severe headache or visual changes
Conservative management	One or more of the following: Controlled hypertension Urinary protein > 5000 mg/24h Oliguria (< 0.5 ml/kg per hour) that resolves with routine fluid or food intake AST or ALT > 2 x upper limit of normal without epigastric pain or right upper quadrant tenderness

*   Blood pressure persistently ≥ 160 mmHg systolic or ≥ 100 mmHg diastolic despite maximum recommended dose of two antihypertensive medications
** Persistent oliguria (< 0.5 ml/kg per hour) or a rise in serum creatinine of 1 mg/dl over baselines levels

sessment of the risk of regional anaesthesia in the presence of platelets dysfunction or prophylactic anticoagulant therapy.

In the post-partum period, the time of onset of manifestations ranges from few hours to seven days, with the majority developing within 48 hours postpartum. According to some authors' these patients are at increased risk for the development of pulmonary oedema and acute renal failure. The differential diagnosis in these patients should include exacerbation of systemic lupus erythematosus, thrombotic thrombocytopenia purpura and haemolytic uremic syndrome.

Patients with delayed resolution of HELLP syndrome should be referred to a tertiary care centre and initial management should be finalised to stabilise maternal conditions, particularly coagulation abnormalities [10].

Sepsis

The American College of Chest Physicians and the Society of Critical Care Medicine held a Consensus Conference in 1991 to standardise definition for sepsis. They proposed systemic inflammatory response syndrome (SIRS) to describe the inflammatory process that can be generated by infectious or non infectious causes. The response is manifested by two or more of the following conditions: temperature above 38°C or below 36°C, heart rate more than 90 beats per minute, respiratory rate more than 20 breaths per minute or $PaCO_2$ below 32 mmHg, white blood cell count more than 12,000 mm^3 or less than 4,000 mm^3 or > 10 per cent band forms. Sepsis is SIRS due to infection. Severe sepsis is sepsis associated with organ dysfunction, hypoperfusion, or hypotension.

Septic shock is defined as sepsis induced hypotension despite adequate fluid resuscitation with the presence of perfusion abnormalities that may include, but are not limited to, lactic acidosis, oliguria, or an acute alteration in mental status.

Many infections may result in septic shock in obstetric patients, but endometritis, chorioamnionitis, and pyelonephritis are the most common causes. Significant risk factors for septic shock include prolonged rupture of membranes, retained products of conception, and instrumentation of the genito-urinary tract. A significant increase in post-caesarean section infection is seen in indigent patients.

Other infections developing in obstetric patients include pneumonia, appendicitis, septic abortion, toxic shock syndrome, septic pelvic thrombophlebitis and endocarditis.

Obstetric infections are usually caused by organisms normally found in the genital tract and thus are often polymicrobical (Escherichia Coli, Klebsiella, Enterobacter, Pseudomonas, Serratia, Chlamydia Tracomatis, Neisseria Gonorrhoeae).

During the 1960s and 1970s, Gram-negative bacteria were the most common cause of septic shock. Now the Gram-positive microbes, in particular Staphylococcus Aureus and Enterococci, account for 40 to 50% of nosocomial infections.

Treatment of septic shock requires general supportive measures, including restoration of intravascular volume and often inotropic support. Adequate oxygenation is essential. Antibiotic therapy for sepsis should be tailored directly to the suspected source guided by information obtained by gram-stain. Failure of the patient to respond promptly to simple volume resuscitation must be followed by a transfer to an intensive care setting [11].

The *toxic shock syndrome* (TSS) has been reported to occur in association with vaginal delivery, spontaneous abortion, caesarean section, and mastitis. The exact incidence is unknown, but mortality is estimated to be about 5%. Typical signs are high fever, diffuse macular erythrodermal rash with desquamation, hypotension, and evidence of multiple organ system involvement caused by the absorption of exotoxin (produced by the Staphylococcus Aureus). A prompt treatment provides aggressive fluid replacement to correct systemic hypotension and a precise antibiotic therapy. ICU transfer is necessary in many instances.

Suppurative pelvic thrombophlebitis (SPT) is a condition of thrombosis of the pelvic veins. Trauma of the surface of the genital tract is often the initiating factor preceding thrombosis and infection. Diagnosis is often difficult and made by exclusion. Treatment begins with intravenous heparin and if medical therapy is unsuccessful or pulmonary infarction additionally occurs, surgical therapy (embolization or ligation of the inferior vena cava and or of both ovarian veins) is indicated.

Necrotizing fascitis is a rare but deadly complication in obstetrics due to a suppurative bacterial infection of superficial and deep fasciae. Treatment consists in surgical removal of necrotic tissue, drainage and parenteral antibiotics.

Cardiac diseases

In pregnancy significant haemodynamic alterations occur since 5 weeks of gestation (increasing of heart rate, increasing of blood volume and of plasmatic volume, increased cardiac output, decreased peripheric resistances). The pregnant patient with normal cardiac function undergoes to these physiological changes without difficulty; however, the presence of a significant cardiac disease makes the pregnancy extremely dangerous, resulting in decompensation and even death. It is estimated that about one third of the indirect maternal deaths are due to cardiac disease [12].

Focusing on the right diagnosis is not easy at all, because some symptoms presented during pregnancy (dyspnea, orthopnea, palpitations, chest pain, syncope) must be differentiated from others associated to heart disease; these are listed in Table 5 [13].

Table 5. Maternal mortality risk associated with specific cardiac diseases

Group 1 Mortality < 1%	Group 2 Mortality 5 to 15%	Group 3 Mortality 25 to 50%
Atrial septal defect	Mitral stenosis with atrial fibrillation	Pulmonary hypertension
Ventricular septal defect	Artificial valve	Coartaction of aorta
Patient ductus arteriosus	Mitral stenosis	Marfan with aortic involvement
Pulmonic/tricuspid disease	Aortic stenosis	
Corrected tetralogy of Fallot	Uncorrected tetralogy of Fallot	
Porcine valve	Previous myocardial infarction	
Mitral stenosis (mild)		

Improved medical and surgical treatment have allowed more women with cardiac disease to live to childbearing years. In best circumstances disease is identified before pregnancy so that appropriate counselling regarding risks and outcome can be undertaken.

Congenital condition like Eisenmenger's syndrome and primary pulmonary hypertension have been associated with such high mortality rates that pregnancy is not advised. Patients with mitral stenosis may elect to undergo cardiac catheterization and possible valve replacement earlier in their illness if contemplating pregnancy.

Anticoagulation may be required in individuals with prosthetic valves as well as in those with arrhythmias who may be at risk for an arterial embolus. Patients with mitral stenosis should also be anticoagulated. Pregnancy will influence the type of anticoagulation, that should be chosen after careful weighing of the benefit for the mother against toxic and teratogenic effects for the fetus. Heparin is the preferred anticoagulant as it does not cross the placenta even if it provides a minor efficacy in thromboembolic prophylaxis. Oral anticoagulant are generally contraindicated, because they cross the placenta and reach the fetal circulation exposing the fetus at risk of haemorrhage (for the inhibition of the synthesis of the vitamin K dependent factors). Fetal exposure to coumadin during the first two months of gestation may result in a significant malformation rate (3-4%). In case of warfarin treatment during the third trimester, it should be stopped one week before delivery and replaced by heparin i.v. for at least one week. During breastfeeding it can be assumed again as it is not present in maternal milk.

Some specific cardiac lesions present the need for antibiotic prophylaxis during labour and delivery. Manual removal of the placenta is an absolute indication for antibiotic prophylaxis in patients with structural heart disease. Prophylaxis usually includes the intravenous administration of aqueous penicillin G and an aminoglycoside at the start of true labour, with continuation every eight hours until one dose post-delivery has been given. In patients who are allergic to penicillin, vancomycin may be the substitute.

Occasionally patients with valvular disease may present a deterioration of clinical conditions so that conservative treatment may not be prolonged; in these cases cardiac surgery might be performed, possibly early in the pregnancy.

Open heart surgery has been associated with a low maternal mortality rate and also fetal salvage rate is increasing. It is recommended to avoid perfusion hypotermia, as this might be responsible for the fetal bradycardia observed during cardiopulmonary bypass [14].

Maternal mortality risks associated with specific cardiac disease are indicated in Table 5 [13].

Medical literature reports more than 30 cases of pregnancy in previously heart transplanted women. The outcome resulted fine in all cases but three in which death occurred for rejection and other two who died for a cryptococcic meningitis. No fetal death was observed while intrauterine growth retardation occurred in 20% of cases [15].

Maternal cardiac arrest is rare during pregnancy. The main causes include trauma, pulmonary and amniotic fluid embolism, iatrogenic factors (e.g. $MgSO_4$ overdose), anaesthesia (local anaesthesia toxicity, failed intubation), heart disease. One of the relatively most frequent causes of cardiac arrest in the labour ward is rapid magnesium administration leading to respiratory and cardiac arrest. Calcium gluconate 1 gram i.v. will competitively antagonise magnesium. Response to resuscitation may be invalidated by the gravidic status: the uterus rises out of the pelvis and causes aorto-caval obstruction with resulting decreased venous blood return to the heart. Left uterine displacement must be kept. Epinephrine increases the uterine artery resistance decreasing the flow. External cardiac compression provides about one third of the normal CO, thus the fetal supply of blood and oxygen is reduced. Open chest cardiac compression provides 70% of CO, but it is not recommended. If resuscitation continues, a peri-mortem caesarean section should be performed [10].

Malignant disease

While cancer is the second most common cause of death for women in their reproductive years, only about 1 in 1,000 pregnancies is complicated by cancer. Approximately one-third of the recorded deaths are secondary to co-existing malignancies.

Delays in diagnosis are common for a number of reasons: many of the presenting symptoms of cancer are often attributed to pregnancy; many of the physiologic and anatomic alterations of pregnancy can compromise the physical examination; many serum tumour markers (β-hCG, α-fetoprotein, CA125, and others) are increased during pregnancy; physician's ability to perform either imaging studies or invasive diagnostic procedures is often altered and limited during pregnancy [16].

The malignancies most commonly encountered in the pregnant patient are: breast cancer (1/1,300 to 1/3,300 pregnancies), cervical cancer (1/2,200 pregnancies), melanoma (2,8/1,000 deliveries), ovarian cancer (incidence ranging from 1/9,000 to 1/25,000), thyroid cancer, leukaemia (1/75,000 pregnancies), lymphoma (from 1/1,000 to 1/6000), colorectal cancer (1/100,000 pregnancies), central nervous system tumours, and urinary tract cancers (50 cases of renal cell carcinoma reported).

Table 6 shows the factors impacting management of the pregnant patient with malignancy.

Table 6. Factors impacting management of the pregnant patient with a malignancy

The gestational age- fetal viability
The stage of the cancer and associated prognosis
The potential for cancer treatment to have adverse effect on the fetus, including the potential for long-term occult problem
The risk to the mother of delaying therapy to permit fetal viability
The risk to the fetus of early delivery to allow more timely cancer therapy
The possible need to terminate an early pregnancy to allow an optimal opportunity to treat and cure the malignancy

Conclusions

Although only about one per cent of obstetric patients require intensive care, these units offer several benefits:

1. intensive observation and organisation allows for prevention or early recognition and treatment of complications;

2. familiarity with invasive haemodynamic monitoring permits personnel to exert prompt rational treatment of haemodynamically unstable patients; and,

3. continuity of care is improved before and after delivery.

Significant improvements have been made reducing maternal mortality particularly from cases related to anaesthesia; this shifts the focus on hypertensive disorders, thromboembolism and haemorrhage. Obstetric units that have not access to a series of facilities that range from simple monitoring to nitric oxide therapy and extracorporeal membrane oxygenation put their patients at a disadvantage, representing a significative cause of mortality; for this reason the provision of such organised centres and the need of a transfer without delay are extremely important as at present most obstetrician-gynecologists do not have adequate specific skills in intensive care. In present circumstances it would be hoped for the formation of an obstetric intensive care unit in order to improve patient care and education of doctors and nurses and respectful of the balance between resources and costs.

References

1. James DK, Stirrat GM (1988) Pregnancy and risk: The basis for rational management. John Wiley and Sons, p 45
2. Capogna G, Celleno D, Frigo MG, Fusco P (1997) High risk patients and ICU management. In: Gullo A (ed) Anaesthesia, pain, intensive care and emergency medicine. Springer, Berlin, pp 543-548
3. Perinal Audit (1996) A report produced for The European Association of Perinatal Medicine. Dunn PM, Mc Ilwaine G (eds) Parthenon, London
4. Duerbeck NB, Chaffin DG, Covey P (1987) Platelet and hemorrhagic disorders associated with pregnancy. A review. Part I. Obstet Gynecol Surv 53(9):575-584
5. Cosmi EV, Di Renzo GC (eds) (1994) Current progress in perinatal medicine. Parthenon, Lancaster, p 980
6. Herczeg J (1998) Post-partum hemorrhage. In: Kurjak A (ed) Textbook of perinatal medicine. Parthenon, London, pp 1836-1840
7. Margaria E, Gollo E, Mutani C, Petruzzelli P (1998) Coagulation disorders in the obstetric patients. In: Gullo A (ed) Anaesthesia, pain, intensive care and emergency medicine. Springer, Berlin, pp 535-542
8. Di Renzo GC, Luzi G (1996) Management of intrauterine growth retardation. In: Chervenak FA, Kurjak A (eds) Current perspectives on the fetus as a patient. Parthenon, New York, pp 527-538
9. Steegers EAP, van den Post JAM (1998) Hypertensive disorder in pregnancy. In: Kurjak A (ed) Textbook of perinatal medicine. Parthenon, London, pp 1901-1902
10. Zakowsky MI (1997) Decision making in high risk obstetric patients. In: Gullo A (ed) Anaesthesia, pain, intensive care and emergency medicine. Springer, Berlin, pp 530-534
11. Didy GA, Cotton DB (1992) Trauma, shock, and critical care obstetrics. In: Reece EA, Hobbins JC, Mahoney MJ, Petrie RH (eds) Medicine of the fetus and mother. Lippincott, Philadelphia, pp 883-924
12. Lyons C (1997) Risk factors and maternal mortality. In: Gullo A (ed) Anaesthesia, pain, intensive care and emergency medicine. Springer, Berlin, pp 523-528
13. Clark SL (1987) Structural cardiac disease in pregnancy. In: Clark SL, Phelan JP, Cotton DB (eds) Critical care obstetrics. Medical Economic Books
14. Landon MB (1996) Cardiac and pulmonary disease. In: Gabbe S, Nyebil, Simpson IL (eds) Obstetrics normal and problem pregnancies. Churchill, Livingstone, pp 997-1013
15. Williams D, de Swiet M (1998) Cardiac disease in pregnancy. In: Kurjak A (ed) Textbook of perinatal medicine. Parthenon, London, pp 1928-1945
16. Schwartz PE (1992) Cancer in pregnancy. In: Reece EA, Hobbins JC, Mahoney MJ, Petrie RH (eds) Medicine of the fetus and mother. Lippincott, Philadelphia, pp 1257-1281

Complications of Obstetric Anaesthesia

G. Lyons

Obstetric anaesthesia encompasses general anaesthesia, intrathecal analgesia and anaesthesia, and epidural analgesia and anaesthesia. J Selwyn Crawford, reviewing 27,000 obstetric epidurals, chose to classify complications according to severity, acknowledging life threatening, serious and minor complications [1]. This form of classification will be used for this review. Sources of information range from reports of maternal mortality, through large follow up studies of complications to single case reports. Comprehensive coverage is not possible and this review will focus on issues that are both relevant and topical.

General anaesthesia

Successive Confidential Enquiries into Maternal Mortality in the United Kingdom report that airway difficulties together with the pulmonary aspiration of gastric contents account for most maternal deaths associated with general anaesthesia [2, 3]. The incidence is so small that most anaesthetists will not have first hand experience in a working lifetime. The incidence of failed tracheal intubation at caesarean section is 1:250, and in 1:10 of these ventilation will be impossible. The use of an algorithm to manage intubation problems has not reduced the incidence of failed intubation but use of a failed intubation drill has ensured that, although this is a life threatening complication, women survive with no or minor morbidity. Perhaps the key to survival is to limit suxamethonium to a single dose [4].

Serious and minor complications associated with general anaesthesia for caesarean section in St James' University Hospital, Leeds include bronchospasm (3%), awareness (1%), and myalgia attributed to suxamethonium (15%) (Table 1). Awareness has now been abolished by using thiopentone 5-7 mg/kg, and by maintaining end tidal isoflurane at 1% until delivery and at 0.5% thereafter [5]. Postoperative neurological deficit has been reported after general anaesthesia, though not in relation to caesarean section [6].

Table 1. Complications associated with caesarean section performed with general anaesthesia. Incidences are those recorded at St James' University Hospital, Leeds, United Kingdom between 1981 and 1997

Life threatening:	
Pulmonary aspiration of gastric contents	1:6400
Failed intubation	1:250
Serious:	
Bronchospasm	3:100
Awareness	1:250
Minor:	
Suxamethonium myalgia	15:100

Intrathecal analgesia and anaesthesia

Intrathecal techniques are chiefly used for anaesthesia for caesarean section, but in recent years there has been a vogue for intrathecal analgesia in labour. Advances in catheter design have led to new interest in continuous subarachnoid techniques for analgesia in labour. This has been the subject of a recent review [7], and is not dealt with here.

Intrathecal analgesia

Despite increasing popularity there have been no deaths reported in the UK as a result of intrathecal anaesthesia for caesarean section, although one death in a woman 30 weeks pregnant has been reported following surgery for a Bartholin's cyst [3]. Hypotension and post dural puncture headache are well reported problems in the obstetric population, and information on neurological complications can be found in a number of postoperative audits involving thousands of surgical patients. This topic has been critically reviewed in a recent editorial [8]. There have been reports of neurotoxicity from intrathecal local anaesthetics, and meningitis following combined spinal/epidural techniques, and these will also be considered. Because post dural puncture headache is common to intrathecal and epidural procedures, it will be dealt with later.

Serious complications

Hypotension

If hypotension is defined as a fall in pressure greater than 20% of the baseline, then approximately 50% of women receiving crystalloid preload will experience hypotension [9]. Prophylactic ephedrine and colloid infusion will reduce but not abolish this incidence [10]. Spinal anaesthesia for elective caesarean section is associated with a small and unpredictable incidence of neonatal acidosis that does not seem to be important clinically [11]. A reduction in cardiac output has been blamed for this [10], and whether this should be taken into account when choosing the anaesthetic technique for a compromised foetus is unclear.

Neurotoxicity

Neurotoxicity attributed to intrathecal local anaesthetics was first described sixty years ago [12]. More recently, the use of hyperbaric 5% lignocaine has been linked with transient lumbosacral pain and tingling [13] and there has been a single report of cauda equina syndrome following an overdose of lignocaine 2% [14]. While the continued use of the hyperbaric 5% solution is in question, the use of clinical doses of the 2% plain solution and all forms of bupivacaine are acceptable.

Meningitis

Both aseptic and bacterial meningitis have been reported after needle through needle combined spinal/epidural techniques [15]. Chemical components of either the drugs or the solution used for skin cleansing are thought to cause the former, and the introduction of bacterial contaminants of the skin or the circulation into the CSF is thought to be responsible for the latter. Coincidental viral infection is another potential cause [16]. Meningism is not exclusive to regional anaesthesia and has also been seen after propofol anaesthesia, though not in obstetric practice [17]. The administration of nonsteroidal anti inflammatory analgesics has also been associated with aseptic meningitis [16].

Epidural anaesthesia and analgesia

In the United Kingdom there have been 15 maternal deaths during epidural anaesthesia and analgesia, between 1973 and 1993, due to a variety of causes [2, 3]. By comparison, in the United States, between 1973 and 1983, at least 24 deaths were reported following the accidental intravenous injection of bupivacaine [18]. The causes of epidural deaths in the UK are shown in Table 2. Failure to recognise unintentional subarachnoid block together with failure to resuscitate suggests poor practice. Use of regional blockade in the presence of cardiac conditions dependent on preload, and in women with anterior placenta praevia and uterine scar will always be hard to justify in the event of a maternal death.

Scott & Tunstall report two cardiac arrests during epidural analgesia, one of which was due to amniotic fluid embolism [19]. It is important to be aware that when cardiac arrest occurs it is not always due to a defective regional block. Peripartum cardiomyopathy in particular is a condition that can present with collapse with any form of anaesthesia [20].

Table 2. Causes of maternal deaths during epidural analgesia and anaesthesia in the UK between 1973 and 1993

Cause of death	N	Comment
Total spinal	4	Avoidable
Cardiac	3	Pulmonary hypertension [2], aortic valve disease [1]
Haemorrhage	2	Placenta praevia postpartum haemorrhage
Pulmonary embolism	1	
Proteinuric hypertension	1	
Others	3	Performed by obstetrician [1], poor practice [1]

Serious complications

Permanent lesions are likely to be neurological in origin and include epidural abscess, which may be linked to regional blockade, epidural haematoma, which can arise spontaneously, and the coincidental central nervous system tumour [21]. These conditions may require surgical intervention. Bromage makes the point that the diagnosis has to be made, and treatment begun within 6 to 12 hours of onset of symptoms if paraplegia is to be avoided. Magnetic resonance imaging is vital to this process [8].

Some serious complications are associated with dural puncture, accidental or intended, and headache is likely to be the first presenting symptom.

Headache

The presence of a fronto-occipital headache, often involving the neck, that disappears in the supine position is typical of post dural puncture headache. While a number of factors influence the severity, the most important factor is the diameter of the needle responsible for the dural breach. Studies of needle point in relation to headache suffer from lack of control group [22], poor statistical analyses [23], and low power [24]. Despite the widespread belief that pencil point needles are kinder than Quincke, meta analysis shows that this is only true for a given gauge [24].

CSF loss causes traction on the intracranial meninges that rarely results in rupture of a venule and progression to subdural haematoma. The same traction can also cause neuropraxis of the 6th cranial nerve and diploplia. Changes in auditory acuity can also occur [25].

Cauda equina syndrome

Symptoms are confined to areas innervated by the lumbosacral nerves, with both weakness and sensory disturbance, loss of sphincter control and autonomic dysfunction. The commonest cause is neurotoxicity from pooling of local anaesthetics.

Anterior spinal artery syndrome

This results in permanent paraplegia. Despite the fact that there is no clear aetiology linking interruption of the cord blood supply to the practice of regional blockade, the latter is likely to be blamed. The syndrome has been described as a complication of obstructed labour in the absence of regional block. Fortunately it is an extremely rare problem [25].

Arachnoiditis

This is responsible for a debilitating process that involves progressive sensory and motor dysfunction with sphincter involvement that often requires surgical decompression of spinal structures. Linked to the epidural injection of irritant solutions, by the time that symptoms are apparent, it is often no longer possible to identify the cause. The preservative methylparaben has been implicated [26]. Preservatives are not generally present in sealed ampoules but are frequent components of rubber capped bottles intended for multiple use.

Obstetric mononeuropathies

These are of note because they are not complications of regional block, but nevertheless the anaesthetist will be expected to take the blame. Neuropraxis of the lumbosacral nerve trunk caused by the foetal brow during rotation by forceps, and damage to the common peroneal nerve from squatting or stirrups, will both cause foot drop. A palsy of the femoral nerve, caused by compression when the thigh is flexed on the abdomen, leads to loss of sensation in the anterior leg, and difficulty climbing stairs. Similarly, meralgia paraesthetica, diminished sensation on the anterior thigh, is caused by compression of the lateral cutaneous nerve as it crosses the inguinal ligament. Recovery takes place in days for minor problems and weeks for the remainder.

Palsy of the 7th cranial nerve is more common in pregnancy, as is carpal tunnel syndrome. More rarely peripartum stroke can occur, particularly from cortical venous thrombosis. The tendency to attribute postpartum neurological pathology to regional block must be resisted because unmasking the real diagnosis may well be delayed. Epidural analgesia may be responsible for one problem in 13,000 procedures, but the overall frequency is 1:2530 deliveries. This makes epidural analgesia an unlikely cause [27].

The claim that long term backache is caused by epidural analgesia in labour has troubled anaesthetists in the UK for some years, while in the US, allegations that epidural analgesia significantly increases the chance of caesarean delivery have stimulated debate.

Backache

A postnatal survey conducted by an epidemiologist found a link between long term backache and epidural analgesia for labour, but not for elective caesarean section. This prompted a prospective study that eventually reported that 7% of women experienced new long term backache postpartum irrespective of the method of pain relief selected. It now seems that women tend to forget that they had backache before delivery, and when this is taken into account differences disappear [28].

Caesarean delivery

An obstetrician randomised women in labour to two pain relief regimes, and found that those receiving epidural analgesia had a significantly increased incidence of caesarean delivery [29]. Critics of this study point out that the results were analysed as the study progressed, that the obstetricians involved in the study were also responsible for the clinical decision, both introducing a source of bias. There has been no interest in this debate in the UK, and the conclusion is still awaited.

Legal considerations

High risk situations should be identified, and discussed as part of the process of informed consent, and the best strategy adopted. Even with the best care problems are inevitable, and should be expected. When they occur, a perusal of the literature will provide useful information. Some neurological problems no longer feature in many of the general texts in Obstetrics and Anaesthesia, and specialist texts [30] are more helpful when dealing with the ill informed. Anaesthetists should take note that the North American closed claims experience showed that 42% of regional anaesthetic claims against anaesthetists were rejected, compared with 27% of general anaesthetic claims. When claims were settled, regional claims were less serious and less expensive than general anaesthesia. The best protection against a legal suit is a well informed caring approach to the women and their clinical problems [31].

References

1. Crawford JS (1985) Some maternal complications of epidural analgesia for labour. Anaesthesia 40:1219-1225
2. Report on Confidential Enquiries into Maternal Deaths in England and Wales 1973-75 (1979), 1976-78 (1982), 1979-81 (1986), 1982-84 (1989). Her Majesty's Stationery Office, London
3. Report on Confidential Enquiries into Maternal Deaths in the United Kingdom 1985-7 (1991), 1988-90 (1994), 1991-93 (1996). Her Majesty's Stationery Office, London
4. Hawthorne L, Wilson R, Lyons G et al (1996) Failed intubation revisited: 17 year experience in a teaching maternity unit. Br J Anaesth 76:680-684
5. Lyons G, Macdonald R (1991) Awareness during caesarean section. Anaesthesia 46:62-64
6. Schreiner EJ, Lipson SF, Bromage PR et al (1983) Neurological complications following general anaesthesia. Anaesthesia 38:226-229
7. Gamlin FMC, Lyons G (1997) Spinal analgesia in labour. Int J Obstet Anesth 6:161-172
8. Bromage PR (1997) Neurological complications of subarachnoid and epidural anaesthesia. Acta Anaesthesiol Scand 41:439-444
9. Rout CC, Rocke DA, Levin J et al (1993) A re-evaluation of the role of crystalloid preload in the prevention of hypotension associated with spinal anesthesia for elective caesarean section. Anesthesiology 79:262-269
10. Robson SC, Boys RJ, Rodeck C et al (1992) Maternal and fetal haemodynamic effects of spinal and extradural anaesthesia for elective caesarean section. Br J Anaesth 68:54-59
11. Hodgson CA, Wauchob TD (1994) A comparison of spinal and general anaesthesia for elective caesarean section: effect on neonatal condition at birth. Int J Obstet Anesth 3:25-30
12. Critchley M, MacDonald, AD, Ferguson FR et al (1937) Discussion on the neurological sequelae of spinal anaesthesia. Proc R Soc Med XXX:1007-1032
13. Schneider M, Ettlin T, Kaufman M et al (1993) Transient neurological toxicity after hyperbaric subarachnoid anesthesia with 5% lidocaine. Anesth Analg 76:1154-1157
14. Drasner K, Rigler ML, Sessler DI et al (1992) Cauda equina syndrome following intended epidural anesthesia. Anesthesiology 77:582-585
15. Harding SA, Collis RE, Morgan BM (1994) Meningitis after combined spinal-extradural anaesthesia in obstetrics. Br J Anaesth 73:545-547
16. Burke D, Wildsmith JAW (1997) Meningitis after spinal anaesthesia. Br J Anaesth 78:635-636
17. Hughes NJ, Lyons JB (1995) Prolonged myoclonus and meningism following propofol. Can J Anaesth 42:744-746
18. Lagasse RF, Marx G (1997) Lessons learned from the bupivacaine experience. Int J Obstet Anesth 6:217-219
19. Scott DB, Tunstall ME (1995) Serious complications associated with epidural/spinal blockage in obstetrics: a two year prospective study. Int J Obstet Anesth 4:133-139
20. Hawthorne L, Lyons G (1997) Cardiac arrest complicating spinal anaesthesia for caesarean section. Int J Obstet Anesth 6:126-129
21. Scott DB, Hibbard BM (1990) Serious non-fatal complications associated with extradural block in obstetric practice. Br J Anaesth 64:537-541
22. Sprotte G, Schedel R, Pajunk H et al (1987) Eine ataumatische Universalkanule fur einzeitige Regionalanaesthesien. Regional-Anaesthesie 10:104-108
23. Snyder GE, Person DL, Flor CE et al (1989) Headache in obstetrical patients; comparison of Whitacre needle versus Quincke needle. Anesthesiology 71:3A;860
24. Fritz T, Crews J, Mathieu A (1994) Relative effectiveness of three spinal needles in minimising postdural puncture (PDPH) and other outcomes. A meta-analysis. Anesthesiology 81:3A;1216
25. Russell IF (1997) Postpartum neurological problems. In: Russell IF, Lyons G (eds) Clinical problems in obstetric anaesthesia. Chapman and Hall, London, pp 149-160

26. Sklar EML, Quencer RM, Green BA et al (1991) Complications of epidural anesthesia: MR appearance of abnormalities. Radiology 81:549-554
27. Holdcroft A, Gibberd FB, Hargrove RL et al (1995) Neurological complications associated with pregnancy. Br J Anaesth 75:522-526
28. Russell R, Dundas R, Reynolds F (1996) Long term backache after childbirth: prospective search for causative factors. Br Med J 312:1384-1388
29. Thorp JA, Albin RM, McNitt J et al (1993) The effect of intrapartum epidural analgesia on nulliparous labor: A randomised, controlled, prospective trial. Am J Obstet Gynecol 169: 851-858
30. Donaldson JO (1988) Neurology of pregnancy. WB Saunders, London
31. Chadwick HS, Posner K, Caplan RA et al (1991) A comparison of obstetric and nonobstetric anesthesia malpractice claims. Anesthesiology 74:242-249

Anaesthesia for Emergency Caesarean Section

G. Capogna, D. Celleno, R. Parpaglioni

The main problem with emergency caesarean section is the rapid induction of anaesthesia in a potentially unstable and unknown patient.

Routine pre-delivery maternal evaluation can predict over 80% of emergency caesarean deliveries [1]. Institution of epidural analgesia in early labor may also allow the rapid extension of a preexisting epidural block in case of an emergency, reducing the risk of maternal aspiration of gastric contents and failed intubation.

Emergency caesarean section for distressed foetus is one of the most rush-decision making situation, however the term "foetal distress" is unfortunately imprecise, non-specific and of little predictive value [2]. Most neonates delivered for fetal distress have normal Apgar scores, are not distressed and do not suffer foetal asphyxia. In addition, electronic foetal heart rate monitoring is an imprecise tool to diagnose foetal distress. However, once the obstetrician declares the need for emergency caesarean section, the anaesthesiologist should rapidly consider the following questions and give the best appropriate answers:

- Can the intrauterine environment be improved enough to decrease the urgency of the caesarean section?
- Does the patient have an epidural catheter which can be used to extend rapidly the block?
- Are there contraindications to general anaesthesia?
- Are there contraindications to spinal anaesthesia?
- Which anaesthesia is best for the distressed foetus?

Can the intrauterine environment be improved enough to decrease the urgency of the caesarean section?

Changing maternal position, administering supplemental oxygen and stopping oxytocin infusion can improve placental perfusion.

Left uterine displacement or maternal full lateral position improves foetal blood flow by relieving aorto-caval compression or umbilical cord compression.

One should also remember that maternal blood pressure measured in the arm may be normal despite significant aorto-caval compression [3].

Maternal hyperoxia improves oxygen delivery to the foetus if uterine hypoperfusion, umbilical cord compression or uterine hypertonus have not affected foetal blood flow. Supplemental oxygen by high flow via a face mask increases maternal and foetal oxygenation [4]. Although the rise of foetal PaO_2 may seem small, foetal haemoglobin lies on the step portion of its oxyhaemoglobin dissociation curve and also a small increment in PaO_2 greatly increases oxygen saturation and content. The increase in umbilical venous oxygen saturation from 65% to 87% can provide significant oxygen reserve and may improve the physiologic reserve of the stressed foetus. Of course, oxygen administration to the mother is not useful if foetal blood supply is interrupted.

Because of limited placental reserve, the stressed foetus cannot tolerate significant reductions in uterine blood flow. For this reason, when a non-reassuring FHR tracing exists during labor, immediately stop oxytocin administration.

Hypotension caused by sympathetic block during regional anaesthesia may be avoided by using very low diluted local anaesthetic/opioid mixtures for epidural labor analgesia or by an incremental titration of the more concentrated local anaesthetic in case of caesarean section. It is very important to avoid and treat maternal hypotension with adequate fluid infusion, left uterine displacement, and ephedrine, if necessary.

Does the patient have an epidural catheter which can be used to extend the block rapidly?

If the parturient has an epidural catheter for labor analgesia, this may be used in order to extend rapidly the epidural block for an emergency caesarean section. A pH-adjusted solution of 2% lidocaine with epinephrine 1:400.000 may be used and a T4 block may be achieved in few minutes.

Are there contraindications to general anaesthesia?

The main contraindication to a rapid sequence induction of general anaesthesia is an airway examination indicating a high probability of failure to intubate the parturient. The incidence of failed intubation is eight times higher in parturients than in general surgery patients [5] and is even more likely in pre-eclamptic oedematous patients. In the UK over 75% of maternal anaesthetic deaths are associated with an emergency caesarean section under general anaesthesia [6]. Failed intubation and inhalation of gastric contents are the leading cause of maternal mortality and morbidity.

Are there contraindications to spinal anaesthesia?

Uncorrected profound maternal hypotension is a relative contraindication to spinal anaesthesia since maternal hypovolaemia may produce intractable hypotension. Preeclampic patients may become severely hypotensive after spinal anaesthesia. Systemic infections are also an absolute contraindication to spinal anaesthesia and chorioamnionitis is the most frequent common systemic infection in parturients. Coagulopathy is also an absolute contraindication to regional anaesthesia. We perform spinal anaesthesia to a parturient with no clinical evidence of bleeding and a platelet count greater than 70,000 mmc.

Which anaesthesia is the best for the distressed foetus?

Anaesthesiologists often use general anaesthesia for emergency caesarean section, however the little data available suggest that neonates born after a rapidly induced regional anaesthesia are in better clinical condition than infants delivered by rapid-sequence general anaesthesia [7]. In the animal model, uterine blood flow decreases transiently following intravenous thiopental, laringoscopy and tracheal intubation [8].

The choice between general and spinal anaesthesia is often also a problem related to the organization of the labor and delivery suite, the staff training and the anaesthesiologist's experience.

In Table 1 are indicated the anaesthetic choices for emergency caesarean section during the year 1997 in our Hospital.

Table 1. Percentage of parturients receiving different anaesthesia techniques for emergency caesarean section

	Epidural	Spinal	General
Foetal distress	36%	40%	22%
Not reassuring FHR	35%	42%	21%
Cord prolapse	57%	28%	14%
Abruptio placentae	–	70%	29%

Ntot = 135, representing 13% of all caesarean deliveries performed during the year 1997

References

1. Morgan BM, Magni V, Goroszenuik T (1990) Anesthesia for emergency cesarean section. Br J Obstet Gynaecol 97:420
2. Frigoletto FD, Nadel AS (1988) Electronic fetal heart rate monitoring: Why the dilemma? Clin Obstet Gynecol 31:179
3. Eckstein KL, Marx GF (1974) Aortocaval compression and uterine displacement. Anesthesiology 40:92
4. Hanowell L et al (1992) Effect of maternal inspired oxygen concentration on fetal umbilical venous oxygen tension. Reg Anesth 17:S38
5. Samsoon GTL, Young JRB (1987) Difficult tracheal intubation: a retrospective study. Anaesthesia 42:487
6. Report on confidential inquiries into maternal deaths in England and Wales. On behalf of Department of Health Welsh Office (1982) Her Majesty Stationery Office, UK, p 84
7. Marx GF, Luykx WM, Cohen S (1984) Fetal-neonatal status following cesarean section for fetal distress. Br J Anaesth 56:1009
8. Palhaniuk RJ, Cumming M (1977) Foetal deterioration following thiopentone-nitrous oxide anaesthesia in the pregnant ewe. Can Anaesth Soc J 24:367

Obstetric Complications: Consumption Coagulopathy

C.T. PETROVITCH

Many disorders unique to pregnancy are associated with the development of disseminated intravascular coagulation (DIC). These conditions include preeclampsia, placental abruption, septic abortion, fetal death in utero, and amniotic fluid embolus. Although the basic underlying clinical entities are very different, the same basic haemostatic problem develops. The normal mechanisms which control and regulate coagulation are disrupted. Thrombin production becomes excessive and rampant clot formation proceeds. In defense, the fibrinolytic system is activated, producing excess quantities of plasmin, in an attempt to lyse the fibrin clots. The action of plasmin leads to the production of fibrin degradation products and further disruption of coagulation. The patients' clinical manifestations of this haemostatic disorder, DIC, will depend on a combination of several factors: 1) the patient's basic underlying disease process, 2) the rate and duration of the coagulation system activation, and 3) the dominance of either the coagulation or fibrinolytic process. In order to diagnose and treat such patients who develop DIC, it is most helpful to review the basic pathophysiologic mechanisms that lead to disseminated intravascular coagulation. Once this basic foundation for understanding the process of DIC is established, the diagnosis and treatment of DIC and the unique problems associated with each clinical entity can be addressed.

The haemostatic mechanism

The hemostatic mechanism must regulate the procoagulant and anticoagulant as well as the fibrinolytic and antifibrinolytic forces within the bloodstream. The haemostatic mechanism maintains a dynamic equilibrium which allows blood to circulate in a liquid form throughout the body under normal circumstances and to be transformed into a fibrin clot at sites of vascular injury. Intricate control mechanisms must interact to orchestrate this balance between liquid blood and a solid clot and to ensure that clot formation takes place only at sites of vascular injury and not uncontrolled "disseminated" throughout the blood stream. The syndrome of DIC represents, in essence, the loss of these control mechanisms. Coagulation proceeds rampantly throughout the blood stream, depleting the natural inhibitors to coagulation and stimulating the fibrinolytic forces. The patient may die from excess coagulation which leads to ischaemic necrosis and tissue injury or from an overactive fibrinolytic system which produces fibrin degradation products at a rate that can not be cleared from the patient's blood stream. These FDPs lead to the disruption of primary haemostasis and coagulation and the patient may bleed to death.

Primary haemostasis

Primary haemostasis basically involves the interaction of blood vessels and platelets. In response to vascular injury, the vessel vasoconstricts, shunting blood flow away from the site of vascular injury and the platelets aggregate together to form a friable platelet plug. This reaction essentially arrests bleeding until the coagulation process can occur to form a tough fibrin clot. It is endothelial damage that sets the haemostatic mechanism in motion. When the endothelial layer of the blood vessel is denuded, platelets circulating in the blood stream are exposed to collagen in the subendothelial layers. The platelets adhere to the collagen surface and spread along the denuded vessel wall until they come into contact with normal endothelial cells [1]. The platelets which adhere to the collagen surface undergo a process of platelet activation which involves several reactions, designed to enlarge the growing platelet plug. The platelets undergo *a shape change* from a flattened disc to a spheroid and they express many pseudopods on their spherical surface [2, 3]. They undergo *a release reaction* in which the platelets release the contents of their cytoplasmic granules. From the dense granules platelets release ADP which serves as a potent platelet activator and a chemical messenger which summons more and more platelets to the platelet plug [4]. With platelet activation, the platelets undergo a synthetic reaction which produces thromboxane A_2. This powerful prostaglandin causes the blood vessel to vasoconstrict and it also promotes further release of ADP and consequent platelet aggregation [5]. The activated platelets also expose a new phospholipid surface called platelet factor 3 (PF3). This phospholipid surface plays a major role in localizing clot formation. Many of the coagulation reactions which follow require the presence of a phospholipid surface. Because these surface-mediated reactions occur on the platelet factor 3 surface, clot formation is localized to the site of vascular injury where the platelets are activated.

Normal endothelial cells secrete a prostaglandin called prostacyclin. Prostacyclin has actions opposite those of thromboxane A_2. Prostacyclin is a potent vasodilator and decreases the release of ADP [6]. The action of prostacyclin is potentiated by endothelium-dependent relaxing factor (EDRF, nitric oxide). The EDRF or nitric oxide helps to regulate vascular tone as well. The opposing actions of prostacyclin secreted by normal endothelial cells, prevent the growth of the platelet plug onto endothelialized vascular surfaces. In fact, it is the balance of these two prostaglandins, thromboxane A_2 and prostacyclin, that controls primary fibrinolysis and localizes the platelet plug [7].

The endothelial layer also expresses ADPases on the surface which serve to decrease the concentration of ADP and therefore decrease platelet aggregation [8]. It is convenient that these haemostatic control mechanisms are orchestrated by the endothelial layer. It is this layer that provides the "non-wettable" surface or the nonthrombogenic lining of our vascular tree.

Coagulation

The coagulation process takes place essentially concurrently with the process of primary haemostasis. While the platelets are adhering to the denuded endothelial surfaces and becoming activated, the coagulation process is producing minute amounts of thrombin which will be incorporated into the platelet plug along with fibrinogen and plasminogen. Ultimately fibrin strands will be produced that will cross-link and form the tough fibrin clot.

Coagulation proceeds by a cascade of reactions, some of which require the presence of a phospholipid surface. This surface can be provided by activated platelets, called platelet factor 3, or platelet phospholipid. Because all of the components of this coagulation pathway are intrinsic to blood, the pathway is referred to as the intrinsic pathway of coagulation. When tissue damage occurs, a second phospholipid can be released into the bloodstream. This phospholipid is known as tissue phospholipid or tissue factor and the coagulation pathway that proceeds on this surface is referred to as the tissue factor pathway or the extrinsic pathway because a substance extrinsic to blood, tissue factor, is required for these reactions [9].

In looking at the overall process of coagulation, several broad principles are helpful in understanding the normal coagulation process and the mechanisms which serve to regulate or control coagulation. First, most of the clotting factors circulate in an inactive form. The successive activation of clotting factors serves as a protective mechanism to prevent excess clot formation. If the clotting factors circulated in an active form, poor blood flow, or simply the compression of a blood vessel could lead to the interaction of multiple activated clotting factors and the inappropriate formation of a blood clot. Instead, the factors must undergo successive activation and even when clotting factors are activated, often rapid blood flow will dilute the factors or "wash them away" preventing abnormal clot formation. Also activated clotting factors are picked up by the reticuloendothelial system.

Most of the clotting factors are synthesized in the liver, with the possible exception of clotting factor VIII. Four of the clotting factors are said to be vitamin K dependent, Factors II, VII, IX, and X. This is because these clotting factors undergo a final enzymatic reaction in their synthesis which requires the presence of vitamin K. These clotting factors are carboxylated. It is this "carboxyl tail" which allows these factors to bind to phospholipid surfaces.

Two of the clotting factors, factors V and VIII, do not become active cleavage enzymes. Instead these two factors serve as cofactors in reaction complexes which take place on phospholipid surfaces and which require the paired binding of two clotting factors in a particular spatial arrangement. Together these two clotting factors, an active cleavage enzyme and its cofactor, will activate the next clotting factor in the coagulation pathway. Because these reactions require the presence of a phospholipid surface, coagulation will only take place where platelets expose platelet phospholipid or where tissue phopholipid is distributed.

Control of coagulation is also seen in some feedback mechanisms which depend upon the activation or deactivation of the two cofactors, factors V and VIII. When thrombin is present in low concentrations, it accelerates the activity of the two cofactors to increase its own production. When thrombin is present in high concentrations, it inhibits factors V and VIII. The inhibitory reactions are somewhat complex. Thrombin, produced in quantity near the endothelial surface, becomes bound by a molecule expressed on the endothelial surface called thrombomodulin. This bound thrombin can then bind protein C (together with its cofactor, protein S) to inhibit the action of factors V and VIII.

Ultimately if there is sufficient thrombin production, thrombin will convert fibrinogen to fibrin. When the fibrinogen is cleaved by thrombin, "fibrin monomers" are released into the circulation. These fibrin monomers aggregate end to end and side by side to form a fibrin polymer or fibrin S (soluble) which is held together by hydrogen bonds. Factor XIII (activated by thrombin and Ca^{++}) will cause covalent peptide bonds to form, crosslinking the fibrin strands and forming the stable fibrin clot (insoluble). Clearly thrombin again plays a critical role in controlling the coagulation process since the action of Factor XIII is dependent upon thrombin activation.

Finally, natural anticoagulants such as antithrombin III circulate in the blood to prevent excess coagulation. Antithrombin III, as its name implies, binds to thrombin, inactivating this enzyme. Antithrombin III also binds to other activated factors in the intrinsic pathway, slowing the production of fibrin. The action of antithrombin III can be magnified by the presence of heparin. Man-made heparin improves the binding of antithrombin III to thrombin by 100 to 1000 fold [10]. This then provides for powerful anticoagulant effects. It is interesting to note that the luminal surface of the endothelium is covered by a coating of mucopolysaccharide which contains a "heparan sulfate" [11]. This heparan weakly stimulates antithrombin III.

In summary control of coagulation occurs by many mechanisms. The clotting factors circulate in an inactive form. Those that are activated are diluted by rapid blood flow and preferentially removed from the blood stream by the reticuloendothelial system. Coagulation requires the presence of a phospholipid surface provided by platelet phospholipid and tissue factor. Several feedback mechanisms exist modulated through thrombin to either speed up or slow down the production of fibrin. Finally, natural anticoagulants like antithrombin III circulate in the blood to control fibrin production.

Fibrinolysis

Quite simply, the fibrinolytic process involves the conversion of plasminogen to plasmin by the action of tissue plasminogen activator. It is convenient that this enzyme is produced by the vascular endothelial cells. Plasminogen preferentially binds to fibrin during clot formation [12]. Then when converted to plasmin, the fibrinolytic enzyme can degrade the fibrin clot until it is released into the blood stream. Antiplasmins, which circulate in concentrations 10 times that of plasmin will rapidly hydrolyze the plasmin and limit the fibrinolytic process. Because plasmin can attack fibrin which is uncross-linked, fibrin which is cross-linked or fibrinogen, the result will be a family of degradation products, FDPs [13]. Under normal circumstances, FDPs are removed from the blood by the liver, kidney and reticuloendothelial system. Their normal half-life is approximately nine hours. However, if the fibrinolytic system is very active and these FDPs should accumulate in blood, they disrupt the haemostatic balance. The FDPs impair platelet function, inhibit thrombin, and prevent the normal cross-linking of fibrin strands [14]. This last action results in a clot that is more readily soluble by plasmin. The ultimate result is a disruption of primary haemostasis and coagulation by the FDP inhibitors and a patient who bleeds profusely.

DIC

Although many entities are associated with DIC, the pathophysiology of DIC in each condition is similar in concept. A triggering event initiates the uncontrolled exposure of phospholipid (either platelet phospholipid or tissue factor) and a powerful procoagulant force ensues [15]. In preeclampsia, vessel wall damage leads to the activation of platelets and exposure of platelet factor 3 (platelet phospholipid). Release of tissue thromboplastin into the circulation occurs in many of the other obstetric conditions such as amniotic fluid embolism or abruptio placenta. With the production of large quantities of thrombin, fibrinolysis is activated and plasmin produced. Both thrombin and plasmin circulate in the bloodstream. Thrombin catalyzes the formation of fibrin clots which are scattered throughout the bloodstream and lead to tissue ischemia. The natural anticoagulants become consumed. With plasmin degrades fibrinogen and fibrin producing FDPs. The patient becomes thrombocytopenic, develops platelet dysfunction due to the FDPs, and may have deficiencies of several clotting factors consumed in the coagulation process.

Various presentations of DIC

Because many conditions can lead to DIC, it is not surprising that the clinical picture which results can vary greatly as well as the laboratory findings [16]. Patients who have widespread deposition of micro thrombi throughout their vascular tree may suffer tissue hypoxia and ischaemic necrosis leading to significant end-organ damage. Extensive thrombosis may occur in many organ systems including the cardiac, renal, hepatic, pulmonary and central nervous systems [16]. The patient may suffer large subcutaneous haematomas, deep tissue bleeding, petechiae and purpura. Or, the patient may exhibit signs of haemorrhage and may bleed from multiple sites. Often these patients require heroic volume resuscitation and inotropic support.

When DIC is suspected, most practitioners order a PT, PTT, fibrinogen level, FDP, platelet count, and a peripheral smear. The PT and PTT may be prolonged, the platelet count decreased, and the peripheral smear may show schistocytes. The presence of FDPs is a sign of fibrinolysis, but is not specific for DIC. The fibrinogen level more often than not will be decreased. Many physicians prefer to measure the level of D-dimer present in the blood. Because D-dimer is a breakdown product of cross-linked fibrin, its presence confirms that fibrinolysis followed coagulation and was not a primary event. Antithrombin III levels will usually be depleted early in the DIC process [17].

Patients with "compensated DIC" may have normal coagulation tests and only exhibit elevated FSPs.

Treatment of DIC

The underlying disorder which triggered the DIC must be the primary focus of treatment. In some way the underlying disorder had to lead to either 1) the activation of platelets and diffuse exposure of platelet phospholipid throughout the bloodstream or 2) to the massive exposure of tissue phospholipid. To prevent further rampant coagulation, the source of the phospholipid must be contained. If a placental abruption has led to the ongoing dissemination of tissue phospholipid into the blood stream, the placenta must be delivered. If tissue factor or tissue phospholipid is liberated due to a fetal death in utero, the mother's uterus must be evacuated.

Some patients will require component therapy until the primary disorder can be treated. Most patients with DIC bleed due to three reasons: 1) thrombocytopenia, 2) the presence of elevated levels of FDPs which act as inhibitors to coagulation, and 3) clotting factor deficiencies. Platelet transfusions and the use of FFP may be necessary. Cryoprecipitate is usually given to treat severe fibrinogen deficiencies. Guidelines for the replacement of blood products include maintenance of normovolaemia and a Hct of 25%, normal urine output, platelet count greater than 20,000 mm^3, and a fibrinogen level greater than 100 mg/dl.

In addition, some practitioners advocate the use of antithrombin III administration to help combat the DIC process. Antithrombin III is available in fresh frozen plasma but is also available as a purified concentrate. Heparin therapy remains controversial.

References

1. Wu KK (1992) Endothelial cells in hemostasis, thrombosis, and inflammation. Hosp Pract (Off Ed) 27:145-50;152:163-166
2. Brandt JT (1985) Current concepts of coagulation. Clin Obstet Gynecol 28:3-14
3. Ellison N (1987) Hemostasis and hemotherapy. In: Barash PG, Cullen BF, Stoelting RK (eds) Clinical anesthesia. JB Lippincott, Philadelphia, pp 707-710
4. Rubin BG, Santoro SA, Sicard GA (1993) Platelet interactions with the vessel wall and prosthetic grafts. Ann Vasc Surg 7:200-207
5. Bennett JS, Kolodziej MA (1992) Disorders of platelet function. Dis Mon 38:577-631
6. Mackie IJ, Pittilo RM (1985) Vascular integrity and platelet function. Int Anesthesiol Clin 23:3-21
7. Freiberger JJ, Lumb PD (1987) How to manage intraoperative bleeding. In: Vaughan RW (ed) Perioperative problems/catastrophes, 1st edn. JB Lippincott, Philadelphia, pp 161-172
8. Stormorken H (1987) The hemostatic mechanism: The role of platelets in physiology and bleeding states. Scand J Gastroenterol [Suppl]137:1-10
9. Broze GJ Jr (1992) The role of tissue factor pathway inhibitor in a revised coagulation cascade. Semin Hematol 29:159-169
10. High KA (1988) Antithrombin III, protein C, and protein S. naturally occurring anticoagulant proteins. Arch Pathol Lab Med 112:28-36
11. Wight TN (1980) Vessel proteoglycans and thrombogenesis. Prog Hemost Thromb 5:1-39
12. Diethorn ML, Weld LM (1989) Physiologic mechanisms of hemostasis and fibrinolysis. J Cardiovasc Nurs 4:1-10
13. Bone RC (1992) Modulators of coagulation. A critical appraisal of their role in sepsis. Arch Intern Med 152:1381-1389
14. Bick RL (1994) Disseminated intravascular coagulation. Objective laboratory diagnostic criteria and guidelines for management. Clin Lab Med 14:729-768
15. Kitchens, Craig S (1995) Disseminated intravascular coagulation. Curr Opin Hematol 2: 402-406
16. Orlikowski CE, Rocke DA (1998) The coagulopathic parturient. 16:349-373
17. Ostlund E (1998) Soluble fibrin in plasma as a sign of activated coagulation in patients with pregnancy complications. Acta Obstet Gynecol Scand 77:165-169

Perioperative Management of Hypertension

M. ZAKOWSKI

Hypertension in pregnancy

The perioperative management of hypertension is important not only for the elderly patient but also for the parturient. Maintenance of homeostasis and the prevention of extremes of blood pressure will prevent morbidity and mortality in both the mother and the neonate. Parturients may acquire hypertensive disorders that are unique in etiology. These different causes of hypertension, their etiology and treatment will be elucidated. The pharmacodynamics of antihypertensive agents and special physiologic considerations during pregnancy will also be emphasized.

Physiology of pregnancy

The physiologic changes during pregnancy, labor and delivery are important to consider when administering vasoactive agents. Pregnancy is a hyperdynamic state characterized by an increase in heart rate (HR) by 15%, stroke volume (SV) by 30%, cardiac output (CO) by 40% and blood volume by 35% with concomitant decreases in systemic vascular resistance (SVR) by 15% and mean arterial pressure (MAP) by 15 mmHg. During labor CO further increases 15% during the latent phase, 30% during the active phase and 45% during the expulsive stage. Increases in HR and SV account for the increased CO. Each uterine contraction returns 300 mL of blood to the central circulation and may increase CO 15%, SV 20-30% and HR 5-10%. Immediately after delivery blood return from the legs and the uterus leads to the peak CO during pregnancy of 80% above pre-labor values [1].

Obstetric anaesthesia is unique in caring for two lives at once. Any haemodynamic alteration in the parturient must consider the effects on the fetus. Since the uterine artery is maximally dilated under normal conditions, the delivery of blood and oxygen to the uterus and placenta is dependent upon the maternal blood pressure. If a vasopressor is needed, a β-adrenergic agonist or mixed β- and α-adrenergic agonist is preferred over a pure α-adrenergic agonist. In hypertensive disorders, the uterine artery becomes constricted. Treatment of hypertension during pregnancy must be oriented toward lowering the maternal blood pressure while maintaining uterine perfusion and oxygen delivery. Thus the primary haemodynamic goal is to maintain or increase cardiac output. Remember that CO = SV*HR and BP = CO*SVR. An antihypertensive agent that lowers blood pressure by decreasing cardiac output via decreased contractility or decreased venous return will decrease uterine artery perfusion. The second haemodynamic goal is to keep uterine artery vasodilated via epidural or SVR. Thus, antihypertensive agents which reduce SVR and increase CO are physiologically ideal (e.g. hydralazine).

Measurement/prediction of hypertension

Accurate measurement of blood pressure (e.g. correct cuff size) is important. Blood pressure should be measured in the same position and by the same methodology in order to accurately assess changes or response to therapy. There have been significant discrepancies between directly measured radial arterial pressure, automated blood pressure reading and manual mercury sphygmomanometer. In severe preeclamptics, automated blood pressure machines underestimated systolic, mean and diastolic pressure by 11-18 mmHg, while manual mercury sphygmomanometer was closer to arterial pressures [2].

Classically the obstetric patient is predisposed to supine hypotensive syndrome (aortocaval compression by the uterus). However, in a recent study the mean arterial pressure (MAP) was greater in the supine compared to lateral positions [3]. Aortic arch pressure was similar in supine and lateral positions and equaled the mean of the MAP from each arm. Automated blood pressure measurements were a better predictor of the development of severe hypertension within 2 weeks of assessment [4]. Plasma fibronectin was elevated early in pregnancy and indicates a higher risk for developing a pregnancy induced hypertensive disorder [5]. Serum nitric oxide (NO) products were significantly reduced during pregnancy in patients with preeclampsia and chronic hypertension with superimposed preeclampsia [6].

Types of hypertension

There are many different causes of hypertension (Table 1). This review will focus predominantly on the common obstetrical problems related to hypertension. Hypertension during pregnancy is classified into one of the following categories:

1. *Chronic hypertension* is present before pregnancy or diagnosed within the first 20 weeks of gestation. Hypertension is a blood pressure greater than 140/90 mmHg. Elevated blood pressure diagnosed beyond the 20th week of gestation and that persists 6 weeks postpartum is also considered chronic hypertension.

2. *Preeclampsia-eclampsia* is defined as elevated blood pressure beyond 20 weeks gestation on two readings taken 6 hours apart. The blood pressure is at least 140/90 mmHg or elevated 30 mmHg above the systolic or 15 mmHg above the diastolic baseline. Alternatively, a mean pressure of 105 mmHg or an increase of 20 mmHg from baseline may also be considered as hypertensive. Proteinuria is present and occurs when 0.1 g/L of protein or 0.3 g/L of protein is measured in a 24 h urine collection. Oedema may occur in the upper parts of the body. Hypertension usually resolves in 24-48 h post-partum but may take a week or longer.
   Severe preeclampsia occurs with one or more of the following: blood pressure above 160/110 mmHg, proteinuria of 5 g/24 hours, oliguria (< 500 mL/24 hour), cerebral or visual disturbance, epigastric pain, pulmonary oedema or HELLP (haemolysis, elevated liver enzymes, low platelets) syndrome. Eclampsia is the occurrence of seizures. Symptoms may start as late as 24 h after delivery.

3. *Preeclampsia superimposed upon chronic hypertension.* Increases of blood pressure as in preeclampsia (see above) with proteinuria and generalized oedema. In parturients with chronic hypertension, a baseline 24 hour urine creatinine clearance and protein excretion from early pregnancy are helpful in distinguishing chronic hypertension from superimposed preeclampsia.

4. *Transient hypertension* is an elevated blood pressure during pregnancy or within the first 24 hours following delivery without other signs of preeclampsia or chronic hypertension.

5. *Unclassified hypertension* is an elevated blood pressure not consistent with one of the above categories.

Table 1. Etiology of hypertension

Primary (essential or idiopathic) hypertension
Secondary hypertension
Renal disease
Endocrine disease
Pheochromocytoma
Cushing's syndrome
Primary aldosteronism
Thyroid storm
Pregnancy induced hypertension
Mechanical (coarctation of aorta, renal artery stenosis)
Neurogenic (increased intracranial pressure)
Adverse physiologic conditions
hypoxia, hypercarbia,
myocardial ischaemia
pain
Drug abuse (cocaine)

Physiology of preeclampsia

Preeclampsia is a hypertensive disorder of pregnancy occurring more frequently in first pregnancies, chronic hypertension, multiple gestation, diabetes, and previous history of preeclampsia. The incidence of preeclampsia is 7% in primiparous women, but is superimposed in 20% of women with chronic hypertension. Multiparous women with eclampsia had a 50% incidence of recurrent hypertension in a subsequent pregnancy. The etiology of preeclampsia is probably an immunologic response against the placenta, resulting in a secondary imbalance of prostacyclin and thromboxane. The blood vessels are constricted resulting in hypertension and intravascular volume depletion.

The kidneys are adversely affected during preeclampsia. Renal biopsy showed glomeruloendotheliosis in 70% of primigravidas with preeclampsia. Multiparous women with preeclampsia had this lesion only 14% of time, with 43% showing some signs of pre-existing renal or vascular disease. Vasospasm causes proteinuria as well as leakier membranes and endothelial damage.

The vascular endothelium serves to modulate coagulation as well as vascular tone. The endothelium is injured in preeclampsia, and releases fibronectin, growth factors, factor VIII antigen into the circulation. Serum from preeclamptic women will even affect endothelium function in vitro.

Women with preeclampsia are more sensitive to endogenous and exogenous vasopressors. They are more sensitive to angiotension II than non-pregnant women while pregnant women are the least sensitive. Preeclamptics have increased sensitivity to epinephrine, norepinephrine and vasopressin compared to normal parturients.

In the late 1800's, the maternal mortality rate for eclampsia was 20-30%, with immediate delivery of the neonate the only treatment available. Expectant management was used in the early 1900's and the maternal mortality rate declined to 10-15%. Magnesium administration was introduced in the 1920-30's and resulted in a further decline of the mortality rate to 5%. When magnesium therapy was combined with hydralazine for control of blood pressure in preeclampsia, the maternal mortality rate dropped to less than 1%. The perinatal mortality rate remains the highest for preeclampsia superimposed on chronic hypertension [7]. Severe preeclampsia resulted in elective delivery in 53%, cesarean section in 61%, and perinatal death in 4% [8].

Magnesium sulfate, a competitive calcium antagonist, is administered to prevent seizures, and has been found to be more effective than phenytoin [9]. Magnesium also has effects on the vascular system and may produce vasodilatation. Following a 4 g loading dose, maternal blood pressure may decrease. In gravid ewes, pretreatment with $MgSO_4$ resulted in a greater decrease in maternal MAP following epidural anaesthesia compared to the control group. However, there was no significant differences in cardiac output or uterine blood flow between groups [10]. Hypermagnesaemia also results in a decreased response to vasopressors and may interact with other antihypertensive agents, calcium channel blockers in particular. In gravid ewes receiving $MgSO_4$, both ephedrine and phenylephrine restored maternal blood pressure. However, ephedrine was significantly better at restoring uterine blood flow [11].

Chronic hypertension

Women with chronic hypertension are at increased risk for complications, with a 20% incidence of superimposed preeclampsia. Maternal morbidity and mortality rates are greater in superimposed preeclampsia than in preeclampsia. Blood pressure elevation is greater, increasing the chance of intracranial haemorrhage. While eclampsia usually occurs in first pregnancies, most maternal deaths occurred in multiparous women in which underlying hypertension is a common disposing factors [12]. Compared to preeclampsia, chronic hypertension was more like to results in fetal death, prematurity and intrauterine growth retardation than preeclampsia [13].

The perinatal mortality rate is higher in hypertensive women. The risk increases as the blood pressure increases with women possessing a BP of 200/120 mmHg having a 50% rate of fetal loss. The perinatal mortality rate is higher for superimposed preeclampsia than for preeclampsia. There is also a higher chance of placental abruption. Superimposed PE appears earlier in gestation than PE.

Antihypertensive therapy reduces maternal mortality for > 105 mmHg diastolic [7]. A diastolic blood pressure > 90 mmHg should be an indication for treatment in people with chronic hypertension. Antihypertensive therapy started early or prior to pregnancy delayed or prevented the appearance of superimposed preeclampsia [14]. The perinatal mortality rate is lower for mildly hypertensive women given antihypertensives. Therapy reduces the maternal risks of markedly elevated blood pressures, delays or prevents the onset of preeclampsia if begun prior to or early in pregnancy, and appears to reduce the rates of perinatal mortality and morbidity. However, antihypertensive therapy begun after 30 weeks gestation has no proven beneficial effects for the fetus.

Unknown hypertension

Although rare, pheochromocytoma should be investigated in parturients with unexplained hypertension, especially escalating and severe in natures. Urinary catecholamines and vanillyl-mandelic acid (VMA) will aid in the diagnosis. The immediate management of pheochromocytoma is to treat the hypertension with α-adrenergic blockers (e.g. phentolamine) [15, 16].

Obstetric management

The obstetric management of hypertensive patients may influence the perioperative anaesthetic management. While delivery is always the definitive therapy for preeclampsia/eclampsia, is the neonate more likely to survive in-utero or ex-utero? The pathophysiologic changes of preeclampsia are present long before the clinical criteria are met. Changes in vascular reactivity, plasma volume and renal function precede the changes in blood pressure, protein secretion and sodium retention. Lowering the blood pressure does not alleviate many of the important pathophysiologic changes [7]. Proteinuria is at least partially caused by vasospasm and partly by glomerular damage due to phagocytosis of abnormal circulating proteins by the glomerulocapillary endothelial cells. If the maternal condition is stable, delivery is indicated by signs of abnormal fetal function. If the maternal condition is unstable, delivery is indicated for maternal signs and because the fetal environment is also deteriorating. Hepatic rupture has a 65% mortality rate. Thus, women with hepatic capsular distention manifested by hepatomegaly, liver tenderness and abnormal LFT should be delivered immediately.

If blood pressure is still elevated after $MgSO_4$ administration, antihypertensive agents may be required. Hypertension can increase postoperative haemorrhage and third-space losses. Increases in intracranial pressure, cerebral oedema, intracranial haemorrhage, and intraocular pressure may also occur [17]. Enhanced sympathetic nervous system activity is a frequent cause of postoperative hypertension. Expansion of blood volume can increase cardiac output and blood pressure. However, there is no evidence that the acute administration of antihypertensive agents have beneficial fetal effects. It has not been proven that lowering blood pressure reduces the risk of seizures. Therefore, lowering blood pressure is to prevent extreme hypertension causing intracranial haemorrhage and other morbidity.

Treatment

Antihypertensive therapy should be started during labor for blood pressure > 160/110 mmHg or a MAP > 105 mmHg. Diastolic blood pressure in the 90-100 mmHg range may be watched closely, and > 100 mmHg should be treated. For chronic hypertension, a diastolic > 90 mmHg is usually an indication to start therapy.

Acutely, the goal is to reduce blood pressure to 140-150/80-90 mmHg only. Antihypertensive therapy is aimed at achieving preoperative baseline levels since "normal" blood pressure for pregnancy (e.g. 110/60) may cause hypoperfusion of vital organs in patients who have autoregulated to a higher blood pressure [17]. The choice of antihypertensive drug should be guided by the pathophysiology of the individual's history with the goal to maintain or increase cardiac output as a means of assuring adequate uterine artery flow.

Epidural analgesia or anaesthesia may be an aid in controlling the blood pressure. Antihypertensive agents should not be given until after the regional anaesthetic has taken effect or profound hypotension may ensue. β-adrenergic blockade may produce paradoxical hypertension by unopposed α-adrenergic induced vasoconstriction in patients with an increase in circulating catecholamines (e.g. pheochromocytoma). In this case, blockade of α-adrenergic receptors should occur prior to β-adrenergic receptor blockade.

Factors which may contribute to hypertension should be investigated. Recent cocaine use will cause hypertension and may cause placental abruption. In the peri-operative period, secondary causes of hypertension must be investigated and treated (e.g. hypercarbia, hypoxia). A sedate patient may be tired following delivery or from narcotic administration.

Drugs (Table 2)

Alpha-methyldopa is a centrally acting false neurotransmitter. Methyldopa is metabolized in the brain to methylnorepinephrine, which acts in the brain to inhibit adrenergic neuronal outflow from the brain stem, through α_2-agonism. Cardiac output and renal blood flow are maintained while SVR decreases. This drug has been used for chronic hypertension in pregnancy for many years and has the best documented safety profile. The onset of action is 20 min, with a peak effect perhaps as late as 6-8 hours, with a duration of up to 24 hours. When given intravenously, the dose is usually 250-500 mg i.v. every 6 hours [18]. Long term follow-up studies of methyldopa use in pregnancy showed no neurologic or somatic effects in children up to 7 years later [7].

Clonidine is a centrally acting vasodilator via α_{-2} adrenergic agonism. The decreased sympathetic outflow results in decreased myocardial contractility, heart rate while maintaining renal blood flow. Clonidine 150 mcg i.v. works in 20-30 min. However, experience is limited in preeclampsia.

Dexmedetomidine is also a centrally acting agent, a more specific agonist for the α_{-2} adrenoreceptor. Like clonidine, it will decrease blood pressure, heart rate and anaesthetic requirement. Administered i.m. or i.v. infusion in 0.25-2 mcg/kg, sedation is a major side effect. Use during pregnancy has not been documented.

Hydralazine is the classic antihypertensive agent used during labor. It is a direct arteriolar vasodilator which causes reflex tachycardia, thus increasing cardiac output and uterine blood flow. Side effects may be headache and epigastric pain. The onset is 5-10 minutes, with peak effects in 15-20 minutes, lasting for 2-6 h.

Sodium nitroprusside is metabolized by smooth muscle cells to nitric oxide (NO), causing vasodilatation. Thus, both arterioles and venules are dilated. Usually GFR is maintained with a modest increase in HR (less than hydralazine, diazoxide). Toxicity from cyanide occurs only at very high doses (> 5 mcg/kg/min) or if used for greater than 24 hours. Toxicity in the neonate does not occur unless the mother is also toxic [19].

Diazoxide is a thiazide analog with no diuretic effects. Diazoxide hyperpolarizes smooth muscle cells by activating ATP-sensitive K^+ channels, thus causing relaxation of the vascular smooth muscle. The reflex tachycardia results in an increased CO, with side effects of maternal and neonatal hypoglycaemia and sodium retention. With a long duration of 4-12 hours, diazoxide may produce uterine hypoperfusion and fetal acidosis.

Trimethaphan is a ganglionic blocking agent. Cardiac output, contractility and uteroplacental perfusion are reduced. Trimethaphan camsylate i.v. infusion at .3-5 mg/min onset 5 min duration 15 min. Side effects include paralytic ileus, dry mouth and blurred vision.

Calcium channel blockers are also commonly used for hypertension during pregnancy. Sublingual nifedepine 10 mg has been commonly used in the United States for acute lowering of blood pressure, with onset in 10 min an maximal effect in 30-40 min. Recently the Food and Drug Administration issued a warning against using sublingual nifedepine, stating that the absorption was erratic and may cause hypotension. In addition, calcium channel blockers may interact with magnesium, a calcium antagonist, resulting in profound hypotension.

Reserpine is another ganglionic blocking agent, which is no longer widely used. Reserpine causes nasal stuffiness in the neonate, which may cause respiratory difficulties in the newborn, an obligate nose breather. Meconium ileus may be another unwanted side effects.

Diuretics are usually not indicated and may produce a small but significant increase in perinatal mortality rate when receiving it for non-medical (weight loss) reasons. Increases in uric acid may make obscure the diagnosis of preeclampsia. Diuretic treatment of hypertension is counterproductive and may adversely affect fetal outcome because plasma volume is already reduced. Diuretics may be helpful postpartum in patients who are intravascularly fluid overloaded.

β-adrenergic receptor antagonists reduce heart rate, myocardial contractility, cardiac output and decrease renin (and thus angiotension II) release. Most β-blockers cross the placenta and produce neonatal effects such as blunting the response to hypoxia. Esmolol used at time of delivery may produce neonatal bradycardia. Women who received atenolol for chronic hypertension during pregnancy had infants who weighed 500 g less than the control group.

Labetalol is a commonly used drug which is safe during pregnancy and labor. The dose for acute treatment of hypertension is 20 mg i.v., repeated every 10 min. The dose can be doubled each time until desired effect is reached (maximum 300 mg total). Labetalol possesses a mixed β- and α-adrenergic blocking effect in a 7:1 ratio when given i.v. Labetalol is a mixture of 4 stereoisomers of which one is an α_1- and another a β-adrenergic antagonist.

α-adrenergic receptor antagonist (prazosin, trerazosin, doxtazosin, ketanserin). The α_1-adrenergic receptor antagonism reduces arteriolar resistance and venous capacitance, initially resulting in reflex tachycardia.

Angiotensin converting enzyme (ACE) inhibitors are contraindicated in pregnancy. Captopril use during pregnancy caused fetal death in animals and neonatal renal dysfunction in humans.

Table 2. Antihypertensive agents

Drug	Dose (i.v.)	Onset	Duration	Side effects
Diuretic				
Furosemide	10-49 mg	5 min	4 h	K^+, hypovolaemia
Sympatholytics				
Alpha-methyldopa	250-500 mg	30 min	24 h	peak up to 6 h, sedation, hepatitis
Clonidine	150 mcg	20 min	?	sedation, dry mouth, withdrawal
Vasodilators-Arterial				
Hydralazine	5-10 mg	15 min	4-6 h	tachycardia
Sodium nitroprusside	0.25+ mcg/k/min	30 sec	3 min	tachycardia, cyanide toxicity, increased cerebral blood flow
Diazoxide	50-100 mg	30 sec	5-12 h	decreased cerebral blood flow
Vasodilator - venous/mixed				
Nitroglycerin i.v.	1-4 mcg/kg/min	2 min		decreased venous return, headache
Nifedepine	10 mg SL	10 min	4 h	less negative inotropy, potent vasodilator
Verapamil	5 mg	3 min	4-6 h	heart block, myocardial depression, vasodilator, reflex tachycardia
Alpha adrenergic blockers				
Phentolamine	2-5 mg			tachycardia, hypotension
Mixed adrenergic blocker				
Labetalol	0.25 mg/kg	3 min	4-6 h	7:1 Beta:alpha blocker i.v., repeat ≥10 min

Modified from [17, 18]

Anaesthetic management

The anaesthetic management of the parturient may have a great effect on maternal blood pressure and the need for antihypertensive agents. Following magnesium therapy in laboring parturients, adequate analgesia is the next step. Pain causes the release of catecholamines and increases in blood pressure. Epidural analgesia is the most effective means of pain relief during labor, decreasing the release of catecholamines and stress related hormones [20]. Indeed, by providing segmental sympathectomy and vasodilatation, epidural analgesia improves uterine blood flow in preeclamptics [21]. Blood pressure must be closely monitored for exaggerated decreases following regional anaesthesia in hypertensive patients.

The anaesthetic choice for caesarean delivery may greatly influence the blood pressure. Spinal anaesthesia has been listed as relatively contraindicated in preeclampsia because of its rapid onset and sometimes profound hypotension in this class of patients with intravascular hypovolaemia. Spinal anaesthesia may be associated with a greater incidence of foetal acidaemia in caesarean deliveries [22].

General anaesthesia for caesarean delivery will also produce haemodynamic alterations. Intubation is very stimulating and will produce an increase in blood pressure, especially in preeclamptics and those whose blood pressure is already elevated. Labetalol has been described as preventing hypertension during laryngoscopy [23]. However, following uterine incision and only moderate bleeding, blood pressure usually declines. Thus, a long acting drug may not be the best choice. Esmolol has been used for prevention of hypertension with laryngoscopy, but also produced bradycardia in the neonate. In spite of a high metabolism by serum cholinesterase (9 minutes half life), esmolol crossed the placenta rapidly, producing fetal bradycardia. Currently, my first choice for preventing hypertension during laryngoscopy is nitroglycerin. A bolus of 200 mcg of nitroglycerin following the thiopental and succinylcholine during induction prevents hypertension during laryngoscopy and is effervescent before blood loss is a potential problem.

References

1. Cheek TG, Gutsche BB (1993) Maternal physiologic alterations during pregnancy. In: Shnider SM, Levinson G (eds) Anesthesia for obstetrics. 3rd edn. Williams & Wilkins, Baltimore, pp 3-18
2. Penny JA, Shennan AH, Halligan AW et al (1997) Blood pressure measurement in severe preeclampsia [letter]. Lancet 349:1518
3. Goldkrand JW, Jackson MJ (1997) Blood pressure measurement in pregnant women in the left lateral recumbent position. Am J Obstet Gynecol 176:642-643
4. Penny JA, Halligan AW, Shennan AH et al (1998) Automated, ambulatory, or conventional blood pressure measurement in pregnancy: Which is the better predictor of severe hypertension? Am J Obstet Gynecol 178:521-526
5. Paarlberg KM, de Jong CL, van Geijn HP et al (1998) Total plasma fibronectin as a marker of pregnancy-induced hypertensive disorders: A longitudinal study. Obstet Gynecol 91:383-388
6. Garmendia JV, Gutierrez Y, Blanca I et al (1997) Nitric oxide in different types of hypertension during pregnancy. Clinical Science 93:413-421
7. Roberts JM (1994) Pregnancy related hypertension. In: Creasy RK, Resnik R (eds) Maternal fetal medicine: Principles and practice. 3rd edn. WB Saunders, Philadelphia, pp 804-844

8. Peek MJ, Horvath JS, Child AG et al (1995) Maternal and neonatal outcome of patients classified according to the Australasian Society for the Study of Hypertension in Pregnancy Consensus Statement. Med J Australia 162:186-189

9. Lucas MJ, Leveno KJ, Cunningham FG (1995) A comparison of magnesium sulfate with phenytoin for the prevention of eclampsia. NEJM 333:201-205

10. Vincent RDJ, Chestnut DH, Sipes SL et al (1991) Magnesium sulfate decreases maternal blood pressure but not uterine blood flow during epidural anesthesia in gravid ewes. Anesthesiology 74:77-82

11. Sipes SL, Chestnut DH, Vincent RDJ et al (1992) Which vasopressor should be used to treat hypotension during magnesium sulfate infusion and epidural anesthesia? Anesthesiology 77:101-108

12. Neutra R, Neff R (1975) Fetal death in eclampsia: II. The effect of non-therapeutic factors. Br J Obstet Gynaecol 82:390-396

13. Jain L (1997) Effect of pregnancy-induced and chronic hypertension on pregnancy outcome. J Perinatology 17:425-427

14. Arias F, Zamora J (1979) Antihypertensive treatment and pregnancy outcome in patients with mild chronic hypertension. Obstet Gynecol 53:489-494

15. Hull CJ (1986 Dec) Phaeochromocytoma. Diagnosis, preoperative preparation and anaesthetic management. Br J Anaesthesia 58:1453-1468

16. Zakowski M, Kaufman B, Berguson P et al (1989) Esmolol use during resection of pheochromocytoma: report of three cases. Anesthesiology 70:875-877

17. Lawson NW (1992) Autonomic nervous system physiology and pharmacology. In: Barash PG, Cullen BF, Stoelting RK (eds) Clinical anesthesia. 2nd edn. JB Lippincott, Philadelphia, pp 319-384

18. Gates JA (1996) Antihypertensive agents and the drug therapy of hypertension. In: Hardman JG, Limbird LE, Molinoff PB, Ruddon RW, Goodman Gilman A (eds) Goodman & Gilman's The pharmacological basis of therapeutics. 9th edn. McGraw-Hill, New York, pp 362-382

19. Naulty J, Cefalo RC, Lewis PE (1981) Fetal toxicity of nitroprusside in the pregnant ewe. Am J Obstet Gynecol 139:708-711

20. Shnider SM, Abboud TK, Artal R et al (1983) Maternal catecholamines decrease during labor after lumbar epidural anesthesia. Am J Obstet Gynecol 147:13-15

21. Jouppila P, Jouppila R, Hollmen A et al (1982) Lumbar epidural analgesia to improve intervillous blood flow during labor in severe preeclampsia. Obstet Gynecol 59:158-161

22. Roberts SW, Leveno KJ, Sidawi JE et al (1995) Fetal acidemia associated with regional anesthesia for elective cesarean delivery. Obstet Gynecol 85:79-83

23. Ramanathan J, Sibai BM, Mabie WC et al (1988) The use of labetalol for attenuation of the hypertensive response to endotracheal intubation in preeclampsia. Am J Obstet Gynecol 159:650-654

Maternal and Foetal Mortality Rates During Pregnancy, Delivery and Puerperium

E. Margaria, E. Gollo, G. Sortino

Pregnancy, delivery and puerperium are physiological events; nevertheless, in the world 585.000 women every year die because of causes connected to pregnancy and delivery.

Maternal mortality data are worrying: approximately 99% of the maternal deaths occur in the Third World, while 1%, equal to 5.800 women, every year die in the developed countries in spite of the available means and advanced technologies.

In order to define "maternal mortality", the Confidential Enquiries into Maternal Death of the United Kingdom (CEMDUK) [1] uses the international diseases classification: "death during pregnancy or 42 days from the pregnancy end, determined by every pertinent cause or aggravated by pregnancy itself or treatment, but not by accidental or incidental causes".

"Late deaths" are defined cases in which death occurs after a much longer period, from pregnancy or delivery related causes.

The percentage of maternal mortality is estimated around 10/100.000 births in the developed countries [2]. In our data too [3] (Fig. 1), the rate is more-or-less the same. According to OMS, these data are underestimated by about 50%. Most of the authors who work on this topic are of the same opinion.

The Maternal Mortality Collaborative (USA) [4] emphasises that we cannot obtain precise data from the most advanced countries. It is difficult to verify if the proposed and adopted solutions obtain the desired results, in terms of mortality and morbility reduction.

In order to diminish maternal morbility and mortality, we can characterize two risk categories where it is possible to operate (apart from accidental or incidental causes, which are difficult to prevent).

In the first group (non-specific pregnancy-related complications) we should include:

- underestimated preexisting pathological conditions;
- known pathologies in women who did not respect advice against pregnancy;
- advanced age;
- poor cultural, social and economic conditions;

patients   deliveries

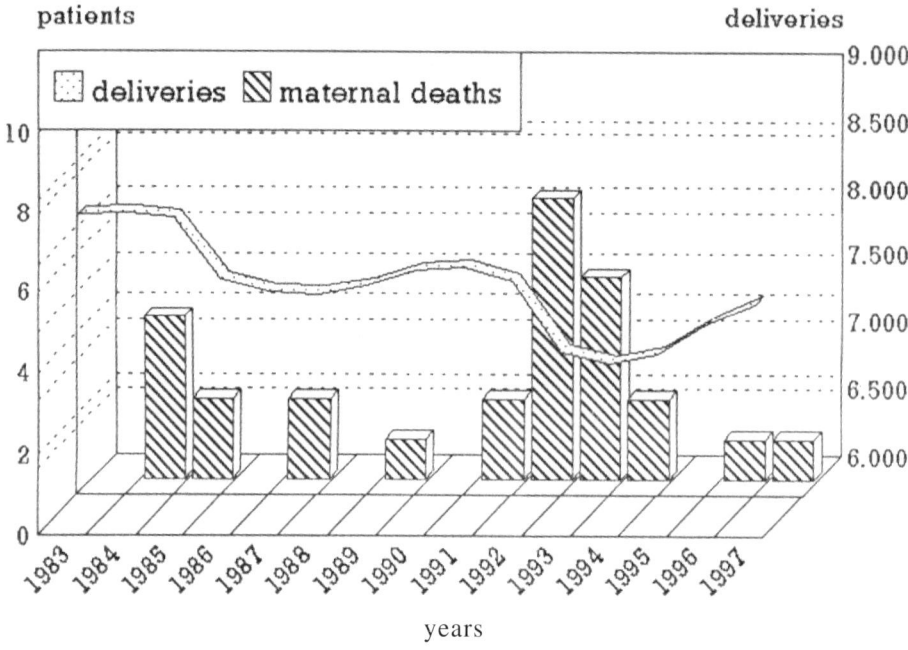

years

Fig. 1. Maternal mortality

- obesity, anorexia;
- surgical delivery, especially in emergency;
- inadequate assistance, lack of experience on the part of operators (surgeons, anaesthetists).

    The second group (specific pregnancy-related complications) involves:

- abortions;
- ectopic pregnancies;
- multiple pregnancies;
- FIVER pregnancies;
- preeclampsia and complications (eclampsia, HELLP syndrome, DIC, ...);
- pulmonary oedema;
- haemorrhage;
- thrombosis;
- pulmonary embolism.

Materials and methods

In order to establish maternal mortality incidence in our centre and to investigate and verify exactly the most prevalent causes, an analysis has been done from January 1983 to June 1998 (including 15 years, 120.000 deliveries and 29 maternal deaths).

The patients, all treated at St. Anna Hospital of Torino, have been divided into three groups:

Group A: 25 patients died during pregnancy, delivery or puerperium from January 1983 to December 1994 (before ICU opening);

Group B: 4 patients died during pregnancy, delivery or puerperium from January 1995 to June 1998;

Group C: 498 pregnant patients treated at the Obstetric ICU from January 1995 to June 1998.

Every patient in the 3 groups has been examined regarding:

1. hospitalization or death cause
2. age and parity
3. gestational age
4. pregnancy-related complications
5. type of delivery
6. anaesthesia
7. newborn outcome

Results

Group A: In the period 1983-1994, out of a total of 93.534 deliveries 25 patients died (equal to 0.026%). As regarding the cause of death the pre-existing pathologies (8 patients, 32%) were: gastric cancer, cardiopathy, splenic art. aneurism, anorexia, leukemia, connectivitis. The pregnancy-related pathologies (10 preeclamptic patients, 40%) are the widest group. In this group we can verify the presence of complications such as HELLP syndrome, pulmonary oedema, cerebral haemorrhage, pulmonary embolism, DIC, etc.

Three patients (12%) had preeclampsia overwhelming other pathologies.

At delivery 5 fatal anaesthesiological and/or surgical accidents (20%) occurred.

In puerperium pathologies such as haemorrhage and pulmonary embolism were 5 (20%).

The age trend exactly imitates that of the control group formed by normal obstetric patients assisted in the same period. First pregnancy represents an important risk factor as 21 were primiparae (90.5%), while 2 (9.5%) were pluri-parae. Over 50% of the patients were at term of pregnancy.

Concerning the type of delivery, 19 (73.91%) patients underwent caesarean section, 5 (21.73%) delivered spontaneously, one patient (4.34%) had an abortion.

Out of the 24 patients who had undergone general anaesthesia, only one had regional anaesthesia.

As regards the newborns, 25 children were born from 22 mothers, 21 (84%) born alive, 4 (16%) still born.

Group B: This group involves 4 patients who died from January 1995 to June 1998, out of 26.000 deliveries (0,015%).

For what concerns the causes of death out of the 4 patients who died, 3 (75%) had different pre-existing pathologies: aspergillosis (respiratory failure), diabetes and dead foetus (post-partum shock), obesity and varicosity (cerebral thrombosis). Only one (25%), with severe preeclampsia had been hospitalized during eclamptic access; she had come from another hospital and died of cerebral haemorrhage.

The patients mean age was 35.2 years, 2 were primiparae, 2 pluriparae; one patient delivered at the end of pregnancy, the others at 29th, 33rd, 35th week.

Three of them underwent caesarean section (2 in general, 1 in epidural anaesthesia); 1 spontaneously delivered a dead foetus, the other children are alive and healthy.

It is interesting to observe that a careful screening of the obstetric patients, together with a prophylactic and therapeutical treatment in ICU, leads to a reduction of the pregnancy-related complications and of maternal mortality in general.

Group C: This group involves 498 obstetric patients treated in ICU from January 1995 to June 1998 (during this period there were 26.000 deliveries). Out of these, 43 women had come from other hospitals.

Actually, approximately 10% of the hospitalizations are to be attributed to patients who had come from other obstetric centres.

In this group 2 patients died, one of massive cerebral haemorrhage, and one after being transferred to a respiratory unit.

In all, 2 of 498 patients died, equal to 0.40% of the obstetric patients who were treated in ICU.

The intern patients mortality, regarding patients who delivered in our hospital and who needed intensive care (2% of total deliveries), is 1 out of 455, equal to 0.22%.

Among patients coming from other hospitals, 1 out of 43 died, equal to 2.3%. It is clear that recovery is influenced by the clinical situation on admission (SAPSO) [5].

If pregnancy is over 30th week and surgery is promptly performed, the outcome of the newborns is satisfactory (100% surviving).

As regards perinatal mortality in general, the rate is high in Italy if compared with other European countries (1-3%). Data from St. Anna Hospital are similar (1.25% in 1993, 0,7% in 1998).

The reduction of perinatal mortality in those years is more evident for newborns with higher weight (> 1000 gr). But it is still high for newborns of lower weight, and it is nearly around 90% for the very small babies (< 500 gr).

On the other hand, it is more difficult to evaluate the incidence of cerebral palsy and neurological damage of variable degree, which can appear in the first months of life [6].

Conclusions

Maternal mortality at St. Anna Hospital of Turin has decreased in the last years ('83-94 = 0.026%, '95-98 = 0.015%): this is probably related to the opening and functioning of the Obstetric ICU, in which different specialists take care of high risk patients, before, during and after delivery.

Patients who need intensive care are 2% of the deliveries. Mortality rate among these patients is today 0.0038% of all deliveries.

It is evident that all pre-existing pregnancy pathologies can be elements of risk and aggravate eventual emergency situations. Nevertheless, preeclampsia represents, for the so-called normal pregnant women, the most important risk factor. But if it is early recognized and appropriately treated, this specific and peculiar pathology cannot get worse or influence maternal and foetal outcome [7].

Other risk factors are primiparity, multiple pregnancy, surgical delivery, emergency operation, general anaesthesia and, for the most recent patients, advanced age.

References

1. Hibbard BM, Anderson MN, Drife JO et al (1996) Report on confidential enquiries into maternal deaths in the United Kingdom 1991-1993. Her Majesty's Stationery Office, London
2. Lyons G (1997) Risk factors and maternal mortality. In: Gullo A (ed) Anaesthesia, pain, intensive care and emergency medicine. Springer, Berlin Heidelberg New York
3. Margaria E, Fanzago E, Mutani C (1996) La mortalità materna in ostetricia. Atti 50° Congresso
   Nazionale SIAARTI. Min Anest 62[Suppl 1]
4. Roger W et al (1988) Maternal mortality in the United States: Report from maternal mortality
   collaborative. 72(1)
5. Margaria E, Gollo E, Castelletti I (1994) Which patient must be admitted in ICU? Anésthèsie-
   Rèanimation en Obstétrique 3 Arnette JEPU 175-183
6. Margaria E, Castelletti I, Gollo E et al (1994) Primary resuscitation of the newborn. Recent advances in obstetric analgesia and anesthesia. 1st European Congress, Firenze
7. Palieri L, Segaliari S, Bertolino E et al (1997) Protocolli di trattamento pre e postpartum in TIO
   di pazienti affette da IGI. Min Anest 63[Suppl 1]9

ACID-BASE DISORDERS, DIAGNOSIS AND TREATMENT

Dimension of Fluid Compartments in Severely Ill Patients

H.J. ADROGUÉ

Substantial deviations from the normal dimension of body fluid compartments or spaces occur in severely ill patients. These abnormalities include changes in the absolute size of a given compartment, in its relative size with respect to other spaces or to total body water, or the development of non-functional compartments [1]. Since the consequences of fluid space abnormalities can be life-threatening, it is most important to recognize their presence, interpret properly their pathogenesis, and implement measures aimed at correcting these disorders. We describe below the most relevant disorders of fluid compartment dimensions in critically ill patients.

Extracellular fluid volume disorders

Water accounts for 45% to 75% of body weight in humans and the major determinants of this wide range are age and gender [2, 3]. The water content of a newborn, an adolescent or a middle-aged individual, and an elderly one are ~75%, 60%, and 50%, respectively. Females generally have 2% to 10% lower water content than males. The gender effect develops after puberty, and differences in water content between males and females are largely dependent on per cent of body fat stores. Women have a higher per cent of fat and therefore less body water in relation to their weight (nonobese adult males ~16 ± 2% and females ~24 ± 2% body fat).

Body fluid is contained in two major compartments, within the cell and outside of it, and it is known as intracellular and extracellular fluid, accordingly (ICF and ECF, respectively). The terms intracellular water (ICW) and extracellular water (ECW) are also used to refer to ICF and ECF, respectively. The transcellular fluid could be considered as a small third compartment comprising the digestive, cerebrospinal, intraocular, pleural, peritoneal, and synovial fluids [2]. The ICF contains approximately 60 per cent of total body water (TBW) and the remaining 40 per cent is held in the ECF. The latter is further subdivided into the interstitial and the intravascular compartments which have two-thirds and one-third, of the water contained in the ECF, respectively.

   Changes in the ECF volume are most relevant in severely ill or surgical patients and include volume contraction (depletion) and expansion [4]. In the normal state, rapid equilibration occurs between the interstitial and vascular spaces,
governed by Starling forces at the capillary level. However, in some disease
states, the effective circulating blood volume and the interstitial fluid volume
are reduced because of fluid sequestration into a "third space". Third spacing
occurs with abdominal accumulation (intestinal obstruction, pancreatitis, peritonitis, rapid re-accumulation of ascites), bleeding, crush injury, skeletal fractures, and obstruction of a major venous system. A characteristic feature of a
"third space" is the tendency toward progressive fluid accumulation within it,
depleting the intravascular compartment and leading to circulatory failure [2].
"Third space" lacks the rapid equilibration processes that characterize the exchange of water and solutes between the interstitial and intravascular compartments. Thus ECF volume depletion can result from fluid sequestered into a
"third space" (in the absence of actual body losses of fluid) or from fluid loss
(e.g., renal losses, extrarenal losses). Renal losses may occur in the presence of
normal intrinsic renal function (e.g., diuretics, osmotic diuresis including gluco-
suria or urea diuresis, and adrenal insufficiency) or in acute and chronic renal
disease (e.g., recovery phase of acute renal failure, salt-wasting renal diseases).
Extrarenal losses include those from the gastrointestinal tract (e.g., vomiting, diarrhoea, gastrointestinal suction, fistulas), and those from the skin (sweat, burns,
extensive skin lesions). Replacement of fluid loss (e.g., several liters) caused by
third-space sequestration leads to repletion of the extracellular and intracellular
fluid spaces and weight gain. Fluid administration in severe volume deficit re-
plenishes intravascular volume restoring haemodynamic status and corrects cellular and interstitial volume deficits. In addition, fluid therapy halts catecholamine release due to circulatory collapse and improves tissue perfusion, decreasing the risk of cerebrovascular accidents, myocardial infarction and acute
renal failure, that occasionally complicate severe volume depletion. However,
fluid administration, if excessive, can be harmful and potentially life-threatening. An overly generous supply of fluids might produce pulmonary oedema and,
occasionally, symptomatic brain swelling; the latter occurring most frequently
in patients with head trauma or in the recovery of diabetic ketoacidosis [2].

   Volume expansion represents a common fluid disorder in severely ill patients
[5]. The administration of NaCl-containing solutions in excess of volume loss is
largely responsible for this condition. Fluid retention is facilitated in patients
with renal failure, heart failure, liver cirrhosis, and nephrotic syndrome. Table 1,
Case A, presents the body composition of a female patient with mitral valve disease and congestive heart failure. She had severe fluid overload manifested by a
TBW/B.Wt. of 67% (predicted normal 53%) with ECF volume expansion
(ECW/TBW 63%, predicted normal 48%) and reduction in the cell compartment (ICW/TBW 37% for a predicted normal of 52%). Volume expansion was
also marked in Case B, Table 1, with ECW/TBW of 81% and a predicted normal of 49%.

Table 1. Body composition in patients with mitral valve disease with congestive heart failure (A), Hodgkin's sarcoma (B), and uncontrolled sepsis (C)

Case	A	B	C
B.Wt. (kg)	45 (45)	42 (42)	59 (59)
TBW (L)	30 (24)	32 (22)	30 (28)
TBW/B.Wt. (%)	67 (53)	76 (52)	51 (47)
ECW/TBW (%)	63 (48)	81 (49)	69 (48)
ICW/TBW (%)	37 (52)	19 (51)	31 (52)
BCM (kg)	13 (16)	11 (14)	12 (19)

Case A: 54-year-old woman; case B: 66-year-old woman; case C: 55-year-old woman
( ) Predicted normal values are indicated in parenthesis
Modified from [5]

Endogenous water released from cells of up to 500 mL/day is commonly overlooked as a source of fluids and can contribute to a state of fluid overload. Considering that during the catabolic period severely ill patients are expected to lose about 0.5 lb/day, absence of weight loss indicates the presence of a positive fluid balance [6].

Intracellular fluid volume disorders

The ICF compartment approximates the body cell mass (BCM) that comprises the potassium-rich, oxygen-consuming, and work-performing tissues [5]. Because of the relative stability of the intracellular potassium concentration in severely ill patients, BCM in grams can be estimated as the total exchangeable potassium in mEq multiplied by the coefficient 8.33 (7 to 10 range). Thus a 70-kg adult male has a BCM of approximately 28 kg. Other estimations of BCM are based on the assumption of an average potassium-nitrogen ratio of 3 mEq of potassium per gram of cellular tissue. BCM represents the skeletal muscle and visceral parenchyma and accounts for approximately 35% body weight in women and 40% body weight in men in the normal state [5]. Whereas the skeletal muscle mass shrinks markedly in response to disease or disuse, the visceral parenchyma does not decrease in size during wasting diseases. The per cent contribution of various tissues within an adult subject to the total body weight are as follows: skeletal muscle 30%, fat 25%, viscera 10%, skin plus skeleton 10%, and ECW 25%.

Severely ill patients in the course of their disease experience changes in the body fluid compartments that resemble states of fasting, catabolism, or repair [6-8]. Fasting leads to body water loss at a rapid rate in the first 5 days, diminishing thereafter; the pattern of water loss is similar in obese subjects but quantitatively larger. About two-thirds of the early water loss originates in the ECF

(~2 L in 5 days) and the lumen of the gastrointestinal tract, plasma volume also decreasing up to 20 per cent.

The BCM in severely ill catabolic patients releases water bound to glycogen and proteins within the intracellular fluid, as well as produces water from oxidation of endogenous triglyceride and protein. A 70-kg subject contains approximately 13 kg of protein distributed as follows: skin plus skeleton 50%, skeletal muscle 35%, viscera 12%, plasma proteins 3% [9]. Glycogen consumption in the liver and muscle releases about 400 mL and 600 mL of bound water, respectively, in the first 2 to 3 days of fasting or acute severe illness. The oxidation of cellular protein also releases bound intracellular water in a ratio of 3 gm of water for each 1 gm of protein. Daily protein catabolism amounts to about 75 gm (i.e., 12 gm nitrogen excretion) in the first few days of fasting or severe injury, with smaller values observed in females and obese subjects; thereafter daily nitrogen losses tend to decrease significantly. Consequently, cell water loss derived from protein amounts to approximately 225 mL/day in the early phase of fasting or injury, and largely explain the observed decrease in BCM or ICW that occurs in response to such stress. Fig. 1 depicts the estimated cumulative cell water and nitrogen losses in a severely catabolic patient. As shown in the figure, a progressive reduction in ICW develops in association with the large negative nitrogen balance [5].

In addition to the previously mentioned loss of bound intracellular water, a sizable volume of water is produced daily in severely ill subjects from oxidation of endogenous components including the skeletal muscle and fat stores. Body fuel stores in a 70-kg normal subject amounts to 160,000 calories in fat deposits, 30,000 calories in skeletal muscle, and 900 calories in glycogen deposits. Whereas glycogen stores are rapidly and completely consumed, only a fraction

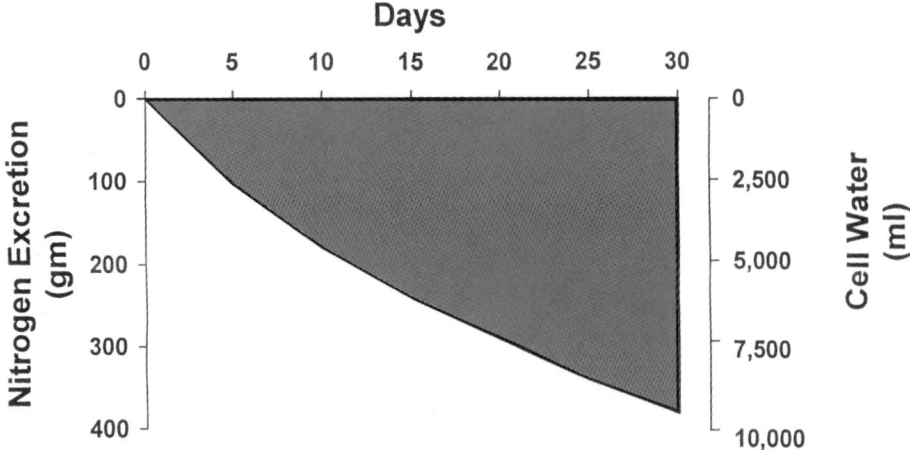

Fig. 1. Estimated cumulative cell water and nitrogen losses in a severely catabolic patient

of the total calories stored in the remaining deposits are burned in caloric deprivation states. Daily energy expenditures amount to about 1800 calories in lean individuals and 2500 calories in the obese, but a larger amount is spent in catabolic patients. The oxidation of fat produces about 150 mL/day of water in lean subjects and 300 mL/day in those obese. Glycogen consumption releases about 90 mL/day of water in the first 2 days of fasting or severe injury. In addition, protein catabolism generates 0.4 gm of water per 1 gm of protein, thus about 20 mL/day of water is derived from protein oxidation. Consequently, a substantial amount of water derived from the cellular compartment enters the ECF in these conditions, and unless excreted by renal or external routes, will result in volume expansion [10, 11].

Severely ill patients as a result of trauma, sepsis, surgery, or other major injury, develop an initial catabolic phase that precedes their recovery (early and late anabolic phases). As previously explained, during the catabolic phase the patient manifests obligatory increases in energy expenditure and nitrogen excretion; his/her metabolic environment prevents the efficient oxidation of nutrients promoting the erosion of vital protein pool. Consequently, critical organ failure can develop in response to a prolonged protein catabolic process without effective specific therapy and nutritional intervention. Whereas the minimum daily urinary nitrogen excretion in adults with elective surgery is about 10 gm, the corresponding value for multiple trauma or severe infection is 15 gm, and in patients with 70% burns amounts to 20 gm. Nitrogen excretion in excess of 15 gm/day indicates rapid depletion of tissue proteins. It is most important to recognize that cellular protein losses are necessarily associated with changes in the dimension of body fluid compartments.

During the wasting process of severe injury a gradual loss of BCM is observed, in which the loss of cellular water is proportional to the severity of potassium loss; most often there is also loss of body weight and total body water [1, 7]. Although the reduction in BCM is a constant feature, body weight and total body water can remain constant or even increase because of the presence of major ECF volume expansion or a large "third space". Table 1, Case B, depicts the body composition of a 66-year-old woman with advanced Hodgkin's sarcoma, massive fluid overload with TBW/B.Wt. 76% (predicted normal 52%), reduction in BCM to 11 kg (predicted normal 14 kg), and extreme decrease in ICW/TBW (19% vs predicted normal 51%). By contrast, Table 1, Case C, presents data of a patient with uncontrolled sepsis whose TBW/B.Wt. was 51%, a value close to the predicted normal (47%). Yet, BCM was greatly reduced to 12 kg (predicted normal 19 kg) and ICW/TBW was 31% (predicted normal 52%); consequently, the major reduction in ICW was balanced with a major similar expansion of ECW, resulting in a relatively normal TBW.

The most destructive processes observed in severely ill patients combine severe injury, invasive sepsis, and starvation, conditions in which BCM melts away [5]. In these patients ICF and total body potassium decreased drastically, and a reduction of the ratio of ICF to total body water is observed. Protein-calorie malnutrition is present in this state and results in a loss of intracellular ions, such as potassium, magnesium, and phosphorus, and most commonly, a body gain in sodium and water.

The major reduction of ICW observed in patients with severe sepsis or major trauma should not be interpreted as a manifestation of cellular dehydration [5]. In fact BCM shrinks as a consequence of the catabolic state in the presence of either adequate or excessive state of hydration. Further support for the absence of cellular dehydration includes the demonstration of the normalcy of cellular [K+] in association with normal or high ECF volume. The decrease in total body potassium observed in severely ill patients is an expression of the reduced BCM [1]. Other investigators have proposed that the massive proteolysis observed in critically ill patients is triggered and maintained by cell shrinkage secondary to "cellular dehydration" [12]. We do not support this concept, which in our view does not have adequate scientific basis. Yet, reduction in ICW appears to be a reliable simple index of moderate or severe nutritional depletion.

Body cell mass recovers during the anabolic phase and studies have documented an increase in ICW after proper nutrition [5]. Table 2 depicts sequential data on the body composition of a patient with ulcerative colitis with dramatic recovery of body composition in a 6-month period. It should be noted that the recovery of body weight from 52 kg to 65 kg was accompanied with only 3 liters gain in TBW. Thus, the recovery of BCM from 18 kg to 25 kg was accompanied with a reduction in ECW from an initial level of 66% to a final value of 46% of TBW. This point also becomes evident examining the ICW/TBW that increased from 34% to 54% and the TBW/B.Wt. that decreased from 63% to 55%. In addition, administration of growth hormone or selected amino acid preparations can help correction of the decreased BCM associated with a major catabolic state.

Table 2. Data demonstrating anabolic recovery in a 50-year-old man with ulcerative colitis

Day	1	23	77	175
B.Wt. (kg)	52	55	58	65
TBW (L)	33	34	34	36
TBW/B.Wt. (%)	63	62	58	55
ECW/TBW (%)	66	57	51	46
ICW/TBW (%)	34	43	49	54
BCM (kg)	18	19	22	25

Modified from [5]

Expanded ECF volume is commonly observed in wasting diseases and critically ill patients, in association with reduced ICF (Table 1). Multiple factors including the excessive administration of saline solutions and the use of intravenous glucose infusion as sole caloric source participate in the pathogenesis of this fluid disorder.

Monitoring of body fluid compartments

Measurement of body fluid compartments require methodology that is not currently available in intensive care units [11]. Tritium dilution is used to estimate total body water (TBW) and [35] S-sodium sulfate or bromide for measurement of ECW volume. ICF is calculated as the difference between TBW and ECF. Bioelectrical impedance analysis can be used to assess TBW and to identify abnormal fluid distribution in severely ill patients. Whole body neutron activation analysis allows assessment of total body protein and counting γ emissions from natural K-40 permit measurement of total body potassium. As indicated above, unfortunately, none of these techniques is currently available for the care of severely ill patients. Therefore fluid monitoring at this time rests on information obtained with other methods including: patient's physical examination, chest radiographs and haemodynamic monitoring, input-output balance charts, daily body weight with electronic bed scales, and estimation of insensible/sensible and catabolic losses [2, 11]. We believe that with adequate training of all members of ICU team, reliable data on the patient's body fluid volume can be obtained with currently available methods.

References

1. Greco BA, Jacobson HR (1996) Fluid and electrolyte problems with surgery, trauma, and burns. In: Kokko JP, Tannen RL (eds) Fluids and electrolytes. WB Saunders, Philadelphia, pp 729-758
2. Adrogué HJ, Wesson DE (1994) Salt & Water. Blackwell's basics of medicine, vol 3. Blackwell Scientific, Boston
3. Adrogué HJ, Madias NE (1997) Aiding fluid prescription for the dysnatremias. Intensive Care Med 23:309-316
4. Elwyn DH, Bryan-Brown CW, Shoemaker WC (1975) Nutritional aspects of body water dislocations in postoperative and depleted patients. Ann Surg 182:76-85
5. Moore FD et al (1963) The body cell mass and its supporting environment. WB Saunders, Philadelphia
6. Hood VL (1996) Fluid and electrolyte disturbances in starvation states. In: Kokko JP, Tannen RL (eds) Fluids and electrolytes. WB Saunders, Philadephia, pp 759-785
7. Bergstrom JP, Larsson J, Nordstrom H et al (1987) Influence of injury and nutrition on muscle water and electrolytes: effect of severe injury, burns and sepsis. Acta Chir Scand 153:261-266
8. Gatzen C, Scheltinga MR, Kimbrough TD et al (1992) Growth hormone attenuates the abnormal distribution of body water in critically ill surgical patients. Surgery 112:181-187
9. Blackburn GL, Bothe A (1978) Assessment of malnutrition in cancer patients. Cancer Bull 30:88-93

10. Pichard C, Fitting JW, Chevrolet JC (1998) Nutritional monitoring. In: Tobin MJ (ed) Principles and practice of intensive care monitoring. McGraw-Hill, New York, pp 1099-1124
11. Farber MO (1998) Monitoring of fluid balance. In: Tobin MJ (ed) Principles and practice of intensive care monitoring. McGraw-Hill, New York, pp 1077-1084
12. Haussinger D, Roth E, Lang F et al (1993) Cellular hydration state: an important determinant of protein catabolism in health and disease. Lancet 341:1330-1332

Pathophysiology of Acid Base Regulation

H.J. ADROGUÉ

The need for the existence of multiple mechanisms involved in acid-base regulation stems from the critical importance of the hydrogen ion (H^+) concentration on the operation of many cellular enzymes and function of vital organs, most prominently the brain and the heart [1]. The task imposed on the mechanisms that maintain acid-base homeostasis is large since metabolic pathways are continuously consuming or producing H^+, and the daily load of waste products for excretion in the form of volatile (carbonic acid) and fixed acids is substantial. The equilibrium reaction of water and CO_2, the end product of oxidative metabolism, results in the daily formation of large amounts of carbonic acid, approximately 15,000 mEq/day [2]. The acceptance of the H^+ derived from carbonic acid by haemoglobin results in the transformation of carbonic acid into bicarbonate, and this ion transports $\sim 80\%$ of the CO_2 added to the blood from the peripheral tissues to the lungs. As red cells reach the lungs and oxygen is taken up by haemoglobin, H^+ is released decomposing bicarbonate into CO_2 that diffuses into the alveoli for final excretion. The presence of carbonic anhydrase in red cells facilitates bicarbonate generation in peripheral tissues and decomposition in the lungs, speeding up the mechanisms of blood CO_2 loading and unloading.

The net daily production of fixed acids, commonly referred to as "endogenous acid production" is approximately 70 to 100 mEq/day (~ 1.0 to 1.5 mEq of H^+/kg body wt/day) and are removed from body fluids by the kidney according to the classic interpretation [2]. Consequently, the daily production of volatile acid is ~ 200-fold that of fixed acids and explains the development of severe acidaemia resulting from CO_2 retention within minutes of a respiratory arrest, whereas it takes days to reach a comparable deviation of acidity as a result of retention of fixed acids in the absence of renal function.

Proton generation and consumption

The endogenous acid production is mostly composed of waste products and other substances derived from the intermediate metabolism of energy-rich compounds. The relatively small net daily production of acids (70 to 100 mEq/d) in the normal state occurs in the presence of a large proton generation and proton consumption in major metabolic pathways of carbohydrates, lipids, and proteins. Glycolysis is the proton producing pathway from carbohydrates, leading to the synthesis of lactic or pyruvic acids. Conversely, regeneration of glucose from lactic acid or complete oxidation of the latter to CO_2 and water consumes hydrogen ions (Table 1). It has been estimated that approximately 1,300 mmol of lactate and H^+ enter the circulation in a resting 70 kg subject every 24 hours and an almost identical amount of this organic acid is removed by the tissues, mostly the liver [3]. A large imbalance between synthesis and consumption of lactic acid is responsible for the development of various forms of lactic acidosis.

Lipolysis in peripheral tissues produce fatty acids, which in turn can undergo partial oxidation leading to the formation of ketoacids. Proton production through these pathways amounts to about 300 mmol/day in normal individuals, and an almost identical quantity of these acids is consumed with the synthesis of triglyceride and fatty acids (Table 1). However, a large imbalance between degradation and synthesis of body fats is observed in states of diabetic, alcoholic, or starving ketoacidosis [4].

Table 1. Overview of H^+ producing and H^+ consuming pathways in the metabolism of carbohydrates, fats and proteins (i.e., amino acids)

H^+ producing pathways		H^+ consuming pathways
Carbohydrates	Glucose $\rightarrow$ 2 Lactate + 2 H^+ Lactate + NAD^+ $\rightarrow$ Pyruvate + NADH + H^+	2 Lactate + 2 H^+ $\rightarrow$ Glucose 2 Lactate + 2 H^+ + 6 O_2 $\rightarrow$ 6 CO_2 + 6 H_2O
Fat stores	Triglyceride $\rightarrow$ 3 Fatty acid anions + 3 H^+ Palmitate + 6 O_2 $\rightarrow$ 4 Ketone anions + 3 H^+ + 2 H_2O	3 Fatty acid anions + 3 H^+ $\rightarrow$ Triglyceride 4 Ketone anions + 3 H^+ + 2 H_2O $\rightarrow$ Palmitate Ketone anions + H^+ $\rightarrow$ CO_2 + H_2O
Proteins	2 NH_4^+ + CO_2 $\rightarrow$ Urea + 2 H^+ + H_2O (neutral AA: 1 NH_4^+; dicarboxylic AA: 1 NH_4^+; basic AA: 2 NH_4^+)	Amino acids (AA) $\rightarrow$ HCO_3^- (neutral AA: 1 HCO_3^-; dicarboxylic AA: 2 HCO_3^-; basic AA: 1 HCO_3^-)

AA: amino acids

Disposal of ammonium (NH_4^+) during oxidation of amino acids in an individual with a 100 g of dietary protein intake generates approximately 1,000 mmol/day of H^+ by the liver in the process of urea synthesis [3]. However, an identical H^+ load is consumed in body tissues with complete oxidation of the carbon skeletons of amino acids if the protein entirely consists of neutral amino acids. During oxidation, dicarboxylic amino acids (glutamate and aspartate) generate 2 HCO_3^- for each NH_4^+, whereas basic amino acids (e.g., lysine) generate 2 NH_4^+ for each HCO_3^- (Table 1). Excess protons are also produced during degradation of sulfur-containing amino acids by the oxidation of sulfur. In well-fed subjects the type of proteins in the diet largely account for differences in the net daily production of fixed acids. Conversely, in starved subjects the utilization of endogenous proteins determine the net acid production from this energy source. An imbalance between the proton load generated by urea synthesis and the bicarbonate production from oxidation of the carbon skeletons of amino acids can lead to a deviation of the normal acid-base status [3]. Furthermore, states of abnormal acid-base composition have a major influence on proton generation and consumption in major metabolic pathways, as described below.

Acidaemia of both metabolic and respiratory origin inhibits glycolysis, whereas alkalaemia stimulates it [5]. This effect is mediated, at least in part, by the pH-sensitive enzyme phosphofructokinase, that plays a key rate-limiting role in glycolysis. Acidaemia also stimulates renal lactate utilization, but inhibits hepatic lactate utilization. In addition, acid-base balance alters ketoacid metabolism in a comparable manner to that of lactic acid. A low systemic pH inhibits ketoacid production, whereas a high pH stimulates it [5, 6]. Consequently, there is a pH feedback control of endogenous acid production. Under conditions of excessive lactic or ketoacid production, the resultant acidaemia feeds back to inhibit the rate of endogenous acid production, thereby serving as a protective mechanism.

Similarly, amino acids oxidation is significantly altered in response to changes in systemic acidity. Hepatic urea synthesis and its associated proton generation (two H^+ are generated per molecule of urea synthesized) is inhibited by a low systemic pH. Conversely, alkalaemia stimulates urea synthesis and therefore leads to increased proton generation facilitating correction of the altered systemic acidity. Acidaemia also has a direct effect on the kidney that increases urinary NH_4^+ excretion, thereby facilitating nitrogen disposal and promoting proton excretion [3]. A synopsis of the direct and indirect effects of acidaemia on the liver and kidney is depicted in Table 2.

Table 2. Effects and consequences of acidaemia on H^+ producing pathways from oxidation of protein (i.e., amino acids)

Direct effect	Indirect effect	Consequences
Kidney: Increases urinary NH_4^+ excretion	→ Liver: Reduces supply of NH_4^+ for urea synthesis →	Alkalinizing effect secondary to decreased H^+ production
Liver: Alters nitrogen disposal pathways: Augments glutamine synthesis delivering substrate to kidney	↑ → Kidney: Increased urinary NH_4^+ excretion	
Decreases urea synthesis		→ Alkalizing effect secondary to decreased H^+ production

Acid-base disorders

Clinical acid-base disorders are conventionally defined from the vantage point of their impact on the carbonic acid/bicarbonate buffer system. This approach is justified by the abundance of this buffer pair in body fluids; its physiologic preeminence; and the validity of the isohydric principle in the living organism, which specifies that all the other buffer systems are in equilibrium with the carbonic acid/bicarbonate buffer pair [7]. Thus, as indicated by the Henderson equation, $[H^+] = 24 \times PaCO_2 / [HCO_3^-]$ (the equilibrium relationship of the carbonic acid/bicarbonate system), the hydrogen ion concentration of blood (expressed in nEq/L) at any moment is a function of the prevailing ratio of the arterial carbon dioxide tension ($PaCO_2$, expressed in mmHg) and the plasma bicarbonate concentration ($[HCO_3^-]$, expressed in mEq/L). As a corollary, changes in systemic acidity can occur only through changes in the values of its two determinants, $PaCO_2$ and plasma bicarbonate concentration [8]. Those acid-base disorders that are initiated by a change in $PaCO_2$ are referred to as respiratory disorders, whereas those initiated by a change in plasma bicarbonate concentration are known as metabolic disorders. Each of the four cardinal acid-base disturbances – respiratory acidosis, respiratory alkalosis, metabolic acidosis, and metabolic alkalosis – can be encountered by itself, as a simple disorder, or can be a part of a mixed disorder, defined as the simultaneous presence of two or more simple acid-base disturbances [2]. The secondary response to a simple acid-base disorder should not be taken as one of the components of a mixed acid-base disorder. Mixed acid-base disorders are frequently observed in hospitalized patients, especially in the critically ill.

Metabolic acidosis is the acid-base disturbance initiated by a decrease in the $[HCO_3^-]_p$. Because the metabolic component of acid-base equilibrium might also be quantified by such terms as the standard $[HCO_3^-]_p$, buffer base, or base excess of the blood, a primary decrease in any of these parameters constitutes metabolic acidosis. The decrease in the metabolic component observed in metabolic acidosis is initiated by a gain in nonvolatile or fixed acid or by a loss of base. It is accompanied by a secondary decrease in the $PaCO_2$ of body fluids.

Assessment of the plasma unmeasured anion concentration (anion gap) is a very useful, first step in approaching the differential diagnosis of unexplained metabolic acidosis [1]. The plasma anion gap (A^-) is calculated as the difference between sodium concentration and the sum of chloride and bicarbonate concentrations. Under normal circumstances, the plasma anion gap is primarily composed of the net negative charges of plasma proteins, predominantly albumin, with a smaller contribution from many other organic and inorganic anions. The normal value of plasma anion gap is 12 ± 4 (mean ± 2 SD) mEq/L. However, recent introduction of ion specific electrodes has shifted the normal anion gap to approximately the 6 ± 3 mEq/L range. In one pattern of metabolic acidosis, the fall in bicarbonate concentration is offset by a rise in the concentration of chloride, plasma anion gap remaining normal. In the other pattern, the decrease in bicarbonate is balanced by an increase in the concentration of unmeasured anions (i.e., anions that are not measured routinely), plasma chloride concentration remaining normal [2, 7].

A normal anion gap (hyperchloraemic) metabolic acidosis may reflect a primary loss of HCO_3^- as such, a failure to replenish HCO_3^- stores depleted by the daily production of fixed acids, or the addition of HCl (Table 3). In turn, a primary loss of HCO_3^- might result from urinary or intestinal losses of alkali. Proximal renal tubular acidosis (type 2 RTA) is caused by excessive loss of bicarbonate by the kidney. Intestinal alkali losses occur in diarrhoea, surgical drainage of the intestinal tract, or with gastrointestinal fistulas, that cause losses of fluid rich in HCO_3^-. Such losses may also occur in patients whose ureters have been attached to the intestinal tract. The alkali of intestinal secretions is decomposed by titration with acid urine; ionic exchanges across the intestinal mucosa that include Na^+/H^+ and HCO_3^-/Cl^- also contribute to this acid-base disorder [7].

Clinical examples of normal anion gap metabolic acidosis that result from failure to replace HCO_3^- stores depleted by the daily production of fixed acids include the classic and hyperkalaemic distal renal tubular acidoses (types 1 and 4 RTA, respectively). In these conditions, the daily net acid excretion by the kidney falls short of the daily acid production, leading to metabolic acidosis due to depletion of endogenous HCO_3^- stores. Hypoaldosteronism or aldosterone resistance are the underlying mechanisms of hyperkalaemic distal RTA [1, 2].

There are two major mechanisms responsible for the development of high-anion-gap metabolic acidosis (Table 3). First, an excessive load of non-HCl acid (whether endogenous or exogenous) can overwhelm the normal capacity of the body either to process or to excrete it. Second, a diminished capacity of the kidney to extract the normal load of endogenous fixed acids is responsible for uremic acidosis.

The absolute or relative lack of insulin in patients with diabetic ketoacidosis (DKA) prevents their insulin-sensitive cells from utilizing glucose as an energy source [9]. Instead, the patient's metabolism is modified to generate large amounts of ketoacids as well as new glucose from noncarbohydrate sources. As a result, the composite clinical picture in full-blown DKA includes hyperglycaemia with metabolic acidosis due to accumulation of ketoacids. This process results in an increment of unmeasured plasma anions and accounts for the classic acid-base pattern of metabolic acidosis associated with an increased plasma anion gap. In uncomplicated DKA, the increment in plasma anion gap above its normal value should be approximately equal to the decrement in plasma bicarbonate. Thus the ratio of excess anion gap to bicarbonate deficit should be about one, or 100%. However, patients admitted with DKA often have a metabolic acidosis with an excess anion gap to bicarbonate deficit ratio quite different from one [10]. A ratio of excess plasma anion gap to bicarbonate deficit that is greater than one suggests that bicarbonate was added to the body fluids or that ketoacids were lost in the urine. For example, vomiting or exogenous bicarbon-

Table 3. Causes of metabolic acidosis

High anion gap	Normal anion gap
Endogenous acid load	*Renal diseases*
Ketoacidosis	Proximal renal tubular acidosis
Diabetes	Classic distal tubular acidosis
Alcoholism	Hyperkalaemic distal tubular acidosis
Starvation	Interstitial nephritis
Uraemia	Urinary tract obstruction
Lactic acidosis	Early renal failure
Exogenous toxins	*Gastrointestinal loss of bicarbonate*
Osmolar gap present	Diarrhoea
Methanol	Small bowel losses
Ethylene glycol	Ureteral diversions
Osmolar gap absent	Anion exchange resins
Salicylates	*Drugs*
Paraldehyde	Acetazolamide
	Mafenide
	Amphotericin B
	Amiloride
	Spironolactone
	Toluene ingestion
	Acid infusion
	HCL
	Arginine HCL
	Lysine HCL

ate administration will minimize the bicarbonate deficit in plasma and increase the ratio.

It is common to see a ratio of less than one between the excess plasma anion gap and the bicarbonate deficit. Ketones may be excreted as sodium salts in the urine, decreasing the serum levels of ketoacids and minimizing the anion gap. Alternatively, administration of chloride-rich fluids will decrease the anion gap and make the ratio smaller without affecting serum ketoacid levels [11]. Finally, increased renal losses of bicarbonate due to hypocapnia or to the concomitant presence of renal tubular acidosis would increase the bicarbonate deficit out of proportion to the increase in anion gap.

Conventionally, two broad types of lactic acidosis are recognized: type A, in which there is clinical evidence of impaired tissue oxygenation, and type B, in which no such evidence is apparent [1, 2]. However, the distinction between the two types might occasionally be less than obvious. Thus, inadequate tissue oxygenation can at times defy clinical detection, and tissue hypoxia can be a part of the pathogenesis of certain causes of type B lactic acidosis. Most cases of lactic acidosis are caused by tissue hypoxia arising from circulatory failure. Accumulation of lactate during hypoxia originates from impaired mitochondrial oxida-

tive function that reduces the availability of ATP and NAD$^+$ (oxidized nicoti-
namide adenine dinucleotide) within the cytosol. In turn, these changes cause
cytosolic accumulation of pyruvate as a consequence of both increased production and decreased utilization. Increased production of pyruvate occurs because
the reduced cytosolic supply of ATP stimulates the activity of 6-phosphofruc-
tokinase (PFK) thereby accelerating glycolysis. Decreased utilization of pyruvate reflects the fact that both pathways of its consumption depend on mitochondrial oxidative reactions.

Measurement of serum osmolality may yield an important clue to the presence of alcohol ingestion, a potential cause of high-anion-gap acidosis. Ethanol,
methanol, ethylene glycol, and isopropyl alcohol are all low molecular weight
compounds which accumulate in body fluids at significant concentrations and
thereby increase measured osmolality [2]. Osmolality can be calculated as follows:

$$\text{Osmolality} = 2\text{Na}^+ + \frac{\text{BUN mg/dl}}{2.8} + \frac{\text{glucose mg/dl}}{18}$$

where BUN is the concentration of urea nitrogen in the blood. Usually the
measured and calculated osmolalities will be within 10 mOsm/liter. The presence of alcohol in blood results in measured osmolality greater than that calculated. The magnitude of the osmolality gap is directly proportional to the plasma
alcohol concentration. When the retained alcohol is known, its concentration
may be approximated from the magnitude of the osmolality gap and the molecular weight of the alcohol. For example, a methanol or ethylene glycol level of
100 mg/dl will produce an osmolality gap of 22 mOsm/L and 16 mOsm/L, respectively. Pseudohyponatraemia can spuriously decrease calculated osmolality
leading to an osmolar gap [7].

Metabolic alkalosis is the acid-base disturbance initiated by an increase in
the $[\text{HCO}_3^-]_p$. Because the metabolic component of acid-base equilibrium might
also be quantified by the standard $[\text{HCO}_3^-]_p$, buffer base, or base excess of the
blood, a primary increase in any of these parameters constitutes metabolic alkalosis [2]. The increase in the metabolic component observed in metabolic alkalosis is generated by an augmented loss of nonvolatile or fixed acid or by a gain
in base. Two crucial questions must be answered when evaluating the pathogenesis of a case of metabolic alkalosis [1]. First, what is the source of the excess
alkali? Answering this question addresses the primary event responsible for
generating the hyperbicarbonataemia. Second, what factors perpetuate the hyperbicarbonataemia? Answering this question addresses the pathophysiologic
events that maintain the metabolic alkalosis. The answers to these questions are
outlined in Fig. 1.

The recognition of metabolic alkalosis as being either Cl$^-$ -sensitive (NaCl-
responsive) or Cl$^-$ -resistant (not corrected by increasing NaCl intake) is of criti-

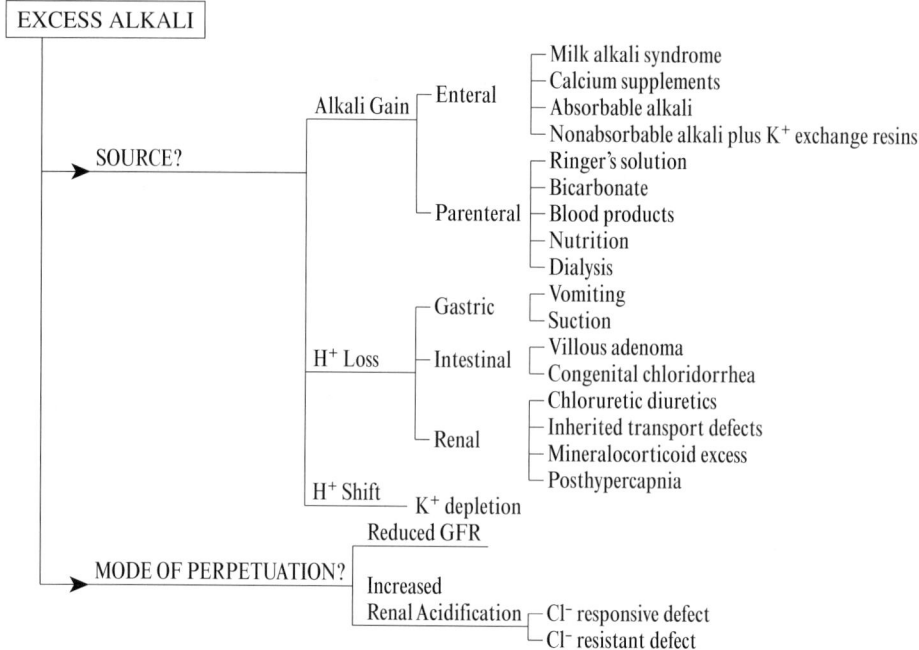

Fig. 1.

cal importance in the management of this acid-base disorder [2]. In Cl⁻ -sensitive or responsive alkalosis, chloride depletion is a critical factor in the pathogenesis of metabolic alkalosis; thus, urine Cl⁻ excretion is markedly diminished, leading to urinary Cl⁻ concentration < 10 meq/L. This category includes gastrointestinal disorders (e.g., vomiting, gastric drainage, villous adenoma of the colon, and Cl⁻ rich diarrhoea), cystic fibrosis, diuretic therapy, excessive skin loss of NaCl, and recovery from chronic hypercapnia. In Cl⁻ -resistant alkalosis, a group of conditions in which chloride depletion is not involved in the pathogenesis of metabolic alkalosis, urine Cl⁻ excretion is within normal limits, with urinary [Cl⁻] concentration > 20 meq/L. This category includes several disorders characterized by excessive mineralocorticoid activity (e.g., hyperaldosteronism, Cushing syndrome, licorice intake, Bartter syndrome) as well as profound K⁺ depletion.

The milk-alkali syndrome comprises the triad of hypercalcaemia, renal insufficiency, and metabolic alkalosis and is caused by the ingestion of large amounts of calcium and absorbable alkali [2, 12]. Although large amounts of milk and absorbable alkali were the culprit in the classic form of the syndrome, its modern version is usually the result of large doses of calcium carbonate alone. Because of recent emphasis on prevention and treatment of osteoporosis with calcium carbonate and the availability of this preparation over-the-counter, the milk-alkali syndrome is currently the third leading cause of hypercalcaemia after primary hyperparathyroidism and malignancy. Another common presentation of the syndrome originates from the current use of calcium carbonate in preference to aluminum as a phosphate binder in patients with chronic renal insufficiency [1, 12]. The critical element in the pathogenesis of the syndrome is the development of hypercalcaemia, which in turn results in renal dysfunction. Generation and maintenance of metabolic alkalosis reflects the combined effects of the large bicarbonate load, the renal insufficiency, and the hypercalcaemia. Metabolic alkalosis contributes to the maintenance of hypercalcaemia by increasing tubular calcium reabsorption. Superimposition of an element of volume contraction caused by vomiting, diuretics, or hypercalcaemia-induced natriuresis can worsen each one of the three main components of the syndrome. Discontinuation of calcium carbonate and the use of normal saline/high-NaCl diet and furosemide result in rapid resolution of the hypercalcaemia and metabolic alkalosis. Although renal function also improves, in a considerable fraction of patients with the chronic form of the syndrome serum creatinine fails to return to its baseline as a result of irreversible structural changes in the kidneys.

The pathophysiology of respiratory acidosis and respiratory alkalosis is discussed in the corresponding chapter of this book. Instead, we shall consider here the entity known as *pseudorespiratory alkalosis* [13, 14]. Arterial hypocapnia does not necessarily imply respiratory alkalosis or the secondary response to metabolic acidosis but can be observed in an idiotypic form of respiratory acidosis. This entity, which we have termed pseudorespiratory alkalosis, occurs in patients with profound depression of cardiac function and pulmonary perfusion but with relative preservation of alveolar ventilation, including patients undergoing cardiopulmonary resuscitation [13, 14]. The severely reduced pulmonary blood flow limits the carbon dioxide delivered to the lungs for excretion, thereby increasing the mixed venous partial pressure of carbon dioxide. By contrast, the increased ventilation:perfusion ratio causes the removal of a larger-than-normal amount of carbon dioxide per unit of blood traversing the pulmonary circulation, thereby creating arterial eucapnia or frank hypocapnia. Nonetheless, the absolute excretion of carbon dioxide is decreased and the carbon dioxide balance of the body is positive – the hallmark of respiratory acidosis –. Such patients may have severe venous acidaemia (often due to mixed respiratory and metabolic acidosis) accompanied by an arterial pH that ranges from the mildly acidic to the frankly alkaline. Furthermore, the extreme oxygen deprivation prevailing in the tissues may be completely disguised by the reasonably preserved values of arterial oxygen. To rule out pseudorespiratory alkalosis in a patient with circulatory failure, blood gas monitoring must include sampling of mixed (or central) venous blood [13, 14]. The management of pseudorespiratory alkalosis must be directed toward optimizing systemic haemodynamics.

References

1. Adrogué HJ, Wesson DE (1994) Acid-base. Blackwell's basics of medicine. Blackwell Science, Boston
2. Cohen JJ, Kassirer JP (1982) Acid/base. Little, Brown, Boston
3. Cohen RD (1995) The liver and acid-base regulation. In: Arieff AI, DeFronzo RA (eds) Fluid, electrolyte, and acid-base disorders. Churchill Livingstone, New York, pp 777-790
4. Adrogué HJ, Madias NE (1998) Management of life-threatening acid-base disorders. Part I. N Engl J Med 338:26-34
5. Hood VL, Tannen RL (1983) pH control of lactic acid and ketoacid production: A mechanism of acid base regulation. Miner Electrolyte Metab 9:317-325
6. Hood VL, Tannen RL (1994) Maintenance of acid base homeostasis during ketoacidosis and lactic acidosis: Implications for therapy. Diabetes/Metab Rev 2:177-194
7. Madias NE (1995) Fluid, electrolyte and acid-base disorders. In: Jacobson HR, Striker GE, Klahr S (eds) The principles and practice of nephrology. Decker, Philadelphia, pp 864-963
8. Schwartz WB, Relman AS (1963) A critique of the parameters used in the evaluation of acid-base disorders: "whole-blood buffer base" and "standard bicarbonate" compared with blood pH and plasma bicarbonate concentration. N Engl J Med 268:1382-1388
9. Alberti KGMM (1990) Diabetic acidosis, hyperosmolar coma, and lactic acidosis. In: Becker KL (ed) Principles and practice of endocrinology and metabolism. Lippincott, Philadelphia, pp 1175-1187
10. Adrogué HJ, Wilson H, Boyd AE et al (1982) Plasma acid-base patterns in diabetic ketoacidosis. N Engl J Med 307:1603-1610
11. Adrogué HJ, Barrero J, Eknoyan G (1989) Salutary effects of modest fluid replacement in the treatment of adults with diabetic ketoacidosis. JAMA 262:2108-2113
12. Adrogué HJ, Madias NE (1998) Management of life-threatening acid base disorders. Part II. N Engl J Med 338:107-111
13. Adrogué HJ, Rashad MN, Gorin AB et al (1989) Assessing acid-base status in circulatory failure. Differences between arterial and central venous blood. N Engl J Med 320:1312-1316
14. Adrogué HJ, Rashad MN, Gorin AB et al (1989) Arteriovenous acid-base disparity in circulatory failure: Studies on mechanism. Am J Physiol 257:F1087-F1093

Fluid and Electrolyte Management in Intensive Care

F. Bobbio Pallavicini, G. Verde, P. Tosi

Despite great variability in water and electrolyte intake, circulating intravascular volume, electrolyte composition of various body fluids, and serum osmolality remain remarkable constant in health.

Conversely, disorders of fluid electrolyte balance are a daily occurrence in the intensive care unit (ICU) because patients often have multiple coexisting organ system failures, are administered medications that disturb fluid and electrolyte status, and are usually denied self-regulation of water balance.

Serum electrolytes

Sodium

Sodium is the extracellular prominent cation. Extracellular sodium represents 98 per cent of the body's sodium (5000 mmol), still osmotically active (measuring) sodium only accounts for one third of body's sodium. The remaining sodium constitutes sodium reserves, but only one half of them may be exchangeable with osmotically active sodium. Extracellularly, the sodium concentration is 142 mmol/L in plasma and 134 mmol/L in the interstitial fluid. Because sodium is the predominant osmotically active extracellular cation, serum osmolality is determined largely by the relative proportions of water and sodium. Reductions in osmolality are virtually reflected in the sodium concentration. Increases in serum osmolality result in thirst and augmented antidiuretic hormone (ADH) secretion. ADH then acts on the medullary collecting duct of the kidney to stimulate water resorption. ADH in combination with renin-angiotensin-aldosterone system restores circulating volume in response to depletion. When plasma osmolality declines, ADH release is inhibited and excess water is lost in an attempt to return osmolality toward normal [1].

Chloride

Chloride is the body's principal anion, the predominant extracellular base. Chloride is responsible for 100 of the 300 mosm/L of extracellular fluid tonicity. Extracellularly, the chloride concentration is 104 mmol/L in plasma and 117 mmol/L in interstitial fluid. Intracellularly, concentrations range from 2 mmol/L in skeletal muscle, 20 mmol/L in various epithelial cells, 40 mmol/L in lymphocytes, and 90 mmol/L in erythrocytes. In cerebrospinal fluid chloride concentration is higher because of the absence of most of the organic anions. The major categories of hyperchloraemia (> 105 mmol/L) encountered in the critically ill patient are artifactual, accompanying respiratory alkalosis, intravascular volume depletion, and hyperchloraemic metabolic acidosis. Hypochloraemias (< 95 mmol/L) seen most often in the ICU are due to dilution, loss from gastrointestinal (GI) tract or kidney (diuretics), secondary to chronic respiratory disease, accompanying hypokalaemia, and as a result of corticosteroid therapy [2].

Potassium

Potassium is the most prominent intracellular soluble cation. About 95 per cent of the total body potassium is intracellular, but extracellular potassium concentration critically influences neuromuscular function. Because a small minority of the body's potassium is in the extracellular compartment, hypokalaemia signals total body depletion of potassium. However, because the intracellular space must be accessed via the small extracellular compartment, potassium therapy (especially intravenous replacement) can lead to potentially harmful hyperkalaemia [3]. Once hypokalaemia (< 3.5 mEq/L) manifests, the average potassium deficit approximates 250-300 mEq. Because of the large influence of systemic pH in the potassium concentration of extracellular compartment, wide and rapid shifts of potassium in exchange for H^+ can surface. This occurs without variations in total body's potassium [4]. A 0.1-unit decrease in pH produces an average 0.6 mEq/L increase in potassium (range 0.4-1.3 mEq/L). However, changes in serum potassium are more sensitive to change in serum bicarbonate than to pH itself. Therefore, respiratory acidosis has relatively little effect on potassium, whereas metabolic acidosis exerts a potent effect. Potassium levels decline 0.1-0.4 mEq/L for each 0.1-unit increase in pH. In turn, hypokalaemia increases renal bicarbonate absorption, perpetuating alkalosis. A number of mechanisms may facilitate potassium entry into cells to produce hypokalaemia. High insulin levels, whether exogenous or induced (e.g., continuous TPN or tube feedings) increase cellular uptake. Hypokalaemia often occurs within 48 hrs of treating vitamin B12 or folate deficiency, as potassium is massively incorporated into newly formed red cells and platelets. Such patients routinely experience reduction in serum potassium of approximately 1 mEq/L, a potentially life-threatening change.

Calcium

Calcium is essential for normal cellular function. Calcium is a major regulator coupling receptor activation to intracellular metabolic events. As such, it plays an important role in maintaining cellular and organ integrity. The extracellular-to-intracellular gradient for calcium is approximately 10,000:1. Calcium enters the cell via diffusion, slow-channel activation, and sodium-calcium exchange. Since uncontrolled increases in free intracellular calcium can activate destructive processes (e.g.: lipases, proteases, nucleases, free-radical generation, prostaglandin release), free intracellular calcium concentrations are normally maintained within narrow limits through energy requiring processes which pump calcium out of the cell or into the sarcoplasmatic reticulum. Failure of these pumps during ischaemia and sepsis leads to increased free intracellular calcium and cellular damage [5].

Calcium circulates in the blood in three forms: a protein-bound form (50%), a chelated form (10%), and a ionized form (40%). The ionized form is the active calcium fraction and is the form that is physiologically regulated. Most hospital laboratories measure total serum calcium concentrations (8.5 to 10.5 mg/dL or 4.25 to 5.25 mmol/L or 2.12 to 2.62 mM). However, the total serum calcium value is frequently a poor indicator of ionized calcium status in critically ill patients. Total calcium is influenced by factors that alter protein-bound and chelated calcium, irrespective of ionized calcium. Acidosis decreases calcium binding to albumin, while alkalosis increases binding. Thus, changes in acid-base status may also alter total and ionized calcium values. For example, acute hyperventilation acutely lowers ionized calcium (calcium shifts on-to the albumin molecule) without affecting total calcium concentrations. The addition of circulating chelators (e.g., citrate, phosphates, lipids) also influences calcium measurement. Ionized calcium measurement of anaerobic blood specimens is the only clinically available, accurate method for assessing physiologic values of circulating calcium. Circulating calcium concentrations are maintained within normal ranges primarily through the actions of parathyroid hormone (PTH) and vitamin D on bone. Dietary calcium is not required for maintenance of a normal circulating calcium level, provided the parathyroid-vitamin D axis is functioning. PTH secretion is regulated by circulating calcium, magnesium, and calcitriol concentrations. Ionized hypocalcaemia stimulates PTH secretion while hypercalcaemia suppresses secretion. Mild hypomagnesaemia stimulates PTH while moderate-to-severe hypomagnesaemia (e.g., magnesium < 1 mg/dL) and hypermagnesaemia suppresses PTH secretion. PTH stimulates calcium mobilization from the bone, resorption from the renal tubule, and absorption from the gut (via effects on vitamin D). About 30% to 35% of dietary calcium is normally absorbed. Calcium is lost from the body in the urine (average 150 mg/day) and stool (average 150 to 200 mg/day). Excretion of calcium in the urine is increased during hypercalcaemia and helps to limit the increase in blood calcium concentrations [6].

Magnesium

Magnesium is the most important intracellular cation after potassium. Extracellular magnesium concentrations (0.5 to 0.6 mmol/L) are 10 to 15 times lower than intracellular concentrations (18 mmol/L). Usually, serum variations of magnesium concentrations match the changes of kalaemia. Magnesium ions are important modulators of cellular and physiologic processes, including ion channel regulation and signal trasduction, enzyme activation, neurotransmission, bioenergetics, and smooth muscle tone and reactivity. Under normal circumstances, the gut and kidney work in concert to tightly regulate serum magnesium levels. Like calcium ion, magnesium depends on its ionized form for biologic action, and total serum concentration do not accurately reflects bioactivity [5, 6].

Renal and gastrointestinal handling of electrolytes

The kidney plays a central role in the body's handling of sodium and chloride. Normally, 80% of the sodium filtered by the glomerulus is resorbed accompanied by chloride and 20% is exchanged for potassium and hydrogen. In the ascending loop of Henle, chloride is actively resorbed [7], while in the distal nephron, chloride assists in the regulation of bicarbonate secretion [8] via a luminally located chloride-bicarbonate exchanger. When bicarbonate is resorbed, chloride is exchanged and excreted in its place. Normally, 135 ± 5 mmol of chloride is excreted daily. In extracellular fluid volume depletion, increased proximal chloride resorption leads to its decreased delivery to the distal nephron and bicarbonate secretion may not occur. The kidney also ritains bicarbonate in state of ineffective circulating volume. If excess bicarbonate were excreted, it would require concurrent sodium loss to maintain electroneutrality, further exacerbating volume depletion. Under these circumstances, the increase of bicarbonate resorption occurs in the distal nephron. In chloride depletion (not necessarily accompanied by volume depletion), urine chloride may be negligible, with less available chloride for resorption throughout the nephron. Concomitantly, less sodium is resorbed proximally and more delivered distally for exchange with hydrogen and potassium. As metabolic alkalosis and hypokalaemia evolve, even less sodium can be resorbed and extracellular fluid volume depletion develops. This extracellular fluid volume depletion stimulates aldosterone secretion, perpetuating renal losses of hydrogen and potassium [2].

The GI tract is capable of both absorbing and excreting chloride. The colon is able to both absorb chloride and secrete bicarbonate. Of the total chloride absorption by the colon, 25% is matched by the secretion of bicarbonate and 75% is coupled to sodium resorption [2]. Stool electrolytes are collected in a 24hr specimen, with the following reference range: chloride 16 mmol/L; sodium 32 to 40 mmol/L; potassium 75 to 90 mmol/L; bicarbonate 30 to 40 mmol/L. Cholera produces a profound secretory diarrhoea that is isotonic with plasma but with concentrations of bicarbonate and potassium greater than plasma. Congenital and acquired chloride diarrhoeas are characterized by increased fecal chloride, metabolic alkalosis, decreased serum electrolytes, and nearly absent urine chloride.

Urine electrolytes

Urine electrolyte values help in the elucidation of a wide variety of clinical disturbances but they must be assessed relative to the clinical setting. Since sodium and chloride are excreted in parallel, their values should reflect extracellular fluid volume status if there is a simultaneous acid-base disturbance that alters the renal handling of sodium and may falsely imply increased renal avidity for sodium. Therefore, a low urine chloride (< 10 mmol/L) confirms that a low urine sodium is consistent with extracellular fluid volume depletion. However, when extracellular fluid volume contraction is accompanied by hyperchloraemic metabolic acidosis (e.g., diarrhoea), there is urine excretion of amonium ion (NH4+) plus chloride yielding a low urine sodium with a high urine chloride [9]. Both a high urine chloride (> 20 mmol/L) and high urine sodium occur during tubular necrosis. In hypokalaemic states the knowledge of urinary potassium and chloride concentrations, and acid-base status may be useful in assessing the cause of hypokalaemia [9, 10]. When urinary potassium levels are low (< 20 mEq/L), the extrarenal mechanism is the etiology, like decreased dietary intake or excessive intestinal loss. A high urinary loss of potassium accompanied by acidosis usually is due to diabetic ketoacidosis or renal tubular acidosis. In alkalaemic patients a low urinary chloride concentration (< 10 mEq/L) is indicative of diuretic use, vomiting or nasogastric suctioning, which produce a combination of sodium deficiency, extracellular fluid volume contraction, and aldosterone release, all promoting renal wasting of potassium. If urinary chloride is high (> 10 mEq/L), it is indicative of mineralocorticoid excess. Diuretics are frequently administered to critically ill patients and complicate the evaluation of urine electrolytes. The most commonly prescribed loop diuretics (furosemide and bumetanide) inhibit active chloride transport in the thick ascending limb and are predominantly chloruretic. Intravenous furosemide acts within minutes and produces a diuresis in 1 hr that can last for 6 to 8 hrs, with distortion of urine electrolyte measurements during that time.

Urine anion gap

The urine anion gap (UAG) is similar in concept to the serum anion gap, in that it represents the difference between measured cations and anions. Urine anions (UA) that are normally present, although not routinely measured, include bicarbonate, sulphate, phosphate, and organ anions. Unmeasured cations (UC) include NH4+ (the predominant unmeasured ion), calcium, and magnesium. Chloride, sodium and potassium are routinely measured in the urine according to the following formula: $Cl^- + UA = Na^+ - K^+ + UC$; or, in a rearranged form: $UA - UC = Na^+ + K^+ = UAG$ [11]. The unmeasured ions in the serum consist of anions, while the gap in the urine is composed of cations. Therefore, the anion gap is negative in serum and positive in the urine (this can also be termed "a cationic gap"). The urine anion gap decreased whenever the sum of unmeasured anions decreases or the sum of unmeasured cations increases (usually NH4+). Conversely, the urine anion gap increases with an increase in unmeasured anions (usually bicarbonate) or with a decrease in unmeasured cations. The ability of the normal kidney to increase NH4+ excretion, in response to endogenous or exogenous acid loading, gives the urine anion gap clinical utility. The urine anion gap (as a rough index of urine NH4+) is most useful in the differential diagnosis of hyperchloraemic metabolic acidosis. A large negative UAG (high urine NH4+ excretion) suggests gastrointestinal bicarbonate loss, a positive or small negative UAG (usually low urine NH4+ excretion) suggests altered distal urine acidification. Factors invalidating the urine anion gap include renal excretion of bicarbonate or excretion of other anions (ketoacids, salicylic acid, lactic acid, and carbenicillin), which falsely lower the gap while excretion of other cations in large amounts spuriously increase the gap.

Serum anion gap

The anion gap is the difference between the measured anions and the measured cations. Measured cations routinely exceed measured anions and an apparent gap created by the laboratory, reflecting the presence of the unmeasured anions [12]. The anion gap is generally estimated as the serum sodium concentration minus the sum of the serum chloride and bicarbonate concentrations, which average 12 ± 2 mmol/L: serum anion gap (SAG) = $Na^+ - (Cl^- + HCO_3^-)$. The unmeasured anions are composed of serum proteins (predominantly albumin), phosphate, sulphate, lactate, ketoacids, and other unmeasured compounds (e.g., drugs). Knowledge of the anion gap may be quite valuable in distinguishing the etiology of metabolic acidosis. The addition of unmeasured anions elevates the anion gap (e.g., HCl administration does not increase the anion gap because CL^- is a measured anion). The anion gap should be adjusted for hypoalbuminaemia, which tends to reduce it by -2.5 mEq/L per gm/dL reduction in albumin concentration. As a rule, the larger the anion gap, the easier it is to determine the cause of the acidosis. Anion gaps > 30 mmol/L invariably reflect the accumulation of organic acids such as lactic acid or ketoacids [2]. Anion gaps between 20 and 29 mmol/L reflect organic acidosis in only 2/3 of cases. The anion gap may not be helpful when two acid-base disturbances occur simultaneously. For example, diabetic ketoacidosis usually presents with an increased anion gap acidosis, with profound losses of both water and electrolytes. However, both a hyperchloraemic acidosis (especially during recovery) and a normal anion gap may be seen. Very high serum levels of anionic salicylate molecules may directly elevate the anion gap, but salicylates also rise the anion gap by interfering with carbohydrate metabolism and O_2 use, thereby inducing lactic acidosis. There may also be spurious increases of anion gap. If the serum sample is left exposed to the air then water and CO_2 are lost, with a resultant decrease in bicarbonate and increase in sodium, chloride and potassium. The anion gap increase by about 3 mmol/L at 1 hr and up to 6 mmol/L at 2 hrs. There are also several causes of increased or decreased anion gaps that are not associated with an acidosis. Hypokalaemia, hypocalcaemia, and hypomagnesaemia decrease the amount of unmeasured cations and, therefore, increase the anion gap. The converse is true for hyperkalaemia, hypercalcaemia, and hypermagnesaemia. Nitrate, formate, penicillin, carbenicillin, and hyperalbuminaemia increase unmeasured anions and increase the gap. If the creatine, keton, and lactate levels are all normal in the setting of a high anion gap, a toxic ingestion becomes the most likely etiology. In such patients, comparing the calculated osmolality to measured serum osmolality proves particularly helpful (an osmolal gap usually indicates some form of alcohol toxicity: ethylene, glycol, ethanol, or methanol). Other drugs that can cause an anion gap acidosis include isoniazid, iron, and paraldehyde.

Life-threatening electrolyte disorders

Hyponatraemia

Hyponatraemia can be defined as a serum sodium lower than 125 mEq/L, and is one of the most common electrolyte disorders. Symptoms of hyponatraemia span the spectrum from muscle cramps, nausea, vomiting, and anorexia to confusion, lethargy, coma, and seizures [1]. The manifestations are generally proportional to the magnitude of the abnormality and the speed with which it develops. A thorough history and physical examination, the urine sodium concentration, the serum glucose, and the serum and urine osmolality provide essential data to determine the etiology. Measurements of serum osmolality help to separate hyponatraemia into three distinct categories, thereby guiding appropriate intervention:

a) *Isotonic hyponatraemia*. This type of hyponatraemia occurs when osmotically active solutes such as proteins (e.g., Waldenstrom's macroglobulinaemia), expand the plasma volume diluting the serum sodium concentration. This reduction in serum sodium can be viewed as a form of "pseudohyponatraemia". Isotonic hyponatraemia also may occur during the administration of large volumes of isotonic, non-salt-containing, solutions, such as glucose, mannitol, glycine.

b) *Hypertonic hyponatraemia*. Hyponatraemia with increased serum osmolality results from the infusion or generation of (non sodium) osmotic substances with extracellular partitioning. Extracellular hypertonicity draws cellular water to the extracellular space lowering the sodium concentration and causing cellular dehydration. The cause of hypertonic hyponatraemia usually can be diagnosed by measuring serum glucose concentration and by reviewing the list of patient's drugs. Hyperglicaemia is rarely of consequence for sodium levels until the plasma glucose exceeds 300 mg/dL.

c) *Hypotonic hyponatraemia.* It is the most common type of hyponatraemia. On the basis of the intravascular status, hypotonic hyponatraemia can be subclassified into one of three categories. Knowledge of the patient's circulating volume status is the key to determining etiology and treatment. Of importance, hypotonic hyponatraemia almost never develops unless the patient has unrestricted access to water or is administered a hypotonic fluid.

–   Hypovolaemic hypotonic hyponatraemia results from replacing losses of salt containing plasma with hypotonic fluid. Volume depletion is a potent stimulus for ADH release that overcomes competing osmotic stimuli (hypotonicity) for ADH suppression. Intake of hypotonic fluid combined with decreased free water clearance (ADH release) causes hyponatraemia. Thirst and postural hypotension are the most objective and reliable signs. Bleeding, diarrhoea, and vomiting are the common and usually apparent non renal causes, being third space losses less obvious non renal mechanism. Renal causes include diuretic use, mineralocorticoid deficiency, salt-wasting nephropathy, and osmotic diuresis from glucose, mannitol, urea, or ketones. Bicarbonaturia from renal tubular acidosis or metabolic alkalosis may also deplete volume and produce hyponatraemia. Because hypovolaemia reduces renal blood flow and tubular flow, urea may "back-diffuse" into the bloodstream. Conversely, because creatinine cannot back-diffuse, its excretion is less severely impaired and the BUN/creatinine ratio rises. Small volumes of hypertonic urine with very low sodium concentration reflect intense conservation of sodium and water. In primary adrenal insufficiency, the urine sodium concentration and the urine osmolality are elevated. If renal salt wasting is the etiology, the urine sodium concentration is high and urine osmolality normal.

–   Hypervolaemic hypotonic hyponatraemia is a syndrome in which water is retained in excess of sodium, and oedema is the hallmark. A 12 to 15 L of total body water must be present before sufficient interstitial fluid accumulates to cause detectable oedema. The basic problem is the reduced sodium and water clearance, that can result from intrinsic renal disease (any form of acute or chronic renal failure) or conditions that limit kidney blood flow (CHF, cirrhosis, hepatic failure). In the last conditions there is intense conservation of salt and water with very low urinary sodium concentrations (< 10 mEq/L), low urine volumes, and high urine osmolality. In the former conditions, urine electrolytes and osmolality are more variable and less helpful.

–   Isovolaemic hypotonic hyponatraemia results from a slight, clinically undetectable, excess of total body fluid (approximately 3 to 4 L). The two most frequent mechanisms are the inappropriate secretion of ADH (SIADH) and the water intoxication. In patients with a variety of underlying problems (e.g., cirrhosis and tuberculosis) a "reset" of the osmostat may be seen. This "reset" phenomenon may be distinguished from SIADH by normal responses to water loading or deprivation, despite hypo-osmolality.

Treatment

As above pointed out, hyponatraemia primarily affects the CNS. Unfortunately, rapid correction of hyponatraemia is also associated with serious neurologic sequelae: central pontine myelinolysis (CPM) may result. Risk factors include not only the rate of hyponatraemia correction but also advanced age, preexisting liver or CNS disorders, diuretic use, and alcoholism. Correction of hyponatraemia must be skillful, balancing the competing risks of cerebral oedema from too slow rapid repair. As general rule, the rate of correction should be proportional to the speed with which the disorder developed. Most hyponatraemic patients should have the sodium corrected to an initial level of 120-130 mEq/L over a 12 to 24-hour period, at an hourly rate not to exceed 2 mEq/L. Slower correction (0.5 mEq/L/hour) is prudent in patients with chronic hyponatraemia. In hypervolaemic hyponatraemia, salt and fluid restriction are the mainstays of the therapy. In hypovolaemic hyponatraemia, normal or hypertonic (3%) saline should be used to restore circulating volume. Diuretics or dialysis may be required when renal function is impaired. Patients with severe hyponatraemia may require hypertonic saline and diuretics to achieve a safe serum sodium with adequate speed.

Hypernatraemia

Hypernatraemia, defined as a serum sodium level higher than 150 mEq/L, usually is the result of restricted access of free water or absence of the sensation of thirst. Hypernatraemia is primarily a disease of patients who are unable to obtain and drink water (infants, elderly, and bedridden), particularly those simultaneously sustaining increased water losses. Hence, hypernatraemia is relatively common in the ICU setting. Hypernatraemia implies hyperosmolality, the major mechanism of toxicity. Dehydration may result solely from increased insensible losses. Regardless of cause, the common symptoms of hypernatraemia are thirst, nausea, vomiting, agitation, stupor, and coma. All of these symptoms are non specific, and often unrecognized. The history and physical examination typically lead to the correct diagnosis, which is usually water deprivation-dehydration [1].

Renal losses of free water may occur from intrinsic kidney diseases or from deficient-ineffective ADH. Osmotic diuretics (glucose, mannitol, etc.) may exaggerate free water clearance. Salt loading (primary hyperaldosteronism, hypertonic saline, sodium bicarbonate therapy) is a rare cause. Diabetes insipidus (DI) produces hypernatraemia by preventing appropriate water handling by the kidney. Central DI results from insufficient hypothalamic-pituitary release of ADH secondary to MS trauma, surgery, tumor, stroke, or granulomatous diseases. It is important to note that the diagnosis of DI may be missed if free water losses have progressed to the point that profound intravascular volume depletion has occurred. In such cases, the classic "tip off" of massive urine output usually is absent, and the fulfilment of a "water deprivation test" may prove harmful. A better strategy is to replete circulating volume and provide an empiric trial of ADH. When haemodynamics is stable, a water deprivation test may be safely performed.

Although hypernatraemia usually does not provide a diagnostic challenge, the urinary osmolarity can be a particularly helpful diagnostic test if the etiology is unclear. The kidney may also fail to respond fully to secreted ADH in the setting of chronic renal insufficiency, hypercalcaemia, hypokalaemia, or sikle cell disease, or in the presence of some drugs such lithium, loop diuretics, or demecyclocine.

Treatment

The treatment of hypernatraemia consists of the replacement of free water, with frequent evaluation of electrolytes and osmolity. Correction of the defect at a rate of approximately 2 mEq/L/hour is an appropriate target. Like hyponatraemia, very rapid correction can precipitate CPM. If endogenous ADH is deficient or ineffective, it may be replaced with DDAVP, an ADH analog.

Hypochloraemia and metabolic alkalosis

Hypochloraemia seen most often in the ICU are due to dilution, losses from GI tract or kidney (diuretics), secondary to chronic respiratory disease, accompanying hypokalaemia, and as a result of corticosteroid therapy.

Chloride depletion (independent of volume depletion) can produce and maintain metabolic alkalosis [2]. Metabolic alkalosis is the most common acid-base disturbance that confronts the intensivist and carries a 40% mortality rate when the pH is > 7.55. Metabolic alkalosis that are responsive to i.v. sodium chloride are the most common type encountered in the ICU. A low urine chloride < 10 mmol/L is a hallmark of these processes. Chloride administration alone can correct metabolic alkalosis in the presence of both volume depletion and low glomerular filtration rate. An abundant supply of chloride is an important element to allow a normal kidney to retain hydrogen. If both sodium and chloride are available, they are resorbed to maintain electroneutrality. If no chloride is available, sodium will be resorbed with bicarbonate or exchanged for another cation if no anion can be resorbed. The only other cations available for exchange are potassium and hydrogen. Potassium is rapidly depleted and the kidney then excrets hydrogen in exchange for sodium, thus perpetuating the alkalosis. The physical findings associated with chloride depletion metabolic alkalosis suggest volume depletion. Metabolic alkalosis produces multisystemic effects but the CNS is most affected. Hypochloraemia with a proportionate increase in bicarbonate, associated hypokalaemia, hypocalcaemia, and hypophosphataemia is present. Therefore, metabolic alkalosis may first present with symptoms and signs reminescent of hypocalcaemia. Neuromuscular complications are more common in patients with chronic hypocalcaemia (malabsorption, chronic renal failure), preexisting seizure disorder, and cerebrovascular disease. Cardiovascular problems are more common in patients receiving mechanical ventilation. Alkalaemia may worsen digitalis toxicity, even in the presence of normokalaemia.

When chloride depletion is generated and maintained by the kidneys, a sodium-chloride unresponsive alkalosis develops. This disorder is associated with normal or slightly increased extracellular fluid volume, high urine chloride (> 20 mmol/L), and is less common than sodium chloride responsive alkaloses. A renal-mediated alkalosis occurs due to the action of endogenously produced mineralocorticoids and glucocorticoids. These compounds induce maximal resorption of sodium and bicarbonate and an excessive loss of chloride in the urine.

Treatment

Extracellular fluid volume can be restored using normal saline, although potassium, as potassium chloride, may be required if concomitant hypokalaemia is present. The availability of chloride is essential in correcting metabolically driven alkaloses. The amount of chloride to be infused can be calculated using the equation: (0.2 L/kg) x (body weight in kg) x (desired chloride – measured chloride). The initial dose of chloride should not exceed 4 mmol/kg, and thereafter replacement should proceed using the serum chloride as a guide.

Chloride allows the kidney to retain hydrogen ion and potassium. Correcting the underlying metabolic alkalosis may require compounds that increase bicarbonate excretion or generate hydrogen chloride. Sodium chloride, potassium chloride, and acetazolamide require normal renal function to increase excretion excess bicarbonate. Arginine, lysine, and ammonium chloride require intact hepatorenal function. A 10% arginine hydrogen chloride solution contains 47.5 mmol/dL of chloride and should be infused over 4 to 6 hrs, with a maximum single dose of 140 mmol. On rare occasions, exogenous acid may be necessary to facilitate correction of metabolic alkalosis. Intravenous hydrogen chloride does not require renal or hepatic metabolism, and diluted hydrogen chloride has the advantage of simultaneously correcting deficits in hydrogen and chloride. It is reserved for severe life-threatening metabolic alkaloses, which are often accompanied by compensatory hypercapnia, mild hypoxaemia, cardiac arrhythmias, and neurologic disturbances. In critically ill patients with multiple system failure, i.v. hydrogen chloride may be considered the treatment of choice. Hypochloraemic metabolic alkalosis can be treated using the formula above reported, and infused in 12 hrs. In instances of uraemia or normochloraemic metabolic alkalosis, the following formula may be used: (0.5 L/kg) x (body weight in kg) x (measured bicarbonate – desired bicarbonate). The use of 0.25 normal solution (250 mmol of hydrogen chloride ions/L) of hydrogen chloride to correct metabolic alkaloses unresponsive to sodium chloride and potassium chloride infusions infused at a rate of 100 mL/hr via a central vein successfully corrected the pH, bicarbonate, and chloride.

Hypokalaemia

Diuretic use is the most common cause of hypokalaemia, and simultaneous use of two or more diuretics having actions at different sites in the nephron, can produce massive potassium losses. If urinary chloride is high (> 10 mEq/L) is indicative of mineralocorticoid excess. A certain number of patients experience hypokalaemia without acid-base and urinary chloride inbalance [13]. Examples include high-dose sodium penicillin therapy, aminoglycoside administration, use of amphotericin, and cisplatin therapy. A high sodium load in the distal renal tubule with accentuate tubular exchange of sodium for potassium is the mechanism.

Virtually, any arrhythmia may occur during hypokalaemia [1]. Hypokalaemia lowers the threshold for ventricular fibrillation, promoting the re-entry phenomenon. Mild hypokalaemia delays ventricular repolarization and is manifest by the ST segment depression, diminished or inverted T waves. When hypokalaemia is severe (< 2.5 mEq/L), P wave amplitude, PR interval, and QRS duration increase. Severe hypokalaemia may also cause profound, life threatening respiratory muscle weakness, quadriplegia, and rhabdomyolysis. Even moderate degrees of hypokalaemia may impair smooth muscle function, producing ileus, pseudo-obstruction, or decreased ureteral motility. Because of increased ammonia production by the kidney during hypokalaemia, a worsening encephalopathy can surface in patients with hepatic failure. Furthermore, hypokalaemia may cause polyuria and polydipsia by injuring the renal tubular epithelium or diminishing responsiveness to ADH.

Treatment

Because the intracellular space must be accessed via the small extracellular compartment, potassium therapy must be cautious and closely monitored to avoid potentially lethal hyperkalaemia. As a general rule, potassium should not be infused more quickly than 40 mEq/hr. It is better to administer intravenous potassium diluted in non-glucose-containing solutions, because of the insulin stimulation by the glucose with the subsequent rapid incorporation of potassium into cells that can further aggravate hypokalaemia. Because hypomagnesaemia aggravates the physiologic effects of hypokalaemia and renders deficit correction difficult, checking serum magnesium levels is reasonable. Possibly the most difficult situation occurs when hypokalaemia and acidosis coexist. In this unusual case, consideration should be given to the use of potassium bicarbonate rather than the more common potassium chloride. When possible, potassium deficits should be replaced with oral (enteral) preparations. Enteral administration provides an effective, safe alternative to i.v. infusion at substantially lower cost and actually allows larger doses to be administered. However, many liquid potassium preparations contain sorbitol, a poorly absorbed sugar, which often precipitates diarrhoea.

Hyperkalaemia

It is difficult for healthy subjects to develop hyperkalaemia because even minimally functional kidneys efficiently excrete excess potassium. Therefore, potassium handling is greatly impaired in patients with diabetes and renal insufficiency. Potassium-sparing diuretics, angiotensin-converting enzyme inhibitors and less commonly, nonsteroidal anti-inflammatory agents can induce hyperkalaemia, especially in patients with baseline reductions in glomerular filtration rate or intrinsic renal diseases. The basic mechanisms that contribute to hyperkalaemia are three: increased potassium intake, shifts of potassium from the intracellular to extracellular compartment, and decreased excretion [1]. Increased potassium intake is very rare in the normal patient. Conversely, iatrogenic potassium overloading is often seen in hospitalized patients with limited excretory power. The potassium source may be an unmodified standing order for potassium replacement or other unsuspected therapy (e.g., potassium penicillin G contains 1.6 mEq of potassium for each 10^6 units of penicillin). Acidosis is the most common cause of shift-related hyperkalaemia. Renal insufficiency is the most common cause of hyperkalaemia, and concomitant drug therapy often is a complicating factor. Acidosis induced by the renal failure further impairs the ability of the kidney to excrete potassium and promotes potassium shift out of the cells. In renal failure of abrupt onset, serum potassium tends to rise before the BUN or creatinine [13]. Adrenal insufficiency should be strongly considered in patients with hyperkalaemia and prominent fluid deficits.

Hyponatraemia, hypocalcaemia, hypermagnesaemia, and acidosis potentiate the neuromuscular effects of hyperkalaemia. Therefore, levels of sodium, calcium, and magnesium ions should be evaluated and corrected concurrently. Functional impairment of skeletal muscle rarely surfaces at potassium levels lower than 7.0 mEq/L. Hyperkalaemia usually spares the respiratory muscles, proximal lower extremity weakness is the most common symptom. The most devasting effects of hyperkalaemia are cardiac arrhythmias. The pump-impairing and vasodilatatory effects of severe hyperkalaemia may cause refractory hypotension.

Treatment

The aggressiveness with which hyperkalaemia is treated should parallel the severity of the clinical manifestations [1]. The ECG is the key diagnostic test in determining the urgency with which hyperkalaemia should be addressed. If the elevated potassium is the culmination of a progressive process in a patient with risk factors for hyperkalaemia (e.g., renal insufficiency) and significant clinical or ECG manifestations are present, immediate treatment is indicated. Conversely, the unexpected discovery of an isolated, elevated potassium value in an asymptomatic patient should be approached with some skepticism. In such cases, the assay should be repeated before treatment is undertaken. In approaching hyperkalaemia treatment, continuous ECG monitoring should be initiated, followed by specific medical interventions:

a) stop all potassium;

b) begin replenishing circulating volume in dehydrate patients;

c) administer drugs to shift potassium into the cellular compartment:
   - $NaHCO_3$, 1-2 ampules over 5-10 minutes,
   - glucose and insulin, 10 U.I. regular insulin add D50W 1-2 ampules in normoglycaemic patients; only insulin in hyperglycaemic patients;

d) stabilize neuromuscular and cardiac function with calcium, if indicated;

e) remove potassium from the body:
   - furosemide 40-80 mg,
   - potassium-binding resins: kayexalate 50 g p.o. or rectally in 100 mL sorbitol,
   - dialysis: it is most often required in patients with renal insufficiency, severe hyperkalaemia, or high potassium loads that result from multiple trauma or tumor lysis.

Hypercalcaemia

Most cases of significant hypercalcaemia encountered in the ICU will be the result of malignancy [14]. Although symptoms are poorly correlated with calcium levels, severe manifestations of toxicity (e.g., coma) are rare unless levels exceed 14 mg/dL. The signs and symptoms of hypercalcaemia are nonspecific but most commonly result from the two major pathophysiologic derangements: dehydration and depressed neuromuscular function. Hypercalcaemia induces an osmotic diuresis resulting in polyuria and polydipsia. Unfortunately, because of the decreased gut motility (nausea, vomiting, constipation, abdominal pain) the possibility to compensate increased fluid losses with increased fluid intake is denied. The most common manifestations of hypercalcaemia are neuromuscular disturbances (lethargy, agitation, coma, fatigue, and weakness). Renal stones and renal insufficiency may result. Skin deposits may induce pruritus.

Treatment

Like hyperkalaemia, the simplest and most rapid method to reduce calcium in the dehydrated patients is to expand circulating volume with isotonic saline. This treatment is often critical in reducing symptoms [15]. In volume replenished patients, furosemide are rapidly effective in lowering serum calcium concentration if good urine flow is established (200 mL/hr). Although, mithramycin (25 µg i.v.) is helpful in acute severe cases, side effects (hepatic, renal, and marrow toxicity) usually prohibit chronic use. Because of 1-2 days of action delay, the drug is usually a second-line therapy. Glucocorticoids are most useful in the malignancy hypercalcaemia, especially lymphoma and breast carcinoma. By inhibiting gut absorption of calcium, steroids are also effective in sarcoidosis and vitamin D intoxication. In symptomatic, severe hypercalcaemia, doses of calcitonin high as 8 units given every 12 hrs can produce prompt (4-6 hrs) reduction in serum calcium levels. Calcitonin is more effective in combination with steroids. Diphosphonates currently are used for the treatment of Paget's disease and malignancy-related hypercalcaemia but are effective only in a minority of patients.

Hypocalcaemia

Total serum calcium levels are low in 70% to 90% of ICU patients, but the occurrence rate of ionized hypocalcaemia is more variable (15% to 50%), depending on type of patients. Ionized hypocalcaemia develops when calcium cannot be mobilized from the skeleton fast enough to meet ongoing losses. Thus, ionized hypocalcaemia may result from four causes: failure of PTH secretion or action; failure of vitamin D synthesis or action, failure of bone to respond to PTH and vitamin D, or calcium chelation/precipitation [16]. Primary hypoparathyroidism is rare, while secondary hypoparathyroidism is a more common cause of ionized hypocalcaemia. It is frequently seen in patients after neck surgery, and as a result of sepsis, pancreatitis, or rhabdomyolysis.

Renal synthesis of vitamin D is impaired in the same circumstances. Citrate-induced decreases in ionized calcium concentrations are usually small and transient in most normothermic individuals with normal organ function. Ionized calcium values returned to normal within 15 mins of transfusion termination.

Citrate is metabolized by temperature-dependent enzymes in the tissues and excreted by the liver and kidney. The metabolism of citrate is impaired during hypothermia and renal or hepatic failure.

Mild degrees of hypocalcaemia (ionized calcium > 0.8 mmol) are usually asymptomatic in the critically ill patient. Symptomatic ionized hypocalcaemia (< 0.8 mmol) usually presents with signs of neuromuscular irritability and muscle weakness, such as paraesthesias, hyperactive reflexes, muscle spasms, Trousseau's sign, Chvostek's sign, laryngeal spasm, bronchospasm, seizures, and tetany. Cardiovascular features of ionized hypocalcaemia include bradycardia, heart block, cardiac arrest, heart failure and hypotension. Hypocalcaemia should be considered in patients with hypotension refractory to fluids and pressor agents.

Treatment

It is current policy not to treat patients with ionized calcium > 0.8 mmol, however, ionized calcium should be monitorized. Conversely, if they develop clinical features of hypocalcaemia or if ionized calcium concentration decrease to < 0.8 mmol, calcium treatment will be instituted. Slow infusion of 10-20 mL of 10% calcium gluconate is the preferred method of supplementation. Such dosing provides approximately 10 mg of elemental calcium per milliliter. Concomitant vitamin D deficiency should be treated. Because thiazides increase renal tubular calcium reabsorption, they are useful adjuncts to increase serum calcium.

Hypomagnesaemia

Hypomagnesaemia is one of the most common electrolyte abnormalities in hospitalized patients [17, 18]. Hypomagnesaemia almost always results from excessive renal and GI losses. Because magnesium is predominantly absorbed in the small bowel, inflammatory bowel disease, chronic diarrhoea, and malabsorption are common precipitants. Malnutrition (particularly in alcoholism) decreases magnesium by limiting intake. Although any form of renal disease may produce magnesium wasting, it most commonly results from the use of diuretics. More importantly, by encouraging potassium egress from the cells and calcium egress from the bone, over the long run, hypomagnesaemia may induce hypocalcaemia and hypokalaemia [19]. Because of the frequency of concurrence of the disorders, magnesium depletion should be considered in patients with hypokalaemia, hypocalcaemia, and hypophosphataemia. Like hypocalcaemia, hypomagnesaemia's most frequent clinical effects are neuromuscular and cardiac. Hypomagnesaemia seems to predispose patients to almost all types of arrhythmias (particularly Torsades de Pointes and those of digitalis toxicity). Hypomagnesaemia should be suspected when the ECG demonstrates prolonged QT and PR intervals and long flat T waves.

Treatment

For patients with normal renal function, magnesium is safe, even in large doses [1]. In life-threatening hypomagnesaemic crises, magnesium can be administered as magnesium solphate (1-2 g) i.v. over 2-3 min. Rapid i.v. magnesium infusions can produce hypotension and, therefore, should be avoided except in emergent circumstances.

Hypophosphataemia

It is the depletion of the intracellular PO_4^{-3} store that produces clinical symptomatology, imperfectly reflected by depressed serum values. Although PO_4^{-3} is easily depleted from skeletal muscle and erythrocytes, level tends to be well preserved in most other tissues, such as the cardiac muscle. Factors predisposing total body phosphate depletion include malnutrition, alcoholism, hypomagnesaemia, renal tubular dysfunction (nonoliguric acute tubular necrosis), and GI losses (diarrhoea, suctioning, antacid binding). It is important not to equate hypophosphataemia with intracellular PO_4^{-3} depletion [20]. Extracellular to intracellular transfer occurs during anabolism, insulin administration, correction of metabolic acidosis, recovery from diabetic ketoacidosis, and during hyperventilation. In many such patients, hypophosphataemia does not reflect pathologic phosphate depletion. As a rule, serum PO_4^{-3} must fall below 1.0 mg/dL before overt symptoms surface [1]. Dysfunction of the cellular elements of the blood, muscle weakness, GI upset, neural dysfunction, and (rarely) tissue breakdown are the major clinical consequences. Depletion of 2,3-DPG diminished the ability of red cells to unload oxygen to the tissues. Thrombocytopenia, platelet dysfunction, and impaired leukocyte killing have been shown experimentally. Skeletal muscle dysfunctions is of major clinical interest in the setting of ventilatory failure. A PO_4^{-3}-related sensorimotorneuropathy is occasionally observed 4-7 days after PO_4^{-3}-poor hyperalimentation is started. Very rarely, severe phosphate depletion can produce haemolysis, rhabdomyolysis, or congestive cardiomyopathy especially when generous re-feeding is abruptly initiated.

Urgent correction should be reserved for situations in which clinical symptoms accompany a serum $PO_4^{-3} < 1.0$ mg/dL. As with potassium repletion, PO_4^{-3} must traverse the small extracellular compartment to reach its intracellular target, so repletion must be cautious. An i.v. infusion of 2.5-5.0 mg/kg as potassium or sodium phosphate over 6 hrs is safe. Oral supplementation usually will suffice when serum phosphate level is only modestly reduced (> 1.0 mg/dL), and should continue for 5-10 days after reestablishing a normal serum level.

References

1. Marini JJ, Wheeler AP (1997) Fluid and electrolyte disorders. In: Zinner SR (ed) Critical care medicine the essentials, 2nd edn vol. 13. Williams and Wilkins, pp 223-240
2. Koch SM, Taylor RW (1992) Chloride ion in intensive care medicine. Crit Care Med 20 (2):227-240
3. Kruse JA, Carlson EW (1990) Rapid correction of hypokalemia using concentrated intravenous chloride infusions. Arch Intern Med 3:529
4. Brown RS (1986) Extrarenal potassium homeostasis. Kidney Int 30:116
5. Zaloga GP, Chernow B (1988) Divalent ions-calcium, magnesium and phosphorus. In: Chrnow B (ed) The pharmacologic approach to the critically ill patient, 2nd edn. Williams and Wilkins, Baltimore, pp 603-636
6. Ladenson JH, Lewis JW, Boyd JC (1978) Failure of total calcium corrected for protein, albumin, and pH to correctly assess free calcium status. J Clin Endocrinol Metab 46:986-993
7. Burg MB, Green M (1973) Function of the thick ascending limb of Henle's loop. Am J Physiol 224:659-668
8. Klahr S, Weiner ID (1990) Disorders of acid-base metabolism. In: Chan JC, Jill JR (eds) Kidney electrolyte disorders. Churchill Livingstone, New York, pp 1-58
9. Halperin ML, Goldstein MB (1988) Fluid, electrolyte, and acid-base emergencies. WB Saunders, Philadelphia, pp 163, 239-241, 290-293
10. Harrington JT, Cohen JJ (1975) Measurement of urine electrolytes-Indications and limitations. N Engl J Ned 293:1241-1243
11. Goldstein MB, Bear R, Richardson RMA et al (1986) The urine anion gap: A clinically useful index of ammonium excretion. Am J Med Sci 292:198-202
12. Oh MS, Carrol W (1977) The anion gap. N Engl J Med 297:814-817
13. Kunau RT, Stein JH (1977) Disorders of hypo and hyperkalemia. Clin Nephrol 7:173-190
14. List A (1991) Malignancy hypercalcemia: Choice of therapy. Arch Intern Med 154:437

15. Roswell RH (1987) Severe hypercalcemia: Causes and specific therapy. J Crit Illness 2:14
16. Baldwin TE, Chernow B (1987) Hypocalcemia in the ICU: Coping with the causes and consequences. J Crit Illness 2:9
17. Chernow B, Bamberger S, Stoiko M et al (1989) Hypomagnesemia in patients in postoperative intensive care. Chest 95:391-397
18. Ryzen E, Wgers PW, Singer FR et al (1985) Magnesium deficiency in a medical ICU population. Crit Care Med 13:19-21
19. Reinhart RA (1988) Magnesium metabolism: A review with special reference to the relationship between intracellular content and calcium levels. Arch Intern Med 148:2415
20. Knocher JP (1977) The pathophysiology and clinical characteristics of severe hypophosphatemia. Arch Intern Med 137:203-220

Respiratory Acidosis and Alkalosis

H.J. ADROGUÉ

Deviations of systemic acidity in either direction can have adverse consequences and, when severe, can be life-threatening. Therefore, it is essential for the clinician to be able to recognize and properly diagnose acid-base disorders, understand their impact on organ function, and be familiar with their treatment and the potential complications of treatment [1]. Respiratory disorders, that is abnormalities of acid-base equilibrium initiated by a change in blood carbon dioxide tension (PCO_2), are frequently encountered in clinical practice, especially in critically ill patients [2]. In the present chapter, we will focus on clinical diagnosis and management of respiratory acidosis and respiratory alkalosis.

Respiratory acidosis (primary hypercapnia)

Respiratory acidosis is the acid-base disturbance initiated by an increase in carbon dioxide tension of body fluids. The secondary increment in plasma bicarbonate observed in acute and chronic hypercapnia should be viewed as an integral part of the respiratory acidosis [3]. On average, $[HCO_3^-]_p$ increases by about 0.1 mEq/L for each 1 mmHg acute increment in $PaCO_2$ and about 0.3 mEq/L for each 1 mmHg chronic increment in $PaCO_2$. Whole body CO_2 stores are increased and the level of arterial carbon dioxide tension ($PaCO_2$) is higher than 45 mmHg in patients with simple respiratory acidosis, who are at rest and at sea level. An element of respiratory acidosis may still occur with lower levels of $PaCO_2$ in patients with metabolic acidosis in whom a normal $PaCO_2$ is inappropriately high for this primary metabolic disorder. Another special case of respiratory acidosis is the presence of arterial eucapnia or even hypocapnia occurring in the company of severe venous hypercapnia in patients having an acute, profound decrease in cardiac output but relative preservation of respiratory function. This disorder is known as "pseudorespiratory alkalosis" and is discussed under respiratory alkalosis [4, 5].

Etiology and pathogenesis

The ventilatory system is responsible for maintaining $PaCO_2$ within normal limits by adjusting alveolar minute ventilation ($\dot{V}_A$) to match the rate of CO_2 production. The main elements of ventilation are the respiratory pump, which generates a pressure gradient responsible for air flow, and the loads that oppose such action. The inspiratory decrease in pleural pressure caused by the respiratory pump must be sufficient to counterbalance the opposing effect of the combined loads, including the airway flow resistance, and the elastic recoil of the lungs and chest wall.

The determinants of carbon dioxide retention can be viewed as factors imposing an imbalance between the strength of the respiratory pump and the weight of the respiratory loads. When the respiratory pump is unable to balance the opposing load, respiratory acidosis develops. Decreases in respiratory pump strength, increases in load, or a combination of the two, can result in carbon dioxide retention [6]. Respiratory pump failure can occur because of depressed central drive, abnormal neuromuscular transmission, or respiratory muscle dysfunction. Higher load can be caused by increased ventilatory demand, augmented airway flow resistance, and stiffness of the lungs or the chest wall. A reduction in pulmonary perfusion can also result in CO_2 retention leading to the condition referred to as "pseudorespiratory alkalosis". Respiratory acidosis is categorized into acute and chronic forms, taking into consideration the usual mode of onset and duration of the various causes (Tables 1 and 2). Life-threatening acidaemia of respiratory origin can occur during severe, acute respiratory acidosis or during respiratory decompensation in patients with chronic hypercapnia [3].

Acute respiratory acidosis develops as a consequence of upper- or lower-airway obstruction, status asthmaticus, severe alveolar defects such as those occurring in pneumonia or pulmonary oedema, central nervous system depression, neuromuscular impairment, and ventilatory restriction (as in patients with rib fractures with flail chest) (Table 1).

Chronic hypercapnia results from many conditions, including chronic obstructive or restrictive pulmonary diseases, upper-airway obstruction, central nervous system depression, neuromuscular impairment, and abnormal chest-wall mechanics [3]. Respiratory decompensation in patients with these conditions, commonly resulting from infection, use of narcotics, or uncontrolled oxygen therapy, superimposes an acute element of carbon dioxide retention and acidaemia on the chronic, background disorder (Table 2).

The following equation presents the simplified form of the alveolar gas equation at sea level and when breathing room air (FiO_2, 21%):

$$P_AO_2 = 150 - 1.25 \, PaCO_2$$

where P_AO_2 is alveolar oxygen tension in mmHg. Examination of this equation demonstrates that the major threat to life from CO_2 retention in patients breathing room air is the associated obligatory hypoxaemia. In the absence of supplemental oxygen, patients suffering respiratory arrest develop critical hypoxaemia within a few minutes, long before severe hypercapnia occurs. The constraints of the alveolar gas equation establish that patients breathing room air cannot reach

Table 1. Causes of acute respiratory acidosis

Increased load	Depressed pump
Increased ventilatory demand	*Depressed central drive*
High carbohydrate diet	General anaesthesia
High carbohydrate dialysate	Sedative overdose
(peritoneal dialysis)	Head trauma
Sorbent-regenerative haemodialysis	Cerebrovascular accident
Pulmonary thromboembolism	Central sleep apnea
Fat, air pulmonary embolism	Cerebral oedema
Sepsis	Brain tumor
Hypovolaemia	Encephalitis
Augmented airway flow resistance	Brain-stem lesion
Upper airways obstruction	*Abnormal neuromuscular transmission*
Coma-induced hypopharyngeal obstruction	High spinal cord injury
Aspiration of foreign body or vomitus	Guillain-Barré syndrome
Laryngospasm	Status epilepticus
Angiooedema	Botulism; tetanus
Obstructive sleep apnea	Crisis in myasthenia gravis
Inadequate laryngeal intubation	Hypokalaemic myopathy
Laryngeal obstruction postintubation	Familial periodic paralysis
Lower airways obstruction	Drugs or toxic agents (e.g., curare,
Generalized bronchospasm	succinylcholine, aminoglycosides,
Airways oedema, secretions	organophosphorus)
Severe episode of spasmodic asthma	*Muscle dysfunction*
Bronchiolitis of infancy and adults	Fatigue
Lung stiffness	Hyperkalaemia
Severe bilateral pneumonia or bronchopneumonia	Hypokalaemia
Acute respiratory distress syndrome	Hypoperfusion state
Severe pulmonary oedema	Hypoxaemia
Atelectasis	Malnutrition
Chest wall stiffness	
Rib fractures with flail chest	
Pneumothorax	
Haemothorax	
Abdominal distension	
Ascites	
Peritoneal dialysis	

$PaCO_2$ levels much greater than 80 mmHg because the degree of hypoxaemia that would occur at greater values is incompatible with life. Thus, extreme hypercapnia occurs only during oxygen therapy, and severe CO_2 retention is often the result of uncontrolled oxygen administration.

The relationship between the severity of the hypoxaemia and the level of $PaCO_2$ differs in the two major clinical forms of respiratory insufficiency [6]. Patients with respiratory pump failure exhibit the pattern of "pure alveolar hypoventilation", in which the alveolar-arterial gradient for oxygen ($P(A-a)O_2$) remains normal and the increase in $PaCO_2$ is accompanied by an equivalent

Table 2. Causes of chronic respiratory acidosis

Increased load	Depressed pump
Augmented airway flow resistance	*Depressed central drive*
Upper airways obstruction	Sedative overdose
Tonsillar and peritonsillar hypertrophy	Methadone/heroin addiction
Paralysis of vocal cords	Sleep disordered breathing
Tumor of the cords or larynx	Brain tumor
Airways stenosis postprolonged intubation	Bulbar poliomyelitis
Thymoma, aortic aneurysm	Hypothyroidism
Lower airways obstruction	*Abnormal neuromuscular transmission*
Airway scarring	Poliomyelitis
Chronic obstructive lung disease	Multiple sclerosis
(e.g., bronchitis, bronchiolitis,	Muscular dystrophy
bronchiectasis, emphysema)	Amyotrophic lateral sclerosis
Lung stiffness	Diaphragmatic paralysis
Severe chronic pneumonitis	Myopathic disease (e.g., polymyositis)
Diffuse infiltrative disease	*Muscle dysfunction*
(e.g., alveolar proteinosis)	Myopathic disease (e.g., polymyositis)
Interstitial fibrosis	
Chest wall stiffness	
Kyphoscoliosis, spinal arthritis	
Obesity	
Fibrothorax	
Hydrothorax	
Chest wall tumors	

decrease in arterial oxygen tension (PaO_2). This type of respiratory pump failure is caused by disorders without parenchymal lung disease, in which the alveolar gas exchange is normal. By contrast, abnormalities in the lung parenchyma produce the so-called "hypoxaemic respiratory failure". In the latter condition, also referred to as "lung failure", the reduction in PaO_2 is a constant finding, whereas $PaCO_2$ is commonly decreased if sufficient ventilatory reserve is present, although hypercapnia can ensue.

Treatment

As previously noted, carbon dioxide retention, whether acute or chronic, is always associated with hypoxaemia in patients breathing room air. In fact, hypoxaemia, not hypercapnia or acidaemia, is the most critical factor that determines morbidity and mortality of patients with acute or chronic respiratory acidosis. Consequently, oxygen administration represents a critical element in the management of respiratory acidosis [3, 6].

Whenever possible, treatment must be directed at removing or ameliorating the underlying cause. Immediate therapeutic efforts should focus on securing a patent airway and restoring adequate oxygenation by delivering an oxygen-rich inspired mixture. Mechanical ventilation must be initiated in the presence of apnea, severe hypoxaemia unresponsive to conservative measures, or progressive respiratory acidosis ($PaCO_2 > 80$ mmHg). Management of respiratory decompensation depends on the cause, severity, and rate of progression of carbon dioxide retention. Vigorous treatment of pulmonary infections, bronchodilator therapy, and removal of secretions can offer considerable benefit. Naloxone will reverse the suppressive effect of narcotic agents on ventilation. Avoidance of tranquilizers and sedatives, gradual reduction of supplemental oxygen (aiming at a PaO_2 of about 60 mmHg), and treatment of a superimposed element of metabolic alkalosis will optimize the ventilatory drive [3]. Whereas an aggressive approach that favors the early use of ventilator assistance is most appropriate for patients with acute respiratory acidosis, a more conservative approach is advisable in those with chronic diseases that limit pulmonary reserve, because of the great difficulty often encountered in weaning such patients from ventilators. However, if the patient is obtunded or unable to cough, and if hypercapnia and acidaemia are worsening, mechanical ventilation should be instituted. Minute ventilation should be raised so that the $PaCO_2$ gradually returns to near its long-term base line and excretion of excess bicarbonate by the kidneys is accomplished (assuming that chloride is provided) [7]. By contrast, overly rapid reduction in the $PaCO_2$ risks the development of posthypercapnic alkalosis, with potentially serious consequences. Should posthypercapnic alkalosis develop, it can be ameliorated by providing chloride, usually as the potassium salt, and administering the bicarbonate-wasting diuretic acetazolamide at doses of 250 to 375 mg once or twice daily. Noninvasive mechanical ventilation with a nasal or facial mask is being used with increasing frequency to avert the possible complications of endotracheal intubation.

Traditionally, the goal of treatment with mechanical ventilation had been to restore $PaCO_2$ and arterial blood pH to the normal values of 40 mmHg and 7.40, respectively. This strategy had led to the widespread use of tidal volumes of 10 to 15 ml/kg body weight [7]. However, large tidal volumes often lead to alveolar overdistension and volutrauma. Therefore, an alternative approach that uses a protective-ventilation strategy and allows $PaCO_2$ to rise, called "permissive hypercapnia" (or controlled mechanical hypoventilation), is undergoing evaluation [6, 8]. In this form of treatment, lower tidal volumes of less than 6 ml/kg body weight and lower peak inspiratory pressures are used. Further, $PaCO_2$ is allowed to rise but rarely exceeds 80 mmHg, and blood pH can decrease to as low as 7.00 to 7.10, while maintaining adequate oxygenation. The increased respiratory drive associated with permissive hypercapnia causes extreme discomfort, making sedation necessary. Because the patients commonly require neuromuscular blockade as well, accidental disconnection from the ventilator can cause sudden death. Furthermore, after the neuromuscular-blocking agent is discontinued, there may be weakness or paralysis for several days or weeks. There are several contraindications to the use of permissive hypercapnia, including cerebrovascular disease, brain oedema, increased intracranial pressure, and convulsions; depressed cardiac function and arrhythmias; and severe pulmonary hypertension. Notably, most of these entities can develop as adverse effects of permissive hypercapnia itself, especially when hypercapnia is associated with substantial acidaemia [9, 10]. In fact, some experimental evidence indicates that correction of acidaemia attenuates the adverse haemodynamic effects of permissive hypercapnia [11]. It appears prudent, although still controversial, to keep the blood pH at approximately 7.30 by administering intravenous alkali when controlled hypoventilation is prescribed [12].

Respiratory alkalosis (primary hypocapnia)

Respiratory alkalosis is the acid-base disturbance initiated by a reduction in carbon dioxide tension of body fluids [13]. The secondary decrement in plasma bicarbonate observed in acute and chronic hypocapnia should be viewed as an integral part of the respiratory alkalosis. The $[HCO_3^-]_p$ falls by approximately 0.2 mEq/L for each 1 mmHg acute decrement in $PaCO_2$ and 0.4 mEq/L for each 1 mmHg chronic decrement in $PaCO_2$. Whole body CO_2 stores are decreased and the level of $PaCO_2$ is less than 35 mmHg in patients with simple respiratory alkalosis, who are at rest and at sea level. An element of respiratory alkalosis may still occur with higher levels of $PaCO_2$ in patients with metabolic alkalosis in whom a normal $PaCO_2$ is inappropriately low for this primary metabolic disorder.

Etiology and pathogenesis

Respiratory alkalosis is the most frequent acid-base disorder encountered, since it occurs in normal pregnancy and with high-altitude residence [14]. It is also the most common acid-base abnormality in critically ill patients, occurring either as the simple disorder or as a component of mixed disturbances; indeed, in such patients, its presence constitutes a grave prognostic sign, especially if $PaCO_2$ levels are below 20-25 mmHg. The presence of hypocapnia signifies excessive alveolar ventilation relative to the prevailing carbon dioxide production, thus leading to negative carbon dioxide balance; it might result from increased alveolar ventilation, decreased carbon dioxide production, or both. Primary hypocapnia might also originate from the extrapulmonary elimination of carbon dioxide by a dialysis device or extracorporeal circulation (e.g., heart-lung machine).

Table 3 lists the major causes of respiratory alkalosis [13]. Most are associated with the abrupt appearance of hypocapnia, but in many instances the process might be sufficiently prolonged to permit full, chronic adaptation to occur. Consequently, no attempt has been made to separate these conditions into acute and chronic categories. In the vast majority of cases, primary hypocapnia reflects

Table 3. Causes of respiratory alkalosis

Hypoxaemia or tissue hypoxia	*Drugs and hormones*
Decreased inspired O_2 tension	Nikethamide, ethamivan
High altitude	Doxapram
Bacterial or viral pneumonia	Xanthines
Aspiration of food, foreign body, or vomitus	Salicylates
Laryngospasm	Catecholamines
Drowning	Angiotensin II
Cyanotic heart disease	Vasopressor agents
Severe anaemia	Progesterone
Left shift deviation of HbO_2 curve	Medroxyprogesterone
Hypotension	Dinitrophenol
Severe circulatory failure	Nicotine
Pulmonary oedema	*Miscellaneous*
Pseudorespiratory alkalosis	Pregnancy
Central nervous system stimulation	Gram-positive septicaemia
Voluntary	Gram-negative septicaemia
Pain	Hepatic failure
Anxiety-hyperventilation syndrome	Mechanical hyperventilation
Psychosis	Heat exposure
Fever	Recovery from metabolic acidosis
Subarachnoid haemorrhage	Haemodialysis with acetate dialysate
Cerebrovascular accident	
Meningoencephalitis	
Tumor	
Trauma	
Pulmonary diseases with stimulation of chest receptors	
Pneumonia	
Asthma	
Pneumothorax	
Haemothorax	
Flail chest	
Acute respiratory distress syndrome	
Cardiogenic and noncardiogenic pulmonary oedema	
Pulmonary embolism	
Pulmonary fibrosis	

alveolar hyperventilation due to increased ventilatory drive. The latter might represent signals arising from the lung, the peripheral chemoreceptors (carotid and aortic), the brainstem chemoreceptors, or influences originating in other centers of the brain. The response of the brainstem chemoreceptors to carbon dioxide can be augmented by systemic diseases (e.g., liver disease, sepsis), pharmacologic agents, volition, and other influences. Hypoxaemia is a major stimulus of alveolar ventilation, but PaO_2 values lower than 60 mmHg are required to elicit consistently this effect. Not uncommonly, alveolar hyperventilation is the result of maladjusted mechanical ventilators. Potential mechanisms of respiratory alkalosis due to decreased carbon dioxide production in the presence of constant alveolar ventilation (i.e., mechanical ventilation) include a reduction in physical activity (e.g., sedation, skeletal muscle paralysis) or a reduction in the basal metabolic rate (e.g., hypothermia).

In sharp contrast with respiratory acidosis, which always reflects a serious condition, some causes of respiratory alkalosis are benign. Since blood pH levels do not exceed 7.55 in most cases of primary hypocapnia, severe manifestations of decreased systemic acidity are usually absent [13, 14]. Severe alkalaemia, however, may be produced, particularly with maladjusted ventilators, some psychiatric conditions, and lesions involving the central nervous system.

In states of severe circulatory failure, arterial hypocapnia may coexist with venous, and therefore with tissue, hypercapnia; however, the body CO_2 stores have been enriched, and respiratory acidosis rather than respiratory alkalosis is present. This entity, which we have termed pseudorespiratory alkalosis, develops in patients with profound depression of cardiac function and pulmonary perfusion but relative preservation of alveolar ventilation, including patients with advanced circulatory failure and those undergoing cardiopulmonary resuscitation [4, 5, 14]. The severely reduced pulmonary blood flow limits the CO_2 delivered to the lungs for excretion thereby increasing the venous PCO_2. On the other hand, the increased ventilation-to-perfusion ratio causes a larger than normal removal of CO_2 per unit of blood traversing the pulmonary circulation thereby giving rise to arterial eucapnia or frank hypocapnia. A progressive widening of the arteriovenous difference in pH and PCO_2 develops in these two settings of cardiac dysfunction, namely circulatory failure and cardiac arrest. Severe oxygen deprivation prevails in the tissues in these two conditions, and it can be completely disguised by the reasonably preserved arterial oxygen values. Appropriate monitoring of acid-base composition and oxygenation in patients with advanced cardiac dysfunction requires mixed (or central) venous blood sampling in addition to the sampling of arterial blood.

Treatment

Because chronic respiratory alkalosis poses little risk to health and produces few or no symptoms, measures at treating the acid-base disorder itself are not required [13, 14]. On the other hand, severe alkalaemia caused by acute primary hypocapnia requires corrective measures that depend on whether serious clinical manifestations are present. Such measures can be directed at reducing plasma bicarbonate concentration, increasing $PaCO_2$, or both. Even if baseline plasma bicarbonate is moderately decreased, reducing it further can be particularly rewarding in this setting, as this manoeuvre combines effectiveness with relatively little risk [15]. For patients with the anxiety-hyperventilation syndrome in addition to reassurance or sedation, rebreathing into a closed system (e.g., a paper bag) might prove helpful by interrupting the vicious cycle that can result from the reinforcing effects of the symptoms of hypocapnia.

Respiratory alkalosis resulting from severe hypoxaemia requires oxygen therapy. The oral administration of 250-500 mg of acetazolamide (Diamox) can be beneficial in the management of signs and symptoms of high-altitude sickness, a syndrome characterized by hypoxaemia and respiratory alkalosis. Of course, patients undergoing mechanical ventilation lend themselves to an effective correction of hypocapnia (whether due to maladjusted ventilator or other causes) by resetting the device.

References

1. Adrogué HJ, Madias NE (1998) Arterial blood gas monitoring: acid-base assessment. In: Tobin MJ (ed) Principles and practice of intensive care monitoring. McGraw-Hill, New York, pp 217-241
2. Adrogué HJ, Wesson DE (1994) Overview of acid-base disorders. In: Adrogué HJ, Wesson DE (eds) Blackwell's basics of medicine. Acid-base. Blackwell Science, Boston, pp 49-133
3. Adrogué HJ, Madias NE (1998) Management of life-threatening acid-base disorders. Part I. N Engl J Med 338:26-34
4. Adrogué HJ, Rashad MN, Gorin AB et al (1989) Assessing acid-base status in circulatory failure. Differences between arterial and central venous blood. N Engl J Med 320:1312-1316
5. Adrogué HJ, Rashad MN, Gorin AB et al (1989) Arteriovenous acid-base disparity in circulatory failure: studies on mechanism. Am J Physiol 257:F1087-F1093
6. Adrogué HJ, Tobin MJ (1997) Management of respiratory failure. In: Adrogué HJ, Tobin MJ (eds) Blackwell's basics of medicine. Respiratory failure, vol 6. Blackwell Science, Boston, pp 311-331
7. Tobin MJ (1994) Mechanical ventilation. N Engl J Med 330:1056-1061
8. Amato MBP, Barbas CSV, Medeiros DM et al (1998) Effect of a protective-ventilation strategy on mortality in the acute respiratory distress syndrome. N Engl J Med 338:347-354
9. Feihl F, Perret C (1994) Permissive hypercapnia: how permissive should we be? Am J Respir Crit Care Med 150:1722-1737
10. Dries DJ (1995) Permissive hypercapnia. J Trauma 39:984-989
11. Cardenas VJ, Zwischenberger JB, Tao W et al (1996) Correction of blood pH attenuates changes in hemodynamics and organ blood flow during permissive hypercapnia. Crit Care Med 24:827-834
12. Gentilello LM, Anardi D, Mock C et al (1995) Permissive hypercapnia in trauma patients. J Trauma 39:846-852
13. Gennari FJ, Kassirer JP (1982) Respiratory alkalosis. In: Cohen JJ, Kassirer JP (eds) Acid-base. Little Brown, Boston, pp 349-376
14. Adrogué HJ, Madias NE (1998) Management of life-threatening acid-base disorders. Part II. N Engl J Med 338:107-111
15. Krapf R, Beeler I, Hertner D et al (1991) Chronic respiratory alkalosis: the effect of sustained hyperventilation on renal regulation of acid-base equilibrium. N Engl J Med 324:1394-1401

Metabolic Acidosis and Metabolic Alkalosis in the Critically Ill

F. Schiraldi, P. Ferraro, F. Paladino

In most cases, the metabolic disorders of acid-base homeostasis are helpful to highlight the main or associated diagnosis in the critically ill. As the physiopathology and the diagnostic aspects are fully covered elsewhere in these proceedings, it seems reasonable to focus here only on the monitoring value of the metabolic derangements of blood gas analysis (BGA) and on some controversial aspects of therapeutics.

Metabolic acidosis

Monitoring

It is perhaps useful to remind that, whatever the etiology of metabolic acidosis, the BGA will show on an arterial sample:

$$
\begin{aligned}
\text{pH} \quad &< \quad 7.38 \\
\text{HCO}_3 \quad &< \quad 24 \text{ mmol/L} \\
\text{PCO}_2 \quad &< \quad 40 \text{ mmHg}
\end{aligned}
$$

In the setting of a simple metabolic acidosis, the PCO_2 must be reduced of 1.2 mmHg for 1 mmol/L reduction of HCO_3 [1-3]: any derangement from this simple rule of thumb will call for a mixed disorder (e.g.: metabolic acidosis plus respiratory acidosis or metabolic acidosis plus respiratory alkalosis).

There is a growing evidence that the venous blood (mixed or central) is a better indicator of the tissues acid-base equilibrium than the arterial one.

Besides, its usefulness in monitoring relies on its time/cost sparing, due to the easier venous blood sampling from a central line instead of the more troublesome serial arterial drawing [4-6].

If the patient we are looking after is a very critical one, the contemporary sampling of mixed/central venous and arterial blood will allow to calculate the V-A gradients (Δ V-A) of pH and PCO_2. Even if some limitations could be found (congenital enzyme defects, global/regional perfusional mismatch...), a strong relationship exists between lactate trends, Δ V-A, O_2 uptake/supply

($\dot{V}O_2/DO_2$) dependency and the prognosis in septic and non-septic critically ill [7, 8]. Interestingly, the timing of pH, PCO_2, Δ V-A is even better than that of lactate trends. As a matter of fact, in the very first minutes of metabolic acidosis linked to hypoperfusion, ATP-hydrolysis ensues (producing H+ and – after cellular buffering – ↑ venous PCO_2) before any significant raising of lactataemia could be demonstrated [9].

Moreover, whatever the causes of the metabolic derangements linked to dysoxia, the venous blood samples drawn from skeletal muscle, brain, liver, kidney, heart are the best indicators of the specific effects on the different organs. Besides, in low flow states, acids and CO_2 concentrations could be much higher in the venous blood (than in arterial samples), due to partial and delayed pulmonary clearance. In such cases, the arterial BGA can just mirror the ventilatory contribute to keep the acid-base metabolism between acceptable limits; on the other hand, a larger than normal pH and/or PCO_2 gradient is a real-time reliable index of the so-called metabolic hypercarbic acidosis (Table 1).

Table 1. Differences between venous hypercapneic and respiratory acidosis

	Hypercapneic metabolic acidosis	Respiratory acidosis
Arterial pH	< 7.35	< 7.35
Arterial PCO_2	normal/high	high
Mixed venous PCO_2	> 5 higher than arterial PCO_2	1-3 higher than arterial PCO_2
Arterial HCO_3	low	elevated
Anion gap	high	normal
Source of excess [H] ions	hydrolysis of ATP lactic acid	carbonic acid
Clinical examples	hypoperfusion, heart failure, cardiac arrest	ventilatory insufficiencies

To summarize these monitoring aspects of the metabolic acidosis in the underperfused patients, if a higher than normal PCO_2 or pH gradient is observed, we can acceptably rely on the "trends" of the Δ V-A to tailor a successful therapeutic approach [10, 11].

Therapy controversies

There are some common effects of acidaemia "per se", which admittedly become clinically relevant only under a blood pH ≤ 7.20, that should be familiar to the intensivist, but never to be overtreated (Table 2).

Aiming to partially correct the acidaemia, intravenous sodium bicarbonate is the mainstay of alkali therapy; the problem arises on which patients should be treated. According to the AHA Advanced Cardiac Life Support (ACLS) guide-

Table 2. Major intrinsic effects of acidaemia

Cardiac
    reduced contractility
    increased arrhythmogenicity
Vascular
    ↓ arterial tone (systemic/pulmonary)
    ↑ venous tone
Respiratory
    ↑ work of breathing
Neurologic
    brain oedema
Metabolic
    hyperkalaemia
    insulin resistance
    ↓ ATP synthesis

---

lines [12], during cardiopulmonary resuscitation (CPR) and almost in every hy-poperfused subject, the alkali therapy is not a first line drug. There is an overwhelming evidence of the detrimental effect of sodium bicarbonate infusions in such setting, due to the massive CO_2 produced by the venous blood buffering, with back-diffusion of CO_2 into the myocardial cells. These experimental and clinical observations led to some trials with different alkalinizing substances as Carbicarb ($NaHCO_3$ plus Na_2CO_3), THAM (0,3 N tromethamine) and DCA (dichloroacetate) in lactic acidosis: none of these compounds demonstrated controlled advantages versus the easily manageable $NaHCO_3$ (13-15).

On the other hand, there are other syndromes (DKA, renal tubular acidoses, some intoxications), in which – being mindful of overtreatment – some partial correction of hypobicarbonataemia could be useful in time-buying, while the primary disease is being corrected [16].

Only in hyperkalaemia, at the same time with calcium chloride (but never to be injected in the same vein!), sodium bicarbonate should be considered as a life-saving drug.

Coming up to the need of quantifying the $NaHCO_3$ to be given i.v., if indicated, it could be summarized as a 4 steps approach:

1. evaluate the distribution space as much as 50% of the body weight;
2. consider as a reasonable target a blood HCO_3 of 12-13 mmol/L;
3. give (12 – X) x 0.5 x body weight (mmoles of HCO_3);
4. after 30 minutes reevaluate arterial BGA, aiming to a pH of about 7.20.

Three caveats should be kept in mind: a) the distribution space could be very smaller than usual in the critically ill, due to underhydration; b) the repair of acidaemia could uncover a potassium/magnesium deficit, partially masked by the low pH; c) whenever $NaHCO_3$ is to be given, some risk arises of sodium/fluids overload, possibly dangerous in heart failure (consider in such cases some dialytic therapeutic approach).

Acidaemias from 7.36 to 7.20 should not be treated

If the acidaemia is due to hypoperfusion, don't give any alkali

Recheck BGA after 30', including K and Mg

Mind the EKG monitoring

Watch out of fluid overload

Metabolic alkalosis

Uncomplicated metabolic alkalosis is easy to memorize as:

$$
\begin{array}{lll}
\text{pH} & > & 7.42 \\
\text{HCO}_3 & > & 26 \text{ mmol/L} \\
\text{PCO}_2 & > & 40 \text{ mmHg}
\end{array}
$$

Interestingly, some metabolic alkaloses in the critically ill could be superimposed to respiratory acidosis (HCO_3 raised more than 0.35 mmol/1 mmHg PCO_2), or to metabolic acidosis (diagnostic clue: the abnormal anion gap) [17-19].

Despite the traditional underevaluation of this acid-base disorder, there are almost two good reasons to be very concerned of the importance of metabolic alkalosis in the critically ill:

a) the alkalaemic disorders are less tolerated by the tissues than the acidaemic ones, due to sizeable electrolyte derangements [20, 21] and linked neurological/myocardial impairment (Table 3);

b) they could be frequently associated to some iatrogenicity, which – if not timely corrected – could negatively affect the outcome.

The potentially very dangerous effects of ↑ blood pH on potassium conductance (gK) and on the ionized fractions of Ca and Mg are depicted in Fig. 1.

Monitoring

In the ICU patients a metabolic alkalosis should firstly arise concern on the "fullness" of the intravascular compartment (the "so-called" contraction alkalosis), due to the overuse of diuretics, the poor fluids infusion or both; the prolonged gastric suction is the third common cause of hyperbicarbonataemia, due to fluids/HCl losses. A practical useful marker of these "underfilling" states is the invariably low chloride urinary excretion fraction (FE Cl, normal value

Table 3. Major intrinsic effects of alkalaemia

Cardiac
    coronary hypoperfusion
    repolarization dispersion (↑ arrhythmogenicity)
Vascular
    arteriolar constriction
Respiratory
    hypoventilation
    unsuccessful weaning
Metabolic
    ↑ anaerobic glycolysis
    ↓ K, Mg^{++}, Ca^{++} plasma concentrations
Neurological
    increased neuroexcitability
    cerebral hypoperfusion

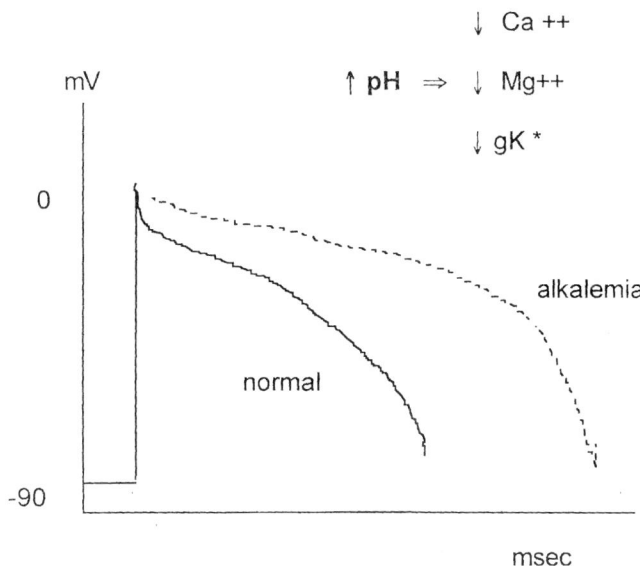

Fig. 1. Arrhythmogenic effects of alkalaemia on the cardiac action potential

> 1%), with absolute Cl urinary excretion less than 20 mmol/L [22, 23]. As the central venous pressure in many critical patients is an unreliable index, due to mechanical ventilation and/or right ventricle impairment, the blood pH and urinary/plasmatic electrolyte monitoring could add useful information on the hydration/perfusional state.

Moreover, a persistent metabolic alkalaemia (the so-called "overshoot alkalosis") is a common finding in overventilated chronically hypercapneic subjects, due to the delayed renal response to the "normalization" of the PCO_2 [24]; once more, in such cases the arterial blood pH monitoring is probably the best guide to set the ventilator.

On the other hand, there are few clinical conditions of metabolic alkalosis and volume expansion ($\uparrow\uparrow$ mineral-corticoid action, Bartter's syndrome, licorice excess), easily detected from the high urinary chloride (i.e. Clu > 20 mmol/L) and associated chronic hypokalaemia.

Controversies in therapeutics

As stated before, two main aspects should be considered about the metabolic alkalosis correction in the critically ill:

– the associated dyselectrolitaemia
– the fluid balance

From this point of view the stoichiometric administration of hydrochloric acid doesn't seem an optimal choice, because it could perhaps, only temporarily, correct the alkalaemia, only partially correcting the dyselectrolitaemia but leaving the hypovolaemia absolutely unchanged. Besides, to avoid local tissue injury, H Cl infusions must be performed through a central catheter and, if injected as ammonium chloride, could be detrimental raising the ammonia concentrations in liver failure [25].

Referring to the hypokalaemia, the potassium chloride amount to be administered should be calculated firstly relying on the difference between a supposed "normal" value and the actual one multiplied by the intracellular body fluids; this theoretical approach could be fostered by some "spot" urinary evaluations of K and Cl concentrations: these latter values are closely related to the total exchangeable pool (the poorer the urinary concentrations, the larger the total amounts to be given) [26, 27].

An associated hypomagnesaemia is likely to be found in such circumstances and should be treated all the same.

Caveats about ionized calcium correction arise in digitalized patients, and should be considered only if a prolonged QT interval isn't going to be corrected after K and Mg administration.

The paramount importance of the electrolyte pattern in metabolic alkaloses is demonstrated by the almost impossible pH correction without the contemporary K/Mg body pool restoration [28].

The correction of intravascular fluid depletion could be cumbersome in heart and renal failure: independently by the colloid/crystalloid ratio, which must be tailored on the single patient, concern arises about the compliance of the cardiovascular system. In some very critically unstable patients, it could be useful the administration of acetazolamide (250 mg twice daily), at the same time of the fluid/electrolytes restitution, to promote bicarbonaturia without any further contraction of the intravascular space [29].

Due to the cardiovascular instability of such subjects, the BGA monitoring should be closely connected to the EKG monitoring: the transmembrane K/Mg fluxes are badly influenced by sudden variation of blood pH, possibly generating life-threatening arrhythmias [30].

If the risk of pulmonary oedema is very high, perhaps the best way to provide an acceptable metabolic environment is a dialytic approach. Reducing the pH of the dialysate will help to achieve a near-normal blood pH, allowing to buy time to correct the primary disease.

Metabolic alkalosis is usually associated with dyselectrolitaemia
Plasma and urine chloride are often the diagnostic clue
Mind the QT interval
Be aware of the mixed alkaloses

References

1. Narins RG, Emmett M (1980) Simple and mixed acid-base disorders: A practical approach. Medicine S9:161-187
2. Narins RG, Jones ER et al (1982) Diagnostic strategies in disorders of fluid, electrolyte and acid-base homeostasis. Am J Med 72:469-512
3. Schiraldi F (1995) Time to abandon base excess as a reliable index in the ICU? Int J Int Care 2:23
4. Zhang H, Vincent JL (1993) Arteriovenous differences in PCO_2 and pH are good indicators of critical hypoperfusion. Am Rev Respir Dis 148:867-871
5. Bircher NG (1992) Acidosis of cardiopulmonary resuscitation: Carbon dioxide transport and anaerobios. Crit Care Med 20;9:1203-1204
6. Van der Linden P, Rausin I et al (1995) Detection of tissue hypoxia by arterio-venous gradient for PCO_2 and pH in anesthetized dogs during progressive hemorrhage. Anesth Analg 80: 269-275
7. Kette F, Weil MH et al (1993) Intramyocardial hypercarbic acidosis during cardiac arrest and resuscitation. Crit Care Med 21:901-906
8. Adrogue HJ, Rashad MN, Gorin AB et al (1989) Assessing acid-base status in circulatory failure. Differences between arterial and central venous blood. N Engl J Med 320:1312-1318
9. Schlitig R, Pinsky MR (1991) Defining the hypoxic threshold. Crit Care Med19:147-149
10. Vincent JL, Dufaye P et al (1983) Serial lactate determinations during circulatory shock. Crit Care Med 11:449-451
11. Mahutte CK, Jaffe MB et al (1991) Cardiac output from carbon dioxide production and arterial and venous oximetry. Crit Care Med 19:1270-1277
12. American Heart Association (1994) Textbook of Advanced Cardiac Life Support
13. Stacpoole PW, Harman EM et al (1983) Treatment of lactic acidosis with dichloroacetate. N Engl J Med 309:390-396
14. Stacpoole PW, Wright EC et al (1992) A controlled clinical trial of DCA for treatment of lactic acidosis in adults. N Engl J Med 327:1564-1569

15. Arieff AI (1993) Managing metabolic acidosis: Update on the sodium bicarbonate controversy. J Crit Illness 8:224-229
16. Rhee K, Toro LO et al (1993) Carbicarb, sodium carbonate, sodium chloride in hypoxic lactic acidosis. Chest 104:913-918
17. Adroguè HJ, Madias NE (1998) Management of life-threatening acid-base disorders. II parts. N Engl J Med 338;1:26-34, 338;2:107-111
18. Gabow P (1985) Disorders associated with an altered anion gap. Kidney Int 27:472-483
19. Smithline N, Gardner KD (1976) Gaps - anionic and osmolal. JAMA 236:1594-1597
20. Faber MD, Kupin WL et al (1994) Common fluid-electrolyte and acid-base problems in the intensive care unit: Selected issues. Semin Nephrol 14(1):8-22
21. Adroguè HJ, Madias NE (1981) Changes in plasma potassium concentration during acute acid-base disturbances. Am J Med 71:456-467
22. Steiner RW (1984) Interpreting the fractional excretion of sodium. Am J Med 77:699-702
23. Laterre PF, Mallie JP (1993) The fractional excretion of chloride instead of sodium indicates hypovolemia: A comparative study of bedside assessment of true or effective intravascular depletion. Clin Intens Care 4:112-115
24. Idris AH, Staples ED et al (1994) Effect of ventilation on acid-base balance and oxygenation in low blood-flow states. Crit Care Med 22:1827-1834
25. Rimmer JM, Gennari FJ (1987) Metabolic alkalosis. J Intensive Care Med 2:137-150
26. Gennari FJ (1998) Current concepts: Hypokalemia. N Engl J Med 339;7:451-458
27. Kamel KS, Ethier JH et al (1990) Urine electrolytes and osmolality: When and how to use them. Am J Nephrol 10:89-102
28. Seldin DW, Rector FC (1972) The generation and maintenance of metabolic alkalosis. Kidney Int 1:306-320
29. Madias NE, Cohen JJ, Adroguè HJ (1990) Influence of acute and chronic respiratory alkalosis on preexisting chronic metabolic alkalosis. Am J Physiol 258:F479-F485
30. Tomsic M, Horvart M (1991) Torsade de pointes associated with combined severe metabolic and respiratory alkalosis. Clin Int Care 2;1:47-50

Differential Diagnosis and Treatment of Acidosis

H.P. Povoas, M.H. Weil

Acidosis may be associated with unrelated disease states and differing mechanisms. Metabolic production of organic acids, respiratory retention of carbon dioxide or renal loss of bicarbonate represent changes in which [H+] of fluids in both extracellular and intracellular compartments may be increased. Excesses of acids and deficits of bicarbonate are defined as metabolic acid base defects and increases or decreases in the CO_2 tension of blood (and tissues) are defined as respiratory acidosis. An important exception is now recognized. During tissue ischaemia, excesses of tissue CO_2 are generated [1]. The resulting hypercarbic tissue acidosis due to tissue hypoxia is therefore a metabolic defect rather than respiratory CO_2 retention [2-5].

Metabolic acidosis caused by overproduction of organic acids is further classified as anion gap acidosis. Anion gaps are characteristic of lactic acidosis, diabetic ketoacidosis, poisonings due to renal failure or ingestion or infusion of organic acids. A gain in hydrogen ions associated hyperchloraemia or a relative loss of bicarbonate in blood, plasma or serum is recognized as hyperchloraemic metabolic acidosis. Clinical classification of currently recognized causes of both metabolic and respiratory acidosis is summarized in Table 1.

For understanding the mechanisms and ultimately the treatment of acid-base abnormalities, a reasonably precise diagnosis of the underlying disease state is required. Special focus should initially be on cardiopulmonary, renal, or endocrine disease. The most common cause of lactic acidosis is impaired tissue perfusion [6]. Respiratory symptoms including apnoea, tachypnoea, stridor or cyanosis may pinpoint alveolar hypoventilation and CO_2 retention and therefore respiratory acidosis.

For practical purposes, acid base disorders may be anticipated based on diagnosis of the underlying disease. However, confirmation and quantitation invariably requires laboratory measurements and especially blood gases. The increasingly wider use of "stat" or "point of care" laboratory tests in which acid base and electrolyte measurements are routinely obtained, more often expose acid base defect before the underlying cause is diagnosed [7]. The laboratory diagnosis of acidosis is based on measurements of blood pH, PCO_2 and HCO_3. Funda-

Table 1. Classification of acid-base disorders

Metabolic acidosis		Respiratory acidosis
Anion gap acidosis	**Hyperchloraemic acidosis**	

Anion gap acidosis	Hyperchloraemic acidosis	Respiratory acidosis
Low flow states	Renal disease	Acute
shock	renal failure	atelectasis
septic	renal tubular acidosis	pneumonia
haemorrhagic	(RTA)	recovery from anaesthesia
traumatic	Gastrointestinal losses	pneumothorax
cardiac arrest	pancreatic and biliary	haemothorax
Hypoxaemia	fistulas	open chest and open heart
Anaemia	Ureterocolic implantation	operations
Diabetic ketoacidosis	Inborn errors of metabolism	thoracic trauma with flail chest
Hepatic failure	carbonic anhydrase	smoke inhalation
Uraemia	deficiency	pulmonary oedema
Neoplasm esp. Leukemia	oxoprolinuria	laparoscopic surgery
D-lactic acidosis	Drugs	Chronic
Surgery	cycloxygenase inhibitors	cardiac failure
cardiopulmonary bypass	β-adrenergic antagonists	chronic bronchitis
aorta cross clamping	angiotensin converting-	pulmonary failure
aortic dissection	enzyme inhibitors	chronic obstructive lung
Drugs	heparin	disease
antibiotics	potassium-sparing diuretics	tobacco smoking
nalidixid acid, isoniazid	trimethoprim-sulfa	bronchiectasis
phenformin related drugs including	digitalis overdose	
metformin		
chemo therapeutic drugs		
5-fluorouracil		
Anti-HIV agents		
zidovudine		
stavudine		
Anticonvulsants		
sulthiame		
topiramate		
Anaesthesia		
propofol		
Salicylates		
5-ASA, mesalazine		
Hypertonic solutions		
laxatives/enemas		
saline/dextran		
Poisoning		
cyanides		
iron		
salicylates		
methanol		
ethylene glycol		
carbamate		
organophosphate		
carbon monoxide		

mental to the understanding of abnormalities in these blood gas parameters, is the Henderson-Hasselbalch equation [8]:

$$pH = pK + \log \frac{[HCO_3^-]}{[CO_2]}$$

It explains the normal physiological buffering mechanism, by which excesses of H^+, conventionally expressed as decreases in pH, represent either decreases in HCO_3^- or increases in arterial PCO_2 ($PaCO_2$).

Metabolic acidosis

Anion gap acidosis

The anion gap is defined as the difference between the cations and anions measured in the plasma:

$$anion\ gap = (Na^+ + K^+) - (Cl^- + HCO_3^-)$$

and a difference exceeding 12 mEq represents an excess of unmeasured anions, as illustrated in Fig. 1. Increases in the anion gap are due to abnormal proteins, excesses of organic anions including hydroxybutirate and aceto-acetate during diabetic ketoacidosis, inorganic phosphates, sulfates and chlorides. Excesses of acids are buffered by bicarbonate, according to the Henderson-Hasselbalch equation such that bicarbonate is decreased. When increases in chloride compensate for the decreases in bicarbonate the anion gap may be unaltered. Renal failure is typically associated with an anion gap because of the accumulation of unexcreted anions including phosphate and sulfate [9].

Lactic acidosis. Lactate is a common and now readily measured biochemical marker. In clinical practice, the L-isomer is measured. Concentrations exceeding 1.5 mmol/l are abnormal. Two types of l-lactate excess are defined as Type A and Type B. Type A represents a failure of O_2 delivery to meet O_2 demand of the tissues or an incapability of tissue to utilize oxygen. In the normal aerobic pathway, pyruvate is metabolized to carbon dioxide and water in the Krebs cycle as shown in Fig. 2. When pyruvate is metabolized aerobically by mitochondria, 36 M of ATP are generated for each mole of glucose. In the absence of oxygen, glucose is metabolized to pyruvate and this pyruvate is "shunted" to lactate. This "emergency pathway" generates only 2 M of ATP for every mole of glucose [10] as shown in Fig. 2. When the oxygen deficit is repaid, lactate is converted back to pyruvate then oxidized through the Krebs cycle to CO_2 and water or converted back to glucose by gluconeogenesis predominantly in the liver. Lactate accumulation and lactic acidosis in this setting represent a failure to sustain the oxygen requirements of tissue either because of decreased supply or increased utilization.

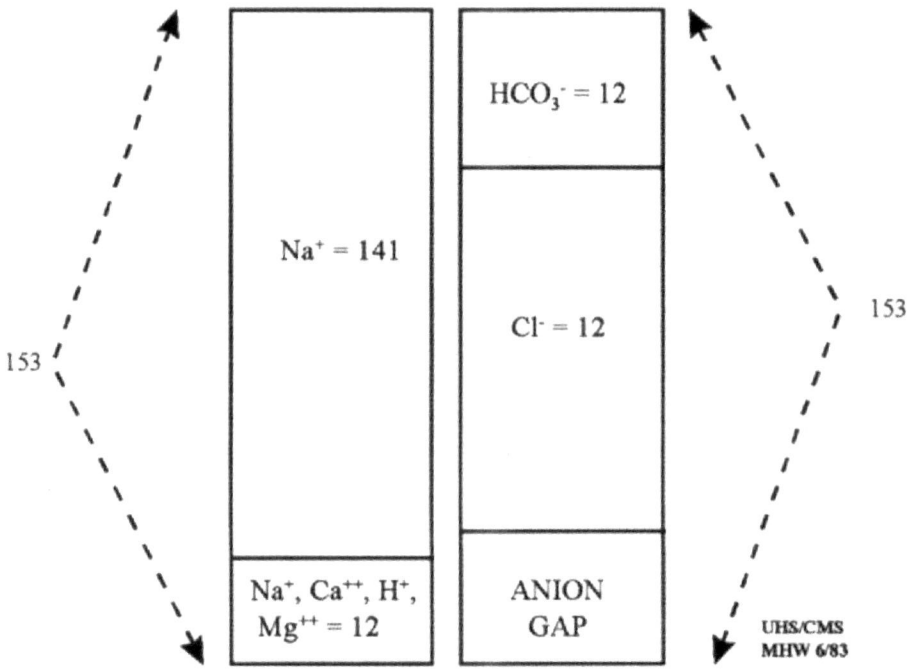

Fig. 1. Anion gap

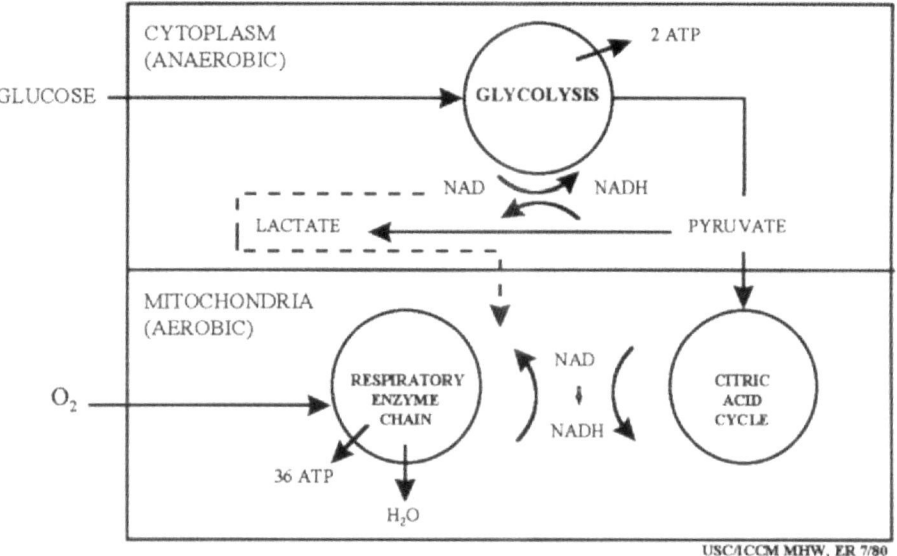

Fig. 2. Cellular metabolism

Circulatory shock states remain the most common causes of pathological Type A lactic acidosis and excesses of lactic acid are highly correlated with the severity of the perfusion deficit [11]. When lactic acidosis occurs in settings unrelated to either excessive oxygen requirements or impaired tissue perfusion, it is defined as Type B lactic acidosis. Type B lactic acidosis is observed uncommonly and in a diversity of clinical disease states. It usually represents metabolic defect in cellular energy metabolism including 1) uncoupling of oxidative phosphorylation, 2) inhibition of mitochondrial respiration and 3) reduced availability of substrates for oxidative metabolism. These abnormalities occur in settings of malignancy, vitamin deficiency, adverse reactions to drugs and toxins, and in rare instances of infection without evidence of circulatory failure. In human patients with septic shock, Gore [12] demonstrated increased pyruvate oxidation refuting the concept of a sepsis-related impairment in pyruvate dehydrogenase activity. HIV-infected patients may manifest lactic acidosis following intravenous infusion of trimethoprim/sulfamethoxazole (TMP/SMX) for treatment of Pneumocystis carinii pneumonia [13]. Acidosis is reversed after the drug infusion is stopped. Investigators have implicated anaesthetic agents including propofol as a cause of Type B lactic acidosis in patients with refractory status epilepticus [14]. However, it is very likely that lactic acidosis in such patients represents oxygen deficits associated with extremes of metabolic oxygen requirements during convulsive seizures. Rare cases of lactic acidosis follow administration of formin oral hypoglycaemic agents including metformin and phenformin, especially when there is coexisting renal failure [15-17]. Chronic use of nucleoside analogs for treatment of HIV-infections including zidovudine, stavudine, didanosine and fialuridine have also been implicated as potential causes of Type B lactic acidosis. The mechanism is likely to be impaired mitochondrial function associated with DNA inhibition [18].

A distinctly different entity in addition to Type A or B lactic acidosis is D-lactic acidosis. D-lactic acid is produced by microorganisms. The D-lactate producing microorganisms include species of lactobacillus, bifidobacterium and eubacterium. D-lactate concentrations are increased to 3 mmol/L or more. The clinical presentation is predominantly neurological with confusion, ataxia and memory disturbances. Metabolic acidosis is characterized by normal L-lactate levels [19]. The abnormalities occur primarily in patients with intestinal diseases in which there is carbohydrate malabsorption, blind loop syndrome after intestinal surgery [20, 21] and in settings of pancreatitis. Though L-lactate is now measured with disarming ease with a lactate electrode [22] or as part of automated chemistry analysis, this does not apply to D-lactate which requires specialized laboratory assays. The management in each instance is that of the underlying cause.

Diabetic ketoacidosis (DKA). DKA is the most common and the most acute life-threatening complication of diabetes. It is responsible for approximately 110,000 emergency hospital admissions annually in the United States [23]. A majority of cases represent Type I insulin dependent diabetes mellitus, but a minority are associated with Type II adult onset diabetes.

The initial metabolic defect is either an absolute or relative deficiency of insulin. Excesses of counterregulatory hormones, especially corticosteroids and catecholamines may be responsible. The metabolic breakdown of fatty acids produces keto and hydroxy acids. Hyperglycaemia induces osmolal diuresis with consequent volume depletion. Accordingly patients present with both acidaemia and dehydration with hypovolaemia. There is an increased anion gap but relative hyperchloraemia may minimize the anion gap. Symptoms include polyuria, polydipsia, nausea, vomiting, abdominal pain and tachypnoea with "fishmouth" breathing. A typical fruity odor of the patient's breath was identified by earlier clinicians. Management includes volume repletion, administration of insulin and concurrent repletion of plasma potassium during reversal of hyperglycaemia. During volume repletion, even small amounts of insulin typically reverse ketoacid production. Volume repletion restores arterial perfusion pressure and cardiac output promoting renal excretion of ketones and excesses of chloride. There is no indication for routine administration of buffer agents, either sodium bicarbonate or sodium lactate because there is no evidence of improved outcomes [24, 25].

Poisoning. Poison and drug intoxication remain important causes of anion gap acidosis in emergency medical settings. Frequent causes are the ingestion of excesses of salicylates or methanol/ethylene glycol. The ingestion of large doses of salicylates produces hyperpyrexia and increased total body oxygen consumption. Salicylates uncouple oxidative phosphorylation in mitochondria. Gastric lavage, activated charcoal and haemodialysis, especially in the presence of renal failure, are current therapeutic options.

Ingestion of as little as 30 ml of methanol or 100 ml of ethylene glycol may be fatal. The toxic effect is not the alcohol itself but the metabolites generated by the action of alcohol dehydrogenase. Methanol generates formic acid and ethylene glycol generates glycolic and oxalic acid. Both produce a profound anion gap acidosis. Visual disturbances usually follow ingestion of methanol and stupor or coma after ethylene glycol. Administration of ethanol provides an appropriate antidote. Alcohol dehydrogenase has 100-fold greater affinity for ethanol than methanol or ethylene glycol. Haemodialysis is also an effective option [26, 27].

Other anion gap acidosis. Enemas. Acidosis may follow phosphate intoxication after use of laxatives or enemas, especially in patients with impaired gut motility, often a complication of diabetes mellitus [28].

Hypertonic solutions. The infusion of excesses of sodium chloride and especially hypertonic solutions such as saline-dextran solutions may produce acidosis, because of the excesses of acidic chloride ions [29].

Hyperchloraemic metabolic acidosis

This type of acidosis occurs in settings of renal failure, especially renal tubular defects with renal losses of bicarbonate, extrarenal losses of bicarbonate, mineralocorticoid deficiency or resistance to the effects of mineralocorticoids.

Renal failure. With a decline in renal function, the kidney's capability to maintain the acid base balance is compromised. Because of decreased ammoniagenesis, less ammonium is secreted from the medullary interstitium into the medullary collecting ducts, reducing ammonium diffusion and active hydrogen ion secretion, which explains metabolic acidosis often with hyperchloraemia.

Renal tubular acidosis (RTA). Both proximal and distal renal tubules normally secrete hydrogen ion [H+] and reabsorb bicarbonate from the luminal fluid. Renal tubular defects account for failure to excrete the normal acid loads resulting in hyperchloraemic acidosis. The renal tubular defects are classified according to the site of involvement. Functional impairment of the distal nephron is classified as a type I defect and of the proximal nephron as a type II defect. Mixed pattern is designated a type III defect. Aldosterone deficiency represents a so-called type IV renal tubular defect [30].

Type I. Distal renal tubular acidosis (DRTA) represents either a defect in secretion of H+ or loss of transport capability of H+ against a concentration gradient between extracellular fluid and urine in the terminal segments of the nephron. This precludes reduction of the urinary pH to less than 5.5 units. In lieu of H+ secretion there is excessive K+ excretion and therefore hypokalaemia. The abnormality is a genetic autossomal dominant defect.

Type II. Proximal renal tubular acidosis is characterized by defects in H+ secretions in the proximal tubule. This accounts for decreased bicarbonate reabsorption, losses of bicarbonate in the urine and decreased serum bicarbonate. Ultimately, there is hypokalaemic and hyperchloraemic acidosis. This disorder is presently managed with replacement therapy.

Type III. These defects were recognized in infants in whom bicarbonate losses and incapacity to lower urine pH coexist with severe acidaemia.

Type IV. This tubular disorder is related to either a lack of aldosterone or failure of aldosterone to stimulate H+ secretion in the cation exchange segment of the distal tubule. Replacement therapy with mineralocorticoids and small doses of bicarbonate is usually effective.

Bicarbonate loss. The most frequent causes of bicarbonate losses that account for metabolic acidosis include diarrhoea, vomiting and pancreatic fistula. All may produce profound hyperchloraemic acidosis [31].

Respiratory acidosis

Respiratory acidosis is diagnosed when PCO_2 concentrations exceed normal ranges when measured on arterial blood. In clinical practice, primary increases in arterial PCO_2 ($PaCO_2$) usually are due to impaired alveolar ventilation. Either or both extra and intra-pulmonary disorders may be implicated. Extra-pulmonary causes due to neuromuscular disorders with decreased respiratory drive, abnormalities of respiratory muscle function, skeletal causes or intrathoracic abnormalities may preclude normal ventilation. Thoracic trauma with flail chest, thoracotomy, sedation, narcosis, anaesthesia and neuromuscular blockade are frequent precipitating events for global alveolar hypoventilation in the absence of primary pulmonary causes. Nevertheless the most common cause is decreased alveolar ventilation due to primary lung disease including chronic obstructive lung diseases, pulmonary oedema, infiltrative lung diseases including pneumonia, and atelectasis. Finally the primary cause may be partial or complete asphyxia due to airway obstruction and rarely due to breathing gas mixtures which have high CO_2 contents.

Failure of carbon dioxide excretion first appears during exercise when large amounts of carbon dioxide are produced and in amounts that fail to be excreted by the lungs. PCO_2 is typically measured in the arterial blood but may also be measured on capillary and venous blood. Because of the high permeability of carbon dioxide gas, increases in arterial PCO_2 are accompanied by tissues hypercarbia. The carbon dioxide in blood and tissues is converted, in part, to H_2CO_3 such as to generate excesses of H^+ with decreases in pH. Accordingly, the severity of acidosis is also related to the bicarbonate concentration.

Two mechanisms for compensation are identified. The first is that of renal retention of HCO_3^- such as to counterbalance the effects of CO_2 by increasing bicarbonate. The implications of such emerge from the Henderson-Hasselbalch equation as shown above. The second is excretion of excesses of hydrogen ions which of themselves result in reabsorption of bicarbonate. The treatment of uncomplicated respiratory acidosis is that of restoring more normal alveolar ventilation by external interventions and especially mechanical ventilation after a patent airway is secured. The ultimate treatment is that of the underlying cause.

Buffer agents

Buffer preparations that have come into clinical use include sodium bicarbonate, sodium lactate and a preparation of Carbicarb®, which is not yet approved for the use in the USA but is used in Europe. Carbicarb® is an equimolar combination of sodium carbonate and sodium bicarbonate. Bicarbonate generates carbon dioxide, Carbicarb® does not. Tromethamine (THAM) is an organic buffer that reduces carbon dioxide tension in tissues and is of special advantage because it does not increase osmolality.

Tromethamine (THAM)

THAM (tris-hydroxymethyl aminomethane) is a biologically inert amino alcohol of low toxicity, which buffers carbon dioxide and acids in vitro and in vivo. THAM supplements the buffering capacity of the blood bicarbonate system, accepting a proton, generating bicarbonate and decreasing the partial pressure of carbon dioxide in arterial blood ($PaCO_2$). Unlike bicarbonate, which requires an open system for carbon dioxide elimination for its buffering effect, THAM is effective in a closed or semiclosed system, and maintains its buffering power in settings of hypothermia. It therefore has theoretical advantages for treatment of acidaemia associated with carbon dioxide retention. However, THAM may also depress respiration and produce hypoglycaemia. Nevertheless it is an appropriate option for acute treatment of salicylate or barbiturate overdose because increases in serum pH favor increased excretion of these drugs. THAM is also an ingredient of cardioplegic solutions and for preservation of liver prior to transplantation. It is also employed for chemolysis of renal calculi [32].

Sodium bicarbonate

Sodium bicarbonate ($NaHCO_3$) is the most widely employed buffer agent. The indications for routine reversal of metabolic acidosis by the intravenous infusion of sodium bicarbonate is a controversial issue. There is a potential disequilibrium of bicarbonate shifts across cell membranes after sodium bicarbonate administration, resulting in "paradoxical" intracellular acidosis [33]. It is also a major cause of hyperosmolar states with resulting cerebral injury, especially in settings of CPR.

Carbicarb®

Carbicarb® (Na_2CO_3 0.33 molar $NaHCO_3$ 0.33 molar), is a carbon dioxide-consuming buffer which was developed to minimize excess CO_2 generation [34]. Comparisons between sodium bicarbonate and Carbicarb®, confirm that Carbicarb® buffers excesses of [H^+] without increasing arterial PCO_2 [35]. However, like sodium bicarbonate Carbicarb® failed to reverse intracellular acidosis including myocardial acidosis, nor improve outcomes during cardiac resuscitation. [36, 37]. Although buffer agents may not improve the success of initial resuscitation when administered during CPR, there is experimental data which indicate that it may ameliorate postresuscitation myocardial dysfunction and thereby improve postresuscitation survival [38].

Carbicarb® has been used for the treatment of hypoxic lactic acidosis. When compared with sodium bicarbonate or sodium chloride, Carbicarb® had a more beneficial haemodynamic effect with respect to increasing cardiac output and arterial perfusion pressure. It also increased cardiac contractility [39]. However, there is currently no persuasive data to favor its clinical use. Neither diabetic ketoacidosis or the acidosis of hypovolaemic shock were improved after administration of Carbicarb® [40].

References

1. Johnson BA, Weil MH 1991) Redefining ischemia due to circulatory failure as dual defects of oxygen deficits and of carbon dioxide excesses. Crit Care Med 19:1432-1438
2. von Planta M, Weil MH, Gazmuri, RJ et al (1989) Myocardial acidosis associated with CO_2 production during cardiac arrest and resuscitation. Circulation 80:684-692
3. Desai VS, Weil MH, Tang W et al (1993) Gastric intramural PCO_2 during peritonitis and shock. Chest 104:1254-1258
4. Sato Y, Weil MH, Tang W et al (1997) Esophageal PCO_2 as a monitor of perfusion failure during hemorrhagic shock. J Appl Physiol 82:558-562
5. Nakagawa Y, Weil MH, Tang W et al (1998) Sublingual capnometry for diagnosis and quantitation of circulatory shock. Am J Respir Crit Care Med 157:1838-1843
6. Astiz ME, Rackow EC, Kaufman B et al (1988) Relationship of oxygen delivery and mixed venous oxygenation to lactic acidosis in patients with sepsis and acute myocardial infarction. Crit Care Med 16:655-658
7. Weil MH, Michaels S, Puri VK et al (1981) The stat laboratory: facilitating blood gas and biochemical measurements for the critically ill and injured. Am J Clin Pathol 76:34-42
8. Henderson LJ (1908) The theory of neutrality regulation in the animal organism. Am J Physiol 21:427-448
9. Ishihara K, Szerlip HM (1998) Anion gap acidosis. Semin Nephrol 18:83-97
10. Weil MH, von Planta M, Gazmuri RJ et al (1988) Incomplete global myocardial ischemia during cardiac arrest and resuscitation. Crit Care Med 16(10):997-1001
11. Weil MH, Afifi AA (1970) Experimental and clinical studies on lactate and pyruvate as indicators of the severity of acute circulatory failure (shock). Circulation 41:989-1001
12. Gore DC, Jahoor F, Hibbert JM et al (1996) Lactic acidosis during sepsis is related to increased pyruvate production, not deficits in tissue oxygen availability. Ann Surg 224:97-102
13. Porras MC, Lecumberri JN, Castrillon JL (1998) Trimethoprim/sulfamethoxazole and metabolic acidosis in HIV-infected patients. Ann Pharmacother 32:185-189
14. Hanna JP, Ramundo ML (1998) Rhabdomyolysis and hypoxia associated with prolonged propofol infusion in children. Neurology 50:301-303
15. Latif MA, Weil MH (1979) Circulatory defects during phenformin lactic acidosis. Intensive Care Med 5:135-139
16. Bell PM, Hadden DR (1997) Metformin. Endocrinol Metab Clin North Am 26:523-537
17. Lalau JD, Lacroix C, Compagnon P et al (1995) Role of metformin accumulation in metformin-associated lactic acidosis. Diabetes Care 18:779-784
18. Sundar K, Suarez M, Banogon PE et al (1997) Zidovudine-induced fatal lactic acidosis and hepatic failure in patients with acquired immunodeficiency syndrome: report of two patients and review of the literature. Crit Care Med 25:1425-1430
19. Uribarri J, Oh MS, Carroll HJ (1998) D-lactic acidosis. A review of clinical presentation, biochemical features, and pathophysiologic mechanisms. Medicine (Baltimore) 77:73-82
20. Kadakia SC (1995) D-lactic acidosis in a patient with jejunoileal bypass. J Clin Gastroenterol 20:154-156
21. Bongaerts GP, Tolboom JJ, Naber AH et al (1997) Role of bacteria in the pathogenesis of short bowel syndrome-associated D-lactic acidemia. Microb Pathog 22:285-293
22. Marbach EP, Weil MH (1967) Rapid enzymatic measurement of blood lactate and pyruvate. Use and significance of metaphosphoric acid as a common precipitant. Clin Chem 13:314-325
23. Brandenburg MA, Dire DJ (1998) Comparison of arterial and venous blood gas values in the initial emergency department evaluation of patients with diabetic ketoacidosis. Ann Emerg Med 31:459-465
24. Okuda Y, Adrogue HJ, Field JB et al (1996) Counterproductive effects of sodium bicarbonate in diabetic ketoacidosis. J Clin Endocrinol Metab 81:314-320
25. Green SM, Rothrock SG, Ho JD et al (1998) Failure of adjunctive bicarbonate to improve outcome in severe pediatric diabetic ketoacidosis. Ann Emerg Med 31:41-48

26. McMartin KE, Ambre JJ, Tephly TR (1980) Methanol poisoning in human subjects. Role for formic acid accumulation in the metabolic acidosis. Am J Med 68:414-418
27. Gabow PA, Clay K, Sullivan JB et al (1986) Organic acids in ethylene glycol intoxication. Ann Intern Med 105:16-20
28. Kirschbaum B (1998) The acidosis of exogenous phosphate intoxication. Arch Intern Med 158:405-408
29. Moon PF, Kramer GC (1995) Hypertonic saline-dextran resuscitation from hemorrhagic shock induces transient mixed acidosis. Crit Care Med 23(2):323-331
30. Batlle D, Flores G (1996) Underlying defects in distal renal tubular acidosis: new understandings. Am J Kidney Dis 27:896-915
31. DuBose TD Jr (1997) Hyperkalemic hyperchloremic metabolic acidosis: pathophysiologic insights. Kidney Int 51:591-602
32. Nahas GG, Sutin KM, Fermon C et al (1998) Guidelines for the treatment of acidaemia with THAM. Drugs 55:191-224
33. Goldsmith DJ, Forni LG, Hilton PJ (1997) Bicarbonate therapy and intracellular acidosis. Clin Sci (Colch) 93:593-598
34. Filley GF, Kindig NB (1984) Carbicarb, an alkalinizing ion-generating agent of possible clinical usefulness. Trans Am Clin Climatol Assoc 96:141-153
35. Sun JH, Filley GF, Hord K et al (1987) Carbicarb: an effective substitute for $NaHCO_3$ for the treatment of acidosis. Surgery 102:835-839
36. Kette F, Weil MH, von Planta M et al (1990) Buffer agents do not reverse intramyocardial acidosis during cardiac resuscitation. Circulation 81:1660-1666
37. Gazmuri RJ, von Planta M, Weil MH et al (1990) Cardiac effects of carbon dioxide-consuming and carbon dioxide-generating buffers during cardiopulmonary resuscitation. J Am Coll Cardiol 15(2):482-490
38. Sun S, Weil MH, Tang W et al (1996) Effects of buffer agents on postresuscitation myocardial dysfunction. Crit Care Med 24:2035-2041
39. Rhee KH, Toro LO, McDonald GG et al (1993) Carbicarb, sodium bicarbonate, and sodium chloride in hypoxic lactic acidosis. Effect on arterial blood gases, lactate concentrations, hemodynamic variables, and myocardial intracellular pH. Chest 104:913-918
40. Beech JS, Williams SC, Iles RA et al (1995) Haemodynamic and metabolic effects in diabetic ketoacidosis in rats of treatment with sodium bicarbonate or a mixture of sodium bicarbonate and sodium carbonate. Diabetologia 38:889-898

Albumin: Is It a Play-Maker, a Carrier or Both?

F. Mercuriali, G. Inghilleri

Albumin is a small highly symmetric, slightly heterogeneous protein weighting 67,000 D with a high cysteine content, composed by 584 aminoacids residues stabilized by 17 internal disulfide bridges. The complete aminoacid sequence maintains high homology through the species [1] and in humans, a relatively high polimorphism is present [2]. In the human genomic it has been found only one copy of the albumin gene on chromosome 4 in bands q11-22 [3].

Albumin contains a large amount of aspartic and glutamic acids and few leucine and tryptophan. This structure explains the high stability of the protein with respect to physico-chemical influences. Albumin's overall charge is negative under physiological conditions and it presents the best solubility characteristics of any plasma protein. At the pH of blood (pH 7.4), the net charge on the albumin molecule, calculated from its aminoacid composition, is −15.

Pharmacokinetics

Albumin is the most important plasma protein in quantitative terms and accounts for the biggest percentage of plasma protein (60%), the plasma concentration being 3.5-5 g/dL. It is synthesized in the liver normally at a rate that is controlled largely by the osmotic pressure of the interstitial fluid.

The synthesis of albumin, that represents about 10% of the liver's protein synthesis activity, is rapid but the hepatic reserves are small [4]. About 15 g of albumin (about 5%) are metabolized and synthesized daily in the normal steady state: besides small amount lost in the gut the removal by circulation occurs in various organs but healthy kidneys. The median half live is about 18 days.

Total body stores in adults approximate 4.5 g/kg of body weight, about 60% of which is extravascular (skin, muscles, guts) and 40% intravascular [5, 6]. Generally the various extravascular pools equilibrate rapidly with the intravascular pool. These pools are part of a complex regulatory process of fluid exchange involving hydrostatic and osmotic forces. Albumin is a dynamic protein and in an hour about 5% of albumin leaves the circulation and after tissue passage, returns through the lymphatics. In one day the entire albumin pool is recycled. The exchange of albumin molecules between the intravascular and extravascular pools occurs by two general processes: endocytosis and a receptor-mediated transcytotic pathway by which molecules are transported through the endothelial cell to the target cell [7].

Functions

The study of albumin reveal a complex picture of this molecule which serves probably more functions than supposed so far.

Albumin has a high water binding capacity of approximately 18 milliliters per gram. This property, together with the rapidity which the extravascular and intravascular pools equilibrate with, determines the physiological importance of albumin in the regulation of water and volume distribution between intravascular and interstitial space. At the normal serum concentration albumin accounts for a colloidosmotic pressure (COP) of 16-18 mmHg, that is from 60 to 70% of the total oncotic pressure at 26-28 mmHg.

Beside the major contribution to the COP in plasma, albumin exerts other biological functions although in patients with hereditary absence of albumin the clinical picture is not seriously compromised and the disease allows to reach old age [8].

Another important function of the albumin molecule, mainly due to the high negative charge, relates to the binding and transport of a large number of compounds including drugs. Albumin is very effective in binding small molecules of many types and for this property is considered a sponge of the circulation. Both cations and anions can be reversibly bound by the albumin molecule. Trace metals, fatty acids, hormones, enzymes, and pharmaceutical products are transported in this manner, and also metabolic product such as bilirubin. Albumin also bind foreign proteins such as protein G of streptococcal cell wall [9]. This property of microbial protein to bind to albumin may contribute to microbial virulence as this association would prevent the identification and the elimination of the microbial agents by specific antibodies and complement [9].

Hypoalbuminaemia

A decrease in measured albumin is found in many situations and often is not a clinical concern. Generally a reduction of COP to about 20 mg/mmHg (corresponding to a total serum protein of 5.2 g/dL) is regarded as a critical value below which patients are in danger. Measuring COP is more useful for judgment of the need for albumin than plasma albumin concentration, as in case of hypoproteinaemia, intravascular albumin shortage is compensated by mobilizing extravascular stock so that an extravascular albumin deficiency may be masked by normal plasma levels [10, 11].

Significant hypoalbuminaemia with intravascular volume depletion, anasarca, ascites and pleural effusions can be observed as a consequence of inadequate synthesis or of excessive loss. Production is decreased in malnutrition, hormonal influences and a wide range of diseases, particularly chronic liver disease. However, in patients with cirrhosis and portal hypertension low levels of albumin are also a consequence of increased plasma volume. Hypoalbuminaemia in malnutrition is the result of a relative or absolute deficiency in calories and proteins. This can be due to inadequate food intake or a result of malabsorption. Deficiency in the aminoacid supply leads to a reduction of albumin synthesis [12]. In malnutrition, refeeding results in the onset of albumin synthesis in minutes in the presence of adequate hepatic function [13].

Infection can depress the synthesis rate of albumin and this can also be frequently observed in inflammatory disorders, as it has been documented clinically and also demonstrated in rats, where upon terpentine-induced inflammation and increased secretion of monocytic inflammatory cytokines, like the interleukin 1, synthesis of albumin is significantly reduced [14]. Excessive loss is seen in nephrotic syndrome, protein-losing enteropathy, burns and massive acute blood loss.

Albumin products

In spite of the fact that in the last period almost all plasma proteins licensed for human use have been cloned and expressed in a biologically active form in animal cells comprising albumin, only two recombinant human factor VIII preparations have been licensed and this is due to the inability to produce these proteins in adequate quantities or in the inappropriate post-translational modification of the recombinant protein [15].

In the absence of large scale introduction of genetically engineered products, albumin is still one of the major products that is produced from human plasma by a manifacturing process defined "fractionation". Cohn's method is the basis for most of the large scale productions of albumin today [16]. The Cohn's process (Fig. 1) is based on differential precipitations of proteins by varying concentrations of alcohol and pH in the cold. Albumin, having the highest solubility and the lowest isoelectric point of all the major plasma proteins, remains in solution as the ethanol concentration is raised in stages from 0% to 40%, with an overall decrease in pH from neutrality to 5.8 and a temperature adjustment to $-5°C$. It is only when the pH is adjusted to 4.8, in the presence of 40% ethanol at $-5°C$, that the bulk of the albumin is finally precipitated in fraction V. After the removal of ethanol and salts, sodium acetyltryptophanate and sodium caprylate are added as stabilizers, and the albumin is filtered and bottled. The vials are then held for 10 hours at 60°C to inactivate any remaining blood-borne virus (pasteurization).

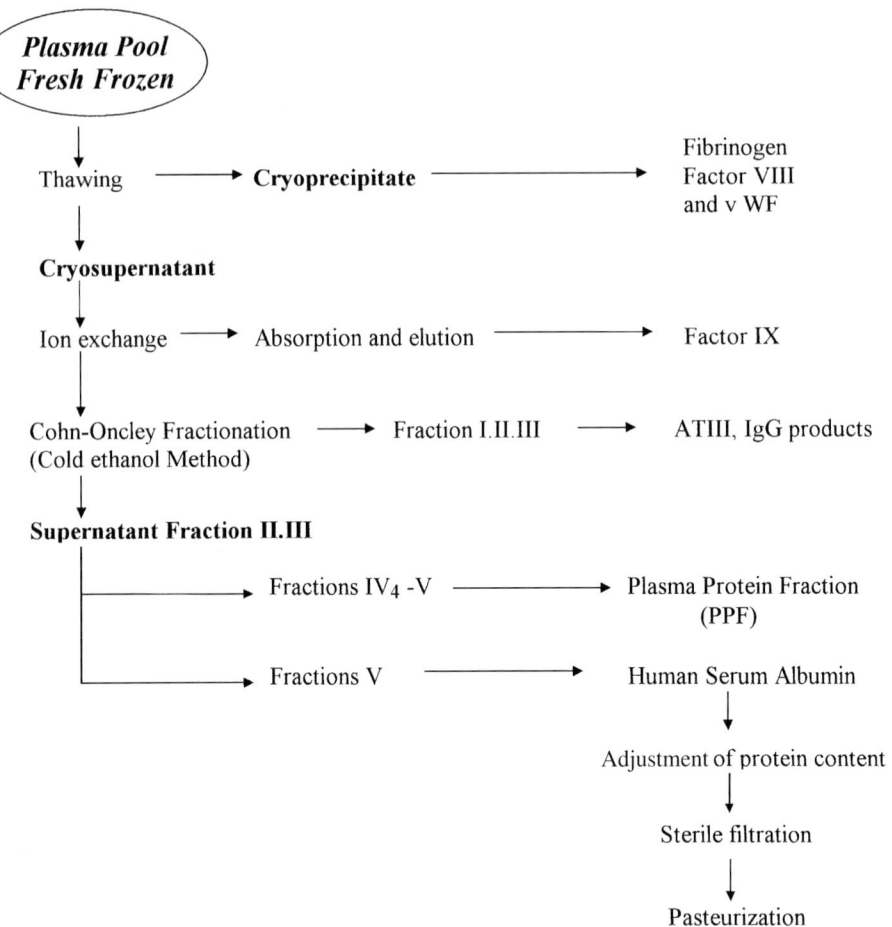

Fig. 1. Plasma fractionation process

The great advantage of the fractionation method lies in its proven safety. The Cohn's fractionation process efficiently inactivates HIV, moreover albumin products withstand virus inactivation by heat.

Three albumin products are currently manufactured: the Albumin (human) 25%, Albumin (human) 5% and plasma protein fraction (PPF). To be designated Albumin, > 96% of the protein content must be albumin. PPF is an albumin product of lower purity, obtained by coprecipitating fraction IV-4 with fraction V. The total protein in PPF must be 83% albumin, with 17% globulins, and 1% γ-globulin. PPF is more economical to produce than albumin, however this product is less safe as the rapid infusion of PPF has been associated with hypotensive episodes.

Albumin 5% is an iso-oncotic infusion solution with normal plasma which increases blood volume by the quantity actually administered. The use of 5% albumin solutions improves the microcirculation by reducing the viscosity of the circulating blood or blood plasma as a result haemodilution. This increases cardiac output.

Albumin 20% is a hyperoncotic infusion solution which creates a volume effect equivalent to approximately 3 or 4 times the quantity administered. This volume effect results in the withdrawal of liquid from the extravascular space. In case of volume deficiency, it must be administered together with another suitable fluid. Albumin 20% is ideally suited for treating hypoalbuminaemia as the volume load remains low.

The alternative to fractionated human serum albumin, unfractionated whole human plasma, is much less useful because the product [1] contains isoagglutinins [2], contains proteins such as fibrinogen, which may be unwanted [3]; and most importantly, cannot be heat sterilized.

Clinical use of albumin products

The lack of transmission of hepatitis virus and HIV has made albumin solutions appealing relative to other blood products [17]. Thus, although albumin was first introduced as a plasma volume expander, a wide variety of other uses were soon proposed for which there was little or no supporting evidence of a benefit. These uncritical uses have led to a number of efforts to define appropriate and inappropriate uses of this product [5, 17, 18].

However, the administration of albumin in the clinical setting continues to be controversial. Availability and cost concerns have forced many hospitals to review their guidelines for albumin administration. Recent studies support the use of albumin only in a limited number of situations.

Blood volume expansion

This is the primary indication for the administration of albumin, because it rapidly restores vascular volume in the setting of trauma, burns, infections and operation. In these circumstances albumin acts by raising colloid oncotic pressure, by forcing fluids to enter the intravascular compartment and to remain there [5]. However, authorities on the management of trauma and shock differ as to its value. Recent studies comparing albumin with crystalloid solutions showed that albumin, titrated to achieve a predetermined albumin concentration or COP, has not been shown to provide benefits beyond those obtained with crystalloid solutions alone when used for intravascular expansion. In addition, crystalloids have been as effective as albumin when the dose of albumin was titrated according to either an empiric formula or haemodynamic stabilization in most patients undergoing surgery [17]. However, albumin may be useful in the elderly population who requires volume expansion, because these patients may not tolerate the large volume of crystalloid solutions often needed for resuscitation.

It can be concluded that normally, in emergency care of hypovolaemic shock, primary volume replacement is provided by crystalloid solutions immediately followed by colloidal plasma expanders which exibit oncotic activity that facilitates the conservation of intravascular volume. It is however still controversial when after blood loss albumin should be used. Some suggest not to use albumin in active haemorrhage because in these cases albumin should be immediately lost, but others advise to use albumin early in order to facilitate the maintenance of correct volaemia through a proper oncotic pressure.

Haemolytic disease of the newborn (HDN)

Bilirubin is bound to albumin by two binding sites of different avidity and some compounds, such as sulfonamides, penicillins, cephalosporins and antimicrobial drugs, can displace bilirubin from high affinity binding site on albumin.

The rationale of the administration of albumin in this condition (1 g/kg of bw daily) is to increase the reserve of albumin binding capacity, as albumin carries a high affinity binding site for bilirubin. The decrease of free bilirubin in the circulation reduces the risks of the complications of HDN and in some occasion the need for exchange transfusion.

A caution in administering albumin in this condition should be observed when the infant is severely anaemic, for the possibility to trigger an acute heart failure [19].

Therapeutic plasma exchange

In therapeutic plasma exchange, different solutions (fresh frozen plasma - FFP, albumin, or other plasma derivatives such as PPF) can be used to provide the colloid necessary to replace the patient's plasma. The optimal replacement fluid varies, depending on the indication for the procedure. Traditionally FFP have been extensively used as an exchange-fluid [17] and it is still the replacement fluid of choice for the treatment of TTP, but because of the risk of infectious disease transmission it has been progressively abandoned and albumin solution or PPF have been more and more utilized.

In order to reduce the use of albumin in our hospital the following exchange protocol has been adopted:

Exchanged plasma (ml)	Fluids utilized	Volume administered (ml)
0-1000	Crystalloid	1200
1000-2000	Colloid (Gelatin o Hespan)	1000
2000-3000	Albumin 4%	1000
Reinfusion to cover dead space	Albumin 20%	100 ml

The protocol has been experimented in 10 reumathoid arthritis patients in whom 88 procedures have been performed. Twelve, not severe, complications episodes have been experienced: hypotension that could be corrected with an increase of reinfusion velocity and 7 episodes of nausea, 4 spontaneously solved in a short time and 3 treated (metorlopramide 10 mg i.v.). No untoward effect due to colloid administration was observed. Serum albumin concentration at the end of the procedure was 3.38 ± 0.58 g/dL vs. 3.5 ± 0.50 at the beginning. The protocol is considered safe as the incidence and type of untoward effect was similar to what observed in patients treated with the standard protocol (exchange fluid = albumin 4%) with a 60% reduction of albumin use.

Critically ill patients

Hypoalbuminaemia is a frequent finding in patients in intensive care units (ICU). The pathophysiology is multifactorial: reduced synthesis due to undernutrishment, impaired liver function, infection and inflammatory episodes that depress the synthesis rate and increase consumption, loss of the molecule through the kidneys and intestine. In these patients hypoalbuminaemia has often been correlated to hospital morbidity. For this reason it has been suggested to rise albumin concentration above 30 g/L, particularly in elderly patients [20].

Paracentesis

Ascites is a frequent and serious complication in patients with cirrhosis of the liver. It can usually be successfully controlled by dietary, Na restriction and carefully monitored diuretic therapy. However, therapeutic paracentesis in association with administration of albumin (6-8 grams per liter of ascitic fluid removed) is a relative safe alternative that have been proven to be effective, in these patients, in preventing acute complications such as hyponatraemia and renal impairment associated with paracentesis and has gained widespread acceptance [21]. Studies are needed to compare the less expensive saline solutions with albumin for the acute stabilization of problems associated with this procedure. The only randomized trial in patients with cirrhosis not undergoing paracentesis found no benefits from the addition of albumin administration to diet and diuretic therapy [17]. However, it has been proven that other plasma expanders offer a cheaper alternative to albumin.

Nephrotic syndrome

Chronic albumin loss, such as in chronic nephrosis (and also in cirrhosis of the liver), are not improved by long term albumin administration. Albumin may be useful in combination with diuretic therapy for patients with oedema secondary to the nephrotic syndrome when diuretics alone have failed. A randomized trial with furosemide titrated to effect or adverse reactions, compared with a combined albumin and furosemide regimen, should be performed. Such a study should include patients with complications related to their oedema [17].

Thermal injuries

Severe burn injuries involving > 10% of body surface including second and third degrees burns represent an accepted indication for the use of albumin. In this situation extensive alterations of the metabolism occur with a substantial elevation of metabolic expenditure, which may exceed the limits of the patient's physiologic reserve. This is followed by hypotension, reduction of cardiac output, hypovolaemia, hypoperfusion and lactic acidosis due to the massive fluid losses in the immediate post burn. These alterations are compensated by a renal sodium retention and tubular water reabsorbtion mediated by the hypersecretion of antidiuretic hormones and aldosterone.

Some authors [22] suggest to utilize in these patients 5% albumin administration. However, when to start albumin administration is still matter of debate. Despite a number of resuscitation formulas that are recommended for patients with thermal injuries, only one randomized trial conducted in humans has compared a crystalloid with a crystalloid and albumin combination. The study found that albumin given within the first 24 hours postburn may increase the lung water level during the following week compared with crystalloid solutions. Comparative studies using albumin and crystalloids after the first 24 hours postburn should be performed because this is the time when colloids are generally used [17].

Other uses of albumin

Albumin has been recommended alone or in conjunction with other therapeutic modalities for a number of uses, including patients with cerebral ischaemia, renal transplantation, and liver resections without definitive evidence of efficacy [17].

The contraindications are: clotting disorders, cardiac insufficiency, pulmonary oedema, renal insufficiency with oliguria or anuria, oesophageal varices, known sensitivity to human proteins and in malnutrition.

Malnutrition

Most patients with severe malnutrition have severe hypoalbuminaemia resulting from relative or absolute deficiency of calories and proteins due to inadequate food intake or as a result of malabsorption. In these cases hypoalbuminaemia may be responsible of oedema. This is particularly evident in children where a deficiency in the aminoacid supply leads to a reduction in the rate of albumin synthesis by as much as 60% after only 2 weeks of low-protein intake. However, albumin should not be used in these patients unless for short periods when acute edematous complications may represent a serious problem [23]. The use of albumin to treat malnutrition is inefficient and expensive and may defer proper measures to restore caloric and amino acid intake. Only about 45 per cent of infused albumin as a total protein source enters the body protein pool of protein-depleted isocaloric patients [24].

Adverse effects

Side effects due to the administration of albumin are very rare, albumin products are inherently safe. Only a few significant adverse effects are reported in the literature. Some of these are due to technical accidents during manufacture. Probably adverse effects are more frequent by inappropriate or incorrect administration [6].

Bacterial contamination

Human serum albumin is a good culture medium for a number of organisms. Not only does it support growth, but it appears to stabilize certain organisms and preserve viability. However rarely, a lot of albumin has been found to be contaminated with bacteria. These lots produced febrile reactions, transient bacteraemia, shock, and possible sepsis in the recipient [5].

Bacterial contamination can occur because pasteurization is very effective to inactivate hepatitis and other viruses, but not to ensure bacterial sterility, which would require autoclaving [5]. Albumin cannot withstand high autoclaving temperatures, and for this reason bacterial contamination can occur and should be considered in any patient who has an episode of fever, particularly with shaking chills, during or shortly after albumin administration. It is important that samples of the administered material and other vials of the same lot be preserved for investigation.

Pyrogenic reactions

Reactions characterized by chills and fever constitute about 75 per cent of all reported reactions. It is difficult to be sure that the cause of these reactions was due to albumin administration or that they were truly pyrogenic in nature. The fact that only a single patient may be reported as reacting to a single lot of albumin suggests that most of such reactions are of other origin. These reactions are rarely severe, but, if they are suspected to be related to albumin product administration, they should be reported to the manufacturer in order to perform appropriate investigations.

Hepatitis and Human Immunodeficiency Viruses

When properly heated and protected from subsequent contamination, albumin and PPF are unable to transmit hepatitis, and this is true also when the fractionated plasma contains high levels of infective HBV. Nevertheless, an outbreak of hepatitis traceable to PPF prepared by one manufacturer occurred in 1973 [25]. It is probable that a defect in the heating process accounted for this episode, but this was never proven. It is interesting that serum albumin products prepared simultaneously by this manufacturer from similar source plasma were not infective. The requirement to screen for hepatitis B surface antigen (HBsAg) and anti-HIV and eliminate those plasma specimens that are positive has resulted in a sharp decline in the amount of HBsAg detectable in albumin products. This may contribute to the safety of the product because it has been demonstrated that the efficacy of the inactivation processes depend upon the infections burden. As HBV is relatively heat-resistant, other less resistant agents will be more easily inactivated by pasteurization.

Fortunately, the Cohn's fractionation process efficiently inactivates HIV [26]. There is not any reported instances of transmission of HIV by transfusion of albumin products. There is however some concern about other clinically important agents (hepatitis A, parvovirus B19) that are more resistant to inactivation. There is no evidence to suggest transmission of prion-type agents caused by any blood product. Recently, the uncertainty of blood product transmitting the agent of Creutzfeldt-Jakob disease has caused the recall of albumin preparations to which a donor had contributed, who subsequently fell sick from this disease.

Hypotension

It has been known for some time that the rapid administration of PPF is frequently associated with transient hypotension. Rarely, lots of human serum albumin had been thought to evoke a similar reaction. This topic was investigated in great detail after an episode in which somewhat more severe hypotension was found to follow the administration of PPF prepared by one manufacturer in 1977. Although this reaction was thought to be due to the presence of bradykinin in trace amounts, these investigations demonstrated that prekallikrein activator (PKA), which is present in PPF and in a few lots of human serum albumin, was responsible. The PKA activates the production of bradykinin from the recipient's own kinin system. This problem has been resolved by changes in the manufacturing process that result in the inactivation of PKA [27].

Other reactions

A number of other reactions have been reported in relation to the administration of albumin products. Of these, urticaria is the most believable. Many such reports may involve coincidences that do not involve a cause-and-effect relationship.

Contamination of albumin preparations with aluminium have been of some concern, particularly for patients receiving large doses, such as is the case in long-term plasma exchanged patients [28]. Aluminium may also be a contaminant of other parenteral solutions [29], and of some buffers and filter materials used for infusable solutions. Moreover, it also may leak from the glass used in the manufacture of the bottles and then reach rather high concentrations of up to 4 mg/l. The low aluminium content of albumin solutions is an important factor, particularly in the treatment of dialysis patients and premature babies, whose kidney function is limited. With the treatment of these patients in mind, health authorities require levels < 200 µg/l, a small residual concentration that appears acceptable.

Risks caused by improper administration

Excessive administration of albumin should be avoided. If the concentration of albumin is raised artificially above about 5.5 g/dl in the plasma, a hyperoncotic state is induced that, in the absence of available extracellular fluid, results in increased albumin catabolism and decreased hepatic synthesis. If there is excessive extracellular fluid, excessive albumin administration will result in a rise in intravascular volume and possible pulmonary oedema. The same effect can occur if excessive amounts of albumin and crystalloid are given simultaneously.

These adverse reactions are more frequent and severe in patients with heart disease who have lowered cardiac functional reserves. Both the rate of administration and amount given are important. Pulmonary oedema can occur in both the clinical context of treatment of hypovolaemia with rapid fluid and albumin administration and in the more leisurely paced treatment of other hypoalbuminaemic state. Careful, frequent evaluation of the patient, with preliminary calculation of the replacement need in both amount and rate, will minimize these adverse reactions.

Guidelines

The use of albumin varies significantly from country to country. The calculation of albumin used in each country is difficult for the following reasons: 1) the statistic of the use of plasma derivatives, that are mainly distributed by pharmacists, are not so accurate as for blood components, distributed exclusively by the blood transfusion services; 2) generally the local production of albumin is known, but the information on the imported products is generally unreliable; 3) in many countries, to lower the costs of treatment, FFP and cryodepleted plasma are used with the same indications of albumin. However, it can be calculated that the use of albumin varies from 200 to 450 kg/million of inhabitants.

Growth of albumin use has been facilitated by the availability of the supply and the producers promoted uses for which there was little or no supporting evidence. However, the high cost of albumin relative to less expensive alternatives, such as nonprotein colloid (e.g., hetastarch, dextran) and crystalloid solutions (e.g., lactated Ringer's solution, various sodium chloride solutions), has intensified clinical use of resuscitation fluids. In response to the controversy, different health authorities developed guidelines for the appropriate clinical use of albumin [5, 30, 31].

Recently published reports suggest that crystalloids solutions (lactated Ringer's and chloride solutions) are the fluids of choice for many conditions as they are equally effective and less costly. The results of a recent consensus [32] on the appropriate and efficient use of albumin, non-protein colloids and crystalloids solutions are summarized in Table 1.

An operational study conducted in 15 academic health centers [33] to assess the appropriateness of albumin and colloids, demonstrated that albumin and colloids were administered mostly in the intensive care (50%) or operating room (31%). The most common prescribers were surgeons (45%) and anaesthesiologists (20%). In 24% of the cases the administration was appropriate (appropriateness based on "model" consensus derived indication guidelines), 62% was unappropriate and 14% unevaluated.

The conclusion of all these efforts can be that for a better use of albumin and other plasma expanders it is important that the guidelines are prepared in each

Table 1. Guidelines for the use of albumin, non protein colloid and crystalloid solution

Indication	Crystalloid	Colloid	Albumin
Haemorrhagic shock	First step	Second step	When Na restriction is required use 25% albumin diluted in 5% glucose
Non haemorragic shock	First step	After 2L of ineffective cristalloids in the presence of capillary leak with pulmonary and peripheral edema	When colloids are contraindicated
Thermal injury	Within the first 24 h	After 24 h > 50% host surface when cristalloid ineffective to maintain volemia	When colloids are contraindicated
Cerebral ischaemia	First choice indication	Only when Hct < 40%	Discouraged
Nutritional intervention			Only when enteral feeding is associated with diarrhoea. Serum albumin < 20 g/L
Cardiac surgery	Fluid of choice (priming solution for CPB pumps)	To avoid interstitial fluid accumulation	Last choice
Cirrhosis and paracentesis	When removal of ascites is < 4L	In association with cristalloids	When removal of ascites is > 4L
Hepatic resection	First step to maintain volaemia when resection is > 40%	Second step when resection is > 40%	When colloids are contraindicated
Nephrotic syndrome			Short term administration. In association with diuretics in acute severe peripheral or pulmonary oedema
Plasmapheresis	First step	Second step	When > 20 ml/kg in one session or per week in repeated sections. Always in association with colloids and/or crystalloids
Liver transplantation			Postoperatively to control ascites or peripheral oedema when albuminaemia < 2.5 g/dL Hct > 30% pulmonary capillary wedge pressure < 12 mmHg
Hyper-bilirubinaemia in HDN	Not indicated	Not indicated	Not conclusive results when used as an adjuvant to exchange transfusion

Modified from [33]

single institution and applied after local review and approval. These guidelines should recommend that patient-specific clinical endpoint be defined before fluid therapy is begun as this step is often overlooked. It is also important that these guidelines indicate the criteria for auditing the prescription, in order to constantly monitor the correct use of the albumin and other resuscitation fluids. The control on the overuse of albumin has significant clinical and economic implications because albumin has periods of short supply and it is generally at least 50% more expensive than colloids and about 20 times than crystalloids. The compliance to guidelines will lead to a cost-efficient use of albumin and of the other resuscitation fluids as recommended particularly in a period of an increasingly cost conscious health care.

References

1. Dugaiczyk A, Law SW, Dennison OE (1982) Nucleotide sequence and the encoded amino acids of human serum albumin mRNA. Proc Natl Acad Sci USA 79:71-75
2. Carlson P, Sakamoto Y, Laurell C et al (1992) Alloalbuminemia in Sweden: Structural study and phenotypic distribution of nine albumin variants. Proc Natl Acad Sci USA 89:8225-8229
3. Peters Jr (1985) The serum albumin. Adv Prot Chem 37:161-245
4. Urban J, Inglis AS, Edwards K et al (1974) Chemical evidence for the difference between albumins from microsomes and serum and a possible precursor product relationship. Biochem Biophys Res Commun 61(2):494-501
5. Sgouris JT, Rene A (eds) Proceedings of the Workshop on Albumin, 1975. Bethesda, Mld, National Heart and Lung Institute 1976, US Dept of Health, Education, and Welfare publication NIH 76-925
6. Tullis JL (1977) Albumin. Background and use. JAMA 237:355-360
7. Simonescu N (1979) The microvascular endothelium: Segmental differentiations; transcytosis, selective distribution of anionic sites. In: Weissmann G, Samuelson B, Paoletti R (eds) Advance in Inflammation Research. Vol 1. Raven Press, NY, p 61
8. Watkins S, Madison J, Galliano M et al (1994) Analbuminemia: Three cases resulting from different point mutations in the albumin gene. Proc Natl Acad Sci USA 91:9417-9421
9. Falkenberg C, Bjork L, Akerstrom B (1992) Localization of the binding site for streptococcal proteins G on human serum albumin. Identification of a 5.5-kilodalton protein G binding albumin fragment. Biochemistry 31:14551-14557
10. Grootendorst AF, van Wilgenburg MG, de Laat PH et al (1988) Albumin abuse in intensive care medicine. Intens Care Med 14:554-557
11. Grunett A (1991) Osmometrie und Onkometrie in der intensivmedizinischen Diagnostik und Therapie. Schweiz. Z Milit Med 68:69-73
12. James WPT, Hay AM (1988) Albumin metabolism: effect of albumin supplementation during parenteral nutrition on hospital morbidity. Crit Care Med 16:1177-1182
13. Rothschild MA, Oratz M, Mongelli J (1968) Effects of a short-term fast on albumin synthesis: Studies in vivo, in the perfused liver, and on amino acid incorporation by hepatic microsomes. J Clin Invest 47:2591
14. Mosnage HJ, Janssen JAM, Franssen JH et al (1987) Study of the molecular mechanism of decreased liver synthesis of albumin in inflammation. J Clin Invest 79:1635-1641
15. Saunders LW, Schmidt BJ, Mallona RL et al (1987) Secretion of human serum albumin from Bacillus subtilis. J Bacteriol 169:2917
16. Cohn EJ, Strong LE, Hughes WL Jr et al (1946) Preparation and properties of serum and plasma proteins. IV. A system for the separation into fractions of the proteins and lipoprotein components of biological tissues and fluids. J Am Chem Soc 68:459

17. Erstad BL, Gales B, Rappaport WD (1991) The use of albumin in clinical practice. Arch Intern Med 151:901-911
18. Swisher SN (ed) Report of Panel 6 on safety and efficacy of blood and blood derivatives. Bureau of Biologics, Food and Drug Administration. The Federal Register 1980
19. Bowman JM (1995) Hemolytic disease of the fetus and newborn. 1995 Conn's Current Ther (Rakel RE, Ed) Saunders, Philadelphia 329-334
20. Grant JP (1994) Nutritional support in critically ill patients. Ann Surg 220:610-616
21. Gines P, Arroyo V, Vargas V et al (1991) Paracentesis with intravenous infusion of albumin as compared with peritoneovenous shunting in cirrhosic with refractory ascites. New Engl J Med 325:829-835
22. Finkelstein JL, Schwartz SB, Madden MR, et al (1992) Pediatric burns: An overview. In: Di Maio (ed) Pediatric emergency medicine. Ped Clin North America 39:1145-1164
23. James WPT, Hay AM (1968) Albumin metabolism: Effect of the nutritional state and the dietary protein intake. J Clin Invest 47:1958-1972
24. Waterhouse C, Bassett SH, Holler J (1949) Metabolic studies on protein depleted patients receiving a large part of their nitrogen intake from human serum albumin administered intravenously. J Clin Invest 28:245
25. Pattison CP, Klein CA, Leger RT et al (1976) Field studies of type B hepatitis associated with transfusion of plasma protein fraction. In: Sgouris JT, René A (eds) Proceedings of the Workshop on Albumin, p 315
26. Wells MA, Wittek AE, Epstein JS et al (1986) Inactivation and partition of T-cell lymphotrophic virus, type III, during ethanol fractionation of plasma. Transfusion 26:210-215
27. Alving BM, Hojima Y, Pisano JJ et al (1978) Hypotension associated with prekallikrein activator (Hageman-factor fragments) in plasma protein fraction. N Engl J Med 299:66
28. Maharaj D, Fell GS, Boyce BF et al (1987) Aluminium bone disease in patients receiving plasma exchange with contaminated albumin. Brit Med J 295:693-696
29. Recknagel S, Bratter P, Crissafidou A et al (1994) Parenteral aluminum loading in critical care medicine part I: Aluminum content of infusion solutions and solutions for parenteral nutrition. Infusionssther Transfusionsmed 21:266-273
30. Development Task Force of the College of American Pathologists (1994) Practice parameters for the use of fresh-frozen plasma, cryoprecipitate, and platelet administration practice guidelines. JAMA 271:777
31. Devine P, Linden JV, Hoffstadter LK et al (1993) Blood donor-, apheresis-, and transfusion-related activities: results of the 1991 American Association of Blood Banks Institutional Membership Questionnaire. Transfusion 33:779
32. Vermeulen LC, Ratko TA, Erstad BL et al (1995) A paradigm for Consensus. The University hospital consortium guidelines for the use of albumin, nonprotein colloid and crystalloid solutions. Arch Intern Med 155:373-379
33. Yim JM, Vermeulen LV, Erstad BI et al (1995) Albumin and non protein colloid solution use in US academic health centers. Arch Intern Med 155:2450-2455

ASSESSMENT OF THE CARDIOPULMONARY FUNCTION IN THE ICU

Capnography

B. ALLARIA, M. DEI POLI, M. FAVARO

The capnographic signal is the end result of a series of passages, each of which in its turn is conditioned by different factors.

The first passage consists of CO_2 production in the tissues, which is influenced in its turn by the type of substrate used in the energy metabolism, by body temperature and any drugs (e.g. sedatives) used.

The second passage consists of CO_2 transport and the factors that influence it above all are the cardiac output and pulmonary flow.

The third passage is the disposal of CO_2 in the lungs: this is affected by lung diseases, respiratory rate, and also by the pulmonary blood flow, and above all by the ventilation/perfusion ratio (V/Q).

An "intelligent" use of the capnographic signal and its relation with the tidal volume and the blood gas analysis data provides important information about the metabolism, the efficiency of the ventilation and the haemodynamic situation.

Capnographic techniques

There are two techniques for measuring CO_2: infrared ray (IR) absorption and colourimetry.

The latter technique is based on the modification of a sensitive paper filter to changes in pH. The CO_2 reacts with the water present as vapour in the exhaled air leading to the production of carbonic acid and a decrease in pH proportional to the quantity of CO_2.

This technique is semi-quantitative and provides rough information about the presence of CO_2, in general with three possible changes in colour corresponding to 3 ranges of different $PetCO_2$: from 0 to 4 mmHg, from 5 to 20 mmHg and > 20 mmHg. These filters are not suitable for prolonged monitoring and can be used to assess the correctness of intubation or the efficacy of a cardiopulmonary resuscitation manoeuvre (a $PetCO_2$ of around 15 mmHg demonstrates efficacious resuscitation manoeuvres and a sudden rise > 20 mmHg accompanies the return to a sufficient autonomous cardiocirculatory activity).

The most widely-used technique for capnographic monitoring in intensive care or the operating room is the one using infrared ray absorption, which has two variations in its turn (according to the different types of sensor):

a) Solid State (with an IR source pulsated at two wavelengths, one not absorbed by CO_2 to provide a reference value, and one absorbed to be used for measurement);

b) Chopper Wheel: a moving fenestrated disk which rotates allowing the infrared rays to come periodically into contact with the sample to be analysed and with a sample with known CO_2 in a sealed cell.

Evidently, since the "Solid State" measurement technique does not contain moving parts, it enables less fragile structures to be created than with the "Chopper Wheel" technique.

Both IR ray techniques can have two variations according to the positioning of the sensor, and of the CO_2 which can be placed along the ventilation channel, generally between the Y of the respirator and the endotracheal tube (mainstream) or remote from the ventilation channel; in general it is attached to the capnograph by means of a small tube (sidestream). In the second case the sampling is done with a suction pump.

The mainstream technique is less influenced by the condensation water and gives a faster response. In general the mainstream capnographic systems give rise to fewer problems, they last a long time and occupy little space. Naturally the mainstream systems are not suitable for non-intubated patients. We shall see later that capnography can also be useful for assessing non-intubated patients. In this case it is essential to use a sidestream system connected to a nasopharyngeal tube.

In the past capnography has supplied precious information based on a sharp or gradual increase and decrease in $PetCO_2$, on the morphology of the capnogram and on the calculation of the gradient between $PaCO_2$ and $PetCO_2$. In modern instruments, the availability of the airway flow combined with capnography makes it possible to monitor the volume of CO_2 produced and the dead space (Fig. 1).

If we make a graph with the $PaCO_2$ on the y axis and the Tidal Volume exhaled on the x axis, we can observe 3 phases (Fig. 2): phase 1 represents the airway dead space; phase 2 represents a mixture of gases without CO_2 coming from the dead space and of gas rich in CO_2 coming from the alveoli; naturally as exhalation continues the mixture increasingly contains alveolar gas rich in CO_2 so a plateau is reached (phase 3), corresponding to the elimination of exclusively alveolar gas.

Using the same graph it is possible to calculate the airway dead space (Fig. 3) and the volume of CO_2 produced with each breath (area X) which multiplied by the respiratory rate gives the volume of CO_2 eliminated per minute (VCO_2).

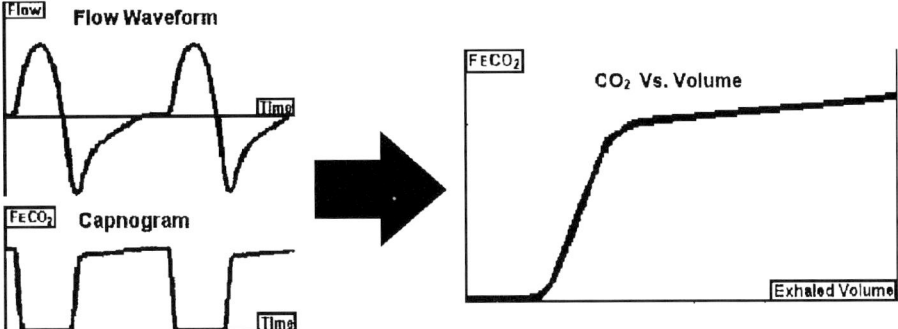

Fig. 1.

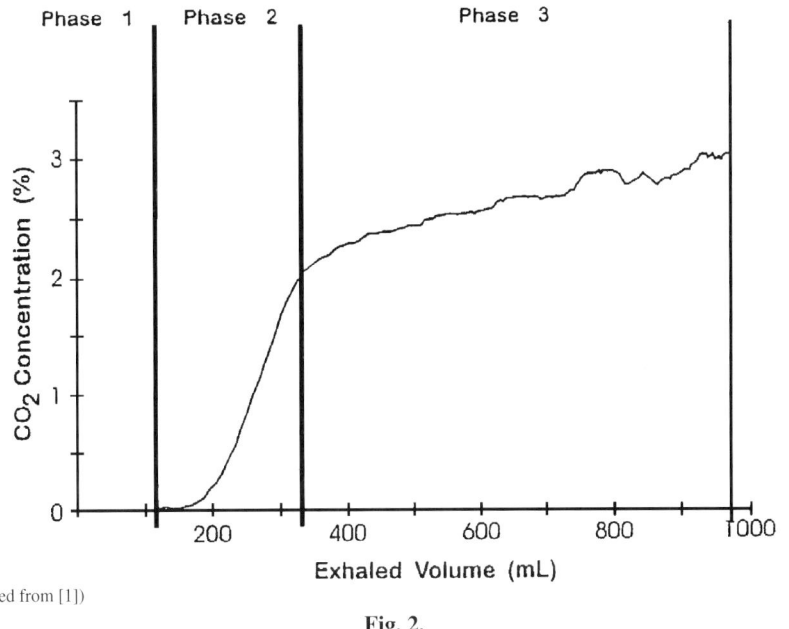

(Modified from [1])

Fig. 2.

The calculation of the dead space is made tracing a tangent to phase 3 and a vertical which intersects the tangent and forms the two equal areas "p" and "q". The part of the tidal volume which reaches the vertical is the dead space.

Knowing the $PaCO_2$ by analysing the arterial blood gas, if we complete the previous graph it is possible to calculate the physiological dead space and the alveolar dead space which compose the airway dead space calculated earlier (Fig. 4).

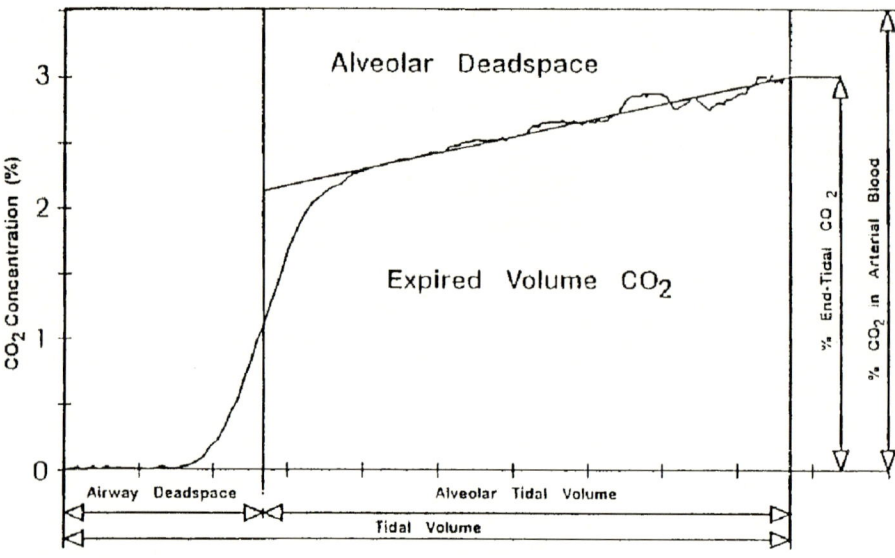

(Modified from [1])

Fig. 3.

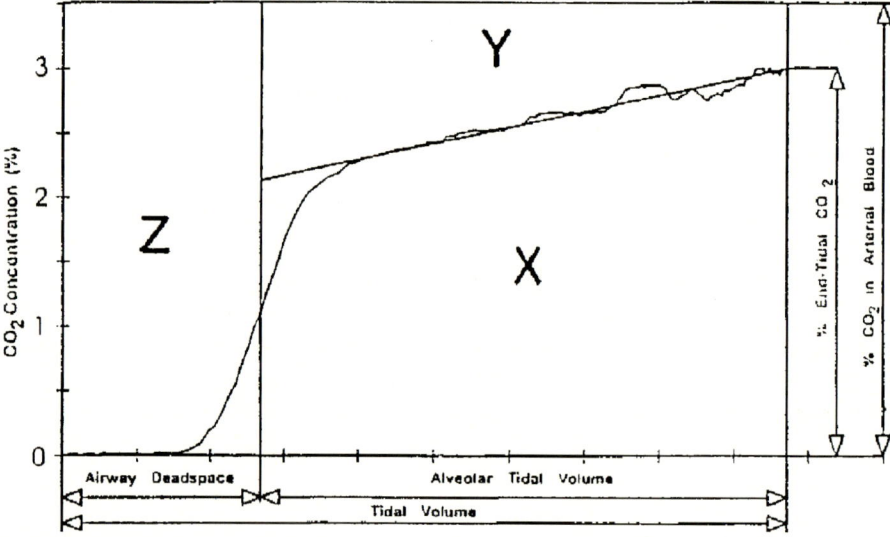

(Modified from [1])

Physiol Vd/Vt $\dfrac{(Y + Z)}{(X + Y + Z)}$

Physiol Vd = (Vd/Vt Physiol) (V+)

Vd alv = Vd Physiol – "Vd vie aeree"

Fig. 4.

It is evident from what has been said up to now that capnography, already precious for the advantages it offered in the past, is becoming a monitoring technique which is able to provide ever more complex data on artificial ventilation, especially when it is associated with measurement of the airway flow (e.g. SMO Plus Novametrics) [1].

Use of capnographic data

The most commonly used information is that regarding $PetCO_2$ which may increase or decrease in particular situations during artificial ventilation.

An increase of $PetCO_2$ may be linked to different factors which appear in Table 1 and which can be metabolic, circulatory, ventilatory or pharmacological.

Table 1. Factors causing an increase in $PetCO_2$

Decrease in ventilation
Improvement of diminished cardiac output
Recovery from cardiocirculatory arrest
Onset of hyperthermia
Shivering or muscular activity (psychomotor agitation)
Bicarbonate infusion
Resolution of bronchospasm

More important from a clinical point of view is the measurement of a fall in $PetCO_2$. Various factors may be responsible in this case too, and they are listed in Table 2, but basically it is the speed with which a fall in $PetCO_2$ occurs. In fact, while gradual decreases do not generally correspond to dramatic events, sharp falls in $PetCO_2$ when ventilation is constant always correspond to major events which cause sharp falls in output with a consequent sharp reduction in pulmonary flow, associated later on with a fall in CO_2 production.

Table 2. Factors causing $PetCO_2$ reduction

Decreased heart output
Pulmonary embolism
Bronchospasm
Alteration of V/Q
Diminished muscular activity (sedatives, curare)
Hypothermia
Increased ventilation

The rapid fall in PetCO$_2$ is defined as "exponential" and haemodynamically significant (when ventilation is constant) when it is halved in 10-15 breaths [2]. Of course the worsening in the haemodynamics may have various causes (blood loss, obstruction of venous return, pulmonary embolism etc.), but it is important to remember that an exponential decrease in PetCO$_2$ is serious when ventilation is constant. Deriaz et al. [3] have demonstrated the link between an exponential fall in PetCO$_2$ and a fall in the CI in anaesthesia with constant ventilation. Similar results are reported by Shibutani et al. [4] in aortic surgery. These authors in particular are able to quantify the foreseeable decrease in the CI knowing the decrease in PetCO$_2$ and establishing a ratio of 1:3 between the decrease in PetCO$_2$ and that of the CI.

There is disagreement about this quantification, indeed other authors have found the ratio higher (1:2) [5].

Another example of the clinical use of capnography is the interpretation of the increase in the PetCO$_2$ during resuscitation manoeuvres in cardiocirculatory arrest. It is necessary to distinguish between the cardiac arrest that occurs in the ICU in a ventilated patient and the cardiac arrest that happens in another place in the hospital or out of hospital, in a patient with spontaneous breathing. In ventilated patients, the interruption of CO$_2$ production and of pulmonary flow is accompanied by a collapse in PetCO$_2$; after this transitional phase, the behaviour of the two types of patient is identical: the PetCO$_2$ is directly proportional to the efficacy of the massage.

Several authors agree about the utility of capnography in improving the possibility of forecasting the success or failure of the resuscitation manoeuvres.

Asplin and White [6] have shown that the PetCO$_2$ of successfully resuscitated patients is higher than the PetCO$_2$ of patients with a negative outcome. Contineau et al. [7] obtained similar results.

According to these authors, PetCO$_2$ values below 10 Torr in the first 20' of cardiopulmonary resuscitation are always accompanied by a negative outcome.

The PaCO$_2$-PetCO$_2$ gradient

The isolated PetCO$_2$ situation gives further precious data if compared with the blood gas analysis data of arterial CO$_2$ (PaCO$_2$). The PaCO$_2$-PetCO$_2$ gradient is normally 2-5 mmHg. It can be imagined that an increase in this gradient means an alteration in the possibility of the lung eliminating CO$_2$. This may happen in very different conditions but they all have the same significance, and that is a change in the ventilation/perfusion ratio which in its turn may be due to a reduced perfusion of the ventilated alveoli (major hypovolaemia, microthrombosis of the pulmonary vessels, lung embolism), alteration in the capillary alveolar barrier, atelectasy (ARDS), incomplete emptying of the alveoli (COPD). It is very important to periodically check the PaCO$_2$-PetCO$_2$ gradient when monitoring a patient under artificial ventilation for acute respiratory failure. In fact the artificial ventilation can itself cause an alteration in CO_2 elimination with the possibility of a very large increase in the gradient. Two examples: ventilation with high PEEP and ventilation with an increased I/E ratio.

It is not unusual, for example in septic patients with ARDS, that in the anxiety about reducing the lung imbibition and achieving better oxygenation, long term use of diuretics is made, with increased I/E ratios, thus contributing to causing an increase in the $PaCO_2$-$PetCO_2$ gradient linked to two factors: hypovolaemia with the resulting fall in pulmonary flow and a fall in duration of the expiratory phase. In these cases gradient increases of as much as 20 mmHg may be seen. The return to a reduced I/E ratio, a better filling of the bloodstream, and when possible an optimisation of the PEEP may make it possible to regain a more normal gradient and therefore a better CO_2 elimination [8]. Also in PEEP optimisation the $PaCO_2$-$PetCO_2$ gradient can play a very useful role [9].

In fact the PEEP may be insufficient for a satisfactory recruitment of the alveoli and in this case the $PetCO_2$ decreases with a consequent increase in the gradient. If the PEEP is excessive, alveolar hyperdistension causes vessel compression and thus a reduced alveolar perfusion with an increase in CO_2 in the vessel which abandons the hyperdistended alveolus and reduction in the $PetCO_2$.

The gradient increases also in this case. The combination of capnographic and oxymetric monitoring enables a graph to be constructed such as in Fig. 5, which enables the most efficacious PEEP to be chosen (10 cm H_2O in the case shown in the figure).

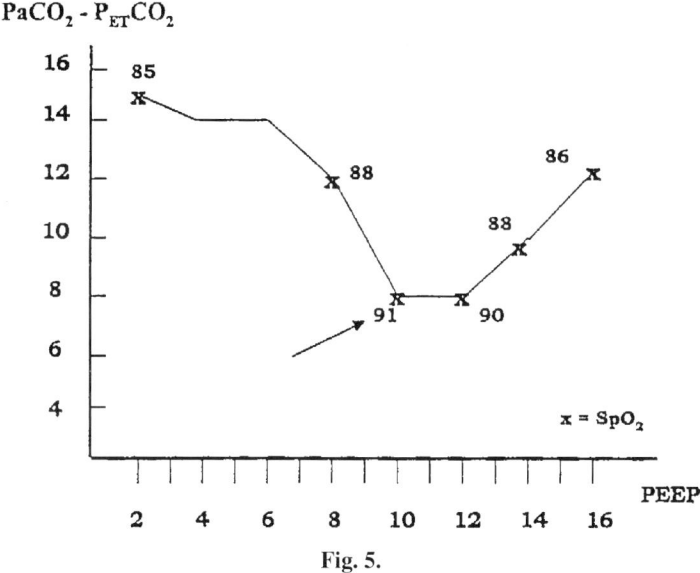

Fig. 5.

On the contrary we do not find the proposals made by others advisable, namely the use of continuous $PetCO_2$ in order to forecast the $PaCO_2$. If it is true for example that when the arterial blood gas analysis shows that the $PaCO_2$-$PetCO_2$ gradient is 4, one simply adds 4 to the $PetCO_2$ to obtain $PaCO_2$, it is also true that the gradient measured is characteristic of the moment in which it was measured and that therefore an estimate of the $PaCO_2$ on this basis can lead to errors in evaluation and above all, it prevents a sudden gradient increase from being noticed, in general it is underestimated. Since as we have said, both a reduced alveolar ventilation and a reduced perfusion cause an increase in the $PaCO_2$-$PetCO_2$ gradient, it becomes difficult to understand if an increase in the gradient is linked to a reduction or to an increase in the V/Q ratio. It is well to remember however that an increase in V/Q (increase in the dead space) has a greater effect on the $PaCO_2$-$PetCO_2$ gradient than a reduction of the same (shunt). If there are any doubts they are settled by observation of the changes in the gradient resulting from the variations in ventilation. A trend such as that described in Fig. 5 is a classical example of an increase in the gradient linked to a decrease in the V/Q ratio, which improves when a more efficacious ventilation is obtained. Finally it must be said that the $PaCO_2$-$PetCO_2$ is greatly influenced by body temperature: a decrease of 1°C increases the gradient by 100% and a decrease of a further degree increases it by another 50% [10] if the $PaCO_2$ is not corrected for the temperature.

Volumetric capnography and capnography of the non-intubated patient

The possibilities offered by volumetric capnography for optimising artificial ventilation and for weaning are extremely interesting. The availability of continuous monitoring of the $PetCO_2$, VCO_2, alveolar ventilation, total dead space in the airways, physiological dead space and alveolar dead space provided by apparatus such as the already-mentioned CO_2 SMO Plus, which also adds fundamental data about the mechanics of breathing to the above-mentioned parameters, makes it possible to manage refined artificial ventilation in all areas of intensive care. In particular in weaning the stability of the VCO_2 and of alveolar ventilation have an important role together with the more commonly used parameters such as haemodynamic stability, the $SpO_2 > 94\%$, respiratory rate < 30 breaths/min, etc.

Capnography has an increasingly important role in non-intubated patients, both in assessing the efficacy of their ventilation and, as we shall see, to acquire non-invasive information about the bloodstream. In order to use capnography on a non-intubated patient, one must use "sidestream" capnography. The sample is obtained using a nasopharyngeal tube, making sure that the catheterised nasal channel is pervious. Improved perviousness can be obtained using a nasal vasodilator spray. During the measurement it is best to interrupt the provision of oxygen therapy if this is underway, in order to avoid diluting the PetCO$_2$ with the fresh gas.

If samples are correctly taken, the PetCO$_2$ shows the PaCO$_2$ well and the Pa-CO$_2$-PetCO$_2$ gradient can be checked with sufficient accuracy [11].

One of the useful applications of non-invasive capnography is in treating patients with asthma attacks. In this case the observation of the morphology of the capnogram and of the absolute PetCO$_2$ value is a useful guide to treatment. The slowing of exhalation caused by bronchospasm leads to an increase in angle "α" and a sloping appearance of the B-C plateau (Fig. 6).

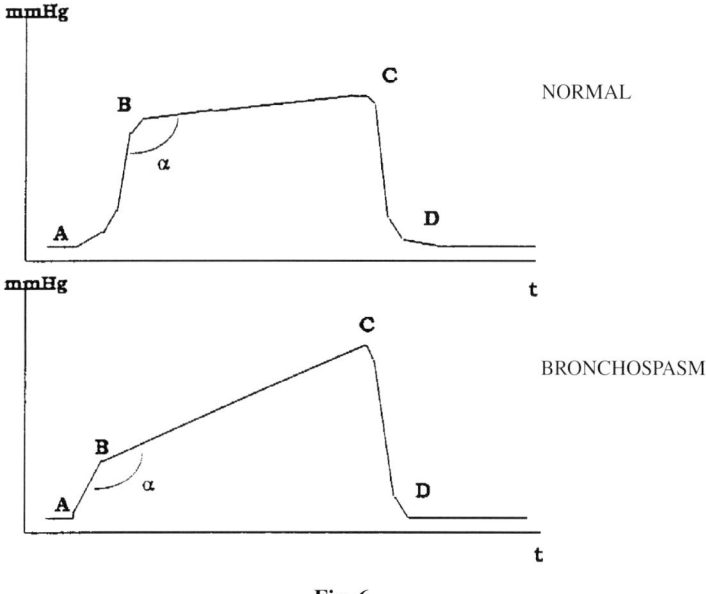

Fig. 6.

If the spray or intravenous bronchodilator treatment has the desired effect, a decrease in angle "α", in PetCO$_2$, and an improvement of the SpO$_2$ will be observed. If these positive changes do not occur, the need for intubation must be considered. Another useful clinical application of capnography in the non-intubated patient consists of the response to bloodstream filling in a patient suspected to have hypovolaemia. Rapid mass administration (250 ml of colloids) in a hypovolaemic patient causes an increase in pulmonary flow with a very modest increase in the CVP. A rapid mass increase improving pulmonary perfusion reduces the number of alveoli ventilated or poorly perfused (thus reducing the alveolar dead space). The result is a sharp increase in PetCO$_2$. In a patient with normal blood volume, with regular alveolar perfusion, a rapid mass administration does not cause a sharp increase in $PetCO_2$, moreover the increased flow to the chambers of the heart which are normally already replete leads to a greater increase in pressure. The patient with a normal blood volume therefore responds to a rapid mass administration with a fair increase in CVP but a modest or zero increase in $PetCO_2$ (Fig. 7).

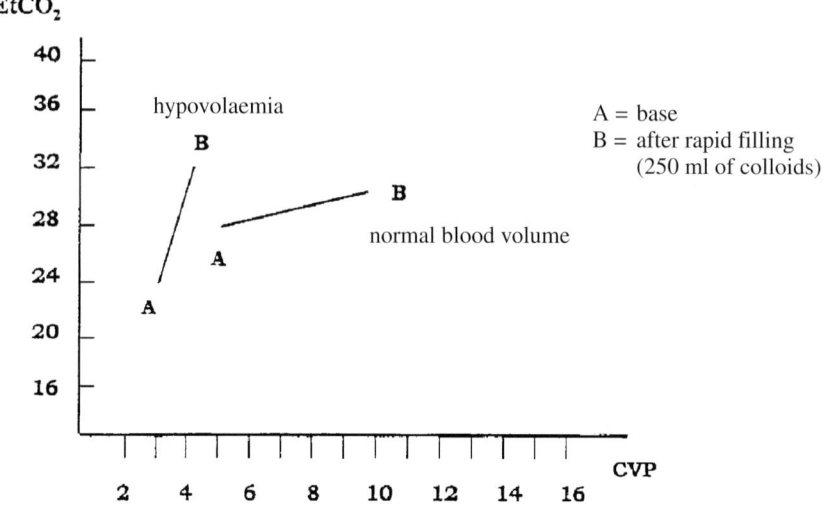

Fig. 7. Filling test with $PetCO_2$ and CVP

We believe that capnography of non-intubated patients may in the future become a very useful means of diagnosis even in non-intensive environments, such as in surgical units, for a simpler evaluation of bloodstream filling, or in hospital wards for a correct definition of the cause of hypotension. It is sufficient to think of the difference between the behaviour of the $PetCO_2$ in a hypotensive patient with vasodilation (normal or even increased $PetCO_2$) and a hypotensive patient with a reduced heart output, whatever the cause (reduced $PetCO_2$). Attempts have been made to distinguish between the cardiac origin (cardiac heart failure, CHF) of acute respiratory failure, and the respiratory origin (chronic obstructive pulmonary disease, COPD/asthma), by using the $PetCO_2$. A very recent work published in Chest [12] appears to show that the situations of serious respiratory failure with a cardiac origin always have a $PetCO_2$ lower than 37 mmHg. However, this finding is not sufficient to establish a correct differential diagnosis. In the above-mentioned work in fact, 22 out of 27 patients with COPD/asthma had a $PetCO_2$ lower than 37 mmHg. It therefore seems possible to affirm that a $PetCO_2$ higher than 37 mmHg is more typical of COPD/asthma patients than of CHF patients, but this may be only indicative. It must be added that in COPD patients the $PetCO_2$ is often poorly representative of the $PaCO_2$ and that to obtain an alveolar $PetCO_2$ it is advisable to use forced expiration ($PemCO_2$) [13].

As a conclusion, we cannot neglect to recommend an extension of the use of capnography to patients not in intensive care. In fact capnography in artificially ventilated patients both in the operating room and in the intensive care unit is sufficiently well-known and utilised, while in other units, where it could be just as useful, its is almost unheard of. Further possibilities will be provided to non-intensive units if the methods of measuring heart output based on the "single breath" CO_2 analysis are clinically validated [14].

References

1. Arnold JH, Thompson JE, Arnold L (1996) Single breath CO_2 analysis: Description and validation of a method. Crit Care Med 24:96-103
2. Allaria B, De Filippi L, Greco S et al (1996) Capnography and circulation. In: Gullo A (ed) 11th Postgraduate Course on Critical Care Medicine. Springer, Berlin Heidelberg New York, pp 169-178
3. Deriaz H, Song Q, Delva F et al (1993) Relationship between cardiac output and end-tidal carbon dioxide tension in anesthetized patients. Anesthesiology 79:A509
4. Shibutani K, Muraoka M, Shirasaki S et al (1994) Do changes in end tidal PCO_2 quantitatively reflect changes in cardiac output? Anesth Analg 79:829-833
5. Isserles SA, Breen PH et al (1991) Can changes in end-tidal $PetCO_2$ measure changes in cardiac output? Anesth Analg 73:808-814
6. Asplin BR, White RD et al (1995) Prognostic value of end-tidal carbon dioxide during out of hospital cardiac arrest. Ann Emerg Med 25:756-761
7. Contineau JP, Lambert Y, Merckx P et al (1996) End-tidal carbon dioxide during cardiopulmonary resuscitation in humans presenting mostly with asistole: a predictor of outcome. Crit Care Med 24:791-796
8. Hyt J (1994) Mechanical ventilation. State of the art. Advances in Anesthesia vol 11 Mosby Yearbook
9. Murrey JP, Modell JH, Gallagher TJ, Barnet MJ (1994) Titration of PEEP by the arterial minus end-tidal carbon dioxide gradient. Chest 85:100-104
10. Sitzwohl C, Kettner S, Reinpecht A et al (1998) The arterial to end-tidal carbon dioxide gradient increases with uncorrected but not with temperature-corrected $PaCO_2$ determination during mild to moderate hypothermia. Anesth Analg 86:1131-1136
11. Barton CW (1994) Correlation of end-tidal CO_2 measurements to arterial $PaCO_2$ in non intubated patients. Ann Emerg Med 23:562-563
12. Brown LH, Gough JE, Seim RH (1998) Can quantitative capnometry differentiate between cardiac and obstruction causes of respiratory distress? Chest 133:323-327
13. Tulon PP, Wallsh SM (1970) Measurement of alveolar carbon dioxide tension at maximal expiration as an estimate of arterial carbon dioxide tension in patients with airway obstruction. Am Rev Resp Dis 102:921-925
14. Arnold JH, Stentz RI, Thompson JE et al (1996) Non invasive determination of cardiac output using single breath CO_2 analysis. Crit Care Med 24:1701-1705

New Insights into Cardiovascular Monitoring: Continuous Arterial Thermodilution and Intrathoracic Blood Volume

A. PEREL, H. BERKENSTADT, E. SEGAL

Cardiac output (CO) by arterial thermodilution

The measurement of cardiac output (CO) is often done when the patient is in need of advanced haemodynamic monitoring. The current method for measurement of cardiac output is by thermodilution and necessitates the insertion of a pulmonary artery catheter (PAC), a procedure which is associated with a number of known complications, including a possible increase in mortality in critically ill patients. In addition, the CO that is derived from the PAC is influenced by the significant respiratory variations, and hence from the phase of the mechanical breath in which the injection is made. Mechanical ventilation was also shown to cause a high incidence of significant tricuspid insufficiency and mild to severe vena caval backward flow, which, like other valvular regurgitations, may reduce the accuracy of CO measured by PAC thermodilution (TD) [1].

CO may also be measured by arterial TD [2, 3], with the injection done through a CVP line, and the change in temperature sensed in a thermistor that is embedded in an arterial catheter. The CO is calculated from an arterial thermodilution curve in the usual way using the Stewart-Hamilton algorithm. The arterial (trans-cardiopulmonary) TD curves are much longer and flatter than the respective PA TD curves. Therefore, these curves are more sensitive to thermal base line drifts and the injectate has to be cold (4°C), and special algorithms are being used for refined analysis of the nature of thermal base line drift and for calculation of true TD curves. The CO measurement is however less affected by the respiratory variations, by the phase of injection within the respiratory cycle, and by valvular problems, since these variations even out during the longer measurement process.

Pulsion Medical Systems offers 2 devices (the COLD and the PiCCO) with which arterial CO can be measured by a CVP line and a 4F thermistor-tipped catheter for the detection of thermo-dilution curve, and a lumen for arterial pressure measurement. The arterial TD CO measured with the PiCCO compares favorably with the simultaneously calculated PAC CO (Table 1).

The results of Wickerts, Hoeft, von Spiegel, and Goedje (Table 1) were all obtained using the COLD system that uses the same algorithms as the PiCCO. Arterial thermodilution is also used in paediatric patients [3, 4]. Weyland et al.

Table 1. Comparisons of CO measured by PA and arterial thermodilution

Authors	Ref	pat/obs	bias CO ARTtd-PACtd	Limits of agreement	r
Lewis et al.	5	18/98			>.9
Bek et al.	2	48/804			.94
Wickerts et al.	6	6 pigs			.93
Hoeft et al.	7	/47			.97
von Spiegel et al.	8	21/48	$-4.7\% \pm 1.5\%$	-13 to 8%	.97
McLuckie et al.	3	9/	$.19 \pm .21$ l/min/m^2	$-.23$ to $.61$ l/min/m^2	
Goedje et al.	9	30/600	$.16$ l/min/m^2	$-.44$ to $.79$ l/min/m^2	.96

found arterial TD to be useful in total cavo-pulmonary anastomosis, where important cardiovascular variables such as CO and pulmonary and systemic vascular resistances usually cannot be assessed directly by the use of a conventional pulmonary artery thermodilution catheter because of the passive pulmonary perfusion after surgical exclusion of the right ventricle [4]. More recently, Tibby et al. [10] used the PiCCO system in children and infants, obtaining an excellent agreement between arterial TD CO and CO measured by the direct Fick method, even at very low CO values (24 patients, range CO 0.24-8.71 l/min, bias .03 ± .48 l/min, $r = .99$).

All these results were obtained with the arterial catheters that were inserted into the femoral artery. We, however, started recently to put these 4F catheters in the axillary artery. A total of 123 measurements were performed in 12 patients. Axillary artery cannulation was successful in all patients and produced good arterial waveforms. The mean COax was 6.75 ± 1.57 l/min and the mean COpa 6.26 ± 1.51 l/min. The correlation coefficient between the two measurements was 0.89 and the mean difference between measurements 0.47 ± 0.72 l/min. The use of the axillary route enables the measurement of CO without a PA catheter in vascular patients or wherever there is reluctance to use the femoral artery.

Continuous CO with the pulse contour method

The PiCCO computes CO continuously by an improved arterial pulse contour analysis, which is calibrated by means of an arterial TD measurement. The corresponding AUC of the arterial pressure waveform is measured by the pulse contour method and divided by the new CO value. The continuous CO is the product of the 30 seconds means of heart rate and stroke volume (SV). Table 2 shows the similarity of PCCO with CO measured with a PAC.

In addition to the continuous display of the CO itself, the instrument displays the maximal and minimal SV values, which are the mean values of the 4 highest

Table 2. Comparison of pulse contour cardiac output (PCCOa) with COpa

Authors		pat/obs	PCCO - COpa bias (l/min)	Limits of agreement min	max (l/min)
Jansen 1990	OR	7/64	0,10 ± 0,5	– 1,0	1,1
Weissmann 1993	OR	11/119	0,06 ± 0,58	– 1,1	1,22
Irlbeck 1995	ICU	20/165	0,09 ± 0,85	– 1,61	1,79
Gratz 1992	OR	127/94	0,02 ± 0,55	– 1,08	1,12
Wesseling 1993	OR	8/68	0,09 ± 0,36	– 0,6	0,8

(Modified from: Jansen JRC, Anaesthesiol. Intensivmed. Schmerzther. S1, 31: 30-34, 96)

and lowest stroke volumes during the last floating 30 sec. The SV variability, termed the stroke volume variation (SVV), seems to be a promising haemodynamic parameter. In patients who are on fully controlled mechanical ventilation, the variability of the SV can be extremely helpful in detecting latent hypovolaemia, or differentiating low preload from decreased contractility. This has been shown before with the variations in the systolic BP during mechanical ventilation. The systolic pressure variation (SPV, the difference between the max and min values of the systolic BP during one cycle of a mechanical breath), and the dDown (the decrease in systolic BP during a mechanical breath), were shown to be sensitive indicators of preload [11-14].

Thus the systolic BP of a hypovolaemic patient will markedly decrease following a mechanical breath, while a patient who is hypervolaemic or in heart failure [12] will have very small changes in the systolic BP during mechanical ventilation. The measurement of mean beat to beat variation in the Velocity Time Integral of the descending aorta blood flow (Doppler) was shown to correlate with the SPV and dDown [15]. Hence, the SVV seems to be a promising tool in the haemodynamic assessment of ventilated patients.

Intrathoracic blood volume (ITBV)

In order to identify and treat a low-flow state we need to have information regarding the cardiac preload or filling. The CVP and PAOP are poor indicators of cardiac preload due to their dependency on the compliance of the heart chambers, the intrathoracic pressure, the cardiac contractility and valvular insufficiency. They have wide normal ranges, inter-individual scatter and frequent inability to predict response to volume loading. The PiCCO system estimates preload by the measurement of volumes rather than pressures.

Central venous injection of a cold bolus results in the cold indicator distributing in an intrathoracic thermal volume (ITTV) which is composed of the intrathoracic blood volume (ITBV) and the extravascular lung water (EVLW). As

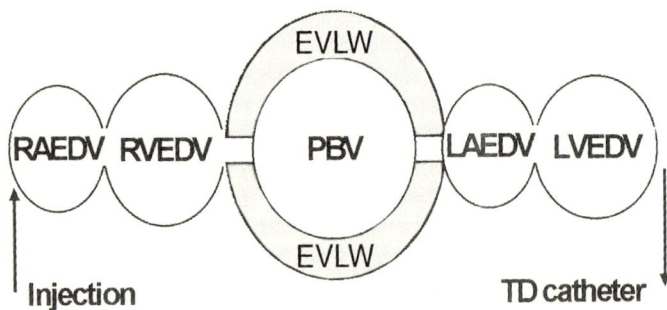

Fig. 1. Schematic description of the indicator mixing chambers of the cardiopulmonary system

can be seen in Fig. 1 the ITBV consists of the sum of all end-diastolic volumes of the atria and ventricles, i.e. the global end-diastolic volume (GEDV), which equals to 2/3 to 3/4 of the ITBV, and the pulmonary blood volume (PBV).

In numerous experimental and clinical studies the ITBV was shown to be an excellent indicator of cardiac preload [16-21]. In an experimental model of severe hypo- and hypervolaemia, Lichtwarck-Aschoff found the ITBV to be a better indicator of cardiac preload compared to CVP, PAOP and RVEDV. He also demonstrated that the ITBV was not dependent on CO, i.e., no relevant mathematical coupling [18]. The same author also found the ITBV to accurately reflect circulatory volume status in mechanically ventilated critically ill patients [19]. Hüttemann et al. could demonstrate that changes of ITBV correlated closely with changes of LVEDA [20], while Preisman et al. found the ITBV to correlate with the SPV and dDown, all three parameters reflecting haemorrhage better than CVP and PAOP [14].

Technique of measurement

Specific volumes can be calculated by multiplying the arterial CO (COart) by transit times determined through the indicator dilution curves (Fig. 2). With the double indicator technique (COLD system) the product of the mean transit time (MTt) of the dye multiplied by the COart equals the ITBV, which is the volume through which the relevant indicator has flown, i.e., the complete volume between the site of injection and the site of measurement. For the cold indicator this is total intrathoracic thermal volume (ITTV); thus the ITTV minus ITBV equals the extravascular lung water (EVLW) (Fig. 1).

The PiCCO, which uses only one (cold) indicator, calculates the mean transit time (MTt) and the exponential downslope time (DSt) of the thermodilution curve (Fig. 2). The result of the product of CO and MTt is the ITTV, while the

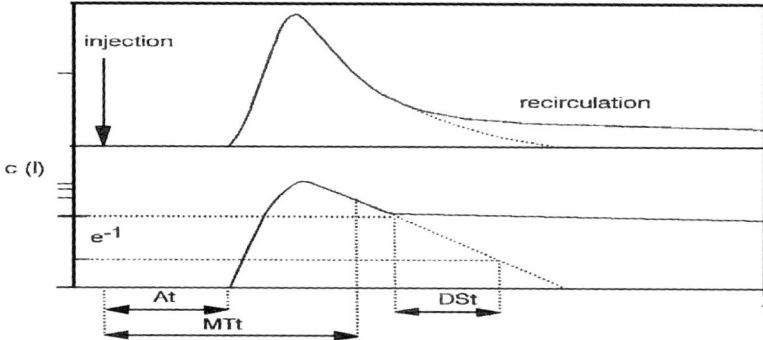

Fig. 2. Schematic depiction of a dilution curve. Note appearance time (At), mean transit time (MTt), and exponential downslope time (DSt)

product of the CO and the DSt is the pulmonary blood volume. The difference between the two is the GEDV (global end-diastolic volume), which correlates closely with ITBV in experimental and clinical studies. By using a structural regression analysis the mathematical relationship between GEDV and ITBV has been analyzed in a large patient population. This regression equation is used to estimate ITBV* from GEDV (ITBV* = a * GEDV + b).

Extravascular lung water (EVLW)

The EVLW is the difference between the intravascular distribution volume of the dye and the total thermal distribution volume. Using the estimated ITBV*, an estimated EVLW* can be calculated as well (EVLW* = ITTV − ITBV*). Thus the PiCCO offers the measurement of lung water using just one indicator. The clinical value of EVLW has been repeatedly shown [5, 22-27] and is of great importance especially in patients with increased pulmonary microvascular permeability.

Normal values (indexed) obtained with the PiCCO:

- CI 3.5-5.0 l/m^2; GEDVI 600-750 ml/m^2; ITBVI 800-1000 ml/m^2;
- EVLWI 4-7 ml/kg; SVI 40-60 ml/m^2; SVRI 1250-1750 $dyn*s*cm^{-5}*m^2$

References

1. Jullien T et al (1995) Incidence of tricuspid regurgitation and in mechanically ventilated patients. A color Doppler and contrast echocardiographic study. Chest 107:488-493
2. Bek JC et al (1989) Cardiac output measurement using femoral artery thermodilution in patients. J Crit Care 4:105-111
3. McLuckie A et al (1996) Comparison of pulmonary and femoral artery thermodilution cardiac indices in paediatric intensive care patients. Acta Paediatr 85:336-338
4. Weyland A et al (1994) Application of a transpulmonary double indicator dilution method for postoperative assessment of cardiac index, pulmonary vascular resistance index, and extravascular lung water in children undergoing total cavo-pulmonary anastomosis: Preliminary results in six patients. J Cardiothorac Vasc Anesth 8:636-641
5. Lewis FR et al (1982) The measurement of extravascular lung water by the thermal-green dye indicator dilution. Ann NY Acad Sci, pp 394-410
6. Wickerts et al (1990) Measurement of extravascular lung water by the thermal-dye dilution technique: Mechanisms of cardiac output dependence. Intensive Care Med 10:115-120
7. Hoeft A (1995) Transpulmonary indicator dilution: An alternative approach for hemo-dynamic monitoring. In: Yearbook of Intensive Care and Emergency Medicine, Springer, pp 594-605
8. von Spiegel T et al (1996) Cardiac output evaluation by means of transpulmonary thermodilution. An alternative to the pulmonary artery catheter? Anaesthesist 45:1045-1050
9. Godje O et al (1998) Reproducibility of double indicator dilution measurements of intrathoracic blood volume compartments, extravascular lung water, and liver function. Chest 113: 1070-1077
10. Tibby SM et al (1997) Clinical validation of cardiac output measurements using femoral artery thermodilution with direct Fick in ventilated children and infants. Intensive Care Med 23:987-991
11. Perel et al (1987) The systolic pressure variation is a sensitive indicator of hypovolemia in ventilated dogs subjected to graded hemorrhage. Anesthesiology 67:498-502
12. Pizov et al (1989) The arterial pressure waveform during acute ventricular failure and synchronized external chest compression. Anesth Analg 68:150-157
13. Coriat et al (1994) A comparison of systolic blood pressure and echocardiographic estimates of end-diastolic left ventricular size in patients following aortic surgery. Anesth Analg 78: 46-53
14. Preisman et al (1997) New monitors of intravascular volume: A comparison of arterial pressure waveform analysis and intrathoracic blood volume. Intensive Care Med 23:651-657
15. Beaussier et al (1995) Determinants of systolic pressure variation in patients ventilated after vascular surgery. J Cardiothoracic Vasc Anesth 9:547-551
16. Hedenstierna G (1992) What value does the recording of intrathoracic blood volume have in clinical practice? Intensive Care Med 18:137-138
17. Hoeft A et al (1994) Bedside assessment of intravascular volume status in patients undergoing coronary bypass surgery. Anesthesiology 81:76-86
18. Lichtwarck-Aschoff M et al (1996) Central venous pressure, pulmonary artery occlusion pressure, intrathoracic blood volume, and right ventricular end-diastolic volume as indicators of cardiac preload. J Crit Care 11:180-189
19. Lichtwarck-Aschoff M et al (1992) Intrathoracic blood volume accurately reflects circulatory volume status in critically ill patients with mechanical ventilation. Intensive Care Med 18: 142-147
20. Huttermann E et al (1996) Intrathoracic blood volume versus echocardiographic parameters in surgical patients. Clin Intens Care Med [Suppl]7:20
21. Pfeiffer UJ et al (1990) Sensitivity of central venous pressure, pulmonary capillary wedge pressure, and intrathoracic blood volume as indicators for acute and chronic hypovolemia. In: Lewis FR, Pfeiffer UJ (eds) Practical applications of fiberoptics in critical care monitoring. Springer, pp 25-31

22. Eisenberg et al (1987) A prospective study of lung water measurement during patient management in the intensive care unit. Am Rev Respir Dis 136:662-668

23. Mitchell JP et al (1992) Improved outcome based on fluid management in critically ill patients requiring pulmonary artery catheterization. Am Rev Resp Dis 145:990-998

24. Schuster DP (1993) The case for and against fluid restriction and occlusion pressure reduction in adult respiratory distress syndrome. New Horizons 1:478-488

25. Sturm JA (1990) Development and significance of lung water measurement in clinical and experimental practice. In: Lewis FR, Pfeiffer UJ (eds) Practical applications of fiberoptics in critical care monitoring, pp 129-139

26. Zeravik et al (1989) Efficacy of high frequency ventilation combined with volume controlled ventilation in dependency of extravascular lung water. Acta Anaesthesiol Scand 33:568-574

27. Zeravik et al (1990) Efficacy of pressure support ventilation is dependent on extravascular lung water. Chest 97:1412-1499

Echo Doppler Monitoring for the Evaluation of Cardiovascular Performances in Anaesthesia and in the Intensive Care Units

R. Muchada, P. Tortoli, F. Gudi

Medical ultrasound imaging has improved considerably because of the development of echo Doppler technics which, nowadays, allow a non invasive exploration of the heart and the large inner mediastinal vessels for diagnostic purpose [1, 2]. The echocardiographic study of the cardiac morphology and its variations provides information on the change of volume, the cardiac chamber dimension and the functional or pathological alterations of the global or regional contractility [3].

The visualization of the valvular system and of the large vessels also allows for both the functional and pathological alterations to be studied [4].

Finally, the sequential or simultaneous integration of a Doppler system broadens the diagnostic possibilities, allowing to appreciate the dynamic variations of the flow at the level of the entry and exit orifices of each cardiac chamber [5, 6], as well as at the level of the main intra-thoracic vascular trunks, especially that of the descending aorta [7].

It is nevertheless necessary to insist on the fact that these explorations are essentially devoted to a functional study for diagnostic purpose [8]. In patients under general anaesthesia or hospitalized in the intensive care area and presenting acute and rapidly evolutive pathologies requiring repeated and punctual therapeutic adjustments, the continuous monitoring of the cardiovascular function is required.

This haemodynamic monitoring has been reduced to its most simple form, by using monitoring techniques which observe the arterial blood pressure (ABP) and the ECG modifications. If we consider that the first invasive measure of the ABP was made by Stephen Hales, in the carotid of his horse in 1776 and that the ECG technology was introduced by Einthoven in 1906, the parameters used for the non invasive monitoring of the cardiovascular function in a continuous way have not made a real progress, except for some improvements regarding the acquisition, the processing and the presentation of signals on today's available devices.

On the other hand, it is interesting to analyze the information obtained.

By definition of its physical principle ABP remains the result of the blood flow multiplied by the vascular resistances. In this way all variations of ABP can be determined by an isolated variation of any of these two parameters or by its concordant and simultaneous variation.

The fact that a pseudo-stability of ABP can be determined by an opposite modification of the same two parameters is even more worrying.

Nevertheless, this pseudo-stability includes a real alteration with a rupture of the haemodynamic physiological equilibrium, which can be dangerous for the patient.

ECG monitoring provides real information about the stimulation and the inner-cardiac electrical conduction.

Today the monitoring of the ST segment could guide the appreciation of the practitioner regarding coronary perfusion and myocardial ischaemia.

Thanks to the quantity of cardiac cycles, we can obtain continuous information about the heart rate (HR). HR is an important parameter since it is one of the determinants of cardiac output, which is the result of HR multiplied by the stroke volume (SV).

The monitoring of HR provides information only about the existence of a brady-, normo- or tachycardia, but in no way about the haemodynamic component of the blood volume ejected in each systole.

Thanks to data obtained by non invasive method and in a continuous way, information on the cardiovascular functions, the current application of the new echo Doppler approach seems to be useful.

Echo Doppler methods and continuous non invasive haemodynamic monitoring

One recent application of the echo Doppler technique has been precisely aimed at measuring the aortic blood flow (ABF) in the descending aorta [9, 10] making it possible to quantify the flow and its variations. This is important because according to Guyton [11], flow variations are important elements to understand the metabolic consequences of some haemodynamic changes.

However, during the follow-up of patients hospitalized in an Intensive Care Unit, all measurements giving quantitative results must be reliable, reproducible, objective. Even when the continuous evolution of each specific parameter is observed, the system must present a correct stability.

The echo Doppler non invasive haemodynamic monitoring cannot escape this rule. For this reason, surveying the blood flow in the descending aorta by ultrasound technique implies a careful methodology and precise steps for its implementation, steps that, if neglected or forgotten, can put at risk some of the real usefulness of the information acquired.

Therefore, we need to take into consideration that:

1. It is necessary to measure the aortic diameter continuously. Only by doing so we can calculate the section of the vessel and obtain the measurement of the blood flow.

2. It is no longer possible to retain the schematic simplification which considers the velocity front of the intra-aortic blood flow to be flat, with a center-axial acceleration and a peripheral dispersion which gradually become slower but homogeneous.

   According to our previous observations, nowadays confirmed by the Multigate Doppler system, developed by the team of Professor P. Tortoli (Florence - Italy) [12, 13] the intra-aortic blood profile of velocity is very often irregular and lateral with respect to the axis. This profile of velocity is not indefinitely constant in the same patient, since it is influenced by phenomena of preload – afterload – contractility, stroke volume, and left ventricle ejection time. Hence, the necessity to obtain a homogeneous insonation of all the transversal sections of the aorta and the integration of all instantaneous velocities to obtain an average value, representative of the real mean intra-aortic velocity.

3. During the diastolic period, the presence of a negative velocity peak is a reality. These negative velocities may be divided into two categories:

   a) Real negative velocities with a retrograde linear displacement, over part of the aorta section.

   b) Forward non linear movement of the red cells stream, with a variation of the angle of incidence-reflection between the Doppler beam and the axis of the movement of the blood column. The resulting velocity vectors are very often oriented in the opposite direction with respect to the real displacement of the front of velocity and the Doppler system assimilates this fact to a negative speed.

These variations are also influenced by haemodynamic modifications (preload and afterload, stroke volume, blood velocity itself) but also by the morphology of the aortic arch, the vascular elasticity and the probable intra-aortic alterations.

A device we daily use for non invasive haemodynamic monitoring is the Dynemo 3000 (Sometec France-USA). It practically complies with all those methodological steps. But if the software included can process the really negative velocity diastolic peaks, some modification must be introduced to correct the probably ABF underestimation when false diastolic negative peaks are present.

Only acquisition and a correct signal processing will allow to present valuable results for ABF that are sufficiently precise to be used during the haemodynamic monitoring in the intensive care services.

The need for a relatively precise measurement of ABF is fundamental, not only for a follow-up of the flow, even if it does not provide, by itself, much information, but also for the calculation of other cardiovascular variables integrating a haemodynamic profile.

For example, the monitoring of ABF and HR allows to calculate the SV indexed to ABF. Obviously, provided that HR is correct, all errors of appreciation of ABF can lead to very important errors in term of systolic work, myocardial O_2 consumption, distribution of the blood flow to the peripheral regions.

In the same way, thanks to the relationship between the mean arterial pressure and ABF, the calculation of total systemic vascular resistances (TSVR) indexed to ABF makes it possible to follow the variation of the arterial pressure by carrying out a differential analysis of each of its components: flow and resistances. But once again any error in the measurement of ABF may lead to an erroneous appreciation of the real situation.

These calculations are interesting because the level of resistances may be assimilated to the notion of afterload, even if this approach is not entirely correct. The result obtained, applied to the clinic evaluation of the patients, provides very interesting information for the preservation of the flow/resistance balance, which generates a correct perfusion pressure and probably homogeneous distribution of SV to the peripheral tissue regions, thereby ensuring a correct tissue perfusion.

Left ventricle performances

The monitoring used to evaluate the contractility of the left ventricle, for diagnostic purposes, is currently obtained with transcutaneous or transoesophageal ultrasound methods [14].

Nevertheless, these techniques are currently rather selectively used: indeed they are applied only under limited circumstances and on particular subjects. Therefore, the correct interpretation of images produced with such techniques proves sometimes difficult [15].

A methodological simplification is commonly applied by users of the Dynemo 3000 system: it makes it possible to continuously measure the systolic time intervals (STI) whose experimental validation [16] opens up interesting prospects for their use when integrated in a haemodynamic profile.

But what can the real interest of such STI measurement be?

Without wanting to be exhaustive, we can evoke the following elements:

1. The function pump of the left ventricle is hardly analyzed in the context of a clinic and continuous haemodynamic monitoring.

2. The price of ejection of the volume during the systolic contraction is the myocardial consumption of energy.

3. This systolic contraction comprises the tension of the myocardial fibers (isovolumetric period). The stroke volume expulsion is ensured by the shortening of myocardiac fibers.

Among other things, the consumption of energy depends on the temporal variation of these two periods and on the volume expelled against a given resistance.

4. The use of cardiovasoactive products for therapeutic purposes (β-mimetics, β-blockers, vasodilators or vasoconstrictors) will directly influence STI as a result of these by action of these drugs or their doses, but also because of the individual reaction of each patient.

    Nowadays it does not seem correct to use cardiovasoactive products if the left ventricle contractility cannot be evaluated.

    According to our personal experience, the decision to use a β-stimulation implies at least the diagnosis of:

    a) a low ABF

    b) a HR under 100 b/min

    c) a pre ejection period indexed to the HR (PEPi) higher than 160 ms.

    Normal or high values for the total systemic vascular resistances, higher than dyn.s.cm^{-5}.

Once a decision has been made to proceed with a β-mimetic perfusion, the dose will be adjusted to the evolution of the cardiovascular parameters, with a special attention devoted to PEPi. When PEPi is lower than 130 ms, and there is no increase in SV, even if ABF increases because of the HR effect, and when the HR exceeds 100 b/min, it is useless to increase the dose of the β-mimetic. Treatment has to be oriented towards other therapeutic options (vascular filling, phosphodisterase inhibitors, products with a pure vascular action and with a short half-life).

Preload information

The directly and continuous information about the preload status is not obtained with the Dynemo device. An indirect way to evaluate the preload is to perform a filling test. When the different parameters of the haemodynamic profile lead to the diagnosis of decreased preload (decreased ABF, increased HR, decreased AP and normal or slightly increased PEPi), the rapid infusion of 200 ml of HM Starch can be carried out under haemodynamic monitoring. If this therapeutic action makes it possible to improve the cardiovascular parameters, the infusion has to be continuous until first an increase and then a plateau of the ABF value are obtained with an increase of AP, a decrease of HR and PEPi. On the contrary if ABF is not improved but PEPi increases, perfusion must not be continued.

If a relationship can be established between ABF and PEPi, a decisional curb (like those concerning CVP or wedge pulmonary pressure and CO) [16] may be used to optimize the amount of volume perfused to correct preload alterations.

Tissue perfusion evaluation

Finally, we have to insist on the fact that all the information provided by the cardiovascular monitoring concerns the haemodynamic modifications only.

Despite this information, it is impossible to evaluate the ultimate function of the cardiovascular system, which is the preservation of the tissue perfusion in the best conditions.

This function would have to be systematically evaluated to ensure the correct evolution of the patient status under the therapeutic measures implemented.

This evaluation has to be rapid, continuous and directly compared to haemodynamic changes.

If some indicators of the tissue perfusion have a real value, like for example the variation of the acid/base balance or the evolution of the diuresis, they have a very long time of reaction, which does not allow for rapid therapeutic adjustments in high risk patients.

Other disputable but useful markers ($\dot{V}O_2$, VCO_2) [17] can currently be monitored with special methods which are unfortunately little used in the clinical field.

If our choice focuses on following the rapid variation of $PetCO_2$ monitored simultaneously with the parameters of a haemodynamic profile, this is done because there is a real relationship between tissue perfusion and CO_2 elimination, when some restrictive observation conditions are respected [18, 19].

Conclusion

To be useful, the non invasive cardiovascular monitoring needs, at least, the acquisition of the information concerning the preload and afterload, the heart rate, the electrical stimulation, the intra-myocardial conduction, the synergy of ventricular contraction and blood flow, without forgetting an indicator of the quality of the tissue perfusion. Actually, all methodologies do not give access to global information, and they can mislead the operator, despite their interpretative ability, and endanger the good evolution of the patient.

A methodological approach is today offered by the system Dynemo 3000, provided that the system is used with all its potential of exploration, $PetCO_2$ trends included.

If sometimes criticism can be levelled at certain aspects of this system, like for example, difficulties related to the measurement of the pseudo-negative diastolic velocity peaks, it must be said that the method offers the possibility of a non invasive, continuous and bedside haemodynamic monitoring.

The analysis of the records obtained with the new Doppler Multigate should help to introduce some modifications in the Dynemo software, allowing this technique to be adjusted even more to a real non invasive bedside, cardiovascular monitoring in anaesthesia and in intensive care patients.

References

1. Hatle L, Angelsen B (ed) (1982) Doppler ultrasound in cardiology: physical principles and clinical applications. Led and Febiger, Philadelphia
2. Visser CA, Koolen SS, Dunning AS (1988) Transesophageal echocardiography: Technique and clinical applications. J Cardioth Anesth 2:74-91
3. Poelaert J, Trouerbach J, De Buyzere et al (1995) Evaluation of transesophageal echocardiography as a diagnostic and therapeutic aid in a critical care setting. Chest 107:774-719
4. Brooks SW, Young JC, Cmolik B et al (1992) The use of transesophageal echocardiography in the evaluation of chest trauma. J Trauma 32:761-766
5. Savage RM, Licina MG, Koch CG et al (1995) Educational program for intraoperative transesophageal echocardiography. Anesth Analg 81:399-403
6. Darmon Ph, Hillel A, Mugtader A et al (1984) Cardiac output by transoesophageal echocardiography using continuous wave Doppler across the aortic valve. Anesthesiology 80:796-805
7. Gueugniaud PY, Muchada R, Moussa M et al (1997) Continuous oesophageal aortic blood flow measurement during general anaesthesia in infants. Can J Anaesth 44:745-750
8. Seward JB, Khandheria BK, Freeman WK et al (1993) Multiplane transesophageal echography: Image orientation, examination technique, anatomic correlations and clinical applications. Mayo Clin Proc 68:523-551
9. Fontaine B, Lenoir B, Stell P, Rourier B (1998) Le Doppler oesophagien: Une alternative hémodynamique. Réan Urg 7:47-49
10. Gueignaud PY, Bertin Maghit M, Abisseror M et al (1998) Myocardial effects of isoflurane in healthy infants and small children. Acta Anesthesiol Scand 42:254-259
11. Guyton AG, Hall JE (ed) (1994) Text book of medical physiology. Overview of circulation. Saunders, Philadelphia 161-169
12. Tortoli P, Guidi G, Berti P et al (1997) An FFT-based flow profile for high-resolution in vivo investigations. Ultrasound in Med & Biol 23:899-910
13. Muchada R, Tortoli P, Guidi F et al (1998) Toward an absolute measurement of the aortic blood flow in anesthesia and intensive care. Eur J Ultrasound 7-1:16
14. Feinberg M, Hopkings W, Davila-Raman V, Barzilai B (1995) Multiplane transesophageal echocardiographic Doppler imaging accurately determines cardiac output measurements in critically ill patients. Chest 107:769-773
15. Muchada R (1997) Systolic time intervals. Experimental validation of a new measurement method. Intensive Med 34-1:91
16. Guyton AG, Hal JE (ed) (1994) Text book of medical physiology. Cardiac output. Venous return and their regulation. Saunders, Philadelphia 239-251
17. Russell JA, Phang PT (1994) The oxygen delivery/consumption controversy. Approaches to management of critical ill. Am J Crit Care Med 149:533-537
18. Petrucci N, Muchada R (1993) End tidal CO_2 come indice predittivo della perfusione regionale e sua relazione con il flusso aortico. Minerva Anestesiol 59:297-305
19. Tournadre JP, Moulaire V, Barreiro G et al (1994) Simultaneous monitoring of non invasive hemodynamic profile and capnography for tissue perfusion evaluation. J Anesth 8:400-405

CEREBRAL HOMEOSTASIS - POLYNEUROPATHY

Pathophysiology of Brain Temperature

S. Rossi, E. Roncati Zanier, N. Stocchetti

The brain is more sensitive than other organs to abnormal temperature. A rise of four or five degrees above normal deeply disturbs brain functions. Indeed it may be that the temperature of the brain is the single most important factor limiting the survival of man and other animals in hot environments. This can be desumed by the sophisticated control of the brain temperature present in mammalian.

The temperature of the brain is dependent upon three main factors: the local heat production, cerebral blood flow, and the temperature of the blood perfusing the brain.

The brain is a big consumer of energy and is a big producer of heat. It uses about 20% of the oxygen and 25% of glucose required by the body at rest (when it weights only 2-3% of the total body weight). It has been assessed that of the carbohydrate consumed by the brain, 95% undergoes oxidative metabolism: 43% of the energy originally held in glucose is captured by the ATP, the remainder is given off as heat [1]. Due to its high metabolic activity, cerebral tissue normally produces a considerable amount of heat, and the temperature of the brain is usually higher than the body core temperature. The perfusing arterial blood usually serves an important function in removing excess heat. It has been demonstrated that evaporation from the nasal and oral cavity during panting represents an effective mechanism of selective brain cooling in dogs and that this mechanism may be enhanced in other species (i.e. sheep), by the presence of a carotid rete which cools the blood directed to the brain inside the cavernous sinus [2, 3]. There is no evidence of the presence of a carotid rete in human; nevertheless it has been demonstrated a local counter current heat exchange between cool blood from the face and head skin in the cavernous sinus and the blood ascending to the brain in the carotid artery [4].

Cerebral temperature and cerebral damage

Experimental data

Hypothermia

Laboratory investigations have highlighted the marked dependence of ischaemic injury on intraischaemic brain temperature [5]. It has been demonstrated that hippocampal pyramidal neurons of the CA1 layer showed extreme grades of histologic damage (many or all neurons affected) in 100% of the hemisphere held at 36C° during ischaemia but only in 20% of those at 34 and in 0% of those held at 33C°. Similarly, ischaemic injury to the dorsolateral striatum, another selectively vulnerable area, was reduced of approximately 80% at 33-34C° and was completely eliminated when intraischaemic brain temperature was 30C° [6]. The classic mechanism proposed for protection by hypothermia is an inhibition of oxygen and glucose consumption sufficient to permit tolerance to prolonged periods of oxygen interruption. Hypothermia decreases the energy requirements of the brain by decreasing both activation metabolism required for neuronal function and the residual metabolism necessary for the maintainance of the neuronal activity. Busto et al. have shown that this pronounced protective effect of mild to moderate brain hypothermia is not explicable only on the basis of alteration in cerebral blood flow and energy metabolites during ischaemia. Further studies employing microdialysis, however, have shown that as intraischaemic brain temperature is lowered from 36 to 33C°, the normally expected sevenfold increase in the release of the excitatory neurotransmitter glutamate into the brain extracellular space, is almost totally suppressed [7]. Besides the extracellular release of dopamine is reduced by 60% [8]. Furthermore, moderate intraischaemic hypothermia has been shown in autoradiographic studies to enhance early post-ischaemic glucose utilisation and blood flow [8]. Evidences suggest that also post-ischaemic induction of moderate brain hypothermia might protect. Nevertheless if the institution of hypothermia is delayed, protection is less pronounced, suggesting the possibility that a narrow post-ischaemic therapeutic window may exist [9].

Hyperthermia

In contrast to hypothermia, brain hyperthermia has been shown to worsen outcome in several animal models of brain injury. For example, in models of cerebral ischaemia intraischaemic hyperthermia has been shown to worsen neuronal and cerebrovascular consequence. Even a delayed post-traumatic hyperthermia (4 days after a fluid percussion injury) significantly increased mortality, blood brain barrier damage and axonal damage [10, 11].

Clinical studies

These experimental evidences were partially confirmed in the clinical setting. Many clinical studies were performed in order to assess the effectiveness of prophylactic and delayed moderate hypothermia for improving neurological outcome and control intracranial hypertension after head injury [12-14]. It seems that moderate hypothermia may improve outcome at 3 and 6 months in patients admitted with a coma score between 5 and 7 [12]. Nevertheless further studies are needed before hypothermia is accepted as a safe and effective treatment in brain damage.

On the other hand it has been demonstrated an association between hyperthermia and initial stroke severity, infarct size, mortality and outcome in 390 patients admitted with acute stroke [15]. Even though it is not proven whether this relation is causal or not, it is surprising the highly significant difference in outcome between hypothermic, normothermic and hyperthermic patients. Also in head injury a consistent relation has been found between duration of pyrexia and poor outcome [16]. Even if in the clinical setting the impact of the modifications of temperature on the evolution of ischaemic lesion is less defined than in the laboratory setting, a marked dependence of ischaemic injury on temperature must be recognized. This dependency suggests that the failure to control brain temperature during the acute phase might affect the neurologic recovery from brain damage.

Brain temperature monitoring

With this background, brain temperature monitoring in patients with acute brain damage has gained increasing interest in the past few years. Continuous monitoring was early performed by introducing a thermocouple in an intraventricular catheter for intracranial pressure (ICP) monitoring [17]. More recently thermometers or thermistors are combined with other probes (for ICP or oxygen and other metabolites measurements) allowing monitoring of brain temperature in the lateral ventricles or in the parenchyma.

Using these techniques gradients were disclosed between different areas of the brain, being the deeper zones at higher temperature compared with the structures on the surface. Besides a consistent gradient was also found when cerebral temperature was compared with internal body temperature. In the majority of patients brain temperature exceeds body temperature. Table 1 provides a list of gradients between the two temperature extrapolated from paper recently published.

Table 1. Differences between cerebral and body (mainly rectal) temperature reported in the literature. Placement refers to the position of the probe inside the intracranial space

Author	# pts	Pathology	Placement	Mean Δ T ($\pm$ sd)	Range
Mellergard et al. (1991) [18]	15	Neurosurgical	Ventricular	0.33C° ($\pm$ 0.18)	−0.5 and 2.3
Mellergard et al. (1989) [19]	7	Neurosurgical	Ventricular	0.68C°	0.4 and 1.0
Zauner et al. (1997) [20]	25	Head injury	Parenchymal	0.3-0.5°C	
Rumana et al. (1998) [21]	30	Head injury	Parenchymal	1.1C° ($\pm$ 0.6)	−0.3 and 3.8
Henker et al. (1998) [22]	8	Head injury	Ventricular	1.06°C	0.32 and 1.8

The range of the differences measured may be quite large varying between different patients and between different phases of the clinical course in the same patient. The reasons of such discrepancies is still far to be completely understood, however many associations between cerebral blood flow (CBF) and metabolism and amplitude of the gradient between brain and systemic temperature have been found. Mellergard et al. described a smaller gradient during impairment of consciousness and in the night in conscious patients, suggesting that the depression of metabolism occurring during coma and (even in a different extension) during sleep may cause a lowering in brain temperature [18]. Other authors found a significant increase of the gradient in case of reduction of cerebral perfusion pressure (CPP) between 50 and 20 mmHg indicating a compromising CBF; nevertheless with a CPP < 20 mmHg, indicating an irreversible impairment of CBF, the gradient was almost suppressed [21]. These data are consistent with the hypothesis that arterial blood flow provides a sort of "wash-out" of the brain heat generated by brain metabolism. Obviously in case of extreme depression of flow and metabolism, as in case of impending brain death, this function is negligible.

Clinical implications

Besides the pathophysiological speculations, in all the quoted studies a considerable individual variation in the brain-systemic gradient was found, and this variation cannot be predicted based on clinical findings. It follows that core temperature may deeply underestimate the value of cerebral temperature.

This observation becomes particularly important in the clinical management, especially in case of fever, which unfavourably affects clinical course and outcome as previously discussed. Moreover the latter is extremely frequent in acute neurosurgical patients. In a population of 112 head injured patients enrolled in a multicentric study only 11 (10%) did not experienced fever during the clinical course in ICU [personal unpublished data].

In the literature the information regarding methods for lowering brain temperature is very sparse but, as far as we are concerned, none of the conventional methods for lowering body temperature showed a specific effectiveness in selectively lowering cerebral temperature [23, 24]. Moreover, it should be kept in mind that pharmacologic agents, frequently used in clinical practice, should be carefully used in acute neurosurgical patients because of their side effect of arterial hypotension which may deeply compromise cerebral perfusion pressure. In this view selective brain cooling was tested, but the author could not find any positive effect in the five patients studied [24]. Selective brain cooling or other innovative methods for controlling cerebral temperature, may deserve further investigation.

References

1. Fitch W (1994) Brain metabolism. In: Cottrell JE, Smith DS (eds) Anesthesia and neurosurgery. Mosby, pp 1-16
2. Baker MA (1972) Influence of the carotid rete on brain temperature in cats exposed to hot environment. J Physiol 220:711-728
3. Baker MA, Hayward NJ (1968) The influence of the nasal mucosa and the carotid rete upon hypotalamic temperature in sheep. J Physiol 198:561-579
4. Cablanc M, Caputa M (1979) Natural selective cooling of the human brain: evidence of its occurrence and magnitude. J Physiol 286:255-264
5. Busto R, Dietrich D (1989) The importance of brain temperature in cerebral ischemic injury. Stroke 20:1113-1114
6. Busto R, Dietrich WD, Globus MY-T et al (1987) Small difference in intraischemic brain temperature critically determine the extent of ischemic neuronal injury. J Cereb Blood Flow Metab 7:729-738
7. Busto R, Globus MY-T, Dietrich WD et al (1989) Effect of mild hypothermia on ischemia induced release of neurotransmitters and free fatty acids in rat brain. Stroke 20:904-910
8. Globus MY-T, Busto R, Dietrich WD et al (1988) Intra-ischemic extracellular release of dopamine and glutamate is associated with striatal vulnerability to ischemia. Neurosci Lett 91:36-40
9. Busto R, Dietrich WD, Globus MY-T et al (1989) Post-ischemic moderate hypothermia inhibits CA1 hippocampal ischemic neuronal injury. Neurosci Lett 101:299-304
10. Dietrich WD, Alonso O, Halley M et al (1996) Delayed posttraumatic brain hyperthermia worsens outcome after fluid percussion brain injury: A light and electron microscopic study in rats. Neurosurgery 38:533-541
11. Clasen RA, Pandolfi S, Laing I et al (1974) Experimental study of relation of fever to cerebral edema. J Neurosurgery 41:576-581
12. Marion DW, Penrod LE, Kelsey SF et al (1996) Treatment of traumatic brain injury with moderate hypothermia. N Engl J Med 336:540-546
13. Metz C, Holzschuh M, Bein T et al (1996) Moderate hypothermia in patients with severe head injury: Cerebral and extracerebral effects. J Neurosurg 85:533-541
14. Shiozaki T, Sugimoto H, Taneda M et al (1993) Effects of mild hypothermia on uncontrollable intracranial hypertension after severe head injury. J Neurosurg 79:363-368
15. Reith J, Jorgensen HS, Pedersen PM et al (1996) Body temperature in acute stroke: relation to stroke severity, infarct size, mortality and outcome. Stroke 347:422-425
16. Jones PA, Andrews PJ, Midgley S et al (1994) Measuring the burden of secondary insults in head injured patients during intensive care. J Neurosurg Anesthesiol 6:4-14
17. Mellergard P, Nordstrom C-H, Christensson M (1990) A method for monitoring intracerebral temperature in neurosurgical patients. Neurosurgery 27:654-657
18. Mellergard P, Nordstrom C-H (1991) Intracerebral temperature in neurosurgical patients. Neurosurgery 28:709-713
19. Mellergard P, Nordstrom C-H (1990) Epidural temperature and possible intracerebral temperature gradients in man. Br J Neurosurg 4:31-38
20. Zauner A, Doppenberg E, Menzel M et al (1997) Relationship of brain temperature to brain metabolism and core temperature in patients with severe head injury. Xth International Symposium on ICP and Neurochemical Monitoring in Brain Injury. Williamsburg USA. Acta PO 2 066
21. Rumana CS, Gopinath SP, Uzura M et al (1998) Brain temperature exceeds systemic temperature in head-injured patients. Crit Care Med 26:562-567
22. Henker RA, Brown SD, Marion DW (1998) Comparison of brain temperature with bladder and rectal temperature in adults with severe head injury. Neurosurgery 42:1071-1075
23. Rossi S, ValerianiVG, Spagnoli D et al (1998) Hyperthermia, antipyretic therapy and cerebral temperature in acute neurosurgical patients. Anesthesia 2000;1:104
24. Mellergard P (1992) Changes in human intracerebral temperature in response to different methods of brain cooling. Neurosurgery 31:671-677

Exploring Cerebral Metabolism by Microdialysis

L. PERSSON, L. HILLERED

Microdialysis (MD) has been widely used for sampling of chemical substances from the interstitial fluid of the brain in experimental research. In the late 1980s, MD was introduced for studies on the human brain and neurochemical sampling was carried out in conjunction with neurosurgical procedures [1-3]. In 1992 we reported the use of intracerebral MD for chemical monitoring of brain injured patients during neurointensive care (NIC) [4]. Since then, there has been a remarkable development in the use of this technique in many neurosurgical centers. One may say that frequent chemical sampling, at the bed side, has brought NIC monitoring from a "physiological level" to a "chemical level", and the term neurochemical monitoring has been coined to describe this development [5].

Prospects for clinical use

A prerequisite for the use of MD for neurochemical monitoring in the NIC is that biochemical markers that reliably reflect the disease process are identified. In principle, the identification of a marker is based on the knowledge of its role in the pathophysiological process. Research during the 1970s and 1980s clarified a number of biochemical mechanisms involved in the development of secondary brain injury, such as lactic acidosis, excitotoxicity, free radical reactions, etc., and new neuroprotective strategies based on this knowledge is currently being developed. In this context monitoring of the biochemistry in the brain specifically reflecting these mechanisms by means of MD clearly make sense and may yield useful information on the disease process which may be used for management decisions and therapy, thereby potentially improving clinical outcome.

MD samples the interstitial fluid of the brain and it is therefore crucial to learn how the disease processes are reflected in this compartment. Previous studies of biochemical processes after brain injury have mainly been based on whole brain homogenate from experimental animals, or in patients, on CSF or blood samples. Findings obtained by such methods may not be directly applicable to clinical MD. The relationship among various patterns of the MD marker concentrations and the disease processes must therefore be studied carefully, and this has been a main theme for our research efforts. A first step was to apply intracerebral MD to experimental models of stroke and TBI. Based on these studies a number of clinical studies have subsequently been conducted to compare the neurochemical changes obtained by MD, to various events occurring after TBI or aneurysmal subarachnoid haemorrhage. Table 1 shows a listing of interstitial markers found to reliably reflect secondary brain ischaemia and infarction in these conditions. Additional markers used by other groups comprise potassium as a marker for membrane depolarization and pH for monitoring of acidosis [6, 7]. Others have also used lactate and glutamate as markers for ischemia and excitotoxicity [2, 4, 8-12]. Markers for energy metabolic disturbances (glucose, lactate, pyruvate, hypoxanthine) and excitotoxicity (glutamate) can be regarded as reliable interstitial markers of energy failure and excitotoxicity, respectively, whereas substances such as glycerol, urea, xanthine, uric acid and allantoin need further validation.

Table 1. Some biochemical markers in brain interstitial fluid

Energy metabolism	Glucose
	Lactate/pyruvate ratio
	Lactate/glucose ratio
	Hypoxanthine
Excitotoxicity	Glutamate
	Aspartate
Membrane degradation	Glycerol
Oxygen radicals	Hypoxanthine, xanthine
	Uric acid and its oxidation products (e.g. allantoin)

Biochemical markers with potential value for clinical use in neurosurgical patients with intracerebral microdialysis. The left column indicates the phenomenon the markers are reflecting

The clinical validation must be based on empirical observations where the MD levels and curve patterns are correlated to various clinical events such as neurological deterioration, increased ICP, decreased CPP, desaturation measured by jugular bulb oximetry or brain tissue PO_2 etc., and the specificity and the sensitivity, as well as predictive values of individual MD markers or combined patters of several markers [13] must be calculated. Moreover, comparison of the MD data and clinical outcome, such as GOS, is crucial. In addition, we are currently trying to establish "brain tissue outcome", as a surrogate end point for assessment of the fate of the brain tissue harboring the probe, by the use of CT and MR obtained in the late phase after acute brain injury [5]. For MD to become a clinical method, bedside monitoring is crucial and currently MD technology is becoming available for bedside use.

Limitations

MD is an invasive technique but the tissue injury caused by probe implantation seems to be negligible from a clinical point of view. However, a tissue reaction detected on the biochemical level is elicited by implantation and this may influence the measurements and the interpretation of data, and these are well described in experimental studies [14, 15]. There is less information from clinical studies, but the current knowledge suggests that the implantation causes less pronounced (neuro)chemical reactions in the human brain where normalization of dialysate metabolite levels seem to occur within approximately 30 minutes [2]. Bleeding and infection are other possible adverse effects following implantation. According to the current experience from many centers including our own, these side-effects do not seem to present much of a problem, although they need to be considered.

The MD probe may cause gliosis which could create a diffusion barrier and thereby blunting the chemical signals. Little is known about gliosis following MD in the human brain, but our own experience from long term measurements suggests that a diffusion barrier does not develop over time, because marked fluctuations in the dialysate levels (related to various clinical phenomena) occur several days (up to 11 days) after implantation [4, 5, 16].

The relative *in vivo* recovery of a MD system is defined as the ratio of the dialysate concentration to the interstitial concentration of a certain substance [15]. The *in vivo* recovery is dependent upon several factors including perfusion flow, membrane surface of the probe, the interstitial diffusion characteristics, the interstitial volume fraction, temperature and the turnover rate for the particular substance [14]. The clinically important implication of this dependency is that the *in vivo* recovery may vary during the course of the disease process and may be caused by changes in blood brain barrier permeability, oedema formation, increased intracranial pressure, as well as episodes of secondary ischaemia, temperature fluctuations and perhaps gliosis.

The problem of controlling for variations of *in vivo* recovery may be approached in different ways. The available methods for *in vivo* calibration of MD probes, e.g. the so-called no-net-flux method described by Lönnroth et al. [17], is reliable, but not suitable for repeated calibrations in the neurointensive care setting. An alternative approach is to use reference compounds, either endogenous (e.g. urea, which is equally distributed in the body fluid compartments) or exogenous compounds administered systemically [18]. We have studied ratios, such as the lactate/pyruvate ratio or the lactate/glucose ratio, and found that these yield clinically relevant information on the ischemic process. Based on the theoretical assumption that these molecules by being structurally and electrically similar, are equally affected by fluctuations of the interstitial diffusion characteristics and thereby independent of the *in vivo* recovery. By varying the perfusion flow (and thus the *in vivo* recovery) we observed that the lactate/pyruvate ratio did not change [19], an observation which thus supports the conclusion that the lactate/pyruvate ratio is uneffected by the *in vivo* recovery.

There is a blood-to-brain gradient for many substances that are being harvested by MD (e.g. glutamate, glycerol) and to control this factor it may sometimes be necessary to do parallel measurements of such substances in blood and CSF to exclude the possibility that leakage over an injured barrier is influencing the MD measurements [16].

It appears to be of fundamental importance for the future success of clinical MD that data from different centers can be directly compared. To achieve this goal it is highly desired that calibration methods become available allowing repeated or continuous estimation of *in vivo* probe recovery and thereby estimation of the true interstitial concentration. Until such methods are available, further evaluation of recovery independent measures such as the lactate/pyruvate ratio and the use of endogenous reference compounds are warranted.

Conclusions

The application of MD for neurochemical monitoring in neurosurgery and neurointensive care is rapidly expanding around the world. In order for MD to become a clinical routine method a number of problems, outlined above, must be solved by the clinical researchers. Regardless of the future success as a routine method, MD has already proven to be an important clinical research tool for years to come, providing new important information on the pathophysiology of acute human brain injury.

Acknowledgments. Financial support for this work was provided by the Swedish Medical Research Council (project no 7888), the Laerdal Foundation for Acute Medicine, the Selander Foundation, the 1987 Foundation for Stroke Research, the Åhlén Foundation, King Gustaf V and Queen Victoria's Foundation, CMA/Microdialysis AB and the Upjohn Company.

References

1. Persson L, Hillered L, Pontén U et al (1989) Intracerebral microdialysis for continuous metabolic monitoring of neurosurgical patients: Preliminary methodological considerations. J Cerebr Blood Flow Metab 9 [Suppl 1]:584
2. Hillered L, Persson L, Pontén U, Ungerstedt U (1990) Neurometabolic monitoring of the ischemic human brain using microdialysis. Acta Neurochir 102:91-97
3. Meyerson BA, Linderoth B, Karlsson H, Ungerstedt U (1990) Microdialysis in the human brain: extracellular measurements in the thalamus of parkinsonian patients. Life Sci 46: 301-308
4. Persson L, Hillered L (1992) Chemical monitoring of neurosurgical intensive care patients using intracerebral microdialysis. J Neurosurg 76:72-80
5. Persson L, Valtysson J, Enblad P et al (1996) Neurochemical monitoring of patients with subarachnoid hemorrhage with intracerebral microdialysis. J Neurosurg 84:606-616
6. Goodman JC, Gopinath SP, Valadka AB et al (1996) Lactic acid and amino acid fluctuations measured using microdialysis reflect physiological derangements in head injury. Acta Neurochir 67[Suppl]:37-39
7. Landolt H, Langemann H, Gratzl O (1993) On-line monitoring of cerebral pH by microdialysis. Neurosurgery 32:1000-1004
8. Bullock R, Zauner A, Myseros JS et al (1995) Evidence for prolonged release of ecitatory amino acids in severe human head trauma. Relationship to clinical events. Ann N Y Acad Sci 765:290-297
9. Hamberger A, Runnerstam M, Nyström B et al (1995) The neuronal microenvironment after subarachnoid hemorrhage. Correlation of amino acid and nucleoside levels with post-operative recovery. Neurol Res 17:97-105
10. Kanthan R, Shuaib A, Griebel R, Miyashita H (1995) Intracerebral human microdialysis. In vivo study of an acute focal ischemic model of the human brain. Stroke 26:870-873
11. Robertson CS, Gopinath SP, Goodman JC et al (1995) $SjvO_2$ monitoring in head-injured patients. J Neurotrauma 12:891-896
12. Säveland H, Nilsson OG, Boris-Möller F et al (1996) Intracerebral microdialysis of glutamate and aspartate in two vascular territories after aneurysmal subarachnoid hemorrhage. Neurosurgery 38:12-19
13. Enblad P, Valtysson J, Andersson J et al (1996) Simultaneous intracerebral microdialysis and positron emission tomography performed in the detection of ischemia in patients with subarachnoid hemorrhage. J Cereb Blood Flow Metab 16:637-644
14. Benveniste H (1989) Brain microdialysis. J Neurochem 52:1667-1679
15. Robinson T, Justice JB (1991) Microdialysis in the neurosciences. Elsevier, Amsterdam
16. Hillered L, Valtysson J, Enblad P, Persson L (1997) Extracellular glycerol as a marker for membrane lipid degradation in the acutely injured human brain. J Neurol Neurosurg Psychiatry (in press)
17. Lönnroth P, Jansson P-A, Smith U (1987) A microdialysis method allowing characterization of intercellular water space in humans. Am J Physiol E253:E228-E231
18. Kehr J (1993) A survey on quantitative microdialysis: Theoretical models and practical implications. J Neurosci Methods 48:251-261
19. Persson L, Hillered L (1996) Intracerebral microdialysis. Letter to the Editor. J Neurosurg 85: 984-985

Epidemiology and Diagnosis of Polyneuropathy in Critical Illness

G. Savettieri, B. Fierro

When sepsis and/or multiple organ dysfunction (MOD) complicate the course of a severe primary illness, a critical illness arises. The frequency of this syndrome has been increasing in the last years mostly because the prolonged survival of Intensive Care Units (ICU) patients due to the advent of modern methods of treatment. The incidence of the syndrome in most of ICU is between 20 and 50%. Bolton [1], in a recent review, hypothesized that infections (through sepsis) or trauma may determine the so called systemic inflammatory response syndrome (SIRS) that, in turn, determines the conditions that lead to nervous system involvement. A detailed description of mechanisms that give rise to SIRS is reported in the paper of Bolton [1]. The nervous system manifestations evolve according to a well-defined pattern [2]. Sepsis induces a septic encephalopathy that can be reverted if the sepsis is successfully treated. The subsequent difficulty in weaning the patient from the ventilator may be caused from neuropathy, myopathy, or both.

Encephalopathy, neuropathy, myopathy are the nervous system manifestations that can complicate critical illness. Septic encephalopathy occurs in 70% of septic patients; in this condition death is usually due to multiple organ failure (MOF); this happens in about 50% of patients [3]. Peripheral nervous system involvement during critical illness has been investigated but frequency, type of involvement, associated factors and natural history of the disease are until now far from an exhaustive knowledge.

Neuromuscular complications in critical illness

Table 1 reports a very long list of conditions that can affect neuromuscular system in critically ill patients. It is quite evident that when a neuromuscular involvement is suspected, systematic electrophysiological studies, metabolic investigations, and muscle biopsy are compulsory for a precise diagnosis and treatment.

When performed in the ICU, electrophysiological studies reveal special problems (i.e. artifacts from imperfect grounding, electrical apparatus attached

Table 1. Neuromuscular disorders in critically ill patients

Neuropathy
    Critically ill polyneuropathy
    Guillain-Barré syndrome
    Thiamine deficiency
    Vitamin E deficiency
    Nutritional deficiency
    Pyridoxyne abuse
    Hypophosphataemia
    Aminoglycoside toxicity
    Penicillin toxicity
    Porphyria
    Motor neuron disease
    Paraneoplastic polyneuropathy
    Entrapment neuropathy
    Diphtheria
Neuromuscular transmission defect
    Anaesthetic drugs
    Aminoglycoside toxicity
    Myasthenia gravis
    Lambert-Eaton syndrome
    Hypocalcaemia
    Hypomagnesaemia
    Organophosphate poisoning
    Wound botulism
    Tick bite paralysis
Myopathy
    Septic myopathy
    Cachexia
    Water and electrolyte disturbances
    Panfascicular fiber necrosis
    Steroid myopathy
    Polymyositis
    Muscular dystrophy
    Acid maltase deficiency

to the patients, mechanical devices such as respirators, intravenous tubing, and so on) [4]. In performing nerve conduction studies, particular attention should be given to recording of distal limbs temperature, which, on average, is higher in septic respect to non-septic patients. Such elevation will decrease both latencies and amplitude of compound action potentials [5]. Patients in ICU may be oedematous due to the "sick cell syndrome" [6]. This oedema moves surface recording electrodes away from underlying nerve and muscle and reduces compound action potential amplitudes. The use of near-nerve recordings may partially overcome this difficulty [7]. Critical illness polyneuropathy (CIP) is the most common polyneuropathy encountered in ICU. In addition, prolonged treatment with neuromuscular blocking agents may induce axonal motor neuropathy, and myositis can be found associated with sepsis.

Critical illness polyneuropathy (CIP): clinical picture and diagnosis

Failure to wean from mechanical ventilation may occur in critically ill patients with sepsis and multi-system organ failure. The reason for this ventilatory problem has been regarded as related to a neuromuscular dysfunction. Critical illness polyneuropathy is the most likely diagnosis in the presence of difficulty in weaning from the ventilator of neuromuscular origin.

Critical illness polyneuropathy has been recognized as an axonal, sensory-motor neuropathy that occurs in the setting of intensive care unit in critically ill patients with sepsis and multi-system organ failure [8, 9]. The very cause of this disorder is uncertain but it is likely that it is related to the systemic inflammatory response associated with sepsis and other pathological conditions including burns and trauma [1]. The earliest sign of peripheral nervous system involvement is difficulty in weaning from the ventilation apparatus; this is due to diaphragmatic weakness. The respiratory neuromuscular system can be investigated by carrying out phrenic nerve conduction studies [10]. Needle electromyography of the diaphragm should not be attempted due to the proximity of lung, liver, and spleen [4]. Phrenic nerve conduction studies revealed compound muscle action potentials from the diaphragm on both sides that are of normal latency and reduced amplitude. Only in severe polyneuropathy an absent bilateral response has been recorded. In a large number of patients signs of denervation of chest wall muscles have been observed on needle electromyography giving some support to the concept that polyneuropathy is a significant contributory factor to difficulty in weaning from the ventilator in these patients [4].

In the stages subsequent to ventilatory problems, distal weakness (mild or severe up to quadriplegia), hypotonia, and loss of deep reflex appear; sensory impairment is generally mild. Cranial nerves are usually spared. A slight increase of cerebro-spinal fluid protein can be found.

In summary, the patients have weak or absent movements of the limbs and, in contrast, normal movements of face, jaw and head. The clinical features described for CIP are indeed not different from those of diffuse myopathy or pan-fascicular muscle fiber necrosis. This is the reason for which electrophysiological studies are essential in the diagnostic evaluation of these patients. As polyneuropathy may be of a primary motor and sensory axonal degenerative type, nerve conduction studies alone may be of little benefit in diagnosis. Measurements of conduction velocities, F-response latencies, distal latencies are near normal; while compound muscle and sensory action potential amplitudes are considerably reduced. Because of technical variability, interpretation of compound action potential may be imprecise, although attention to technical details will reduce this imprecision. Reduction of compound muscle action potential amplitude could also be due to other conditions as motor neuron disease, primary myopathy, so it is important to demonstrate depression of sensory compound action potential amplitudes before a firm electrophysiologic diagnosis of polyneuropathy can be made. These electroneurographic changes are typical of axonal damage and occur within one week from the onset.

Needle electromyography is particularly important. The degree, type, and distribution of electromyographic abnormalities will often provide relevant information to making a specific diagnosis of polyneuropathy. Denervation potentials such as fibrillation and positive sharp waves, predominant in the distal muscles, may not appear until three weeks from the axonal damage. Motor unit potentials, if the patient can voluntarily activate them, are reduced in number, somewhat polyphasic, but not increased in size. In follow-up, this electromyographic abnormalities improved: abnormal spontaneous activity gradually disappears and motor unit activity returns as reinnervation occurs in most patients who survive the critical illness. Interpretation of the electrophysiological neuromuscular changes in critically ill patients is not obvious because the varying presence of neuropathy, myopathy or both. Increased abnormal spontaneous activity and the presence of voluntary motor unit potentials normal or somewhat low amplitude and polyphasic suggest an associated primary involvement of muscles.

Latronico et al. [11] studied 24 comatose patients who developed neuromuscular disease. Electroneuromyography was performed and nerve and muscle specimens were taken. According to electrophysiologic studies 92% of patients had an axonal polyneuropathy, but muscle biopsies revealed a myopathy in 23 of 24 patients. This discrepancy is attributable to the limitations of electroneuromyography in comatose patients. In this setting, in fact, electroneuromyography cannot distinguish between axonal motor neuropathy and myopathy. The reduced amplitudes of the sensory-nerve action potentials in front of normal sensory nerves at biopsy, could be explained by an early impairment of axonal transport and transmembrane potential, easily documented by electrophysiological, but not histological, studies.

Critical illness polyneuropathy shows several similarities to the Guillan-Barré syndrome and, by using electrophysiologic criteria alone, it is impossible to distinguish axonal Guillain-Barré syndrome from critical illness polyneuropathy. One clinical criterion, among others, is that critical illness polyneuropathy improves over months with resolution of critical illness and that intravenous immunoglobulins (IVIG) did not improve recovery [12]. On the other hand, in course of Guillain-Barré syndrome facial weakness and ocular muscles involvement are more frequent. In the most common demyelinating type of Guillain-Barré syndrome, the conduction velocity is much more slowed and, in the early stages, abnormal spontaneous activity of muscles is relatively absent.

Epidemiology

Although the polyneuropathy seems to be very frequent among critically ill patients, its precise incidence is uncertain. What we know about frequency and risk factors comes from anecdotal report, case series studies, and from some prospective investigations.

Incidence

Published incidence estimates give widely differing values raging from 33 to more than 80%. Much of the variation among studies is explained by differences in case definition and inclusion criteria. In addition sampling bias and small numbers are frequently encountered. Witt et al. [13] in a prospective study found that 70% of patients with sepsis and multiple organ failure had electrophysiological evidence of peripheral nerve involvement, but only 30% showed clinical signs of neuropathy.

A prospective study was carried out by Spitzer et al. [14]. This investigation evaluated a cohort of 21 patients with prolonged ventilator dependency to estimate the frequency of neuromuscular dysfunction as cause of the failure to wean. The study, mainly electrophysiologic, found that 62% of patients were affected by a neuromuscular disorder that caused the ventilator dependency. In 24% of patients a neuromuscular disease was a contributory cause of the ventilator dependency. Interestingly, only seven (53%) of the 13 patients with neuromuscular disease had critical illness polyneuropathy. This indicates an incidence of critical illness polyneuropathy of 33%.

Leijten et al. [15] in a prospective study of 18 months, followed a cohort of 38 critically ill patients who had been mechanically ventilated for more than 7 days, without previous signs of or risk factors for polyneuropathy. This well-designed study showed that peripheral nerve dysfunction was present in about 47% of patients.

Nine patients, who fulfilled the criteria for SIRS, thus at risk for critical illness polyneuropathy, were enrolled in a prospective study carried out by Schwarz et al. [16]. Electrophysiological follow-up examinations were performed in all patients. Five of 9 patients (about 55%) developed a critical illness polyneuropathy.

The frequency of the development of polyneuropathy was particularly high in a prospective study carried out by Barek et al. [17]. Patients were included in the study if they had sepsis or SIRS combined with MOF. Incidence was 81.1%, but in more than 30% of the patients signs of neuropathy were detected by electrophysiologic studies alone and no clinical sign was present.

It is evident that the lack of homogeneity in the criteria used for enrolling patients corresponds to different rates of frequency. This fact does not allow a meta-analytic study to extrapolate the frequency of the disorder. In addition a good comparability among studies results problematic due to the small numbers.

Risk factors

As reported above, the etiology and pathogenesis of critically ill polyneuropathy are not well understood. There are evidences that this type of polyneuropathy is mainly associated with sepsis and multiple organ failure.

Five critically ill patients with acute polyneuropathy were studied by Lopez Messa and Garcia [18]. Four of these patients showed organ failure in 3 or more organs. Witt et al. [13] found that 70% of patients with sepsis and multiple organ failure showed electrophysiological evidence of peripheral nerve involvement. Other findings were that the deterioration of peripheral nerve function correlated with the time in the ICU and that increasing blood glucose and decreased serum albumin were directly correlated with decreasing nerve function. These metabolic changes may indeed depend on the sepsis and multiple-organ failure syndrome. Leijten et al. [15] in his cohort study followed 38 patients who were on mechanical ventilation for more than 7 days. After 18 months patients who developed CIP were compared with those without CIP. The conclusion was that CIP was strongly associated with multiple organ dysfunction; total duration of ventilatory support was weakly associated with critical illness polyneuropathy, but the authors do not sustain a cause-effect relationship between these two events. Sepsis was present in 56% of CIP patients and in 40% of non-CIP; the difference was not statistically significant, but the numbers are too small. Mortality was 44% among patients with critical illness polyneuropathy, which is twice higher than that found in the group of patients not affected by CIP. A previous investigation of the same group [19] showed that polyneuropathy was associated with higher mortality and that caused a considerable slowing in rehabilitation program. Latronico et al. [11] report interesting findings concerning epidemiology. In brief, the authors found that sepsis and multiple organ dysfunction, but not drugs, are associated with neuromuscular disease.

Conclusions

The investigations we analyzed in this review, although not homogenous from a methodological point of view, lead us to draw some epidemiological features of critical illness polyneuropathy. The syndrome is very frequent among patients affected by critical illness; the degree of severity is quite variable and sometimes CIP is only an instrumental or bioptic finding. The syndrome is strongly associated with multiple organ dysfunction or failure and at a less degree with the presence of sepsis and duration of ventilator support. In those patients with critical illness the prolonged need for ventilatory support contributes to mortality. The mortality seems in fact to be higher in CIP patients respect to non-CIP critically ill patients.

Finally, we believe that the studies on neuromuscular disorders in critically ill patients so far available are not enough to obtain clear frequency figures, to delineate the natural history of the disease, and to individuate risk or protective factors associated with the disorder. Multicentre, prospective, cohort studies should be designed to investigate neuromuscular disorders in critically ill patients.

References

1. Bolton CF (1996) Sepsis and the systemic inflammatory response syndrome: neuromuscular manifestation. Crit Care Med 24:1408-1416
2. Bolton CF, Young BG, Zochodne WD (1993) The neurological complications of sepsis. Ann Neurol 33:94-100
3. Young CF, Bolton CF, Austin TW et al (1990) The encephalopathy associated with septic illness. Clin Invest Med 13:297-304
4. Bolton CF (1987) Electrophysiologic studies of critically ill patients. Muscle Nerve 10:129-135
5. Bolton CF, Sawa GM, Carter K (1981) The effects of temperature on human compound action potentials. J Neurol Neurosurg Psychiatry 44:407-413
6. Flear CT, Bhattacharya SS, Singh CM (1980) Solute and water exchanges between cells and extracellular fluids in health and disturbances after trauma. J Parental Enteral Nutr 4:98-119
7. Rosenfalk A (1978) Early recognition of nerve disorders by near-nerve recording of sensory action potentials. Muscle Nerve 1:360-367
8. Bolton CF, Gilbert JJ, Hahn AF et al (1984) Polyneuropathy in critically ill patients. J Neurol Neurosurg Psychiatry 47:1223-1231
9. Zochodne DW, Bolton CF, Wells GA et al (1987) Critical illness polyneuropathy. A complication of sepsis and multiple organ failure. Brain 110:819-842
10. Markand ON, Kincaid JC, Rahman AP et al (1984) Electrophysiologic evaluation of diaphragm by transcutaneous phrenic nerve stimulation. Neurology 4:604-614
11. Latronico N, Fenzi F, Recupero D et al (1996) Critical illness myopathy and neuropathy. Lancet 347:1579-1582
12. Wijdicks EF, Fulgham JR (1994) Failure of high dose intravenous immunoglobulins to alter the clinical course of critical illness polyneuropathy. Muscle Nerve 17:1494-1495
13. Witt NJ, Zochodne DW, Bolton CF et al (1991) Peripheral nerve function in sepsis and multiple organ failure. Chest 99:176-184
14. Spitzer AR, Giancarlo T, Maher L et al (1992) Neuromuscular causes of prolonged ventilator dependency. Muscle Nerve 15:682-686
15. Leijten FSS, De Weerd AW, Poortvliet DCJ et al (1996) Critical illness polyneuropathy in multiple organ dysfunction syndrome and weaning from the ventilator. Intensive Care Med 22:856-861
16. Schwarz J, Planck J, Briegel J et al (1997) A single-fiber electromyography, nerve conduction studies, and conventional electromyography in patients with critical-illness polyneuropathy: evidence for a lesion of terminal motor axons. Muscle Nerve 20:696-701
17. Barek K, Margreiter J, Willeit J et al (1996) Polyneuropathies in critically ill patients: a prospective evaluation. Intensive Care Med 22:849-855
18. Lopez Messa JB, Garcia A (1990) Acute polyneuropathy in critically ill patients. Intensive Care Med 16:159-162
19. Lejten FSS, De Weerd AW, Poortvliet DCJ et al (1995) The role of polyneuropathy in motor convalescence after prolonged mechanical ventilation. JAMA 274:1221-1225

Polyneuropathy in Patients Undergoing a Neuromuscular Junction Blockade

D. ØSTERGAARD

Neuromuscular blocking drugs (NMBD) are used extensively in many intensive care units (ICU) in the USA, whereas in Europe they are less frequently used [1, 2]. Often these drugs are used without monitoring the neuromuscular block quantitatively. The NMBD are used in doses which exceed by far those used in the operating room and for a considerably longer period of time in patients who are very different from the healthier patients undergoing general anaesthesia. Most recommendations for the use of NMBD are extrapolated from the short-term use in the operating room and this information is not applicable to the long-term use in critically ill patients. The ICU patients are often haemodynamically unstable: they have reduced organ functions or even organ failure and often receive concomitant medication. Furthermore these patients are immobilised, which might have consequences for the neuromuscular block. The importance of the different structure and pharmacokinetics of the individual NMBD is of special importance in the ICU patients. The long-term use of NMBD is associated with many difficulties and serious complications. Many case reports describe persistent paralysis after long-term use of NMBD to facilitate mechanical ventilation. The incidence of prolonged paralysis is estimated at 20% for the patient receiving NMBD for more than 6 days and 15-40% in patients with asthma receiving NMBD and corticosteroids [1]. It has been suggested that reducing the amount of NMBD administered by monitoring the neuromuscular transmission may decrease the risk of prolonged paralysis. Hence recommendations are necessary on when and how to use NMBD in critically ill patients and how to monitor the neuromuscular block. This is the topic of this presentation.

Indications for the use of neuromuscular blocking drugs

One indication might be to obtain optimal intubation conditions. Due to the rapid onset of succinylcholine, this drug is often used in patients with the risk of aspiration. Succinylcholine, however, has adverse effects which are relevant in the ICU. In patients with burns or excessive trauma, who are already hyperkalaemic, the rise in serum potassium caused by succinylcholine may induce cardiac arrhythmias and even cardiac arrest. In these situations it is preferable to use a non depolarising NMBD with a fast onset (see later). Many patients can be intubated using sedatives only. Once endotracheal intubation is established, succinylcholine is not indicated in the ICU setting.

Another indication for the use of NMBD is to improve mechanical ventilation in patients with adult respiratory distress syndrome or in patients with status asthmaticus [3]. In patients with tetanus NMBD might be indicated to reduce the seizures. However NMBD are seldom indicated in neurological patients or in patients with multiple fractures [4]. Due to the serious complications following prolonged use of NMBD in the ICU, the number of indications for the use of NMBD is rapidly decreasing and mechanical ventilation is often facilitated using adequate doses of sedatives and analgesics.

Complications

The complications of long-term use of NMBD in ICU patients are numerous; persistent neuromuscular block after stopping the administration of NMBD, steroid-associated myopathy, polyneuropathy and combinations of these conditions. Because monitoring is uncommon and dose recommendations are lacking in the critically ill, it is conceivable that many reports refer to excessive dosing of NMBD. Various factors, including the underlying disease with subsequent complications, concurrent administration of drugs (especially corticosteroids), alterations in normal pharmacokinetics and pharmacodynamics, may contribute to the complex aetiology. The first cases presented were due to the use of steroids (pancuronium and vecuronium) [5, 6]. Recently, however, prolonged neuromuscular dysfunction has been described following the benzylisoquinolinium substances, atracurium and cisatracurium [7, 8]. A significant incidence of prolonged weakness has been reported in patients receiving NMBD in combination with corticosteroids during status asthmaticus or organ transplantation [3, 9]. This prolonged weakness is different from the typical critical illness polyneuropathy which is a sensorimotor polyneuropathy and can occur during sepsis in patients who are not treated with NMBD [3]. If NMBD are used for more than 2-3 days, increased dose requirements are observed due to development of tolerance. An increase in the number of extrajunctional receptors has been reported following chronic administration even in the absence of immobilisation [10].

Which drug is to be used in intensive care patients

The properties of the ideal NMBD drug for the intensive care unit patients are specificity for the neuromuscular receptor (no cardiovascular side effects), no histamine releasing effect, organ independent elimination, no active or toxic metabolites (no accumulation). Stability of the drug (infusion) and modest cost are also important. The introduction of intermediate acting drugs has changed the practice of anaesthesia. The use of pancuronium in anaesthesia is rapidly decreasing due to the higher risk of residual curarisation. A large, randomised trial has recently shown that the incidence and the degree of residual curarisation is significantly larger in patients receiving pancuronium and that more patients developed pulmonary complications (16,9% vs 5,4%) following atracurium or vecuronium [11]. NMBD can be classified according to their chemical structure.

NMBD with steroid structure

Pancuronium, pipecuronium, vecuronium, rocuronium and ORG 9487.

The advantage of these drugs is the cardiovascular stability. Furthermore they are devoid of histamine releasing properties. The disadvantage is the organ dependent elimination and, except for rocuronium, the active metabolites.

The long acting drug, *pancuronium*, with high affinity to the neuromuscular receptor, has a moderate vagolytic effect. It is primarily eliminated via the kidney (60-80%) and, to a lower degree, metabolised in the liver to the active 3-desacetyl metabolite, which has 40-50% of the neuromuscular blocking activity of the parent compound and is excreted by the kidney. Plasma clearance of pancuronium is reduced in patients with renal or hepatic disease and this lead to accumulation and a prolonged duration of action.

Pipecuronium is a long acting NMBD resembling pancuronium in its structure, potency, time course of action and pharmacokinetic profile. Unlike pancuronium, pipecuronium does not have any cardiovascular effects. Pipecuronium is more dependent on renal elimination than pancuronium and the elimination is diminished in patients with decreased renal or hepatic function.

Vecuronium has a higher specificity and hence fewer cardiovascular side effect than pancuronium. It is predominantly eliminated (70-80%) through the hepatobiliary pathways. Vecuronium is metabolised in the liver to the 3-desacetyl metabolite which has 50-70% of the potency of the parent compound. The metabolite seems to accumulate in patients with renal failure [5].

Rocuronium is an analogue of vecuronium with lower potency, which means that the onset time is short and optimal intubation conditions can be obtained after 60-90 sec. Its duration of action is the same as vecuronium. Rocuronium has mild vagolytic properties which may cause a dose-related increase in heart rate. The main route of elimination appears to be the hepatobiliary pathway; however, rocuronium does not appear to be metabolized in the liver. Hence rocuronium has no active metabolites. In ICU patients the volume of distribution at steady state is increased, the clearance reduced and the terminal half-life prolonged [12].

A new aminosteroid, *ORG 9487* is undergoing clinical trials in Europe and the US. The drug is less potent than rocuronium and has a shorter duration of action than rocuronium. It seems to have no cardiovascular side effects. If given as a continuous infusion for more than 1 hour, the duration of action changes from short to intermediate. Pharmacokinetic information is limited.

NMBD with benzylisoquinolinium structure

Doxacurium, atracurium, cisatracurium, mivacurium.

The advantage of these drugs is the organ independent elimination. The disadvantage lies in the histamine releasing properties, especially of atracurium and mivacurium. The histamine releasing effect is dose-related and can be reduced if the drug is injected slowly.

Doxacurium is a long acting agent, which has no effect on the cardiovascular system and no histamine releasing effect. The drug is minimally metabolized and is excreted in an unchanged form predominantly in the urine.

The intermediate acting agent *atracurium* was designed to undergo Hofmann elimination and ester hydrolysis, i.e. an organ independent elimination. Hence the elimination is unchanged in children of less than 1 year, in the elderly and in patients with organ failure. Atracurium has no clinically important active metabolites, but one of the elimination products is laudanosine, which has been shown to have cerebral excitatory activity. Laudanosine is excreted in the kidney.

Cisatracurium has the same pharmacokinetic and pharmacodynamic profile as atracurium but is much more potent. Therefore lower doses are used and the production of laudanosine is lower. It does not cause the release of histamine.

Mivacurium has a short duration of action due to rapid hydrolysis by plasma cholinesterase. Mivacurium has no active metabolites. The disadvantage is the slow metabolism in patients with low plasma cholinesterase activity and in patients with abnormal plasma cholinesterase genotype. Renal and hepatic failure is known to influence plasma cholinesterase activity and therefore the duration of action is longer in these patients.

Following this short review of old and new NMBD a question should be asked: is the ideal NMBD for ICU patients available? The answer is no, but the cardiovascular stability and the absence of active metabolites make rocuronium the most appropriate drug with steroid structure. The cardiovascular stability, the absence of histamine releasing properties and the organ independent elimination make cisatracurium the best alternative with benzylisoquinolium structure. These two second generation intermediate acting drugs seem to be superior to the older long and intermediate acting drugs [12, 13]. In a recent study Prielipp et al. [13] report a more rapid recovery following infusion of cisatracurium than following vecuronium in ICU patients. The recovery following pancuronium and doxacurium were compared [14]. A more prolonged and variable recovery was observed following pancuronium.

Today the economic factor is also important. Despite the evident advantages of the new intermediate acting drugs, many departments use pancuronium to reduce the costs. Tobias et al. [15] have emphasised the economies deriving from the use of an inexpensive, long acting drug, pancuronium, instead of more expensive drugs. However, they carefully avoided patients who may be at risk for prolonged neuromuscular block (e.g. renal failure). The economical benefit of using more inexpensive drugs may easily disappear in the case of a few patients with a prolonged paralysis staying in the ICU for a longer period of time. Economies could be achieved by a more rational use of neuromuscular blocking drugs administered to a reduced number of patients.

Why, how and when is the neuromuscular block to be monitored

Is it beneficial to monitor the neuromuscular block? First of all there is a great variation in individual sensitivity in healthy adult patients [16]. This variation may be even greater in ICU patients with decreased organ function, which will influence the pharmacokinetics and pharmacodynamics of NMBD. Often these patients are receiving medication (antibiotics, H_2 antagonists) that might interact with NMBD. Also these patients may have electrolyte and acid-base abnormalities.

Some authors believe that if the neuromuscular block is monitored there would be no prolonged recovery. Studies have been designed to emphasise this point and succeeded [17, 18]. Furthermore, Rudis et al. [19] demonstrated that patients monitored with a nerve stimulator received a lower dose of NMBD than patients not monitored. Prielipp et al. [13], however, concluded that monitoring did not prevent the development of myopathy or polymyopathy. In this study a number of patients had renal failure and some patients received high doses of steroids.

The use of a nerve stimulator can provide useful information on the actual level of the block and provide useful guidelines for the dosing of NMBD. Finally the use of a nerve stimulator can provide valuable information on when it is possible to extubate the patient. Any peripheral nerve may be stimulated. However it must be mentioned that the diaphragm and respiratory muscles are more resistant to NMBD than peripheral muscles [20]. The absence of response at the adductor pollicis does not eliminate the possibility of cough when suctioning. Techniques that monitor the degree of neuromuscular block at the respiratory muscles should perhaps be used. The most suitable stimulation patterns are the train-of-four (TOF) and the post tetanic count (PTC) [21]. Complete neuromuscular block is seldom indicated. NMBD should be administered in order to obtain the neuromuscular block necessary to achieve the maximal benefit (e.g. improved oxygenation, low airway pressure, etc.).

How and when are NMBD to be used

The following guidelines are recommended in the ICU [1]:

– Avoid the use of NMBD by maximal use of sedatives and analgesics and by manipulation of ventilatory parameters.
– Administer NMBD only when required and to achieve a well defined goal.
– Minimise the dose of NMBD.
– Minimise the dose of steroids, the combination of steroids and NMBD should be avoided.
– Monitor the neuromuscular function.

As none of the NMBD is the ideal drug, the choice of which drug should be used in a given situation depends on 1) the indication, 2) the condition of the patient and 3) the chemical structure, route of metabolism and cardiovascular side effects of the NMBD.

The initial doses are similar to the doses used during anaesthesia. After 2-3 days, however, the doses are increased due to the development of tolerance. Long acting drugs are more safely used as intermittent bolus doses, intermediate acting drugs are usually administered as a continuous infusion, which is essential if a constant level of block is necessary. Some advocate changing NMBD selecting different chemical structures in order to avoid tolerance.

References

1. Miller RD (1995) Use of neuromuscular blocking drugs in the intensive care unit patients. Editorial. Anesth Analg 81:1-2
2. Bion JF, Ledingham JI (1987) Sedation in intensive care - a postal survey. Intensive Care Med 13:215-216
3. Meistelman C, Plaud B (1997) Neuromuscular blockade: is it still useful in the ICU? Eur J Anaesth [Suppl 15]:53-56
4. Hsiang JK, Chesnut RM, Crisp CB et al (1994) Early, routine paralysis for intracranial pressure control in severe head injury: Is it necessary? Crit Care Med 22:1471-1476
5. Segredo V, Caldwell JE, Matthay M et al (1992) Persistent paralysis in critically ill patients after long-term administration of vecuronium. N Engl J Med 327:524-526
6. Gooch JL, Suchyta MR, Balbierz JM et al (1991) Prolonged paralysis after treatment with neuromuscular blocking agents. Crit Care Med 19:1125-1131
7. Meyer KC, Prielipp RC, Grossman JE et al (1994) Prolonged weakness after infusion of atracurium in two intensive care unit patients. Anesth Analg 78:772-774
8. Davis NA, Rodgers JE, Gonzales ER et al (1998) Prolonged weakness after cisatracurium infusion: A case report. Crit Care Med 26:1290-1292
9. Nates JL, Cooper DJ, Day B et al (1997) Acute weakness syndromes in critically ill patients - A reappraisal. Anesth Intens Care 25:502-513
10. Hogue CW, Ward JM, Itani S et al (1992) Tolerance and upregulation of acetylcholine receptors following chronic infusion of d-tubocurarine. J Appl Physiol 72:1326-1331
11. Berg H (1997) Is residual neuromuscular block following pancuronium a risk factor for postoperative pulmonary complications? Acta Anaesthesiol Scand 41[Suppl]:156-158

12. Sparr HJ, Wierda MKH, Proost JH et al (1997) Pharmacodynamics and pharmacokinetics of rocuronium in intensive care patients. Br J Anaesth 78:267-273
13. Prielipp RC, Courain DB, Scruderi PE et al (1995) Comparison of the infusion requirements and recovery profile of vecuronium and cisatracurium 51W89 in intensive care unit patients. Anesth Analg 81:3-12
14. Murray MJ, Coursin DB, Scuderi PE et al (1995) Double-blind, randomised, multicenter study of doxacurium vs. pancuronium in intensive care unit patients who require neuromuscular blocking agents. Crit Care Med 23:450-458
15. Tobias JD, Lynch A, McDuffee A et al (1994) Pancuronium infusion for the neuromuscular block in children in paediatric intensive care units. Anesth Analg 81:13-16
16. Katz RL (1967) Neuromuscular effects of d-tubocurarine, edrophonium and neostigmine in man. Anesthesiology 28:327-336
17. Khuehln-Brady KS, Reitslatter B, Sclager A et al (1994) Long-term administration of pancuronium and pipecuronium in the intensive care unit. Anesth Analg 78:1082-1086
18. Frankel H, Jeng J, Tilly E et al (1996) The impact of implementation of neuromuscular blockade monitoring standards in a surgical intensive care unit. Am Surg 62:503-506
19. Rudis MI, Sikora CA, Angus E et al (1997) A prospective, randomised, controlled evaluation of peripheral nerve stimulation versus standard clinical dosing of neuromuscular blocking agents in critically ill patients. Crit Care Med 25:575-583
20. Donati F, Meistelman C, Plaud B (1990) Vecuronium neuromuscular blockade at the diaphragm, the orbicularis oculi and the adductor pollicis muscles. Anesthesiology 73:870-875
21. Viby-Mogensen J (1993) Monitoring neuromuscular function in the Intensive Care Unit. Intensive Care Med 19:S74-S79

Muscular Wasting as a Consequence of Sepsis

N. Latronico, A. Candiani

Muscle involvement in severe disease is known since the dawn of medicine [1], however only in recent years has research focused on this topic. Basic and clinical scientists have made available a rich harvest of clinical, physiological, biochemical and pathological data, and with them the Babel tower problem: "Clinicians face the problem of muscle wasting and weakness; biochemists are confronted with muscle glutamine efflux, physiologists with reduced or absent excitability, pathologists with atrophy and necrosis". Are they simply the same problem seen through different lenses? Do they perfectly overlap, so that clinically observed muscle wasting corresponds to histologically proven myopathy?

This chapter tries to provide the reader with a pathophysiological explanation of commonly encountered clinical, electrophysiological and histological findings.

Analysis of literature indicates that muscle proteolysis is the protagonist around whom all other parts rotate. Therefore, we will depict the causes of muscle proteolysis and will then have a deep insight into its consequences.

Causes of muscle proteolysis

Cytokines have a primary role in causing protein breakdown. Tumor necrosis factor (TNF), interleukin-1 and, to a lesser extent, interleukin-6 have a demonstrated capacity of priming muscle proteolysis [2-7]. Recently a novel molecule with such a capability has been isolated from mice tumors [8]. Furthermore, decreased levels of anabolic hormones (insulin and insulin-like growth factor-1), and increased levels of catabolic hormones (cortisol, cathecolamines and glucagon) together with cytokine generate a powerful catabolic effect, making muscle amino-acids available for key processes (see below).

The ultimate effectors of proteolysis are intracellular proteolytic systems, namely the ubiquitin-proteasome, calpains, lysosomal and non-lysosomal systems [9-14]. Recently, specific proteasome inhibitors have been shown to block the sepsis-induced increase in muscle proteolysis [15].

What are the consequences of muscle proteolysis?

The old adagio that "too much of good is bad" is particularly valid for muscles.

Protein breakdown is in dynamic equilibrium with protein synthesis and represents a physiological process permitting the adaptation to new conditions. By disassembling proteins, it makes amino-acids available to build other proteins, which are important in that particular situation. As cited by Mitch and Goldberg [9], in fasting state enzymes (proteins!) for glucose storage are degraded, while enzymes for gluconeogenesis are synthesized. These adaptive phenomena are rapid: muscle proteolysis increases within hours of an infectious threat [9].

On the light side, muscle proteolysis has a homeostatic role [2, 14, 16]. In fact, proteins are degraded to aminoacids, which are partly transaminated to α-keto acids and oxidised to provide energy. Furthermore, alanine and glutamine are transported to the hepatic lab, where they are converted to glucose (gluconeogenesis), glutathione and acute phase proteins like C-reactive protein, α-acid glycoprotein, fibrinogen, haptoglobin. Amino-acids are also taken up by kidneys, gastro-intestinal tract, endothelial cells, rapidly dividing cells, such as those involved in wound healing, and cells of the immune system. These latter are extremely dependent on plasma glutamine availability "as brain is on blood glucose" [16]. It has been hypothesized that all the muscular proteolytic machinery is activated to provide sufficient amounts of glutamine to maintain immuno-competency [16]. Certainly severe glutamine depletion strongly correlates with poor outcome [17].

On the dark side, it should be remembered that degraded muscle proteins come prevalently from myofibrillar proteins (actin, myosin), which represent 60 to 70 per cent of muscle proteins [9]. In fact, urinary excretion of 3-methylhistidine (3-MH), an amino-acid uniquely contained in myofibrils, is enormously increased in the septic state and myofibrillar breakdown is increased up to 400 per cent [11]. If synthetic processes do not keep up with such a violent catabolism, myofibrillar dysarrangement ensues, and there is evidence that protein synthesis is depressed in sepsis [18]. 3-MH comes from both actin and myosin, however, degradation of myosin thick filaments seems prevalent, as suggested by results of histological studies describing the so-called thick filament myopathy [13, 19]. Further progression leads to structural alteration of the entire muscle fibre with the frequently encountered histologic finding of necrosis [20-22]. Necrosis is usually scattered. However, in some cases described as acute necrotizing myopathy, the necrotic process is extensive and accompanied by a massive increase of plasmatic levels of intracellular muscle enzymes [23]. These forms represent "the extreme end of a spectrum of critical illness-related muscle degeneration" [24].

The efflux of glutamine and other free amino-acids from muscle is accompanied by the osmotic efflux of intracellular water with reduction of cell volume [17]. Atrophy may be the histologic equivalent of this phenomenon, and it could make reason of some cases of very early atrophy (1st-2nd admission day) described by Coacley et al. [21], which we attributed to a limitation of the biopsy technique [25]. Obviously, later in the course disuse atrophy takes place.

The reduction of muscle cell volume, which had been postulated on pathophysiological basis and demonstrated on isolated perfused rat liver and human muscle biopsies [17], has recently been demonstrated in vivo in humans by using sophisticated techniques [26]. As the authors point out, "it is a radical departure from the usual teaching that critically ill patients are overhydrated and exhibit cellular overhydration".

Not only is the muscle cell volume reduced, but also its excitability. The reduction of the resting membrane potential (RMP) in critically ill patients was first demonstrated by Cunningham more than 25 years ago [27] and has then received several confirmations [28-32]. RMP reduction causes partial depolarisation, which in turn reduces muscle excitability. It is worthy of note the fact that both denervation and tumor necrosis factor (TNF) are able to reduce the RMP [30-33]. This may give us an explanation of acute quadriplegic myopathy in septic patients [34, 35]: the combination of sepsis (TNF) and critical illness polyneuropathy (denervation) may well cause muscle inexcitability and thus paralysis in absence of any structural abnormalities. Specialised electrophysiological techniques allowing direct muscle stimulation have demonstrated loss of muscle excitability [35].

It is unclear how TNF and/or other events can alter RMP. Interestingly, Rich et al. have recently showed in an experimental model of acute steroid myopathy that combined denervation and steroids reduce RMP and membrane sodium conductance [33]. Sodium and potassium have a leading role in maintaining RMP and sepsis-related proteolysis is accompanied by massive loss of potassium in the order of 20 per cent of total body potassium [26]. It is attractive to link ionic muscle abnormalities to altered excitability. However, Finn et al. found that intracellular potassium concentration was unchanged [26], and therefore cellular events leading to reduced muscle excitability in sepsis need further research.

Muscle and its neighbours

An acute axonal sensory-motor polyneuropathy is frequently described in septic patients [36, 37]. This so-called critical illness polyneuropathy seems almost invariably associated with critical illness myopathy [10, 24]. Denervation boosts muscle damage, as nerve-derived trophic factors are impeded to reach the muscle [14]. Furthermore, denervation makes muscles very vulnerable to the action of steroids and non-depolarising muscle blocking agents [23, 33, 38].

Microcirculation is not spared by sepsis. Piper et al. have convincingly demonstrated by means of intravascular microscopy that in septic rats the capillaries with absent flow increase over time [39]. This process started within six hours of septic insult. It can explain the observation that high-energy muscle phosphate metabolism was preserved in the early stage of sepsis, at least in absence of other insults. However, superimposition of an ischaemic stress caused dissipation of high-energy muscle phosphate, suggesting an associated microvascular alteration [40]. The interrelation between vascular and cellular events has been recently reviewed by Bolton [37].

Conclusions

Patients with muscle wasting may have or not muscle weakness depending on the ongoing electrophysiological and histological alterations, if any. Function and structure can be normal or near-normal (atrophy): muscle strength is usually preserved or only mildly reduced in these cases. Function can be completely abolished while structure is normal (acute quadriplegic myopathy), or finally both function and structure can be abnormal (necrosis). In this latter case, alterations can be subtle requiring electron microscopy for diagnosis (thick filament myopathy) or they can be visible on optical microscopy, either as sparse or diffuse or even massive lesions (acute necrotizing myopathy). Only in this latter instance will plasma CK levels be increased.

Although several questions are still unanswered, skein is being unraveling and a continuous line can be traced from atrophy to massive muscle necrosis. In fact, from a pathophysiological point of view, muscle proteolysis seems to be the common denominator and, according to others (24), the term "critical illness myopathy" can be proposed as a comprehensive denomination.

Acknowledgements. We are greatly indebted with Frank Rasulo, MD, for his careful English revision.

References

1. Ippocrate (1994) Aforismi e giuramento. TEN Newton Compton, Roma
2. Shapiro L, Gelfand JA (1995) Cytokines. In: Shoemaker, Ayres, Grenvik, Holbrook (eds) Textbook of critical care, 3rd edn. WB Saunders, Philadelphia, pp 154-161
3. Zamir O, Hasselgren PO, Kunkel SL et al (1992) Evidence that tumor necrosis factor partecipates in the regulation of muscle proteolysis during sepsis. Arch Surg 127:170-174
4. Matsui J, Cameron RG, Kurian R et al (1993) Nutritional, hepatic, and metabolic effects of cachectin/tumor necrosis factor in rats receiving total parenteral nutrition. Gastroenterology 104:235-243
5. Costelli P, Carbo N, Tessitore L et al (1993) Tumor necrosis factor mediates changes in tissue protein turnover in a rat cancer cachexia model. J Clin Invest 92:2783-2785
6. Zamir O, O'Brian W, Thompson RC et al (1994) Reduced muscle protein breakdown in septic rats following treatment with interleukin-1 receptor antagonist. Int J Biochem 26:943-950
7. Goodman MN (1994) Interleukin-6 induces skeletal muscle protein breakdown in rats. Proc Soc Exp Biol Med 205:182-185

8. Todorov P, Cariuk P, McDevitt T et al (1996) Characterization of a cancer cachectic factor. Nature 379:739-742

9. Mitch WE, Goldberg AL (1996) Mechanisms of muscle wasting. New Engl J Med 335: 1897-1905

10. Latronico N (1997) Acute myopathy of intensive care. Ann Neurol 42:131-132

11. Tiao G, Fagn JM, Samuels N et al (1994) Sepsis stimulates nonlysosomal, energy-dependent proteolysis and increases ubiquitin mRNA levels in rat skeletal muscle. J Clin Invest 94: 2255-2264

12. Voisin L, Breuillé D, Combaret L et al (1996) Muscle wasting in a rat model of long-lasting sepsis results from the activation of lysosomal, Ca^{2+}-activated, and ubiquitin-proteasome proteolytic pathways. J Clin Invest 97:1610

13. Showalter CJ, Engel AG (1997) Acute quadriplegic myopathy: analysis of myosin isoforms and evidence for calpain-mediated proteolysis. Muscle Nerve 20:316-322

14. Keays R (1998) Skeletal muscle in critical illness. In: Vincent JL (ed) Yearbook of intensive care and emergency medicine. Springer, Berlin Heidelberg New York, pp 599-608

15. Hobler SC, Tiao G, Fischer JE et al (1998) Sepsis-induced increase in muscle proteolysis is blocked by specific proteasome inhibitors. Am J Physiol 274:R30-R37

16. Grimble RF (1990) Nutrition and cytokine action. Nutr Res Rev 3:193-210

17. Haussinger D, Roth E, Lang F et al (1993) Cellular hydration state: an important determinant of protein catabolism in health and disease. Lancet 341:1330-1332

18. Vary TC, Kimball SR (1992) Sepsis-induced changes in protein synthesis: differential effects on fast-twitch and slow-twitch muscles. Am J Physiol 262:C1513-C1519

19. Sher JH, Shafiq SA, Shutta HS (1979) Acute myopathy with selective lysis of myosin filaments. Neurology 29:100-106

20. Helliwell TR, Coacley JH, Wagenmakers AJM et al (1991) Necrotizing myopathy in critically ill patients. J Pathol 164:307-314

21. Coacley JH, Nagendran K, Honavar M et al (1993) Preliminary observations on the neuromuscular abnormalities in patients with organ failure and sepsis. Intensive Care Med 19: 323-328

22. Latronico N, Fenzi F, Recupero D et al (1996) Critical illness myopathy and neuropathy. Lancet 347:1579-1582

23. Ramsay DA, Zochodne DW, Robertson DM et al (1993) A syndrome of acute severe muscle necrosis in intensive care unit patients. J Neuropathol Exp Neurol 52:387-398

24. Leijten FSS (1997) Neuromuscular complications of prolonged critical care. In: Vincent JL (ed) Yearbook of intensive care and emergency medicine. Springer, Berlin Heidelberg New York, pp 774-786

25. Latronico N, Candiani A (1994) Neuromuscular abnormalities in patients with organ failure and sepsis. Intensive Care Med 20:612-613

26. Finn PJ, Plank LD, Clark MA et al (1996) Progressive cellular dehydration and proteolysis in critically ill patients. Lancet 347:654-656

27. Cunningham JN Jr, Carter NW, Rector FC et al (1971) Resting transmembrane potential in normal subjects and severely ill patients. J Clin Invest 50:49-59

28. Gibson WH, Cook JJ, Gatipon G et al (1977) Effect of endotoxin shock on skeletal muscle cell membrane potential. Surgery 81:571-577

29. Trunkey DD, Illner H, Wagner IY et al (1979) The effect of septic shock on skeletal muscle action potentials in the primate. Surgery 85:638-643

30. Tracey KJ, Lowry SF, Beutler B et al (1986) Cachectin/tumor necrosis factor mediates changes of skeletal muscle plasma membrane potential. J Exp Med 164:1368-1373

31. DeMeules JE, Pigula FA, Mueller M et al (1992) Tumor necrosis factor and cardiac function. J Trauma 32:686-692

32. Eastridge BJ, Darlington DN, Evans JA et al (1994) A circulating shock protein depolarizes cells in hemorrhage and sepsis. Ann Surg 219:298-305

33. Rich MM, Pinter MJ, Kraner SD et al (1998) Loss of electrical excitability in an animal model of acute quadriplegic myopathy. Ann Neurol 43:171-179

34. Latronico N, Rasulo FA, Recupero D et al (1998) Acute quadriplegic with delayed onset and rapid recovery. J Neurosurg 88:769-772
35. Rich MM, Bird SJ, Raps EC et al (1997) Direct muscle stimulation in acute quadriplegic myopathy. Muscle Nerve 20:665-673
36. Zochodne DW, Bolton CF, Wells GA et al (1987) Critical illness polyneuropathy. A complication of sepsis and multiple organ failure. Brain 110:819-842
37. Bolton CF (1996) Sepsis and the systemic inflammatory response syndrome: neuromuscular manifestations. Crit Care Med 24:1408-1416
38. Antognini JF, Gronert GA (1996) Extra-junctional receptors and neuromuscular blocking drugs. Curr Opin Anaesth 9:344-347
39. Piper RD, Pitt-Hyde M, Li F et al (1996) Microcirculatory changes in rat skeletal muscle in sepsis. Am J Respir Crit Care Med 154:931-937
40. Gilles RJ, D'Orio V, Ciancabilla F et al (1994) In vivo ^{31}P nuclear magnetic resonance spectroscopy of skeletal muscle energetics in endotoxemic rats: a prospective, randomized study. Crit Care Med 22:499-505

CURRENT STATUS OF CRITICAL CARE

Epidemiology of Trauma

A.J. SUTCLIFFE

Data describing the distribution and determinants of injury are vital for the development of strategies to mitigate its effects. Such strategies include measures to prevent accidents, to control exposure to risk, to reduce the severity of injuries sustained and to improve medical care. They can be implemented by legislative or educational means to modify behaviours and the environment. Successful strategies would be expected to alter the incidence, pattern and outcome of injury. Thus, epidemiological studies of injury need to be repeated at regular intervals in order to assess the current situation. Although injury is a significant cause of morbidity and mortality worldwide [1], there are local differences attributable to the type of injury and the population studied. This chapter reviews some recent epidemiological studies of trauma.

Population studies of injury

Any epidemiological report must be studied with care because the precise nature of the data will influence the conclusions that may be drawn. The following examples demonstrate some variations in reporting and interpretation. A recent study of a large cohort of males from eighteen American cities [2] shows that black males have a higher incidence of injury from accidents and violence than white males but that overall, heart disease and malignancy are more important causes of mortality. Thus, although a good case can be made for targeting injury in black males, government agencies may prefer to use this data to justify expenditure on financing measures to reduce mortality from heart disease rather than injury because the impact on the whole population would be greater. Studies confined to injured patients (Table 1) show national differences in the causes of injury.

Even these studies are not directly comparable because some include all injured patients [5, 6], some include only patients treated by hospitals [3, 7] and some are restricted to patients with major trauma [4]. Nevertheless, the differences are large enough to demonstrate how important it is that behavioural and environmental measures to reduce the incidence or severity of injury are designed specifically to suit the population at risk.

Table 1. National and regional differences in common causes of injury

Cause of injury	Eldoret, Kenya [3]	Victoria, Australia [4]	Alingsas, Sweden [5]	Madras, India [6]	Papua, New Guinea [7]
Assault and violence	40%				31%
Road traffic accidents	18%	61%	11%	16/1000	14%
Falls	17%	19%			
Burns	3%	5%			
Leisure activities			36%		
Sport			18%		
Accidents in the home			18%	57/1000	25%
Accidents at work			17%	19/1000	
Tribal fights					24%

Some reports (Table 2) describe the location of deaths from injury.

Table 2. National and regional differences in location of deaths from injury

Location of deaths and percentage mortality	Mersey & N Wales, UK [8]	California, USA urban [9]	California, USA rural [9]	Auckland, New Zealand [10]	Papua, New Guinea [7]
Prehospital mortality	58.2%	40.5%	72.0%	63%	Unknown
Hospital mortality	41.8%	59.5%	28%	37%	1.8%

The figures show where the majority of deaths are occurring. If deaths are to be prevented, further information is required about the specific population at risk and their injury patterns. Some deaths may be preventable by public health measures such as compulsory use of seat belts or the fitting of airbags to cars [11]. Others may be prevented by improving clinical management or systems organisation. The incidence of hospital preventable deaths is variable and has been quoted as 10% in Italy [12], 32% in Ireland [13], and 7% in Florida [14]. The potential to reduce preventable deaths has been used to justify the development of hospital trauma systems [14] but a greater impact might be made by reducing prehospital deaths; 39% may be preventable according to one British study [15]. At the scene of an accident, simple measures such as airway manipulation and the administration of oxygen can have a dramatic effect in reducing mortality [16]. Deaths are not always preventable by better medical care. In California [9], excess mortality in rural compared to urban patients can be explained by their greater age and comorbidities. Several studies show that the majority of non-preventable hospital deaths are due to overwhelming primary brain injury [17, 18]. Secondary brain injury due to hypoxia and hypovolaemia is, however, preventable [18].

Population studies can also elucidate specific risk factors for injury such as psychopathology [19], alcohol consumption and the use of illicit drugs [19], previous injury [20], extremes of age [21] and occupation [22].

Subpopulation studies of injury

Studies of the type described so far can be used to establish general principles of care such as the probable benefit of a hospital based trauma system or the need to reduce the incidence and severity of road traffic accidents. Subpopulation studies provide more detailed evidence for actions which may be appropriate. For example, an analysis of skiing injuries requiring hospital admission [23] shows that 18% are serious and that about one third of these are due to collisions with various obstacles. Skiers need to be educated to control their speed. Snowboarding causes a different injury pattern with a high incidence of minor injury amongst beginners who may benefit from better basic training [24]. The incidence of injuries caused by diving into swimming pools could also be reduced by better training although improvements in pool design may be needed as well [25]. A study of American occupational injuries shows that decentralised, rural industries such as logging and fishing are most hazardous and that many deaths occur in industries which are outside the jurisdiction of occupational health and safety agencies [23]. The same study, shows that homicide is an important cause of death in taxi drivers and grocery store workers. Clearly, different approaches to prevention are needed for loggers and taxi drivers.

Injury-specific epidemiological studies

Studies of specific injuries may provide data whose relevance is restricted to that injury [18]. Alternatively, they may be more generally applicable. A study of spinal cord injuries [26] shows that, in common with other types of injury, failure to use seat belts and the use of alcohol are important risk factors. Significantly, 74% of injuries are preventable by more rigorous enforcement of existing legislation.

Conclusions

This chapter describes only a small number of the epidemiological studies of injury which have been published in recent years. It illustrates the complexity of trauma epidemiology. Many studies concentrate on fatal injury but the will and ability to implement preventative measures and improve medical care could reduce not only mortality but also morbidity following injury.

Furthermore, conclusions relating to trauma may be more widely applicable. In an emergency department in Singapore, the number of preventable deaths due to injury is small but one third of the non-trauma deaths may be preventable [27]. It could be that the reduction in mortality achieved by the development of trauma systems could be emulated by the development of similar systems to improve the medical care of non-injured patients.

References

1. Nolan JP (1993) Trauma statistics and demographics. In: Grande M (ed) Textbook of trauma anesthesia and critical care. Mosby, St Louis, pp 35-54
2. Smith GD, Neaton JD, Wentworht D et al (1998) Mortality differences between black and white men in the USA: contribution of income and other risk factors among men screened for the MRFIT. Lancet 351:934-939
3. Odero WO, Kibosia JC (1995) Incidence and characteristics of injuries in Eldoret, Kenya. East Afr Med J 72:706-710
4. Cameron P, Dziukas L, Hadj A et al (1995) Patterns of injury from major trauma in Victoria. Aust N Z J Surg 65:848-852
5. Holmdahl L, Ortenwall P (1997) Causes and consequences of trauma in a Swedish county 1989-1992. Eur J Surg 163:83-92
6. Sathiyasekaran BW (1996) Population-based cohort study of injuries. Injury 27:695-698
7. Matthew PK, Kapua F, Soaki PJ et al (1996) Trauma admissions in the southern highlands of Papua New Guinea. Aust N Z J Surg 66:659-663
8. Gorman DF, Teanby DN, Sinha MP et al (1995) The epidemiology of major injuries in Mersey region and North Wales. Injury 26:51-54
9. Rogers FB, Shackford SR, Hoyt DB et al (1997) Trauma deaths in a mature urban vs rural trauma system. Arch Surg 132:376-381
10. Smeeton WM, Judson JA, Synek BJ et al (1987) Deaths from trauma in Auckland: a one year study. N Z Med J 100:337-340
11. Loo GT, Siegel JH, Dischinger PC et al (1996) Airbag protection versus compartment intrusion effect determines the pattern of injuries in multiple trauma motor vehicle crashes. J Trauma 41:935-951
12. Stocchetti N, Pagliarini G, Gennari M et al (1994) Trauma care in Italy: evidence of in-hospital preventable deaths. J Trauma 36:401-405
13. Caldwell MT, McGovern EM (1993) Fatal trauma: a five year review in a Dublin hospital. Ir J Med Sci 162:309-312
14. Thoburn E, Norris P, Flores R et al (1993) System care improves trauma outcome: patient errors dominate reduced preventable death rate. J Emerg Med 11:135-139
15. Hussain LM, Redmund AD (1994) Are pre-hospital deaths from accidental injury preventable? Br Med J 308:1077-1080
16. Ali J, Adan RU, Gana TJ et al (1997) Effect of prehospital trauma life support program on prehospital trauma care. J Trauma 42:786-790
17. Sauaia A, Moore FA, Moore EE et al (1995) Epidemiology of trauma deaths: a reassessment. J Trauma 38:185-193
18. Siegel JH (1995) The effect of associated injuries, blood loss, and oxygen debt on death and disability in blunt traumatic brain injury: the need for early physiologic predictors of severity. J Neurotrauma 12:579-590

19. Poole GV, Lewis JL, Devidas M et al (1997) Psychopathologic risk factors for intentional and nonintentional injury. J Trauma 42:711-715
20. Sayfan J, Berlin Y (1997) Previous trauma as a risk factor for recurrent trauma in rural northern Israel. J Trauma 43:123-125
21. van der Sluis CK, Klasen HJ, Eisma WH et al (1996) Major trauma in young and old: what is the difference? J Trauma 40:78-82
22. Loomis DP, Richardson DB, Wolf SH et al (1997) Fatal occupational injuries in a southern state. Am J Epidemiol 145:1089-1099
23. Furrer M, Erhart S, Frutiger A et al (1995) Severe skiing injuries: a retrospective analysis of 361 patients including mechanism of trauma, severity of injury, and mortality. J Trauma 39: 737-741
24. Pigozzi F, Santori N, Di Salvo V et al (1997) Snowboard traumatology: an epidemiological study. Orthopedics 20:505-509
25. Blanksby BA, Wearne FK, Elliott BC et al (1997) Aetiology and occurrence of diving injuries. A review of diving safety. Sports Med 23:228-246
26. Tyroch AH, Davis JW, Kaups KL et al (1997) Spinal cord injury. A preventable public burden. Arch Surg 132:778-781
27. Seow E, Lau G (1996) Who dies at A&E? The role of forensic pathology in the audit of mortality in an emergency medicine department. Forensic Sci Int 82:201-210

Nitric Oxide in Sepsis and ARDS

H. Zhang, T.E. Stewart, J.-L. Vincent

Septic shock, a major clinical problem with mortality rates of up to 70%, is characterized by systemic hypotension, impaired tissue O_2 extraction capabilities and myocardial depression. Much interest has been focused on the role of nitric oxide (NO) in septic shock during the last decade. Following the discovery of the NO radical it was clear that NO could play a role in the vascular relaxation and hypotension during sepsis and endotoxaemia. *In vitro* studies showed that isolated macrophages produced increased amounts of nitrate and nitrite upon stimulation with lipopolysaccharides [1, 2]. This increase was shown to be caused by the increased production of NO, which was dependent on the presence of L-arginine and could be inhibited by analogs of L-arginine. The NO synthase enzyme responsible for production of NO in macrophages is inducible (iNOS) and differs from the constitutive NO synthase (cNOS) in endothelial cells. The cNOS is calcium and calmodulin dependent and releases small amounts of NO, whereas the iNOS is calcium and calmodulin independent and releases large amounts of NO for a prolonged period of time. The iNOS enzyme shown in macrophages can also be found in neutrophils, hepatocytes, myocardial cells and vascular smooth muscle cells stimulated with endotoxin or cytokines [3-5]. iNOS is expressed under the influence of endotoxin and several cytokines like tumor necrosis factor-α (TNF-α), interleukin-1β (IL-1β) and interferon-γ [4, 6]. In general, one can say that cNOS plays a physiological role in maintaining organ perfusion, whereas iNOS plays a more pathological role (as in sepsis and endotoxaemia) leading to the production of excessive amounts of NO resulting in vascular relaxation and tissue damage [7].

A number of investigators have studied the role of NO by administering NO blockers and NO donors during septic shock. This review will briefly summarize some experimental and clinical data available from the literature on the use of NO antagonists and agonists during septic shock.

Effects of NO blockers

Increased production of NO in sepsis has been well demonstrated both in animals and humans [8-14]. Accordingly, the pharmacological inhibition of NOS may represent a logical therapeutic approach to sepsis. Competitive agents such as N^G-nitro-L-arginine methyl ester (L-NAME), N^G-mono-methyl-L-arginine (L-NMMA), or N$^\omega$-nitro-L-arginine (L-NNA) block both the iNOS and the cNOS, leading to reduced NO production. The beneficial effects of these L-arginine analogs in septic shock have been much debated.

Role of NO in experimental sepsis

Non-selective NOS inhibition

In general, NOS inhibitors consistently increase arterial pressure and systemic vascular resistance, but reduce cardiac output [12, 14, 15]. However, some of these studies were performed in hypodynamic models where the fluid status might have been inadequate for endotoxic shock, and some models were too acute for NO to be produced in high amounts (Table 1).

Table 1. Pre- and post-treatment with NO inhibitors in septic shock

Nitric oxide inhibitors	Object	Pre- or post- treatment	Bene- ficial effects	Reference
L-NMMA	Dog	post-	+	Kilbourn et al. 1990
L-NMMA	Rat	post-	+	Nava et al. 1992
L-NAME	Sheep	post-	+	Meyer et al. 1992
L-NMMA	Rabbit	post-	±	Wright et al. 1992
L-NMMA	Patient	post-	+	Schilling et al. 1993
S-methyl-isothiourea	Rat	post-	+	Szabo et al. 1994
S-methyl-isothiourea	Mouse	post-	+	Szabo et al. 1994
L-NAME	Sheep	post-	+	Landin et al. 1994
L-NAME	Pig	post-	+	Ogura et al. 1994
L-NMMA	Dog	post-	–	Henderson et al. 1994
L-NMMA	Patient	post-	±	Petros et al. 1994
Aminoguanidine	Mouse	post-	+	Wu et al. 1995
Ethyl-isothiourea	Sheep	post-	+	Booke et al. 1995
Aminoethylisothiourea	Rat	post-	+	Thiemermann et al. 1995
L-NMMA	Mouse	post-	+	Rees et al. 1995
L-NAME	Dog	post-	–	Schumacker et al. 1995
L-NAME	Pig	post-	–	Ayuse et al. 1995
L-NAME	Sheep	post-	+	Hinder et al. 1996
L-NMMA	Sheep	post-	+	Booke et al. 1996
Mercaptoethylguanidine	Rat	post-	+	Southan et al. 1996
Guanidinoethyldisulfide	Mouse	post-	+	Szabo et al. 1996
L-NNA	Dog	post-	+	Kaszaki et al. 1996
S-methyl-isothiourea	Rat	post-	+	Aranow et al. 1996
L-NMMA	Rat .	post-	–	Atrand et al. 1997

L-NMMA	Dog	post-	–	Zhang et al. 1997
L-NAME	Sheep	post-	+	Hinder et al. 1997
L-NMMA	Baboon	post-	+	Redl et al. 1997
L-NAME	Patients	post-	+	Kiehl et al. 1997
L-NAME	Patients	post-	±	Avontuur et al. 1998
L-NAME	Mouse	post-	–	Liaudet et al. 1998
L-NAME	Rat	post-	–	Klemm et al. 1998
S-methyl-isothiourea	Rat	post-	+	Rosselet et al. 1998
L-NAME	Sheep	post-	±	Bone et al. 1998
L-NAME	Pigs	post-	–	Cohen et al. 1998
L-NMMA	Mouse	simultaneously	–	Billiar et al. 1990
NAA	Dog	pre-	–	Cobb et al. 1991
L-NMMA	Rabbit	pre-	–	Wright et al. 1992
L-NAME	Rat	pre-	–	Mulder et al. 1994
L-NAME	Mouse	pre-	–	Fukahatsu et al. 1994
L-NAME	Rat	pre-	–	Tiao et al. 1994
L-NAME	Mouse	simultaneously	–	Minnard et al. 1994
L-NMMA	Mouse	simultaneously	–	Nishida et al. 1994
L-NAME	Rat	simultaneously	–	Spain et al. 1994
L-NMMA	Dog	simultaneously	–	Statman et al. 1994
L-NMMA	Dog	simultaneously	–	Cobb et al. 1995
L-NAME	Mouse	pre-	–	Fukatsu et al. 1995
L-NAME	Dog	pre-	–	Mitaka et al. 1995
L-NMMA	Rat	pre-	–	Gardiner et al. 1995
L-NAME	Rat	pre-	–	Wang et al. 1995
L-NAME	Rat	pre-	–	Klabunde and Conton 1995
L-NAME	Piglet	simultaneously	–	Meadow et al. 1996
L-NAME & L-NMMA	Mouse	pre-	–	Fukatsu et al. 1996
L-NNA	Pig	pre-	±	Herbertson et al. 1996
L-NMMA	Rat	pre-	–	Meng et al. 1997
L-NAME	Rat	simultaneously	–	Werner et al. 1997
L-NAME	Hamster	pre-	±	Laniyonu et al. 1997
L-NAME	Rat	pre-	–	Aaron et al. 1998

While an excessive release of NO has been incriminated in the development of sepsis-related myocardial depression [3, 16], the effects of NOS inhibition on endotoxin-induced myocardial depression are still controversial. Studies reporting that NOS inhibitors may improve myocardial contractility usually involved isolated myocardiums [3, 16], but studies involving entire organisms usually failed to observe such effects [17-22]. Keller et al. [21] observed that the NOS inhibitor L-NAME had no effect on ventricular contraction in guinea pigs 4 or 16 h after endotoxin injection. Neither ventricular cNOS nor iNOS activity was affected by endotoxin. Meng et al. [20] studied the effects of L-NMMA on cardiac contractile dysfunction induced by endotoxin in the rat. They found that pretreatment with L-NMMA (30 mg/kg, i.v., –5 min) or the selective iNOS inhibitor S-methylisothiourea sulfate (SMT) failed to prevent the contractile dysfunction. Moreover, infusion of L-NMMA or SMT *in vitro* could not restore contractile function in hearts isolated at 6 h after endotoxin challenge. In contrast, inhibition of NOS with L-NMMA or SMT decreased coronary blood flow both *in vivo* and *in vitro*. Also, Klabunde and Coston [18] reported that L-NNA could alter myocardial function in endotoxic shock in rats. Avontuur and Ince [22] reported that coronary blood flow was reduced by L-NNA, resulting in local areas of myocardial ischaemia in endotoxin-treated, but not in untreated, hearts in rats, suggesting that endotoxaemia can promote myocardial ischaemia in vulnerable areas of the heart after NOS inhibition. Recently, Cohen et al. [23] reported that following endotoxaemia, L-NAME administration restored arterial blood pressure but resulted in worsening pulmonary hypertension, increased right ventricular volumes, and decreased cardiac output, compared with a control group of pigs. This study suggests that the decrease in cardiac output after NOS inhibition in endotoxaemia is due to increased right ventricular afterload. Taken together, these observations question a beneficial effect of NOS inhibition on myocardial function in septic shock.

The pulmonary arterial bed under basal conditions is only minimally regulated by NO, but increased after endotoxin. NO release is critically important to mitigate the increase in pulmonary vascular resistance which is otherwise observed [24]. Several studies have shown that the vasoconstricting effects of L-NMMA were more dramatic in the pulmonary than in the systemic circulation [25-27]. L-NMMA potentiates endotoxin-induced pulmonary hypertension by increasing pulmonary vascular resistance in endotoxic shock [25-27]. On the other hand, Spath et al. [24] found a loss of endothelium-dependent relaxation in pulmonary vessels in endotoxic sheep probably because endothelial cells are damaged in these conditions. The increase in pulmonary artery pressure induced by NOS inhibition may represent a major limitation to their clinical use.

The administration of L-NMMA can decrease regional blood flow in various organs, suggesting that NOS inhibitors may exacerbate regional vasoconstriction and ischaemia. Henderson et al. [28] demonstrated that L-NMMA (25 mg/kg) significantly decreased blood flow in the internal carotid artery (48%), renal artery (34%), mesenteric artery (26%), and distal aorta (34%) during hyperdynamic endotoxic shock in dogs. These changes were reversed completely by the administration of L-arginine. Ayuse et al. [29] reported that hepatic arterial resistance increased after L-NAME under control and endotoxic shock conditions in pigs thus reducing total hepatic blood flow and diminishing venous return across the liver. Mulder et al. [25] partially (0.1 mg) or completely (1 mg) inhibited NOS with L-NNA 30 min before endotoxin challenge in rats. They found that complete, and even partial, inhibition of NOS was deleterious during the first hour of endotoxic shock: the perfusion of especially the pancreas, small and large intestines, and kidney significantly decreased. In a rabbit endotoxic shock model, Pastor and Payen [30] showed that L-NNA reduced portal vein and hepatic artery blood flow. Nishida et al. [31] showed a 33% reduction in liver sinusoidal blood flow after L-NAME administration in endotoxic mice. Wang et al. [32] reported that inhibition of NOS with L-NAME aggravated ischaemia and endotoxin-induced liver injury by 90%, and further impaired microvascular blood flow in rats. NOS inhibition also aggravated small intestinal vasoconstriction in septic rats [33]. L-NAME reduced gut blood flow by increasing gut vascular resistance following endotoxaemia in dogs [34]. Werner et al. [35] demonstrated that L-NAME significantly increased intrapancreatic trypsinogen activation peptides (TAPS), an index of pancreatic injury which correlates with inflammation, necrosis, and mortality. We [27] recently observed that L-NMMA reduced renal blood flow in endotoxic dogs. This is in keeping with the results of Spain et al. [36] indicating that NOS inhibition can further constrict renal vasculature and decrease interlobular artery flow during sepsis.

NO can modulate microvascular permeability to solutes in whole organs, venules, and cultured endothelial cell monolayers [37]. At low doses, NO can protect the endothelial barrier whereas at high doses, it can damage it. Some investigators have reported that NOS inhibition increases microvascular permeability [38-40] and potentiates the effects of several agonists that increase permeability [41, 42]. Rumbaut et al. [42] recently showed that NOS inhibition decreases capillary hydraulic conductivity – an index of the ability of water to pass across the capillary barrier, confirming the role for NO in the modulation of capillary permeability.

NOS inhibition has been suggested to worsen tissue oxygenation. In an awake canine model of hypodynamic endotoxic shock, L-NMMA increased arterial lactate levels and decreased arterial pH [26]. Statman et al. [43] found that L-NMMA in septic dogs significantly decreases oxygen delivery (DO_2) and oxygen uptake ($\dot{V}O_2$). These changes were reversed with the administration of L-arginine. Mitaka et al. [14] demonstrated that L-NNA decreased arterial pH and PaO_2 in the presence or absence of lipopolysaccharide. However, in a dog model of endotoxic shock we found that L-NMMA at a dose of 10 mg/kg/h did not influence tissue O_2 extraction capabilities since neither the critical DO_2 nor the critical oxygen extraction ratio were significantly altered [27].

The deleterious effects of NOS inhibition can be associated with eliciting an inflammatory response under pathological conditions. Kurose et al. [44] demonstrated that L-NAME increases leukocyte adherence, platelet-leukocyte aggregation, mast cell degranulation, and albumin leakage in rat mesenteric venules. NO can also influence the TNF response. Fukatsu et al. [45] observed that pretreatment with L-NAME in mice with gram negative sepsis increased plasma TNF levels and numbers of viable bacteria in both the peritoneal cavity and blood, and decreased survival time, compared with control mice.

Several investigators found that the administration of NOS inhibitors increased the mortality rate during endotoxic shock [7, 45-47, 55]. Laniyonu et al. [48] reported that L-NAME increased mortality by more than 50% in endotoxic hamsters. In mice, Minnard et al. [47] showed that the survival rate after endotoxic shock was reduced to 0% in the group receiving L-NAME compared with

87.5% in controls. The increased mortality rate was associated with an increase in tissue damage in the lung, liver, and kidney [45, 49].

The timing of interventions may be of great importance. Although some studies [9, 50] reported that the rapid (5 to 30 mins) development of hypotension in response to endotoxin *in vitro* and *in vivo* may be mediated by an enhanced release of NO through the constitutive pathway, the bulk of NO release is attributed to the induction of iNOS, which may take several hours [51-54]. The activity of the cNOS of the endothelial cells may even be depressed during the early phase of endotoxaemia, resulting in impaired endothelium-dependent vasodilation [56-59]. Laszlo et al. [60] showed that concurrent administration of L-NAME with endotoxin caused a dose-dependent elevation of plasma leakage in cardiac, pulmonary and renal tissues when determined 2 h later. By contrast, the delayed administration of L-NAME 3 h after endotoxin challenge, dose-dependently inhibited plasma leakage in the heart, lung and kidney. These results support a protective role of cNOS in the early phase of endotoxic shock. Gardiner et al. [61] reported that pretreatment with L-NMMA 1 h before endotoxin infusion did not prevent the early hypotension, but abolished the later (6-8 h) fall in arterial pressure. However, mesenteric and femoral blood flows were decreased. Delaying treatment with L-NMMA until 4 h after the start of endotoxin infusion still reduced mesenteric blood flow. When treatment with L-NMMA was delayed until 24 h after the start of endotoxin infusion, mesenteric blood flow was still compromised. Delayed treatment with L-NAME also caused a marked reduction in mesenteric and femoral blood flow, and alterations in cardiac performance.

The dose of NOS inhibitor is also very important, and may account for some of the differences observed in different studies. A high dose can result in excessive vasoconstricting effects, and is more likely to increase mortality rates [62].

Selective inducible NOS inhibition

Glucocorticosteroids can block the expression of a Ca^{2+}-independent NOS in endothelial cells activated with endotoxin and interferon-γ [63]. This is now well documented for various cells, including vascular smooth muscle cells, macrophages, neutrophils, and hepatocytes [64-67]. Pretreatment with dexamethasone prevents the induction of iNOS and the vascular failure caused by endotoxin in isolated vascular preparations *in vitro* [68] and reduces NOS induction in anaesthetized rats with endotoxic shock [68, 69]. Such an inhibition of induction prevents hypotension and vascular hypocontractility in response to vasoconstrictor agents [50], whereas glucocorticosteroids do not modify the haemodynamic patterns when given after endotoxin [69].

Several agents of different structures have been reported to selectively inhibit iNOS activity, such as aminoguanidine [70], SMT [71-73], and mercaptoethylguanidine (MEG) [74] with a preferential effect on iNOS. Although some authors found that SMT decreased expression of oxygen free radicals, elevated the endotoxin-induced reduction in thiols levels [72] and prolonged survival time in endotoxic rats [73], Vromen et al. [75] recently reported that selective inhibition of iNOS with MEG reduced plasma nitrite/nitrate levels, but did not prevent the development of vascular hyporeactivity, and did not improve survival in a rat model of cecal ligation and puncture. Hence, whether an iNOS inhibition is beneficial remains to be further investigated.

Clinical studies involving inhibitors of NOS and of guanylate cyclase

Evidence for the overproduction of NO in shock in humans comes from reports of increased serum nitrates, a breakdown product of NO, which correlate with systemic vasodilation in sepsis [12, 76, 77]. Petros et al. [78] first described the effects of administering L-NMMA i.v. to two patients in whom the mean blood pressure was maintained at about 65 mmHg by a combination of fluids, dopamine and norepinephrine. In these patients there was a rapid, transient increase in arterial pressure following L-NMMA administration and a marked increase in systemic vascular resistance. One of these patients ultimately died of a combination of recurrent abdominal sepsis, acute respiratory distress syndrome and disseminated intravascular coagulation.

Kiehl et al. [79] investigated the effects of NOS inhibition with L-NAME on haemodynamics and outcome in 10 leukocytopenic (< 1000/µl) patients with severe septic shock requiring strong vasopressor support. Continuous infusion of L-NAME (0.3 mg/kg, i.v.) was administered for a study period of 24 h with prolongation for up to 96 h according to individual requirements. Compared to baseline values, an increase in mean arterial pressure, systemic vascular resistance, and left ventricular stroke work index with a concomitant decrease in vasopressor requirement was observed during the first 24 h of L-NAME treatment. Five patients died during L-NAME treatment at between 28 and 94 hours. In the remaining five patients, L-NAME infusion was stopped after 27 to 84 h when the patients again became responsive to conventional vasopressor drugs. Two of these patients were free of vasopressors on days 6 and 9, respectively. The other three patients died within 53 h of stopping L-NAME due to septic shock, again unresponsive to vasopressor drugs, and without further L-NAME treatment. However, neither exhaled NO nor plasma nitrate and nitrite were measured in this study. Others investigators reported, in neutropenic patients with sepsis syndrome or septic shock, that plasma nitrate levels were lower than in septic patients with normal or elevated numbers of neutrophils [80].

Avontuur et al. [81] investigated prolonged inhibition of NOS in 11 patients with septic shock. Measurements of haemodynamic, haematologic, and biochemical variables were made before, during, and after the start of a continuous intravenous infusion of 1 mg/kg/hr of L-NAME for a period of 12 hrs. Continuous infusion of L-NAME resulted in a direct increase in mean arterial pressure and an increase in systemic vascular resistance, reaching a maximum at 0.5 hr.

Pulmonary arterial pressure was increased at 1 hr, and pulmonary vascular resistance increased at 3 hrs. Paralleling these changes, cardiac output and DO_2 decreased. L-NAME was most effective during the early stages of administration and the effect of L-NAME on blood pressure and vascular resistance tended to diminish throughout the continuous infusion of L-NAME. Seven of 11 patients ultimately died, with survival time ranging from 2 to 34 days. This study indicates that NO appears to play a role in cardiovascular derangements during human sepsis. Despite the fact that prolonged inhibition of NOS with L-NAME may help to maintain vascular tone and blood pressure, the overall clinical condition was not improved and the mortality rate remained high in these patients with septic shock.

Three dose-response, safety studies of NOS inhibitors have been reported in hypotensive patients with septic shock [82]. Blood pressure was restored rapidly in a dose-dependent fashion. A few patients had a complete normalization of blood pressure off all vasopressors for > 24 h, and some patients responded with an increase in systolic blood pressure to > 100 mmHg for 1h. However, none of these trials showed improved survival rate. The results of these clinical studies are summarized in Table 2. A more recent, as yet unpublished, study with L-NMMA in over 200 patients also failed to show a significant improvement in terms of haemodynamic variables and mortality rate. Dose escalation in the sepsis study proceeded to 40 mg/kg. A completed Phase II trial [83] of continuous infusion of L-NMMA as high as 20 mg/kg/h for 8 h showed a decrease in vasopressor requirements in septic patients.

In general, the detrimental effects of such procedures include markedly increased systemic vascular resistance, increased central venous pressure and pulmonary arterial pressure and resistance, decreases in cardiac output and oxygen delivery. Also a decrease in platelet count has been observed in the first phase II trial.

Blockade of the target enzyme of NO, guanylate cyclase, with methylene blue (MB) may present another option, capable of counteracting the haemodynamic effects of NO. In a preliminary report in two patients with septic shock [84], MB increased arterial pressure and systemic vascular resistance and slightly decreased cardiac index, without changing heart rate and pulmonary artery occlusion pressure. MB induced a longer lasting improvement of circulatory failure without deleterious side effects, but did not prevent the occurrence of delayed multiple organ failure or subsequent death. In 14 patients with severe septic shock, Preiser et al. [85] demonstrated that MB administration was followed by a progressive increase in arterial pressure, but pulmonary arterial pressure, cardiac filling pressures, cardiac output, DO_2, and $\dot{V}O_2$ were not significantly affected. Left ventricular stroke work index increased. Eleven of 14 patients subsequently died in this trial. In nine patients with septic shock, Daemen-Gubbels and colleagues [86] observed that after initial fluid resuscitation a single dose of MB transiently increased arterial pressure and $\dot{V}O_2$, associated with an improvement in myocardial function and DO_2. However, MB did not appear to improve survival rate, since eight of the nine patients died in this study.

Table 2. NOS inhibition in clinical shock

Nitric oxide inhibitors	Patient	Response	Reference
L-NMMA/L-NAME	Septic shock (n = 2)	Increased blood pressure	Petros et al. 1991
L-NMMA	Septic shock (n = 1)	Increased blood pressure	Schilling et al. 1993
L-NAME	Sepsis (n = 8)	Increased blood pressure, increased SVR, decreased CI and increased PAP	Lorente et al. 1993
L-NMMA	Septic shock (n = 6)	Increased blood pressure, decreased CO	Petros et al. 1994
L-NMMA	Septic shock (n = 1)	Increased blood pressure	Lin et al. 1994
L-NMMA	Cancer patients with shock (n = 13)	Increased blood pressure and decreased vasopressor requirement	Kilbourn et al. 1995
L-NMMA	Cancer patients with shock (n = 12)	Increased blood pressure and SVR, decreased CO	Kilbourn et al. 1996
L-NMMA	Septic shock (n = 32)	Blood pressure was sustained, allowing norepinephrine to be reduced	Zacardelli et al. 1995
L-NAME	Septic shock (n = 5)	Increased blood pressure, SVR and LVSWI	Kiehl et al. 1997
L-NAME	Septic shock (11)	Increased blood pressure, PAP, SVR and PVR, decreased CO	Avontuur et al. 1998
Methylene blue	Septic shock (n = 2)	increased SVR	Schneider et al. 1992
Methylene blue	Septic shock (n = 14)	Increased blood pressure, improved LVSWI, decreased blood lactate levels	Preiser et al. 1995
Methylene blue	Septic shock (n = 1)	Increased blood pressure, decreased vasopressor support	Brown et al. 1996
Haemoglobin	Critically ill (n = 14)	A 15-100% reduction in vasopressor drug requirement	Rhea et al. 1996

Effects of NO donors

Since NO is responsible for an essential vasodilatory tone and regulates microvascular perfusion it may play an important role in the maintenance of O_2 availability to the tissues [87]. It is intriguing, therefore, to test the hypothesis that NO-releasing compounds may have beneficial effects in septic shock. A number of investigators have studied NO donors, and found that they are protective during septic shock.

One of the important reasons for studying the effects of NO donors during septic shock is based on the underlying concept that cNOS activity is attenuated by endotoxin and cytokines [59-60, 88, 89]. The phenomenon seems to result from an increased degradation rate of endothelial cNOS mRNA [58, 59]. Wang et al. [57] demonstrated that endothelium-derived NO release is depressed during the hyperdynamic and hypodynamic stages of sepsis, not only in large arteries, but also in the microcirculation.

Effects of NO donors in experimental sepsis

We [27] recently studied the effects of the NO donor SIN-1, the vasoactive metabolite of molsidomine currently used as a nitrate compound in the treatment of coronary artery disease, in endotoxic shock in dogs. Although the model was characterized by a low vascular resistance, SIN-1 had no deleterious effect on arterial pressure. The adequate fluid loading of the animal was probably a prerequisite for such good cardiovascular tolerance, as SIN-1 may otherwise reduce venous return to the heart by its effect of venous capacitance. The lack of hypotension was also related to a significant increase in cardiac index associated with an improvement in cardiac function, as reflected by a greater left ventricular stroke work index. Such improvement in cardiac performance following SIN-1 administration, which has been observed previously [87], may be due to an improvement in coronary blood flow, a decrease in myocardial necrosis and endothelial dysfunction [90], or a direct enhancement of myocardial contractility [91, 92].

NO donors have been reported to increase regional blood flow in septic conditions. Mulder et al. [25] showed that splanchnic blood flow is critically dependent on NO during the first hour of endotoxaemia in rats. We observed that SIN-1 administration selectively increased hepatic, portal and mesenteric blood flow in a dog model of endotoxic shock [27]. In endotoxic rabbits, Pastor et al. [93] reported that SIN-1 maintained aortic and portal blood flow, and increased hepatic artery blood flow without effect on arterial pressure. Serum lactate levels increased in the endotoxic animals, and did not change in the SIN-1-treated animals. These findings show that during the early phase of endotoxic shock, and even in the absence of intense fluid resuscitation, SIN-1 administration may be beneficial in maintaining systemic and hepatic perfusion while preventing lactic acidosis. The protective effect of NO donors on the liver in endotoxaemia is associated with an up-regulation of hepatic protein synthesis by NO [94]. Boughton-Smith et al. [95] reported that exogenous supplementation of NO by S-nitro-N-acetyl-penicillamine (SNAP) administration, could preserve gut blood flow and attenuate endotoxin-induced jejunal damage in the rat. These data suggest that, in the early phase of endotoxic shock, NO is insufficiently released to allow adequate hepato-splanchnic perfusion. On the contrary, SIN-1 administration may decrease blood flow to the renal bed [27].

Werner et al. [35] demonstrated that both the NO donor sodium nitroprusside, and L-arginine reduced oedema formation. Evaluations of inflammation and necrosis by histologic scoring confirmed the reduction of pancreatic injury by NO donors. Wang et al. [32] reported that treatment with the NO donor spermine-NONOate or L-arginine reversed L-NAME induced ischaemia, liver injury, and impaired microvascular blood flow in endotoxic rats, suggesting that endogenous NO formation is necessary to limit ischaemic liver injury during reperfusion and endotoxaemia. The protective effects of NO donors on tissue injury may occur partially via a reduction of polymorphonuclear leukocyte infiltration [96]. Nishida et al. [31] reported that L-NAME or L-NMMA resulted in a threefold increase in leukocyte adherence in endotoxic mice. These disturbances were reversed by simultaneous administration of L-arginine. This suggests that NO plays a significant role in stabilizing the hepatic microcirculation during endotoxaemia, thereby helping to protect the liver from ischaemia and leukocyte-induced oxidative injury. Another NO donor, C87-3754, has been reported to attenuate the splanchnic artery occlusion-induced decline in release of endothelium-derived NO, and to improve short term survival in cats [97]. Additionally, C87-3754 significantly decreased polymorphonuclear leukocyte adherence to the superior mesenteric endothelium *in vitro*. Several investigators [98, 99] also reported that the NO donors sodium nitroprusside, spermine-NO, SIN-1, and SNAP significantly reduced microvascular dysfunction during ischaemia/reperfusion, and the protective effects of NO donors may be related to their ability to reduce leukocyte-endothelial cell and leukocyte-platelet interactions and/or mast cell degranulation [99].

Oxygen free radicals such as superoxide anion (O_2^-) can play an important role in the pathogenesis of septic shock. Several studies [100, 101] demonstrated that NO can depress the rate of reduction of cytochrome C by O_2^- released from polymorphonuclear leukocytes or generated from the oxidation of hypoxanthine by xanthine oxidase. These observations indicate that NO can be an important scavenger of O_2^- and provides a chemical barrier to cytotoxic oxygen free radicals. Moreover, Moilanen et al. [102] reported that NO donors, possibly through increased cGMP, inhibit the activation of human polymorphonuclear leukocytes and may thus act as a local modulator in inflammatory processes. Kumins et al. [103] more recently showed that SIN-1 attenuated TNF, IL-1 and IL-6 production in endotoxic mice.

NO release may also have protective effects in trauma. Christopher et al. [104] reported that the NO donor, SNAP prolonged survival time after trauma in the rat, and attenuated the increase in plasma aminonitrogen and tissue myeloperoxidase activities. Moreover, SNAP significantly preserved superior mesenteric artery endothelial function and the vasorelaxation to acetylcholine. These results indicate that NO donors may afford significant protection in traumatic shock by preserving vascular endothelial integrity, inhibiting neutrophil-endothelial interaction and reducing microvascular leakiness.

Inhaled NO in patients with acute respiratory distress syndrome

Inhaled NO therapy is proposed to increase oxygenation and decrease pulmonary artery pressure and perhaps facilitates the resolution of acute lung injury. Three clinical trials [105-107] have been conducted to evaluate the effects of inhaled NO therapy in patients with acute respiratory failure. All three trials concur to indicate the lack of significant effect on outcome. Dellinger et al. [105] recently evaluated the safety and physiologic response of inhaled nitric oxide in patients with acute respiratory distress syndrome (ARDS). This prospective, double-blind trial of inhaled NO in ARDS was the largest study performed to date and the first to use placebo controls. It was the first to use standardized principles of mechanical ventilation support of ARDS, a standardized NO delivery device, and a single type of ventilator. This study confirmed the important effects of NO in acute inflammatory lung disease [105]. PaO_2 was increased by > 20% in 60% of patients receiving NO, allowing clinicians to reduce the FiO_2 (1 day) and to ventilate the patients at a lower oxygenation index including FiO_2, tidal volume and positive end-expiratory pressure (4 days). There was also a consistent reduction in the pulmonary arterial pressure (2 days). A diminished pulmonary artery pressure has been reported to be related to a reduced pulmonary oedema formation [108]. The primary objective of this trial was to evaluate safety and physiologic responses of different doses of inhaled NO (1.25 to 80 ppm). The trial showed no evidence of NO toxicity, although mild methaemoglobinaemia and nitrogen dioxide formation were noted at 80 ppm NO dose level. The study by Dellinger et al. [105] supports the conclusion that NO may be useful to increase PaO_2 in severe hypoxaemia but cannot be considered as a therapeutic agent against acute lung disease.

Conclusions

Inhibition of NOS could be deleterious as tissue perfusion can be altered, and reports published so far have not demonstrated clinical success. The benefits of selective inhibition of iNOS remain to be proven because iNOS expression opposes platelet prothrombotic and leukocyte proadhesive properties induced by sepsis. Since NO donors exert some protective effects it is thus conceivable that an inhibitor of iNOS could be given simultaneously with an NO donor including NO to reverse severe hypoperfusion and oxygenation failure on one hand and to protect tissue function on the other. Other therapeutic approaches could be to inhibit other mediators, such as oxygen free radicals and the cytokine network, which contribute to iNOS expression during sepsis.

References

1. Marletta MA, Yoon PS, Iyengar R et al (1988) Macrophage oxidation of L-arginine to nitrite and nitrate: Nitric oxide is an intermediate. Biochemistry 27:8706-8711
2. Stuehr DJ, Gross SS, Sakuma I et al (1989) Activated murine macrophages secrete a metabolite of arginine with the bioactivity of endothelium-derived relaxing factor and the chemical reactivity of nitric oxide. J Exp Med 169:1011-1020
3. Brady AJ, Poole-Wilson PA, Harding SE, Warren JB (1992) Nitric oxide production within cardiac myocytes reduces their contractility in endotoxemia. Am J Physiol 263:H1963-H1966
4. Geller DA, Nussler AK, Di Silvio M et al (1993) Cytokines, endotoxin, and glucocorticoids regulate the expression of inducible nitric oxide synthase in hepatocytes. Proc Natl Acad Sci USA 90:522-526
5. Moncada S, Palmer RM, Higgs EA (1991) Nitric oxide: Physiology, pathophysiology, and pharmacology. Pharmacol Rev 43:109-142
6. Kilbourn RG, Jubran A, Gross SS et al (1990) N^G-methyl-L-arginine inhibits tumor necrosis factor-induced hypotension: Implications for the involvement of nitric oxide. Proc Natl Acad Sci USA 87:3629-3632
7. Wright CE, Rees DD, Moncada S (1992) Protective and pathological roles of nitric oxide in endotoxin shock. Cardiovasc Res 26:48-57
8. Evans T, Carpenter A, Kinderman H, Cohen J (1993) Evidence of increased nitric oxide production in patients with the sepsis syndrome. Circ Shock 41:77-81
9. Salvemini D, Korbut R, Anggard E, Vane JR (1990) Immediate release of nitric oxide-like factor from bovine aortic endothelial cells by Escherichia coli lipopolysaccharide. Proc Natl Acad Sci USA 87:2593-2697
10. Nakae H, Endo S, Inada K et al (1996) Nitrite/nitrate (Nox) and type II phospholipase A2, leukotriene B4, and platelet-activating factor levels in patients with septic shock. Res Commun Mol Pathol Pharmacol 92:131-139
11. Endo S, Inada K, Nakae H et al (1996) Nitrite/nitrate (Nox) and cytokine levels in patients with septic shock. Res Commun Mol Pathol Pharmacol 91:347-356
12. Gomez-Jimenez J, Salgado A, Mourelle M et al (1995) L-arginine: nitric oxide pathway in endotoxemia and human septic shock. Crit Care Med 23:253-258
13. Wong HR, Carcillo JA, Burckart G, Kaplan SS (1996) Nitric oxide production in critically ill patients. Arch Dis Child 74:482-489
14. Mitaka C, Hirata Y, Ichikawa K et al (1995) Effects of nitric oxide synthase inhibitor on hemodynamic change and O_2 delivery in septic dogs. Am J Physiol 268:H2017-H2023
15. Lorente J, Landin L, De Pablo R et al (1993) L-arginine pathway in sepsis. Crit Care Med 21:1287-1295
16. Finkel MS, Oddis CV, Jacob TD et al (1992) Negative inotropic effects of cytokines on the heart mediated by nitric oxide. Science 257:387-389
17. Decking UKM, Flesche CW, Gödecke A, Schrader J (1995) Endotoxin-induced contractile dysfunction in guinea pig hearts is not mediated by nitric oxide. Am J Physiol 268:H2460-H2465
18. Klabunde RE, Coston AF (1995) Nitric oxide synthase inhibition does not prevent cardiac depression in endotoxic shock. Shock 3:73-78
19. Vincent J-L, Colice G, Grover R (1995) The effects of 546C88 on left ventricular performance in patients with septic shock. Intensive Care Med 21:S20 (abstract)
20. Meng X, Ao L, Brown JM et al (1997) Nitric oxide synthase is not involved in cardiac contractile dysfunction in a rat model of endotoxemia without shock. Shock 7:111-118
21. Keller RS, Jones JJ, Kim KF (1995) Endotoxin-induced myocardial dysfunction: is there a role for nitric oxide? Shock 4:338-344
22. Avontuur JAM, Ince BC (1995) Inhibition of nitric oxide synthesis causes myocardial ischemia in endotoxemic rats. Circ Res 76:418-425
23. Cohen RI, Shapir Y, Chen L, Scharf SM (1998) Right ventricular overload causes the decrease in cardiac output after nitric oxide synthesis inhibition in endotoxemia. Crit Care Med 26:738-747

24. Spath Jr JA, Sloane PJ, Gee MH, Albertine KH (1994) Loss of endothelium-dependent vasodilation in the pulmonary vessels of sheep after prolonged endotoxin. J Appl Physiol 76: 361-369
25. Mulder MF, Van Lambalgen AA, Huisman E et al (1994) Protective role of NO in the regional hemodynamic changes during acute endotoxemia in rats. Am J Physiol 266:H1558-H1564
26. Robertson FM, Offner PJ, Ciceri DP (1994) Detrimental hemodynamic effects of nitric oxide synthase inhibition in septic shock. Arch Surg 129:149-156
27. Zhang H, Rogiers P, Smail N et al (1997) Effects of nitric oxide on regional blood flow and oxygen extraction capabilities in endotoxic shock. J Appl Physiol 83:1164-1173
28. Henderson JL, Statman R, Cunnigham JN et al (1994) The effects of nitric oxide inhibition on regional hemodynamics during hyperdynamic endotoxemia. Arch Surg 129:1271-1275
29. Ayuse T, Brienza N, Revelly JP (1995) Role of nitric oxide in porcine live circulation under normal and endotoxemic conditions. J Appl Physiol 78:1319-1329
30. Pastor CM, Payen DM (1994) Effect of modifying nitric oxide pathway on liver circulation in a rabbit endotoxin shock model. Shock 2:196-202
31. Nishida J, McCuskey RS, McDonnell D, Fox ES (1994) Protective role of NO in hepatic microcirculatory dysfunction during endotoxemia. Am J Physiol 267:G1135-G1141
32. Wang Y, Mathews WR, Guido DM et al (1995) Inhibition of nitric oxide synthesis aggravates reperfusion injury after hepatic ischemia and endotoxemia. Shock 4:282-288
33. Spain DA, Wilson MA, Bar-Natan MF, Garrison RN (1994) Nitric oxide synthase inhibition aggravates intestinal microvascular vasoconstriction and hypoperfusion of bacteremia. J Trauma 36:720-725
34. Walker TA, Curtis SE, King-Van Vlack CE et al (1995) Effects of nitric oxide synthase inhibition on regional hemodynamics and oxygen transport in endotoxic dogs. Shock 4:415-420
35. Werner J, Rivera J, Castillo CF (1997) Differing roles of nitric oxide in the pathogenesis of acute edematous versus necrotizing pancreatitis. Surgery 121:23-30
36. Spain DA, Wilson MA, Bloom ITM, Garrison RN (1994) Renal microvascular responses to sepsis are dependent on nitric oxide. J Surg Res 56:524-529
37. Kubes P, Granger DN (1992) Nitric oxide modulates microvascular permeability. Am J Physiol 262:H611-H615
38. Kurose I, Kubes P, Wolf R (1993) Inhibition on nitric oxide production: mechanisms of vascular albumin leakage. Circ Res 73:164-171
39. Oliver JA (1992) Endothelium-derived relaxing factor contributes to the regulation of endothelial permeability. J Cell Physiol 151:506-511
40. Kubes P (1993) Ischemia-reperfusion in feline small intestine: a role for nitric oxide. Am J Physiol 264:G143-G149
41. Payne D, Kubes P (1993) Nitric oxide donors reduce the rise in reperfusion-induced intestinal mucosal permeability. Am J Physiol 265:G189-G195
42. Rumbaut RE, McKay MK, Huxley VH (1995) Capillary hydraulic conductivity is decreased by nitric oxide synthase inhibition. Am J Physiol 368:H1856-H1861
43. Statman R, Cheng W, Cunningham JN et al (1994) Nitric oxide inhibition in the treatment of the sepsis syndrome is detrimental to tissue oxygenation. J Surg Res 57:93-98
44. Kurose I, Wolf R, Grisham MB, Granger DN (1995) Effects of an endogenous inhibitor of nitric oxide synthesis on postcapillary venules. Am J Physiol 268:H2224-H2231
45. Fukatsu K, Saito H, Fukushima R et al (1995) Detrimental effects of nitric oxide synthase inhibitor (N-ω-nitro-L-arginine-methyl-ester) in a murine sepsis model. Arch Surg 130:410-414
46. Cobb JP, Natanson C, Quezado ZMN et al (1995) Differential hemodynamic effects of L-NMMA in endotoxemic and normal dogs. Am J Physiol 268:H1634-H1642
47. Minnard EA, Shou J, Naama H et al (1994) Inhibition of nitric oxide synthesis is detrimental during endotoxemia. Arch Surg 129:142-148
48. Laniyonu AA, Coston AF, Klabunde RE (1997) Endotoxin-induced microvascular leakage is prevented by a PAF antagonist and NO synthase inhibitor. Shock 7:49-54
49. Fukatsu K, Saito H, Fukushima R et al (1996) Effects of three inhibitors of nitric oxide synthase on host resistance to bacterial infection. Inflamm Res 45:109-112

50. Szabó C, Mitchell JA, Thiemermann C, Vane JR (1993) Nitric oxide-mediated hyporeactivity to noradrenaline precedes the induction of nitric oxide synthase in endotoxin shock. Br J Pharmacol 108:786-792

51. Mitchell JA, Kohlhaas KL, Sorrentino R et al (1993) Induction by endotoxin of nitric oxide synthase in the rat mesentery: lack of effect on action of vasconstrictors. Br J Pharmacol 109:265-270

52. Morris S, Billiar T (1994) New insights into the regulation of inducible nitric oxide synthesis. Am J Physiol 266:E829-E839

53. Salter M, Knowles RG, Moncada S (1991) Widespread tissue distribution, species distribution and changes in activity of Ca^{2+}-dependent and Ca^{2+}-independent nitric oxide synthase. FEBS 291:145-149

54. Wallis G, Brackett D, Lerner M et al (1996) *In vivo* spin trapping of nitric oxide generated in the small intestine, liver, and kidney during the development of endotoxemia: a time-course study. Shock 6:274-278

55. Cobb JP, Natanson C, Hoffman WD et al (1992) N^{ω}-amino-L-arginine, an inhibitor of nitric oxide synthase, raises vascular resistance but increases mortality rates in awake canines challenged with endotoxin. J Exp Med 176:1175-1182

56. Parker JL, Adams HR (1993) Selective inhibition of endothelium-dependent vasodilator capacity by Escherichia coli endotoxemia. Circ Res 72:539-551

57. Wang P, Ba ZF, Chaudry IH (1995) Endothelium-dependent relaxation is depressed at the macro- and microcirculatory levels during sepsis. Am J Physiol 269:R988-R994

58. Lu J-L, Schmiege III LM, Kuo L, Liao JC (1996) Downregulation of endothelial constitutive nitric oxide synthase expression by lipopolysaccharide. Biochem Biophys Res Commun 225:1-5

59. Yoshizumi M, Perrella MA, Burnett JC Jr, Lee ME (1993) Tumor necrosis factor downregulates an endothelial nitric oxide synthase mRNA by shortening its half life. Circ Res 73: 205-209

60. Laszlo F, Whittle BJR, Evans SM, Moncada S (1995) Association of microvascular leakage with induction of nitric oxide synthase: effects of nitric oxide synthase inhibitors in various organs. Eur J Pharmacol 283:47-53

61. Gardiner SM, Kemp PA, Bennett MT (1995) Cardiac and regional haemodynamics, inducible nitric oxide synthase (NOS) activity, and the effects of NOS inhibitors in conscious, endotoxaemic rats. Br J Pharmacol 116:2005-2016

62. Nava E, Palmer RMJ, Moncada S (1991) Inhibition of nitric oxide synthesis in septic shock: how much is beneficial? Lancet 338:1555-1557

63. Radomski MW, Palmer RM, Moncada S (1990) Glucocorticoids inhibit the expression of an inducible, but not the constitutive, nitric oxide synthase in vascular endothelial cells. Proc Natl Acad Sci USA 87:10043-10047

64. DiRosa M, Radomski M, Carnuccio R et al (1990) Glucocorticoids inhibit the induction of nitric oxide synthase in macrophages. Biochem Biophys Res Commun 172:1246-1252

65. McCall TB, Palmer RM, Moncada S (1991) Induction of nitric oxide synthase in rat peritoneal neutrophils and its inhibition by dexamethasone. Eur J Immunol 21:2523-2527

66. Pittner R, Spitzer J (1992) Endotoxin and TNF-α directly stimulate nitric oxide formation in cultured rat hepatocytes from chronically endotoxemic rats. Biochem Biophys Res Commun 185:430-435

67. Rees DD, Cellek S, Palmer RM et al (1990) Dexamethasone prevents the induction by endotoxin of a nitric oxide synthase and the associated effects on vascular tone: An insight into endotoxin shock. Biochem Biophys Res Commun 173:541-547

68. Knowles RG, Salter M, Brooks SL et al (1990) Anti-inflammatory glucocorticoids inhibit the induction by endotoxin of nitric oxide synthase in the lung, liver and aorta of the rat. Biochem Biophys Res Commun 172:1042-1048

69. Paya D, Gray G, Fleming I et al (1993) Effect of dexamethasone on the onset and persistence of vascular hyporeactivity induced by E. coli lipopolysaccharide in rats. Circ Shock 41: 103-112

70. Misko TP, Moore WM, Kasten TP et al (1993) Selective inhibition of the inducible nitric oxide synthase by aminoguanidine. Eur J Pharmacol 233:119-125

71. Szabo C, Southan G, Thiemermann C (1994) Beneficial effects and improved survival in rodent models of septic shock with S-methylisothiourea sulfate, a potent and selective inhibitor of inducible nitric oxide synthase. Proc Natl Acad Sci USA 91:12472-12476

72. Chamulitrat W, Skrepnik NV, Spitzer JJ (1996) Endotoxin-induced oxidative stress in the rat small intestine: role of nitric oxide. Shock 5:217-222

73. Aranow JS, Zhuang J, Wang H et al (1996) A selective inhibitor of inducible nitric oxide synthase prolongs survival in a rat model of bacterial peritonitis: comparison with two nonselective strategies. Shock 5:116-121

74. Southan GJ, Zingarelli B, O'Connor M et al (1996) Spontaneous rearrangement of amino-alkylisothioureas into mercaptoalkylguanidines, a novel class of nitric oxide synthase inhibitors with selectivity towards the inducible isoform. Br J Pharmacol 117:619-632

75. Vromen A, Arkovitz MS, Zingarelli B et al (1996) Low-level expression and limited role for the inducible isoform of nitric oxide synthase in the vascular hyporeactivity and mortality associated with cecal ligation and puncture in the rat. Shock 6:248-253

76. Ochoa J, Curti B, Peitzman A (1992) Increased circulating nitrogen oxides after human tumor immunotherapy correlate with toxic hemodynamic changes. J Natl Cancer Inst 84:864-867

77. Wong H, Carcillo J, Burkart G et al (1995) Increased serum nitrate and nitrite concentrations in children with sepsis syndrome. Crit Care Med 23:835-842

78. Petros A, Bennett D, Vallance P (1991) Effect of nitric oxide synthase inhibitors on hypotension in patients with septic shock. Lancet 338:1557-1558

79. Kiehl MG, Ostermann H, Meyer J, Kienast J (1997) Nitric oxide synthase inhibition by L-NAME in leukocytopenic patients with severe septic shock. Intensive Care Med 23:561-566

80. Neilly IJ, Copland M, Haj M et al (1995) Plasma nitrate concentrations in neutropenic and non-neutropenic patients with suspected septicaemia. Br J Haematol 89:199-202

81. Avontuur JA, Nolthenius RPT, van Bodegom JW, Bruining JA (1998) Prolonged inhibition of nitric oxide synthesis in severe septic shock: A clinical study. Crit Care Med 26:660-667

82. Hibbs J, Westenfelder C, Taintor R (1992) Evidence for cytokine-induced nitric oxide synthesis from L-arginine in patients receiving interleukin-2 therapy. J Clin Invest 89:867-877

83. Zaccardelli D, Grover R, Colice G (1995) Hemodynamic effects of 546C88 (L-N^G-methylarginine HCL) in an open label, dose escalation study of patients with septic shock. Intensive Care Med 21:S21 (abstract)

84. Schneider F, Lutun P, Hasselmann M et al (1992) Methylene blue increases systemic vascular resistance in human septic shock. Preliminary observations. Intensive Care Med 18:309-311

85. Preiser J-C, Lejeune P, Roman A et al (1995) Methylene blue administration in septic shock: A clinical trial. Crit Care Med 23:259-264

86. Daemen-Gubbels CR, Groeneveld PH, Groeneveld AM et al (1995) Methylene blue increases myocardial function in septic shock. Crit Care Med 23:1363-1370

87. Zhang H, Rogiers P, Spapen H et al (1996) Effects of nitric oxide donor SIN-1 on oxygen availability and regional blood flow during endotoxic shock. Arch Surg 131:767-774

88. Greenberg S, Xie J, Wang Y et al (1993) Tumor necrosis factor-alpha inhibits endothelium-dependent relaxation. J Appl Physiol 74:2394-2403

89. Myers PR, Wright TF, Tanner MA, Adams HR (1992) EDRF and nitric oxide production in cultured endothelial cells: direct inhibition by E. coli endotoxin. Am J Physiol 262:H710-H718

90. Siegfride MR, Erhardt J, Rider T et al (1992) Cardioprotection and attenuation of endothelial dysfunction by organic nitric oxide donors in myocardial ischemia-reperfusion. J Pharmacol Exp Ther 260:668-675

91. Pabla R, Buda AJ, Flynn DM et al (1995) Intracoronary nitric oxide improves postischemic coronary blood flow and myocardial contractile function. Am J Physiol 269:H1113-H1121

92. Schluter KD, Weber M, Schraveb E, Piper HM (1994) NO donor SIN-1 protects against reoxygenation-induced cardiomyocyte injury by a dual action. Am J Physiol 267:H1461-H1466

93. Pastor CM, Losser MR, Payen D (1995) Nitric oxide donor prevents hepatic and systemic perfusion decrease induced by endotoxin in anesthetized rabbits. Hepatology 22:1547-1553

94. Frederick JA, Hasselgren PO, Davis S et al (1993) Nitric oxide may upregulate in vivo hepatic protein synthesis during endotoxemia. Arch Surg 128:152-157

95. Boughton-Smith NK, Hucheson IR, Deakin AM (1994) Protective effect of S-nitroso-N-acetyl-penicillamine in endotoxin-induced acute intestinal damage in the rat. Eur J Pharmacol 191:485-488

96. Andrews FJ, Malcontenti-Wilson C, O'Brien PE (1994) Protection against gastric ischemia-reperfusion injury by nitric oxide generators. Dig Dis Sci 39:366-373

97. Carey C, Siegfried MR, Ma X-L et al (1992) Antishock and endothelial protective actions of a NO donor in mesenteric ischemia and reperfusion. Circ Shock 38:209-216

98. Kurose I, Wolf R, Grisham MB, Granger DN (1994) Modulation of ischemia/reperfusion-induced microvascular dysfunction by nitric oxide. Circ Res 74:376-382

99. Gauthier TW, Davenpeck KL, Lefer AM (1994) Nitric oxide attenuates leukocyte-endothelial interaction via P-selectin in splanchnic ischemia-reperfusion. Am J Physiol 267:G562-G568

100. Bubanyi GM, Ho EH, Cantor EH et al (1991) Cytoprotective function of nitric oxide: inactivation of superoxide radicals produced by human leukocytes. Biochem Biophys Res Commun 181:1392-1397

101. Gryglewski RJ, Palmer RMJ, Moncada S (1986) Superoxide anion is involved in the breakdown of endothelium-derived vascular relaxing factor. Nature 320:454-456

102. Moilanen E, Vuorinen P, Kankaanranta H et al (1993) Inhibition by nitric oxide-donors of human polymorphonuclear leucocyte functions. Br J Pharmacol 109:852-858

103. Kumins NH, Hunt J, Gamelli RL, Filkins JP (1997) Molsidomine increases endotoxic survival and decreases cytokine production. Shock 7:200-205

104. Christopher TA, Ma X-L, Lefer AM (1994) Beneficial actions of S-nitroso-N-acetylpenicillamine, a nitric oxide donor, in murine traumatic shock. Shock 1:19-24

105. Dellinger RP, Zimmerman JL, Taylor RW et al (1998) Effects of inhaled nitric oxide in patients with acute respiratory distress syndrome: Results of a randomized phase II trial. Crit Care Med 26:15-23

106. Rossaint R, Falke KJ, Lopez F (1993) Inhaled nitric oxide for the adult respiratory distress syndrome. N Engl J Med 328:399-405

107. Gerlach H, Rossaint R, Pappert D (1993) Time-course and dose-response of nitric oxide inhalation for systemic oxygenation and pulmonary hypertension in patients with adult respiratory distress syndrome. Eur J Clin Invest 23:499-502

108. Gottlieb SS, Wood LD, Hansen DE (1987) The effect of nitroprusside on pulmonary edema, oxygen exchange, and blood flow in hydrochloric aid aspiration. Anesthesiology 67:203-210

Management of Shock Complicating Acute Myocardial Infarction

A. Marn Pernat, M.H. Weil, A. Pernat

Incidence

Cardiogenic shock remains a leading cause of early cardiac death. The mortality rate of cardiogenic shock as a complication of acute myocardial infarction (AMI) exceeds 80%. Large multicenter studies disclose an incidence of 5 to 15% of all instances of AMI admitted to the hospital [1-5]. Cardiogenic shock is in evidence at the time of hospital admission in only minority of patients. Approximately 90% of patients develop shock during the in hospital stay [5].

These patients usually have greater clinical and haemodynamic evidence of an impaired ventricular function at the time of admission to the hospital than those who do not develop cardiogenic shock [2].

Setting

Typically such patients are more often women, are older, and present with a past history of a coronary event or congestive heart failure. They more often manifest recurrent ischaemia characterized by unrelenting chest discomfort, arm pain, jaw pain or nausea. The electrocardiogram typically reveals elevated or depressed ST segments and inverted T waves in affected leads, acute Q waves, and/or bundle branch block.

Cardiogenic shock is characterized by systemic hypotension in which systolic arterial pressure is less than 80 mmHg. In patients with established hypertensive disease, the systolic pressure may exceed 80 mmHg but there is a decline greater than 40 mmHg below prior levels unrelated to effects of vasoactive drugs. In each instance, the haemodynamic abnormalities are accompanied by evidence of end-organ hypoperfusion. These include altered mental status, cold extremities, oliguria and metabolic acidosis. Increases in left ventricular filling or diastolic pressures are clinically associated with pulmonary congestion, orthopnoea and sometimes right ventricular failure with abnormal neck vein distention. Frequently, serum enzymatic markers of infarction indicate extension or reinfarction with a secondary elevation. The preferred marker in our clinic remains creatine kinase MB isoenzyme. For the early detection of myocardial-cell injury in coronary syndromes, cardiac-specific troponin T and troponin I are appropriate alternative markers especially in emergency department settings [6].

Diagnosis and treatment

Immediate haemodynamic, echocardiographic and angiographic evaluations are now routine for patients who present with cardiogenic shock. The focus may be on coronary anatomy and left ventricular contractile function but it is essential that other mechanical complications including right ventricular infarction are identified.

The clinician is alerted to mechanical causes during physical examination in which a new thrill, murmur, or adventitial sound indicate the possibility of mechanical defects. Such complications typically occur during the first week. Transthoracic or, preferably, transoesophageal echocardiography is now employed for more precise diagnosis. Mechanical causes include postinfarction ventricular septal defect, left ventricular free wall rupture, left ventricular aneurysm, and papillary muscle and chordal dysfunction or rupture accounting for acute mitral valve regurgitation. Some mechanical lesions may be confirmed with measurements provided by the Swan Ganz flow-directed, pulmonary artery catheter. In the setting of an acquired ventricular septal defect, an oxygen saturation step-up in the pulmonary artery is detected. Ventricular rupture of the free wall with pericardial tamponade produces equalization of diastolic pressures and pulsus paradoxus. Echocardiographic findings are diagnostic for this life threatening mechanical defect. The primary therapy is operative intervention usually preceded by balloon counterpulsation if time allows. Prompt surgical repair decreases the very high mortality [7, 8].

After primary mechanical causes are excluded, coronary angiography is likely to identify culprit arteries which in turn guides definitive therapy. Such is either "rescue" angioplasty or emergency surgical revascularization.

Cardiogenic shock is characterized by a low cardiac output state in which there is a concurrent increase in left ventricular filling pressure. For purposes of clinical diagnosis, the measurement of pulmonary artery occlusive pressure confirms such if it exceeds 18 mmHg. The cardiac index is typically decreased to less than 2.0 liters/min per m^2. When right ventricular infarction predominates, there is a greater right than left ventricular filling pressure. Echocardiographically, left ventricular dilation with a hypo- or akinetic right ventricle pinpoints right ventricular involvement. With current echo-Doppler methodologies appropriate distinction between primary right ventricular infarction and right ventricular dilation caused by pulmonary thromboembolism or pulmonary hypertension is facilitated.

When a flow-directed pulmonary artery catheter is in place, fluid challenge is utilized to maximize cardiac output and yet prevent excessive increases in left ventricular diastolic pressure as reflected in the pulmonary artery occlusive ("wedge") pressure [9, 10]. Intra-arterial pressure monitoring is now viewed as mandatory because indirect measurements are inaccurate in the vasoconstrictive, low flow state of cardiogenic shock [9, 11].

Medical management

Both pharmacological and mechanical support of the failing heart provide means for stabilizing the haemodynamic state of the patient pending definitive interventions. *Medical management alone has failed to improve outcomes* [12]. In the previously normotensive patient in whom systolic blood pressure declines to less than 80 mmHg, there is a current opinion favoring the administration of dopamine in an initial dose of 5 to 15 µg/kg per minute [9, 13]. Dobutamine may improve cardiac output by its inotropic action but its β-adrenergic effect may also increase myocardial ischaemia and expand the region of infarction. However, dobutamine may increase coronary blood flow in parallel with increased cardiac output and thereby preserve blood flow to the ischaemic but viable myocardium. It also reduces left ventricular filling pressure [14]. There is also an expert opinion favoring administration of norepinephrine in doses ranging from 2 to 10 µg/min such as to maintain diastolic blood pressure above 60 mmHg. Norepinephrine increases diastolic arterial pressure and coronary perfusion and therefore improves contractility. However, it also has β-adrenergic effect by which it increases contractility and cardiac output but also at the expense of increased myocardial oxygen consumption [9, 15, 16]. Current opinion therefore favors mechanical support with minimal vasopressor or adrenergic inotropic interventions in such settings.

In the instance of primary right ventricular infarction intravascular volume expansion with physiological salt solution and/or dobutamine are appropriate interventions [17].

Mechanical support

Intra-aortic balloon pumping is the primary circulatory support option. The intra-aortic balloon is inflated during diastole and therefore increases proximal aortic, coronary, and cerebral perfusion. The balloon is released during systole allowing for reduction of left ventricular afterload. Such support decreases myocardial oxygen demand and therefore preserves myocardial mass in contrast with the effects of adrenergic inotropic drugs [17].

Newer circulatory assist methodologies include prosthetic ventricles, left ventricular turbine which is a catheter-mounted left ventricular assist device, partial or complete extracorporeal circulation and total artificial heart implantation. All are currently viewed as bridges to life-saving surgical interventions including cardiac transplantation [17-20].

It is important to reiterate that mechanical support systems help to stabilize patients but do not improve survival. Invasive procedures, both angioplasty and open heart surgery, may then be performed with greater safety and potentially improved outcomes [21]. Their most important role is to allow time for definitive intervention.

Patients with cardiogenic shock are best transferred to a cardiac catheterization laboratory for urgent angiographic evaluation followed by percutaneous or surgical revascularization. In the GUSTO-I trial, mortality was significantly reduced among the 406 patients who had early angiography and revascularization when compared to 1794 patients who were managed without catheterization (38% vs 68%) [22]. Coronary angiography is also required prior to repair of mechanical complications such that surgically correctable coronary lesions are identified and treated as part of the surgical intervention.

Reperfusion of the ischaemic myocardium

Cardiogenic shock in the absence of a major mechanical cause is associated with massive myocardial muscle loss usually involving more than 40% of the left ventricle [23]. In two-thirds of the patients with shock, extension and expansion of transmural infarction or global endocardial ischaemia with multiple recent infarcts of variable age were documented on postmortem examinations [2, 24]. Because the mass of dysfunctional myocardium has been shown to be the most specific predictor of development of cardiogenic shock, immediate treatment is intended to secure survival of as much myocardium as possible. Accordingly, early restoration of nutritional flow to the ischaemic region of the infarct such as to rescue "stunned" myocardium appears to be the most reasonable treatment [25]. Reperfusion is achieved either by thrombolysis or invasive revascularization.

Thrombolysis

The role of thrombolytic therapy in established shock status is limited. It has been demonstrated that efficacy of thrombolytic drugs is diminished in part because the coronary flow is diminished to the extent that the thrombolytic drug fails to reach the thrombus [26]. Anecdotal reports of successful reperfusion with thrombolytic agents [27] were not sustained by larger randomized studies of thrombolytic treatment in which mortality was very disappointing [4, 5, 28, 29]. Treatment with direct intracoronary infusion of streptokinase [28], intravenous streptokinase [5, 29] and intravenous recombinant tissue-type plasminogen activator (rt-PA) [4] have each failed to improve outcome. Regardless of the thrombolytic agent employed, mortality ranged from 50 to 80% [4, 5, 29]. The lowest 6-week mortality of 51% was reported in the TIMI 2 Trial in which rt-PA was injected peripherally [4]. Although intracoronary administration of streptokinase potentially improves survival only 43% of the patients with shock demonstrated reperfusion of thrombosed coronary arteries [28]. At the time of this writing, we conclude that thrombolysis should be reserved only for those patients who can not be transferred to a regional center for early catheterization and revascularization. Yet, early thrombolytic treatment of acute MI reduces the likelihood that shock will evolve. Minor advantages of rt-PA are currently identified [5, 22, 30].

Emergent revascularization

Urgent revascularization by emergency angioplasty including conventional percutaneous transluminal coronary angioplasty (PTCA) and stents, or coronary artery bypass graft surgery (CABG) have yielded striking improvement in overall survival to as high as 70% [31, 32]. Revascularization should be performed early and preferably within less than 24 hours of the onset of cardiogenic shock. When the time from development of cardiogenic shock to revascularization was within 24 hours, 77% patients survived. There was only 10% survival if revascularization by either or both angioplasty and coronary bypass surgery was delayed for more than 24 hours [33].

Percutaneous transluminal coronary angioplasty

Successful angioplasty yielded survival of between 60-80% compared to less than 20% when angioplasty failed to restore effective coronary blood [13, 18, 34, 35]. Both initial survival and long term survival with return to normal activity followed successful angioplastic revascularization [34].

We now favor aggressive intervention, beginning with angioplasty for patients who are haemodynamically stable. Failing to restore blood flow at the site(s) of major occlusion, we then promptly defer to coronary bypass operations contingent on the angiographic interpretations of the suitability for such. Surgical revascularization is believed to be the intervention of choice in patients with triple-vessel disease even if partial reperfusion of the infarct-related coronary artery has been secured with PTCA [18, 36].

There is nevertheless some continuing controversy on the benefits of rescue PTCA after unsuccessful thrombolysis. Although the TIMI-2 study reported no differences in six-week survival rates of 33% and 31% in patients with and without attempted angioplasty after thrombolysis, only 18 patients in this series had rescue angioplasty following thrombolysis [4].

These reports on failure of balloon angioplasty in the setting of shock must now be reevaluated for poor outcomes with the improved use of newer stenting techniques [37].

Coronary artery bypass graft surgery

Emergency CABG, which may involve bypassing occluded as well as severely obstructed nonoccluded vessels, remains the ultimate option for revascularization. It is the intervention of choice when all three major coronary arteries have luminal obstructions exceeding 70% [38].

DeWood was the first to show 60% survival rate for patients with cardiogenic shock treated with emergency bypass surgery [21] and subsequent studies confirmed this to be superior to medical treatments [39-41]. Quite remarkably, of eighty-nine patients with cardiogenic shock who underwent coronary artery bypass surgery between 1972 to 1992, the 1-year and 10-year survivals were 77 and 60% respectively [40].

The largest of multicenter, prospective, randomized trials on cardiogenic shock [31] are ongoing. The outcomes of emergency revascularization with either PTCA or CABG are compared with delayed revascularization. Early results indicate greater decreases in mortality after CABG. For the present, however, we can not exclude selection bias and we would therefore hesitate to predict the ultimate outcome of this study [31]. For the present, we recommend routine angiography and selection for PTCA or CABG based on the results thereof. In instances of failure of PTCA to reestablish blood flow, patients are treated with surgical revascularization.

Emergency cardiac transplantation

In appropriately selected patients, cardiac transplantation is indicated. Our optimism is in part based on a European report of survival rate of 70% of 15 patients including 9 patients with onset of shock within 3 days and 6 patients within 1 day after acute MI. Cardiac assist devices were used in 6 of the patients as a bridge to transplantation. Early post-transplant mortality was only 20% [20]. Yet, the strategy for securing donor organs is likely to preclude wide application of this option. Some patients are likely to be maintained by temporary mechanical cardiac assist devices. However, the ultimate resolution is likely to be successful development and commercial availability of a permanent artificial heart.

References

1. Scheidt S, Ascheim R, Killip III T (1970) Shock after acute myocardial infarction. Am J Cardiol 26:556-564
2. Hands ME, Rutherford JD, Muller JE et al (1989) The in-hospital development of cardiogenic shock after myocardial infarction: incidence of occurrence, outcome and prognostic factors. J Am Coll Cardiol 14:40-46
3. Goldberg RJ, Gore JM, Alpert JS et al (1991) Cardiogenic shock after acute myocardial infarction. Incidence and mortality from a community-wide perspective, 1975 to 1988. N Engl J Med 325:1117-1122
4. Garrahy PJ, Henzlova MJ, Forman S et al (1989) Has thrombolytic therapy improved survival from cardiogenic shock? Thrombolysis in myocardial infarction (TIMI II) results. Circulation 80[Suppl II]:II-623
5. Holmes DR, Bates ER, Kleiman NS et al (1995) Contemporary reperfusion therapy for cardiogenic shock: the GUSTO-I trial experience. J Am Coll Cardiol 26:668-674
6. Hamm CW, Goldmann BU, Heeschen C et al (1997) Emergency room triage of patients with acute chest pain by means of rapid testing for cardiac troponin T or troponin I. N Engl J Med 337:1648-1653
7. Kishon Y, Oh JK, Schaff HY et al (1992) Mitral valve operation in postinfarction rupture of a papillary muscle: immediate results and long-term follow-up of 22 patients. Mayo Clin Proc 67:1023-1030
8. Lemery R, Smith HC, Giuliani ER et al (1992) Prognosis in rupture of the ventricular septum after acute myocardial infarction and role of early surgical intervention. Am J Cardiol 70:147-151
9. Da Luz PL, Weil MH, Shubin H (1976) Current concepts on mechanisms and treatment of cardiogenic shock. Am Heart J 92:103-113
10. Forrester JS, Diamond G, Chatterjee K et al (1976) Medical therapy of acute myocardial infarction by application of hemodynamic subsets. N Engl J Med 295:1356-1363
11. Cohn JN (1970) Monitoring techniques in shock. Am J Cardiol 26:565-569
12. Antman EM, Braunwald E (1997) Hemodynamic disturbances in acute myocardial infarction. Cardiogenic Shock. In: Braunwald E (ed) Heart disease. A textbook of cardiovascular medicine. WB Saunders, Philadelphia, pp 1233-1245
13. Califf RM, Bengtson JR (1994) Cardiogenic shock. New Engl J Med 330:1724-1730
14. Gillespie TA, Ambos HD, Sobel BE et al (1977) Effects of dobutamine in patients with acute myocardial infarction. Am J Cardiol 39:588-594
15. Weil MH, Shubin H, Carlson R (1975) Treatment of circulatory shock. JAMA 231:1280-1286
16. Mueller H, Ayres SM, Gregory JJ et al (1970) Hemodynamics, coronary blood flow, and myocardial metabolism in coronary shock: Response to L-norepinephrine and isoproterenol. J Clin Invest 49:1885-1902
17. ACC/AHA guidelines for the management of patients with acute myocardial infarction (1996) A report of the American College of Cardiology/American Heart Association Task Force on Practice Guidelines (Committee on Management of Acute Myocardial Infarction). J Am Coll Cardiol 28:1328-1428
18. Gacioch GM, Ellis SG, Lee L. et al (1992) Cardiogenic shock complicating acute myocardial infarction: the use of coronary angioplasty and the integration of the new support devices into patient management. J Am Coll Cardiol 19:647-653
19. Joyce LD, Johnson KE, Toninato CJ et al (1989) Results of the first 100 patients who received Symbion total artificial hearts as a bridge to cardiac transplantation. Circulation 80[Suppl 3]III:192-201
20. Champagnac D, Claudel JP, Chevalier P et al (1993) Primary cardiogenic shock during acute myocardial infarction: results of emergency cardiac transplantation. Eur Heart J 14:925-929
21. DeWood MA, Notske RN, Hensley GR et al (1980) Intraaortic balloon counterpulsation with and without reperfusion for myocardial infarction shock. Circulation 61:1105-1112

22. Berger P, Holmes D, Stebbins A et al (1997) Impact of an aggressive catheterization and revascularization strategy on mortality in patients with cardiogenic shock in the Global Utilization of Streptokinase and Tissue plasminogen Activator for Coronary Arteries (GUSTO-I) Trial. J Am Coll Cardiol 96:122-127

23. Page DL, Caulfield JB, Kastor JA et al (1971) Myocardial changes associated with cardiogenic shock. N Engl J Med 285:133-137

24. Gutovitz AL, Sobel BE, Roberts R (1978) Progressive nature of myocardial injury in selected patients with cardiogenic shock. Am J Cardiol 41:469-475

25. Braunwald E, Kloner RA (1982) The stunned myocardium: prolonged, postischemic ventricular dysfunction. Circulation 66:1146-1149

26. Prewitt RM, Gu S, Garger PJ et al (1992) Marked systemic hypotension depresses coronary thrombolysis induced by intracoronary administration of recombinant tissue-type plasminogen activator. J Am Coll Cardiol 20:1626-1633

27. Mathey D, Kuck KH, Remmecke J et al (1980) Transluminal recanalization of coronary artery thrombosis: a preliminary report of its application in cardiogenic shock. Eur Heart J 1:207-212

28. Kennedy JW, Gensini GG, Timmis GC et al (1985) Acute myocardial infarction treated with intracoronary streptokinase: a report of the society for cardiac angiography. Am J Cardiol 55:871-877

29. Gruppo Italiano per lo Studio della Streptochinasi nell'Infarto Miocardico (GISSI) (1986) Effectiveness of intravenous thrombolytic treatment in acute myocardial infarction. Lancet 1:397-401

30. Holmes DR, Bates E, and the GUSTO investigators (1993) Cardiogenic shock during myocardial infarction. The GUSTO experience with thrombolytic therapy. Circulation 88 [Suppl]:I-253 (abstract)

31. Hochman JS, Boland J, Sleeper LA et al (1995) Current spectrum of cardiogenic shock and effect of early revascularization on mortality. Circulation 91:873-881

32. O'Neill WW (1992) Angioplasty therapy of cardiogenic shock: are randomized trials necessary? J Am Coll Cardiol 19:915-917

33. Moosvi AR, Khaja F, Villanueva L et al (1992) Early revascularization improves survival in cardiogenic shock complicating acute myocardial infarction. J Am Coll Cardiol 19:907-914

34. Lee L, Erbel R, Brown TM et al (1991) Multicenter registry of angioplasty therapy of cardiogenic shock: initial and long-term survival. J Am Coll Cardiol 17:599-603

35. Hibbard MD, Holmes DR, Bailey KR et al (1992) Percutaneous transluminal coronary angioplasty in patients with cardiogenic shock. J Am Coll Cardiol 19:639-646

36. Lee L, Bates ER, Pitt B et al (1988) Percutaneous transluminal coronary angioplasty improves survival in acute myocardial infarction complicated by cardiogenic shock. Circulation 78:1345-1351

37. Webb JG, Carere R, Hilton JD et al (1997) Usefulness of coronary stenting in cardiogenic shock. Am J Cardiol 79:81-84

38. Kirklin JK, Akins CW, Blackstone EH et al (1991) Guidelines and indications for coronary artery bypass graft surgery: a report of the American College of Cardiology/American Heart Association Task Force on Assessment of Diagnostic and Therapeutic Cardiovascular Procedures (Subcommittee on Coronary Artery Bypass Graft Surgery). J Am Coll Cardiol 91: 2335-2344

39. O'Connor GT, Plume SK, Olmstead EM et al (1992) Multivariate prediction of in-hospital mortality associated with coronary artery bypass graft surgery. Circulation 85:2110-2118

40. Sergeant P, Blackstone E, Meyns B (1997) Early and late outcome after CABG in patients with evolving myocardial infarction. Eur J Cardiothorac Surg 11:848-856

41. Lee JH, Murrell HK, Strony J et al (1997) Risk analysis of coronary bypass surgery after acute myocardial infarction. Surgery 122:675-680

Management of Acute Ischaemic Stroke

C. Fieschi

Despite its dramatic incidence and prognosis, until few years ago, stroke was considered as the Cinderella of medicine. For both public and physicians, even neurologists, this pathology was unavoidable and untreatable. Fortunately, in the past decades this nihilistic attitude regarding stroke has been replaced by a more enthusiastic one. This is explained by research advances in pathophysiology of ischaemia and by the greater awareness of economic concerns about this pathology. The aim of experimental and clinical research is now to reduce mortality and stroke morbidity following stroke, and consequently to minimise costs.

Acute ischaemic stroke is caused by the thrombo-embolic occlusion of an intracranial artery in at least 80% of cases [1]. The arterial occlusion and the consequent lowering of cerebral blood flow (CBF) generate a cascade of neuro-chemical events which transform ischaemic tissue into infarction. The tissue survival time after arterial occlusion, the so-called "therapeutic window", depends on the amount of residual CBF through collateral circulation and on selective neuronal vulnerability to ischaemia [2]. The first observations of a viable and preservable portion of non-functioning brain tissue, called "ischaemic penumbra", were made in late 1970s [3]. Moreover, it has been demonstrated that restoring blood flow can protect brain tissue from mechanisms leading to neuronal death [3], but on return of blood flow, interactions between blood and the damaged tissue can be responsible for reperfusion injury. This has further highlighted the key role of very early intervention in stroke patients.

General management

European guidelines for stroke treatment, based on the evidence from stroke research, recommend immediate hospitalization for all stroke patients, if possible in an intensive care unit dedicated to stroke [4]. The non specific management carried out in a stroke unit include support of vital functions, accurate diagnosis, prevention and treatment of deterioration and complications, use of acute therapeutic agents for appropriate patients, rehabilitation, risk factor correction, secondary prevention. The elements necessary to stroke unit include the 24-hour availability of expert stroke neurologists and neuroradiologists, together with

CT scanning and ultrasound equipment, and neurosurgeon or vascular surgeon counselling. Several studies have demonstrated the efficacy of stroke units on reducing early and long term mortality (by 28% in a metanalysis of 10 studies), improving functional outcome and reducing length of hospital stay [5, 6]. Alternatively, organised stroke teams should be created, which can treat patients in any hospital ward.

On the other hand, well-trained and motivated emergency physicians may provide the key to rapid treatment from stroke symptom onset to initiation of therapy. It is also vital to minimise the time taken to perform all the necessary emergency investigations and the time interval between admission and initiation of therapy. Patients eligible for acute treatment must be identified quickly and appropriate therapy administered promptly, while cardiovascular and other complicating factors that adversely affect stroke outcome must be monitored and treated.

Specific management

As regards specific therapies, most results are disappointing even if encouraging. The ideal anti-ischaemic treatment should restore blood flow and counteract the cascade of biochemical events leading from ischaemia to neuronal death. After demonstration by a large randomized US trial, the National Institute of Neurological Disorders and Stroke rt-PA Trial (NINDS) [7], that i.v. thrombolysis improves 3-months outcome, the US FDA has approved the administration of rt-PA in this indication within 3 hours of stroke onset. But a similar European study, the European Cooperative Acute Stroke Study (ECASS) [8], has failed to confirm such an efficacy of rt-PA administered within 6 hours from stroke onset. Thrombolysis appeared efficacious only in a subgroup of patients without extensive early ischaemic signs on CT scan. In remaining patients, the clinical benefits of i.v. rt-PA administration did not overweigh its haemorrhagic risks. European guidelines recommend rt-PA administration in carefully selected patients and in specialized centers by well-trained personnel [4].

The complex chain of biochemical events leading from ischaemic damage to tissue necrosis offers many potential targets for neuroprotective drugs. Although the number of new drugs investigated in acute ischaemic stroke, we do not have any clinical evidence of the effectiveness of neuroprotectant.

In order to increase the stroke population who can benefit from thrombolysis, the next step should be a European trial using t-PA and a neuroprotectant in combination. The very early administration of a safe neuroprotectant could enlarge therapeutic window, increase the amount of cerebral tissue that may benefit from reperfusion and protect tissue from reperfusional injury. This project has received financial support of the Biomed 2 Program of the European Commission and the EMFATAS (European Multicenter Four-Arm Trial in Acute Stroke) Coordinating Group is currently working on the study protocol.

Conclusions

Now stroke must be considered and managed as medical emergency as well as myocardial infarction. If only a small proportion of patients is eligible for specific acute treatment, all stroke patients must benefit from intensive medical care with careful monitoring and management of general and cerebral functions.

Nevertheless, before effectively fighting with this society burden, much obstacles remain to overcome such as public ignorance, general practitioners and emergency care physicians training, and last but not least lack of specific stroke treatment. This new approach of stroke as emergency requires educational programmes directed at the general public, general practitioners and primary and emergency department physicians, to teach the recognition of stroke symptoms and the importance of treating stroke with the same urgency as myocardial infarction.

References

1. Fieschi C, Argentino C, Lenzi GL et al (1989) Clinical and instrumental evaluation of patients with ischemic stroke within the first six hours. J Neurol Sci 91:311-322
2. Ginsberg MD, Pulsinelli WA (1994) The ischemic penumbra, injury thresholds, and the therapeutic window for acute stroke. Ann Neurol 36:553-554
3. Astrup J, Siesjo BK, Symon L (1981) Thresholds in cerebral ischemia - the ischemic penumbra. Stroke 12:723-725
4. The European Ad Hoc Consensus Group (1996) European strategies for early intervention in stroke. Cerebrovasc Dis 6:351-324
5. Langhorne P, Williams BO, Gilchrist W et al (1993) Do stroke units save lives? Lancet 342: 395-398
6. Jørgensen HS, Nakayama U, Raaschou HA et al (1995) The effect of a stroke unit: reductions in mortality, discharge rate to nursing home, length of hospital stay, and cost. A community-based study. Stroke 26:1178-1182
7. The National Institute of Neurological Disorders and Stroke rt-PA Stroke Study Group (1995) Tissue plasminogen activator for acute ischemic stroke. N Engl J Med 33:1581-1587
8. Hacke W, Kaste M, Fieschi C et al (1995) Intravenous thrombolysis with recombinant tissue plasminogen activator for acute hemispheric stroke. The European Cooperative Acute Stroke Study (ECASS). JAMA 274:1017-1025

Role of Heat Shock Proteins in Cytoprotection

H. Zhang, Y.K. Kim, A.S. Slutsky

The heat shock response is a highly conserved stress response which can be activated by a variety of thermal and nonthermal stimuli such as ischaemia, heavy metals, sodium arsenite, ethanol, oxidants, and infection [1-5]. Stress-induced heat shock protein (HSP) accumulation is thought to be cytoprotective. Initial studies focused on thermo-tolerance, the ability to survive an otherwise lethal heat stress; later studies demonstrated tolerance to a variety of stresses, including ischaemia [6], ultraviolet irradiation [7], and cytokines such as tumor necrosis factor-α (TNF-α). The fact that overexpression of various HSPs confers tolerance in the absence of conditioning stress [8] and that inhibition of HSP accumulation through blocking antibodies [9] impairs stress tolerance strongly supports the hypothesis that HSPs themselves confer the stress tolerance. The HSPs are grouped into four classes or families according to their molecular weights. Each class is composed for a number of proteins, and the designation of the class refers to the "round number" approximating the molecular weights of its typical members (i.e., 20, 30, 70, 90 and 100 kDa). Depending on the stimulus and the cell type, different HSPs are expressed [10]. For example, the heme oxygenase is a low-molecular-weight HSP (HSP30) consisting of two isoforms [11]: HO-2 is expressed constitutively, and HO-1 is highly inducible by heme, heavy metals, sodium arsenite, and oxidants [12]. Recent data indicate that heme oxygenase may play an important cytoprotective role against oxidant stress [13]. The HSP70 family, consisting of constitutive (cHSP70) and inducible (iHSP70) isoforms, has been well characterized with regard to ubiquity, regulation, and cytoprotective properties. The last has been demonstrated in cell lines and transgenic animals that constitutively overexpress HSP70 [14]. After HSP expression the cell rapidly exerts protection against injury caused by heat and other noxious conditions [10].

The present review article will focus on the role of HSP in immune response and resistance to inflammation, particularly stimulated with lipopolysaccharide (LPS), a major component of the outer membrane of gram-negative bacilli.

Immune response of HSP to inflammation

HSP induction in inflammation: role of LPS

The HSPs, in particular the HSP70 family are probably one of the best-studied stress proteins found in different cells. Recent studies suggest that HSPs are major antigens of many pathogens. The suggestion is that the stress imposed by the host may lead to increased HSP synthesis by microorganisms. The HSPs become antigens that trigger a major portion of the immune repertoire. In particular, the HSP70 family members are major targets for antibodies and T cells in many bacterial infections.

The iHSP70s are barely detectable at normal temperatures, but become one of the most actively synthesized proteins in the cell following stress [15, 16]. The HSPs can be induced not only by heat, but also by a number of stimuli including LPS [17]. The i.p. administration of LPS resulted in the heat shock response and the production of iHSP70 in peritoneal macrophages of the host mice as determined electrophoretically and immunologically. Because purified LPS was injected, the HSP70 detected was definitively derived from the host cells and not from infectious agents. Therefore, it suggested that LPS is a stressful agent which induces *in vivo* heat shock responses. The administration of TNF-α together with LPS markedly enhanced the expression of HSP70 [17], suggesting a synergistic effect because the *in vivo* administration of TNF-α alone did not cause production of HSP. Oxygen free radicals might also play a role in the enhancement of LPS-induced HSP induction [18, 19]. Another study also reported HSP induction in response to different stresses, including heat, ischaemia, reperfusion injury, and inflammation [19].

HSP expression differs among organs. Meng et al. [20] reported that injection of sublethal doses of LPS to rats resulted in a transient increase in HSP70 mRNA in the heart but not in the kidney. The maximal increases were observed between 6 and 12 hr after treatment, and the HSP70 mRNA level had returned to baseline by 24 h. The increase in total HSP70 mRNA was largely due to the iHSP70 genes, since the cHSP70 gene was minimally inducible [21, 22]. Enhanced expression of HSP70 in the heart is more likely to be an endogenous adaptive process in response to LPS-induced cardiac stress. The time course of enhanced HSP70 mRNA expression appeared to coincide with the onset of contractile depression [20]. Thus, the enhanced expression of the iHSP70 gene may serve as an indicator of LPS-induced myocardial stress.

In *in vitro* systems, the response appears to be more variable. Human monocytes cultured in vitro with LPS showed an increase in *in vitro* HSP70 transcripts and expression of HSP70 [23]. No HSP production was found in nonadherent peritoneal cells, consistent with the observation that thymocytes and spleen cells do not produce HSPs [17]. Also, HSPs may not be induced by LPS in endothelial cells [24]. However, Wang et al. [25] reported that sodium arsenite, which induced HSP70 expression and oxygen free radical in endothelial cells, resulted in endothelial apoptosis, suggesting that the HSP70 may be responsible for human endothelial apoptosis.

Immune resistance of HSP to inflammation

HSP-mediated resistance to acute lung injury

Villar et al. [4] first demonstrated a cytoprotective effect of HSP induction in a rat model of acute lung injury caused by intratracheal administration of phospholipase A2. HSPs was induced in the lungs of experimental animals by subjecting them to 41-42°C core body temperature for 15 min at 18 h before lung injury. Heat-treated animals were significantly resistant to phospholipase A2-mediated acute lung injury and had decreased mortality at 48 h (0 vs. 22%) compared with control (nonheated) animals. Using the same heat stress model, these investigators subsequently demonstrated that induction of HSPs also produced protection against acute lung injury caused by cecal ligation and perforation [5]. Although not defining the mechanisms of protection, or the involvement of HSP70, these studies raised the intriguing possibility that the HSPs induction could have potential applications as a therapeutic strategy to attenuate acute lung injury. In addition, induction of the heat response after LPS challenge was recently demonstrated to be protective [26].

In vitro studies have also demonstrated the role of HSP in protecting lung cells against agents that are commonly involved in the pathophysiology of acute lung injury. Induction of HSP70, by either thermal stress or sodium arsenite, attenuated LPS-mediated apoptosis in cultured sheep pulmonary artery endothelial cells [27]. The mechanisms of cytoprotection may involve an antioxidant effect, since HSP induction was associated with inhibition of LPS-mediated superoxide anion production. Furthermore, HSP70 appears to be directly involved in protection against LPS-induced apoptosis, since transfected cells that overexpressed HSP70 were resistant to LPS-induced apoptosis compared with other cells and cells transfected with a control plasmid [27]. In other studies involving cultured murine lung epithelium and bovine pulmonary artery endothelium, induction of HSP70 by heat stress protected cells against oxidant injury [28, 29]. A recent study demonstrated that overexpression of heme oxygenase protected cultured human respiratory epithelium against hyperoxia [30].

HSP-mediated resistance to sepsis

HSP-associated heat adaptation may also involve endotoxin tolerance. Conditioning stresses that result in HSP accumulation or the overexpression of the HSP70 gene in cells confer tolerance to endotoxins in animals [5, 31, 32] and cells [8]. Klosterhalfen et al. [33] investigated haemodynamic effects with and without induction of the stress response in a porcine model of endotoxaemia. Induction of the stress response was carried out by a pretreatment with Zn^{2+}, a potent inducer of HSP70 expression. After LPS infusion, pretreated animals showed significantly decreased peak pulmonary artery pressure and pulmonary vascular resistance index values, significantly increased systemic artery pressure and systemic vascular resistance index values, and significantly altered hypodynamic/hyperdynamic cardiac output levels.

Meng et al. [20] reported that both LPS and hyperthermia (42°C, 15 min) in rats induced an enhanced expression of HSP70 mRNA in the myocardium, accompanied by the induction of HSP70 in cardiac interstitial cells, including macrophages at 24 h after treatment. In rats pretreated with LPS 24 earlier, subsequent LPS exposure did not depress left ventricular developed pressure. When hyperthermia-pretreated animals were similarly challenged with LPS, myocardial depression at 6 h was also abrogated, although to a lesser extent. In addition, it has been recently reported that isolated hearts from transgenic mice that overexpressed HSP70 exhibited enhanced postischaemic recovery of myocardial function [6, 14], suggesting a role for HSP70 in the recovery of myocardial function.

Of particular interest, induction of HSP70 by hyperthermia has also been associated with reduced mortality in animals exposed to a lethal dose of LPS [5, 14, 31]. Ryan and colleagues [32] demonstrated that the administration of a lethal dose of LPS (20 mg/kg) to rats resulted in 71.4% mortality. In contrast, all rats that had been heat stresses 24 h earlier survived after administration of the same dose of LPS. A study by Hotchkiss et al. [31] reported similar protective effects of heat stress in mice and linked the protective effects of the induction of HSP70 in tissues. In a study from our laboratory [5], we demonstrated that heat-stressed rats exhibited an enhanced expression of HSP70 at 6-18 h after treatment. Pretreatment with heat stress, 18 h before cecal ligation and perforation, reduced lung injury and enhanced animal survival in the face of LPS-induced sepsis. Klosterhalfen et al. [34] also showed that the induction of heat shock response by Zn^{2+} significantly increased the survival rate after LD100 endotoxaemia in rats. An enhanced survival rate in animals pretreated with Zn^{2+} was associated with an increased tissue levels of HSP70, a subsequent decreased release of the proinflammatory cytokines and a significantly decreased rate of apoptosis.

HSP-mediated attenuation of proinflammatory cytokines

HSP-mediated resistance to acute lung injury and sepsis may reflect a direct attenuating effect of cytotoxic mediators such as proinflammatory cytokines. In this regard, macrophages stimulated to produce HSPs show both transcriptional inhibition and decreased secretion of the inflammatory cytokines TNF-α and interleukin-1 (IL-1) [35, 36]. To determine the specific role of HSP70, we exposed *in vitro* primary alveolar macrophages obtained from normal rats to heat stress or sodium arsenite stimulation [37]. Eighteen hours later, the cells were challenged with LPS and TNF-α-levels were obtained. The exposure of alveolar macrophages to heat stress or to sodium arsenite induced the synthesis of HSP70 in a time-related fashion. The stress response attenuated the amount of TNF-α released from the cells under LPS stimulation. Similarly, animals that have undergone a conditioning heat stress sufficient to cause HSP70 accumulation show a decrease in circulating TNF-α after endotoxin exposure [37, 38]. These findings that both animals and cells produced decreased production of TNF-α indicate that the HSP attenuates the pivotal inflammatory mediator in septic conditions. In addition to decreased cytokine production by inflammatory cells and resultant decreases in circulating TNF-α, the cellular accumulation of HSP renders cells resistant to the cytotoxic effects of TNF-α [39, 40]. Finally, TNF-α and IL-1 upregulate the HSPs [41, 42].

Our observations were confirmed by the studies of Klosterhalfen et al. [33, 34] who reported that pretreatment with Zn^{2+} induced an increase in HSP70 expression determined by immunohistochemistry, Western blotting and HSP70 antibodies from the lungs, liver, and kidneys of both rats and pigs. After LPS infusion, pretreated rats showed significantly decreased production of TNF-α, IL-1β and interleukin-6 (IL-6), and peak plasma levels of 6-keto-PGF1α and thromboxane-B2, compared with the untreated control groups.

HSP-mediated resistance to the toxic effects of nitric oxide (NO)

During Gram-negative septic shock, LPS triggers the release of cytokines, which in turn induces the inducible nitric oxide synthase (iNOS), leading to increased production of NO resulting in hypotension [43]. For example, activated macrophages produce NO as a non-specific immune response directed against invading bacteria or microorganisms. The same macrophages that initiate the production of NO also can be affected by NO. Incubation of RAW 264.7 macrophages with LPS and/or interferon-γ (IFN-γ) induced the formation of NO by the activation of iNOS. Treatment of macrophages with ten cycles of nonlethal doses of LPS and IFN-γ resulted in cell resistance to the NO toxicity induced by LPS and IFN-γ. These resistant macrophages showed a 2-fold increase in expression of the HSP70 [44]. Hauser et al. [45] also demonstrated that HSP protects rats from LPS by blocking LPS-induced iNOS, leading to a decrease in the overproduction of NO, thereby reversing LPS-induced vasoplegia and LPS-induced hypotension. De Vera and colleagues [46] demonstrated induced HSP by sodium arsenite or hyperthermia, and then treated the AKN-1 human liver cell line with TNF-α, IL-1β and IFN-γ to stimulate high levels of iNOS mRNA and NO production. They found that cytokine-induced NOS gene transcription was blocked by HSP. Wong et al. [47] have recently reported that induction of HSP by either heating or by sodium arsenite inhibits the IL-1β-mediated iNOS gene expression in cultured rat pulmonary artery smooth muscle cells. Thus HSP induction may block the effects of LPS at several different levels, including attenuation of cytokine release, reduction of cytokine toxicity, and inhibition of iNOS gene transcription and translation [1, 10]. HSP may also alter the metabolism of intracellular calcium and high-energy phosphates [31], as well as the structure and function of many other cellular and moleculars [48], and many of which may affect NOS in septic states.

Mechanisms of HSP-mediated cell resistance to infection

As mentioned above, studies have shown that a preheat treatment of rodents results in a significant improvement in the survival rate in endotoxic or septic shock [5, 31, 32]. Heating increases the level of the iHSP70; however, there is also an increase in catalase enzyme activity [49], and increased expression of other HSPs and related stress proteins [50]. Thus, the observed protective effect by the induction of the heat shock response may not necessarily be solely related to the increase in HSP70.

To answer the question whether the increased expression of the iHSP70 could exert a protective effect against cellular injury induced by exposure to LPS, Shi [8] heated H9c2 cells (43°C for 60 min), allowed them to recover for 8 h, and subsequently exposed them to LPS for 16 h. This preconditioning of H9c2 cells markedly increased the expression of the iHSP70 [50] and was found to render the cells markedly resistant to LPS stimulation. To further investigate the role of the iHSP70 in cross protection against cellular injury caused by LPS, the investigators chose a stably transfected H9c2 single cell-derived clonal cell line (H9/hHSP70/1) which overexpresses the exogenous human HSP70 [50]. They showed that the cell line H9/hHSP70/1 exhibited a significant increase in resistance to cellular injury after exposure to LPS measured by the cell survival assay and by lactate dehydrogenase release into the medium. They also showed that the presence of the exogenous human HSP70 did not alter the level of the other HSPs or of the enzymatic activity of antioxidant enzymes, such as catalase, which potentially might also be involved in protection against cellular injury. This indicates that a major part of the protection conferred by a preheat treatment against a subsequent LPS exposure is most likely attributable to the increased presence of the iHSP70.

HSPs induce protection against a number of stresses distinct from heat shock, including exposure to oxygen free radicals. In the human promonocytic line U937, Polla [19] investigated in whole cells the effects of pretreatment with heating and exposure to hydrogen peroxide on mitochondrial membrane potential, and ultrastructure. Heat shock prevented hydrogen peroxide-induced alterations in mitochondrial membrane potential while increasing expression of HSPs. Protection correlated best with the expression of the HSP70. This study suggested that mitochondria represent a selective target for heat shock-mediated protection against oxidative injury.

It has been also suggested that the mechanism underlying the protective effect of HSPs involves their function as "molecular chaperones" of damaged cellular proteins [1] or interference with oxygen free radical-induced injury [5, 11, 51]. Additional effects of HSP on the inflammatory response can explain the protective effects of HSP induction in septic animals. Heat shock downregulates IL-1β biosynthesis [52], decreases TNF-α transcription and release in LPS-stimulated macrophages [53, 54], and protects cells from TNF-α toxicity [55], probably via inhibition of TNF-α-induced activation of phospholipase A2 [2]. Indeed, we [37, 53, 54] and others [56] have reported that pretreatment of cultured rat macrophages with hyperthermia inhibits the synthesis of TNF in response to LPS.

Elevations in cellular HSP70 are associated with an attenuation in heat-induced permeability of an epithelial monolayer [57]. Thus the association of HSP70 accumulation with the maintenance of epithelial barrier integrity suggests a means to confer heat tolerance in a multicellular system that is associated with HSPs and distinct from thermotolerance. The preservation of the epithelial barrier through a HSP-associated mechanism, possibly through stabilization of the cytoskeleton or through the preservation of important cell-to-cell contacts, may be an important factor in preventing heat-associated LPS translocation across the gut [42, 58].

Another mechanism may be related to the important role of HSPs in the processing of stress-denatured proteins [59, 60]. The maintenance of structural proteins may also be a key in the HSP-associated stress tolerance. In this regard, HSP70, a protein homogolous with α-crystalline, prevents actin microfilament disruption under stress conditions [58]. This effect on the cytoskeleton may be important not only in individual cell tolerance to stress through cytoskeletal stabilization but may also be integral to the protection of the whole organism through the maintenance of endothelial and epithelial barrier functions.

Conclusions

Inflammation results in host immune response leading to release of a number of mediators including proinflammatory cytokines and HSP. In turn, inflammatory cytokines such as TNF-α contribute to the development of severe inflammatory response syndrome, subsequently multiple organ dysfunction and death. Heat stress exerts resistance to inflammatory stimuli by a number of mechanisms. Whether HSP alone directly affects synthesis and/or production of mediators such as cytokines remains to be elucidated. There is a potential place for HSP in the treatment of sepsis and acute lung injury.

References

1. Jaattela M, Wissing D (1992) Emerging role of heat shock proteins in biology and medicine. Ann Med 24:249-258
2. Jaattela M (1993) Overexpression of major heat shock protein hsp70 inhibits tumor necrosis factor-induced activation of phospholipase A2. J Immunol 151:4286-4294
3. Ribeiro SP, Villar J, Downey GP et al (1994) Sodium arsenite induces heat shock protein-72 kilodalton expression in the lungs and protects rats against sepsis. Crit Care Med 22:922-929
4. Villar J, Edelson JD, Post M et al (1993) Induction of heat stress protein is associated with decreased mortality in an animal model of acute lung injury. Am Rev Respir Dis 147:177-181
5. Villar J, Ribeiro SP, Mullen JBM et al (1994) Induction of the heat shock response reduces mortality rate and organ damage in a sepsis-induced acute lung injury model. Crit Care Med 22:914-921
6. Marber MS, Mestril R, Chi S-H et al (1995) Overexpression of the rat inducible 70-kDA heat stress protein in a transgenic mouse increases the resistance of the heart to ischemic injury. J Clin Invest 95:1446-1456
7. Barbe MF, Tytell M, Gower DJ, Welch WJ (1988) Hyperthermia protects against light damage in the rat retina. Science 24:1817-1820
8. Shi S-H, Mestril R (1996) Stable expression of a human HSP70 gene in a rat myogenic cell line confers protection against endotoxin. Am J Physiol 270:C1017-C1021
9. Taggart DP, Bakkenist CJ, Biddolph SC et al (1997) Induction of myocardial heat shock protein 70 during cardiac surgery. J Pathol 182:362-366
10. Morimoto RI, Milarski KL (1990) Expression and function of vertebrae hsp70 genes. In: Morimoto RI, Tissieres A, Georgopoulos C (eds) Stress proteins in biology and medicine. Cold Spring Harbor Laboratory Press. Cold Spring Harbor, NY, p 323-359
11. Otterbein L, Sylvester SL, Choi AMK (1995) Hemoglobin provides protection against lethal endotoxemia in rats: the role of heme oxygenase-1. Am J Respir Cell Mol Biol 13:595-601
12. Keyse SM, Applegate LA, Tromvoukis Y, Tyrrell RM (1990) Oxidant stress leads to transcriptional activation of the human heme oxygenase gene in cultured skin fibroblasts. Mol Cell Biol 10:4967-4969
13. Vile GF, Basu-Modak S, Waltner C, Tyrrell RM (1994) Heme oxygenase 1 mediates an adaptive response to oxidative stress in human skin fibroblasts. Proc Natl Acad Sci USA 91: 2607-2610
14. Plumier J-C, Ross BM, Currie RW et al (1995) Transgenic mice expressing the human heat shock protein 70 have improved post-ischemic myocardial recovery. J Clin Invest 95: 1854-1860
15. Welch WJ, Suhan JP (1985) Morphological study of the mammalian stress response: characterization of changes in cytoplasmic organelles, cytoskeleton, and nucleoli, and appearance of intranuclear actin filaments in rat fibroblasts after heat-shock treatment. J Cell Biol 101: 1198-1131
16. Young RA, Elliott TJ (1989) Stress proteins, infection, and immunosurveillance. Cell 59:5-8
17. Zhang Y-H, Takahashi K, Jiang Guo-Z et al (1994) In vivo production of heat shock protein in mouse peritoneal macrophages by administration of lipopolysaccharide. Infect Immun 62: 4140-4144
18. Muller JM, Ziegler-Heitbrock HW, Baeuerle PA (1993) Nuclear factor kappa B, a mediator of lipopolysaccharide effects. Immunobiology 187:233-256
19. Polla BS, Kantengwa S, Francois D et al (1996) Mitochondria are selective targets for the protective effects of heat shock against oxidative injury. Proc Natl Acad Sci USA 93: 6458-6463
20. Meng X, Brown JM, Ao L et al (1996) Endotoxin induces cardiac HSP70 and resistance to endotoxemic myocardial depression in rats. Am J Physiol 271:C1316-C1324
21. Gunther E, Walter L (1994) Genetic aspects of the hsp70 multigene family in vertebrates. Experientia Basel 50:987-1001

22. Nowak Jr TS, Bond U, Schlesinger MJ (1990) Heat shock RNA levels in brain and other tissues after hyperthemia and transient ischemia. J Neurochem 54:451-458

23. Fincato G, Polentarutti N, Sicca A et al (1991) Expression of a heat-inducible gene of the HSP70 family in human myelomonocytic cells: regulation by bacterial products and cytokines. Blood 77:579-586

24. Rinaldo JE, Gorry M, Strieter R et al (1990) Effect of endotoxin-induced cell injury on 70-kD heat shock proteins in bovine lung endothelial cells. Am J Respir Cell Mol Biol 3:207-216

25. Wang JH, Redmond HP, Watson RWG, Bouchier-Hayes D (1997) Induction of human endothelial cell apoptosis requires both heat shock and oxidative stress responses. Am J Physiol 272:C1543-C1551

26. Chu EK, Riberio SP, Slutsky AS (1997) Heat stress increases survival rates in lipopolysaccharide-stimulated rats. Crit Care Med 25:1727-1732

27. Wong HR, Mannix RJ, Rusnak JM et al (1996) The heat shock response attenuates lipopolysaccharide-mediated apoptosis in cultured sheep pulmonary artery endothelial cells. Am J Respir Cell Mol Biol 15:745-751

28. Wang JR, Xiao XZ, Huang SN et al (1996) Heat shock pretreatment prevents hydrogen peroxide injury of pulmonary endothelial cells and macrophages in culture. Shock 6:134-141

29. Wong HR, Ryan M, Gebb S, Wispe JR (1997) Selective and transient in vitro effects of heat shock on alveolar type II cell gene expression. Am J Physiol 272:L132-L138

30. Lee PJ, Alam J, Wiegand GW, Choi AMK (1996) Overexpression of heme oxygenase-1 in human pulmonary epithelial cells results in cell growth arrested and increased resistance to hyperoxia. Proc Natl Acad Sci USA 93:10393-10398

31. Hotchkiss R, Nunnally I, Lindquist S et al (1993) Hyperthermia protects mice against the lethal effects of endotoxin. Am J Physiol 265:R1447-R1457

32. Ryan AJ, Flanagan SW, Moseley PL, Gisolfi CV (1992) Acute heat stress protects rats against endotoxin shock. J Appl Physiol 73:1517-1522

33. Klosterhalfen B, Hauptmann S, Tietze L et al (1997) The influence of heat shock protein 70 induction on hemodynamic variables in a porcine model of recurrent endotoxemia. Shock 7:358-363

34. Klosterhalfen B, Hauptmann S, Offner F-A et al (1997) Induction of heat shock protein 70 by zinc-bis-(DL-hydrogenaspartate) reduces cytokine liberation, apoptosis, and mortality rate in a rat model of LD100 endotoxemia. Shock 7:254-262

35. Ensor JE, Wiener SM, McCrea KA et al (1994) Differential effects of hyperthermia on macrophage interleukin-6 and tumor necrosis factor-α expression. Am J Physiol 266: C967-C974
Pola BS (1988) A role for heat shock protein in inflammation? Immunol Today 9:134-137

36. Snyder YM, Guthire L, Evans GF, Zuckerman (1992) Transcriptional inhibition of endotoxin-induced monokine synthesis following heat shock in murine peritoneal macrophages. J Leukoc Biol 51:181-187

37. Ribeiro SP, Villar J, Downey GP et al (1996) Effects of the stress response in septic rats and LPS-stimulated alveolar macrophages: evidence for TNF-alpha posttranslational regulation. Am J Respir Crit Care Med 154:1843-1850

38. Kluger MJ, Rudolph K, Soszynski D et al (1997) Effect of heat stress on LPS-induced fever and tumor necrosis factor. Am J Physiol 273:R858-R863

39. Jaattela M, Wissing D (1993) Heat shock proteins protect cells from monocyte cytotoxicity: possible mechanism of self-protection. J Exp Med 177:231-236

40. Landry J, Chretien P, Lambert H et al (1989) Heat shock resistance conferred by expression of the human HSP27 gene in rodent cells. J Cell Biol 109:7-15

41. Freshney NW, Rawlinson L, Guesdon F et al (1994) Interleukin-1 activates a novel protein kinase cascade that results in the phosphorylation of HSP27. Cell 78:1039-1049

42. Saklatvala J, Kaw P, Guesdor F (1991) Phosphorylation of the small heat shock protein is regulated by interleukin-1, tumor necrosis factor, growth factor, bradykinin, and ATP. Biochem J 277:635-642

43. Stoclet JC, Fleming I, Gray G et al (1993) Nitric oxide and endotoxemia. Circulation 87 [Suppl V]:V77-V80

44. Hirvonen M-R, Brune B, Lapetina EG (1996) Heat shock proteins and macrophage resistance to the toxic effects of nitric oxide. Biochem J 315:845-849

45. Hauser GJ, Dayao EK, Wasserloos K et al (1996) HSP induction inhibits iNOS mRNA expression and attenuates hypotension in endotoxin-challenged rats. Am J Physiol 271: H2529-H2535

46. de Vera ME, Wong JM, Zhou J-Y et al (1996) Cytokine-induced nitric oxide synthase gene transcription is blocked by the heat shock response in human liver cells. Surgery 120:144-149

47. Wong HR, Finder JD, Wasserloos K, Pitt BR (1995) Expression of inducible nitric oxide synthesis in cultured rat pulmonary artery smooth muscle cells is inhibited by the heat shock response. Am J Physiol 269:L843-L848

48. Calderwook SK, Bornstein B, Farnum EK, Stevenson MA (1989) Heat shock stimulates the release of arachidonic acid and the synthesis of prostaglandins and leukotriene B4 in mammalian cells. J Cell Physiol 141:325-333

49. Currie RW, Karmazyn M, Kloc M, Mailer K (1988) Heat-shock response is associated with enhanced postischemic ventricular recovery. Circ Res 63:543-549

50. Mestril R, Chi SH, Sayen MR et al (1994) Expression of inducible stress protein 70 in rat heart myogenic cells confers protection against simulated ischemia-induced injury. J Clin Invest 93:759-767

51. Buchman TG (1994) Manipulation of stress gene expression: a novel therapy for the treatment of sepsis? Crit Care Med 22:901-903

52. Schmidt JA, Abdulla E (1988) Down regulation of IL-1β biosynthesis by inducers of the heat-shock response. J Immunol 141:2027-2034

53. Ribeiro SP, Downey GP, Edelson JD, Slutsky AS (1995) Evidence that heat shock protein-72 (HSP70) participates in post-transcriptional control of tumor necrosis factor in alveolar macrophages exposed to the stress response (abstract). Am J Respir Crit Care Med 151:A161

54. Ribeiro SP, Villar J, DeHoyos A et al (1993) Heat stress decreases tumor necrosis factor release in LPS-stimulated alveolar macrophages (abstract). Am Rev Respir Dis 147:A2229

55. Kusher DI, Ware CF, Gooding LR (1990) Induction of the heat shock response protects cells from lysis by tumor necrosis factor. J Immunol 145:2925-2931

56. Moseley PL, Gapen C, Wallen ES et al (1994) Thermal stress induces epithelial permeability. Am J Physiol 267:C425-C434

57. Lavoie J, Gingras-Bertan G, Tanguay RM, Landry J (1993) Induction of Chinese hamster HSP27 gene expression in mouse cells confers tolerance to heat shock. HSP27 stabilization of the microfilament organization. J Biol Chem 268:3420-3429

58. Fouqueray B, Philippe C, Amrani A et al (1992) Heat shock prevents lipopolysaccharide-induced tumor necrosis factor-α synthesis by rat mononuclear phagocytes. Eur J Immunol 22:2983-2987

59. Finkel MS, Oddis CV, Jacob TD et al (1992) Negative inotropic effects of cytokines on the heart mediated by nitric oxide. Science 257:387-389

60. Mizzen L, Welch (1988) Effects on protein synthesis activity and the regulation of heat shock protein 70 expression. J Cell Biol 106:1105-1116

FOCUS ON HYPERBARIC MEDICINE

Evidence-Based Hyperbaric Oxygen Therapy

F. Wattel, D. Mathieu

Medical practice is changing and the change, which involves using the medical literature more effectively in guiding medical practice, is profound enough that it can appropriately be called a paradigm shift. To get rid of the blame being "a therapy in search of disease" [1], hyperbaric oxygen therapy (HBOT) has to prove its effectiveness in comparison with alternative therapeutic procedures, as well as to be technically feasible and safe, with a minimum of possible adverse effects. It is now accepted that virtually no drug – and hyperbaric oxygen must be considered as a drug – can enter clinical practice without a demonstration of its efficacy in clinical trials.

One of the possibilities to give an opinion on the effectiveness of HBO therapy and to help clinicians in treating the patients is to consider the best available evidence from experimental and clinical studies that have been reported in the literature on the subject, using the procedure of the Evidence-Base Medicine (EBM), a new approach to teaching the practice medicine by application of formal rules of evidence evaluating the clinical literature [2]. The approach and tools used by EBM have been well described. They include the use of prospective, randomized, double blind controlled clinical trials to answer specific questions, the use of measures rather than their assessments as the primary end points of clinical trials, the collation of results through the Cochrane collaboration and meta-analysis of multiple clinical trials to resolve variations in results. However, at the moment, inevitably, as in numerous fields of medicine, only a very small proportion of all the issues involved in the cure of patients with HBOT have been assessed in this way.

Each therapeutic procedure has its own requirements. Clinicians should remember the following facts:

- clinical decision making is usually based on the balance of evidence rather than on the level of evidence that would be required to establish proof beyond all reasonable doubt.
- An absence of evidence of benefit does not equal evidence of absence of benefit. That is until an adequate study has been performed, the verdict on usefulness of a procedure or treatment should remain open.

– There is a hierarchy of evidence and that just because multiple large clinical trials have not been performed, it does not mean that there isn't reasonable evidence to support a clinical decision.

Proceedings of recent consensus conferences on hyperbaric medicine [3, 4] demonstrate just how few of procedures commonly used are supported by the highest level of evidence. That's the reason why the scientific committee of the ECHM (European Committee for Hyperbaric Medicine) which is in charge of organizing consensus conferences, had elaborated, before starting the meetings, instructions for experts and juries. It was suggested that a common scale would be used to assess the weight of their recommendations:

a) recommendation based on at least 2 concordant large, double-blind controlled, randomized studies with no or only weak methodological bias;

b) recommendation based on double-blind controlled randomized studies but with methodological bias or concerning only small sample, or only a single study;

c) recommendation based only on uncontrolled studies (historic control group, cohort study...).

As large scale double blind controlled studies are often lacking in HBOT medicine, it was suggested that facts, arguments and recommendations would be divided in three groups (basic studies, animal studies with control group, human studies and clinical trials) and graded as follows:

4. strong evidence of beneficial action (equivalent to a) in the previously exposed classification);

3. evidence of beneficial action (equivalent to b);

2. weak evidence of beneficial action (equivalent to c);

1. no evidence of beneficial action, case report only, methodological or interpretation bias preclude any conclusion.

So HBOT evaluation, conducted from assessment of reported experimental and clinical data according to available medical evidence and using recommendations of experts Committee (cfr UHMS committee report-revised) and conclusions of consensus conference juries leads to recognize the usefulness of HBOT with regards to the weight of recommendation as well:

– type 1 recommendation (1R): HBOT is strongly recommended because it is recognized that HBOT positively affects the prognosis for survival. This implies that the patient is transferred to the nearest hyperbaric facility as soon as possible;

– type 2 recommendation (2R): HBOT is recommended because it is recognized that HBOT constitues an important part of the treatment of that given disease which, even if it may not influence the prognosis for patient's survival, it is nevertheless important for the prevention of serious disorders. This implies that the transfer to a hyperbaric facility is made, unless this represents a danger to the patient's life;

– type 3 recommendation (3R): HBOT is optional because HBOT is regarded as an additional treatment modality which can improve clinical results.

In other situations, where sufficient evidence in favour of HBOT is not available, it is necessary to start evaluation procedures based on multicentric studies and on clearly defined protocols, as approved by a suitable ethical committee. Only after the completion of such studies, will it be possible to accept a new indication.

Acute indications for HBOT

General

Hyperbaric facilities accepting emergency indications in potentially Intensive Care requiring patients should be hospital-based and located in or close the hospital Intensive or Emergency Care Department.

Technical competence and personnel skills at the hyperbaric facility must be adequate. The patient's condition must not interfere with the decision to accept an indication for HBOT.

Hyperbaric oxygen therapy must be seen as a part of a therapeutical continuum, without any interruption of the chain of treatment. It cannot be considered as an isolated treatment modality.

Diving decompression accident and air embolism (DCS and AE)

The need for recompression to decrease bubble size, and elimination of N_2 from the inspired gas to enhance movement of N_2 molecules from tissue to blood and hence to alveolar gas sets HBO as the general treatment of choice for both DCS and AE. However, a large number of questions remain unanswered. Some are very basic whereas others are of simple, practical significance to the patient with DCS or AE. Areas of fundamental science include elucidation of predisposing factors, mechanisms of bubble formation and movement. Areas of applied science include strategies for education and prevention; continuing development and evaluation of adjunctive therapies, especially when chambers are not available; optimization of chamber regimes for treatment; and methods for assessing organ function.

Decompression accidents in recreational diving

Decompression accidents are true medical emergencies that must benefit from treatment in specialized centers as soon as possible. The victims of a decompression accident should be immediately directed from the site of the diving accident to the closest specialized center (type 1 R).

Initial recompression modality

Minor decompression accidents (pain only) should be treated with oxygen re-compression tables at 18 meters depth maximum (type 1 R).

Regarding more serious decompression accidents (neurological and vestibular accidents), there are presently two acceptable protocols, as neither one has been proved better by any scientifically valid study to date: oxygen recompression tables at 2.8 ATA (with possible extension) or hyperoxygenated breathing mixtures at 4.0 ATA.

The choice between the two may depend on personal experience and on local logistics. However, under no circumstance the unavailability of one of the two accepted modalities should delay the treatment (type 1 R).

The following optional treatment modalities may also be considered (type 3 R):

– compression to 6 ATA in case of cerebral arterial gas embolism, with the condition that this compression is performed using hyperoxygenated mixtures and not compressed air and that the delay to treatment is not more than a few hours;
– saturation treatment tables in case of persistent symptoms.

Finally, in water recompression should never be undertaken as the initial re-compression modality for a decompression accident (type 1 R).

Fluid treatment

On site: oral hydration is recommended only if the patient is conscious (type 1 R).

Contraindications to oral rehydration are stringent and include: any con-sciousness abnormality, nausea and vomiting, suspected lesions of the gastro-in-testinal tract. Oral-hydration should be done with plain water, possibly with the addition of electrolytes but with no gas, adapted to the patient's thirst and ac-ceptance.

Venous rehydration should be preferred if a physician is present, using preferably Ringer Lactate as the infusion fluid.

At the hospital, intravenous rehydration is recommended while controlling the routinary physiological parameters: urinary output, haemodynamics, CVP, standard laboratory tests.

Drug treatment

Normobaric oxygen is strongly recommended (type 1 R). The administration of normobaric oxygen allows for the treatment of hypoxaemia and favours the elimination of inert gas bubbles. Oxygen should be administered with an oro-nasal mask with reservoir bag, at a minimal flow rate of 15 l/min, or with CPAP mask circuit, using either a free flow regulator or a demand valve, in such a way to obtain a FiO_2 close to 1. In case of respiratory distress, shock or coma, the patient should be intubated and ventilated with a $FiO_2 = 1$ and setting the venti-lator to avoid pressure and volume trauma. Normobaric oxygen should be continued until hyperbaric recompression is started (with a maximum of 6 hours when the FiO_2 is 1).

Any necessary drug for the support treatment of an intensive care patient (adequate first aid kit) is recommended (type 2 R). The role of specific drugs at this early stage remains unresolved and suitable for further studies, so the use of Aspirin is optional.

Treatment protocol for persistent symptoms after the initial recompression. There are no scientifically valid data to allow for a recommended approach to this issue.

Results

Oxygen first aid and hyperbaric treatment in clinical outcome of 202 DCS cases of the DAN Europe 1989-1993 diving accident database objective total recovery in 176 cases (87.13%) and incomplete or negative in 26 cases (12.87%). Comparing the group of injured divers who receive oxygen first aid (119) with those who dit not (82) the negative results were only 5 (4.2%) in the first group and 25 (30%) in the second non treated group. Difference between the two groups is statistically significant [5].

Gas embolism (AE)

Its origin is mainly iatrogenic and it may happen in surgical setting (neurosurgery, cardiac surgery, laparoscopy) as well as in medical setting (central venous catheterisation, pleural and pulmonary endoscopy or biopsy, haemodialysis...). Whatever the symptomatology of air embolism, morbidity and mortality of AE remain high. All patients (AGE or VGE) with neurological abnormalities should receive recompression treatment: HBOT is strongly recommended. The minimal treatment pressure must not be lower than 3 ATA (type 1 R). The outcome after recompression treatment of AE is good in both animals studies and clinical series [6] with immediate recompression treatment being most effective [7].

Carbon monoxide (CO) intoxication

CO poisoning is actually the first cause of accidental poisoning in Europe and North America. This intoxication remains frequent, severe and overlooked [8]. In addition to hypoxaemic hypoxia (effect on oxygen transport) CO poisoning induces a histotoxic hypoxia (CO binding to myoglobin and to cytochromes). This process is self-worsening, in good agreement with the clinical presentation and experience (heart damage, pulmonary oedema, late neurological sequelae, CO intoxication during pregnancy). Hyperbaric oxygen is well recognized as the treatment of choice due to its effects on accelerated dissociation of CO haemoproteins and its role in preventing reoxygenation injury [9, 10], even if some controversy remains concerning the treatment of poisoning of minor importance and if different HBO profiles should be compared to determine optional treatment for a given set of conditions.

Recommendations

Carbon monoxide intoxications must be treated with normobaric oxygen as a first aid treatment (type 1 R).

Carbon monoxide intoxications presenting with consciousness alterations, clinical neurological, cardiac, respiratory or physiological signs must be treated with hyperbaric oxygen therapy, whatever the carboxyhaemoglobin value may be (type 1 R).

Pregnant women must be treated with hyperbaric oxygen therapy, whatever the clinical situation and the carboxyhaemoglobin value may be (type 1 R).

In minor carbon monoxide intoxication, there is a choice between normobaric oxygen therapy for at least 12 hours and HBO. Until the results of randomized studies are available, HBO remains optional (type 3 R).

Results

In a serie of 774 patients managed with HBO according to these recommendations, results at 1 year objective only 4.4% of patients suffer from persistent manifestations and only 1.6% have major functional impairment (motor or sensory impairment, hypertonia) by comparison with report of 10% or more of immediate gross neurological sequelae and more than 30% of delayed personality deterioration and memory disturbance when patients received inadequate therapy (any oxygen in the emergency treatment, delayed therapy with or without HBO).

Clostridial myonecrosis (gas gangrene) and anaerobic or mixed bacterial necrotizing soft tissue infections (NSTI)

For the onset of gas gangrene two conditions are necessary: the presence of clostridial spores, and an area of lowered oxidation-reduction potential caused by circulatory failure in a local area or by extensive soft tissue damage and necrotic muscle tissue, an area with a low pO_2 where clostridial spores can flourish into the vegetative form.

The clostridial bacteria surround themselves with toxins. Local host defense mechanisms are abolished when the toxin concentration is sufficiently high, and then begins the ever-increasing tissue destruction and further clostridial growth.

The progressive nature of gas gangrene depends on the continuous production of alpha toxin by clostridia. Unless toxin production and bacterial multiplication are stopped, the patient will die.

The local condition of the wound is far more important than the presence of clostridia and can be considered as the clinically deciding factor for the onset of gas gangrene.

Regarding the clinical presentation 3 remarks may be focused:

1. patients who are at risk for infection in general (e.g., patients with predisposing factors such as ischaemia, diabetes mellitus, lowered resistance, foreign bodies, etc.; patients with underlying systemic diseases; elderly people; debilitated patients with gastrointestinal, biliary, or genitourinary tract infection; drug addicts; etc.) are also more vulnerable to gas gangrene.

2. The local picture of gas gangrene is not like that of other pyogenic infections. Signs and symptoms depict an overwhelming process.

3. Extreme severity of the disease is characterized by a toxic psychosis, caused by the direct influence of circulating alpha toxin on the central nervous system, a jaundice partly caused by haemolysis by alpha toxin and partly by hepatic insufficiency, an acute renal failure due to the haemolytic uremic-syndrome and septic shock.

The present treatment for gas gangrene includes surgery, antibiotics, general resuscitative and ancillary measures and hyperbaric oxygen (type 1 R).

The action of hyperbaric oxygen on clostridia and other anaerobes is based on the formation of oxygen free radicals in the absence of free radical degrading enzymes such as superoxide dismutases, and peroxidases. A tissue pO_2 over 250 mmHg can be reached with 100% oxygen breathing at 3 ATA when the patient is at 3 ATA and breathing 100% oxygen, virtually all dangerous alpha toxin has disappeared after 30 min. Moreover, HBO interacts with antimicrobial agents and reinforces the aspecific immune response (phagocytic killing, adherence of leukocytes to the vascular endothelium) [11].

It is very important that hyperbaric oxygen therapy starts as early as possible, because the best treatment results are achieved in the earliest possible stage of the infection: early hyperbaric oxygen is life-saving, limb- and tissue-saving, and clarifies the demarcation between dead and still-living tissue within 24-30h. The recommended treatment profile is 3 ATA pure oxygen for 90 minutes (multiplace chamber), 3 times in the first 24 hours and then twice delay for the next 4-5 days.

A control of the treatment should be done by using transcutaneous and intramuscular pO_2 measurements before, during and after the HBO sessions.

Before hyperbaric oxygen therapy became available, the treatment of gas gangrene was almost entirely surgical. The main objective was to excise or amputate as soon as and as generously as possible so as to remove all diseased tissue. Mortality remained between 20 and 55%. Moreover, patients who lived were often disabled and subjected to long-lasting physical and psychological rehabilitation programs. The incidence of demolitive and seriously disabling amputations is over 60% [12].

Animal experiments and clinical data show that combination of hyperbaric oxygen, local debridement, and antibiotics led to less mortality and morbidity than any of these treatment modalities alone. The incidence of demolitive amputation is reduced to less than 15% and overall mortality to less than 20% [13].

Anaerobic or mixed bacterial necrotizing soft tissue infection (NSTI)

Mechanistically HBO should be helpful in all NSTI. The rationale for using adjunctive HBO and the mechanisms have been outlined extensively by Mader [14]. However, if antibiotic and surgical treatments are generally effective in a type of necrotizing infection, then adjunctive HBO probably is not cost-effective. But when the morbidity and/or mortality of a particular infection is high, then adjunctive HBO may be life-saving as well as cost-effective [15]. Mortality in NSTI is also related to the size of the infectious process [16]. Adjunctive HBO is strongly recommended for compromised hosts with crepitant anaerobic cellulitis and necrotizing fasciitis, including Fournier's disease and cervical necrotizing fasciitis. Patients with non clostridial myonecrosis have also an extreme morbidity and mortality risk. These patients should receive adjunctive HBO. These recommendations (type 1 R) are supported by in vivo and in vitro studies and clinical observations [14, 17-20].

Acute soft tissue ischaemia

HBO therapy has to be considered as an adjunctive treatment modality. Optimal surgery and resuscitation have to be done before or simultaneously.

There is experimental and clinical evidence supporting that HBO act to correct post-traumatic tissue oedema and delayed bone healing [21]. There is some experimental evidence showing a positive effect of HBO in preventing reperfusion injury, but there is not sufficient clinical evidence. However, no study showed a detrimental effect of HBO in increasing the oxidative stress in injured tissue [22]. In prevention of post-traumatic superimposed infections, the procedure of choice is surgery (repeated if necessary), but HBO can be recommended as an adjunctive treatment to enhance antibiotic efficacy, to improve tissue oxygenation and prevent surinfection.

Recommendations of the international jury of the 3rd ECHM Consensus Conference devoted to the role of HBO in acute musculo-skeletal trauma (Milano, September 1996) were as follows:

– In limb crush trauma and reperfusion post-traumatic syndromes, adjunctive HBO is recommended (type 2 R) because in case of severe tissue damage, with dubious vitality, there is experimental and clinical evidence that HBO improves tissue salvage and clinical outcome [23]. In cases of open fractures with extensive soft tissue and/or vascular damage (corresponding with type III/B/C of Gustillo's classification) adjunctive HBOT is recommended (type 2 R). In less severe cases, HBOT adjunctive to surgery can be used in compromized hosts (type 3 R).

– In compromised skin grafts and myo-cutaneous flaps, HBO is recommended (type 2 R). It cannot be overemphasized that patient's selection and the timing of HBO treatment are the keys to a successful outcome for most conditions in plastic surgery. Although HBO research has become more scientific and less anecdotal, there is still a need for further experimental and prospective clinical studies to more accurately define and confirm the specific role of HBO in this field [24].

- In the re-implantation of traumatically amputed limbs, HBO is optional (type 3 R) as in post-vascular surgery reperfusion syndromes.

- In every case the measurement of transcutaneous oxygen pressure under hyperbaric oxygen is needed as an index for the definition of the HBO indication and follow-up (type 2 R).

The cost of the adjunctive HBO will be at least compensated by the decrease in morbidity in these patients (e.g. lower amputation rate).

Burns

Encouraging theoretical and experimental evidence as well as clinical results exist for the adjunctive use of HBO in the acute phase of selected critical thermal burns. However, well-controlled clinical studies are lacking and considerable controversy still exists in the burn surgeon community. Broad-based justification for the use of adjunctive HBO in burns depends on favourable results from well-controlled prospective and randomized clinical trials in burn with HBO capabilities to which patients are taken within a few hours of injury [25].

At the moment, HBO is strongly recommended when the burn is associated with carbon monoxide intoxication and smoke inhalation injury (type 1 R). In the absence of a carbon monoxide intoxication, HBO is optional when burns exceed 20% of body surface, are of 2nd degree or more, or involve critical body parts (face, hands, feet and perineum), consist of circumferential burns of the extremities or are electrical burns (type 3 R). If burned areas are less than 20% of body surface, HBO therapy is not advised.

Post-anoxic encephalopathy - traumatic brain injury

Utilization of adjunctive HBOT in post-anoxic encephalopathy remains controversial. The potential benefit [26] must be balanced against its potential toxicity. Even if HBO was classified as optional (type 3 R) with regard to cerebral anoxia, it may be used under clinical research trial, associated with other therapeutic procedures. HBO modalities (pression level, duration, delay, number of sessions) must be precisely defined and prospective randomized controlled studies are needed [27].

Utilization of HBO in hearing disorders (sudden vascular deafness, objective tinnitus) remains to be objectively evaluated. Clinical reports are very numerous, in favour of efficacy of HBOT according to electrophysiological evaluation, but HBO is often associated with other treatment measures such as haemodilution, and the respective efficacy of the two treatment modalities is not known at the moment. HBO may be classified as optional (type 3 R) before having results of conducted prospective trials.

New frontiers

In the next future, HBO may constitute an adjunctive therapy to antibiotics and drainage in particular form of aeroanaerobic intracranial abcesses, aeroanaerobic lung abscesses, empyema and mediastinitis, intra-abdominal sepsis and peritonitis. Acute coronary insufficiency and myocardial infarction may also constitute a possible indication. If first and anecdotal reports indicate a beneficial action, multicentric randomized prospective and well controlled studies are needed before concluding to recommend HBO as well as further clinical researches may include well-controlled human trials of HBO as a preventive approach in post surgical wound infection.

Chronic indications for HBOT

Defective wound healing and osteoradionecrosis

Defective wound healing (DWH) is a major health problem, with corresponding financial implications. Basic research strongly supports the potential for HBO and clinical studies encourage inclusion of HBO in the management of DWH although controlled, randomized studies are still limited. Oxygen deficiency caused by impaired O_2 delivery is the most common cause of DWH. Wounds fail to heal and become infected when sufficiently hypoxic. DWH is commonly associated with: diabetes, peripheral venous stasis, arterial insufficiency, decubitus pressure, irradiation of tissue, collagen vascular diseases, pulmonary disease, malnutrition, and sickle cell disease. Contributing factors in these diseases include: inadequate blood supply (insufficient oxygenation and nutrient delivery); repeated physical trauma, persistent infection; inadequate inflammatory and/or immunologic responses, and interference with healing by prescribed drugs such as steroids, immunosuppressive agents, and antimetabolites. Additional factors include general debility, malnutrition, and chronic diseases (such as malignancy, anaemia, chronic renal failure, possible AIDS).

Blood flow in normal tissues and the process of vascular regeneration are both sensitive to local PO_2. Measuring oxygen tension in wounded tissue so that HBO can be properly evaluated and determining the upperlimit beyond which further increases in oxygen tension are harmful have been experimentally assessed while concomitant exploration of the microcirculation using laser doppler velocimetry and videomicroscopy have help to understand the role of O_2 in healing process face to the heterogeneity of the local microcirculatory bed. If HBO augments PO_2 but simultaneously reduces local perfusion, the net effects on inflammatory cell accumulation, nutrient supply, metabolite clearance and ultimately wound healing require attention.

At the biochemical level, the key ingredient to successful wound healing (synthesis and deposition of collagen) is O_2 dependent. If collagen is not adequately hydroxylated because of insufficient O_2, it is degraded rather than deposited for wound healing and the result can be DWH. Animal skin grafting studies indicate a beneficial role of HBO on graft survival across a variety of grafting approaches and species [28]. In clinical practice, transcutaneous oxygen pressure measurements and intramuscular oxygen pressure measurements at the wound level have been shown to reflect oxygen delivery to tissues and constitute a very useful and reliable test to predict efficacy of HBO and to follow evolution, when measurement are done under pure hyperbaric oxygenation [29].

In chronic critical leg ischaemia with arteriosclerotic ulcer and in diabetic foot lesions, clinical trials have demonstrated the benefit of adjunctive HBO to surgical debridements and wound dressings, which induces a reduction in the amputation rate statistically significant by comparison with the non HBO treated group [30]. So, in diabetic patients, the use of HBO is recommended in the presence of a chronic critical ischaemia as defined by the European Consensus Conference on critical ischaemia, if transcutaneous oxygen pressure readings under hyperbaric conditions (2.5 ATA, 100% oxygen) are higher than 100 mmHg (type 2 R).

In arteriosclerotic patients the use of HBO is recommended in case of a chronic critical ischaemia, if transcutaneous oxygen pressure readings under hyperbaric conditions (2.5 ATA, 100% oxygen) are higher than 50 mmHG (type 2 R).

A specific focus of HBO is osteoradionecrosis, where it has been shown to be efficacious as part of comprehensive management, including surgery, antibiotics and general care such as nutritional support and local wound toilet [30]. Cost-effectiveness is well documented for HBO in osteoradionecrosis [31]. So, HBO is strongly recommended in osteoradionecrosis (type 1 R). The most frequently adopted treatment protocol implies 20 HBO pre-surgery sessions and 10 post-surgery sessions. HBO is strongly recommended as a preventive treatment for dental extraction in irradiated or osteonecrotic bone (type 1 R). The most frequently adopted treatment protocol implies 20 HBO pre-extraction sessions and 10 post-extraction sessions.

HBO is also strongly recommended in soft tissue radionecrosis such as radionecrotic cystitis (type 1 R), except in radionecrotic lesions of the intestine where HBO has to be considered only as optional (type 3 R).

HBO is optional in spinal cord radionecrosis (type 3 R).

Refractory chronic osteomyelitis

Several early clinical reports describe the benefit of adjunctive HBOT to patients with refractory osteomyelitis. *In vitro* and *in vivo* studies have been designed to quantify and define the value of HBO. A PO_2 of 40 mmHg or more seems necessary for clinical healing of infected bone in experimental settings.

Success rates between 70-85% have been reported when treated with adjunctive HBO [32]. So HBO is recommended in chronic refractory osteomyelitis defined as osteomyelitic lesions persisting more than six weeks after adequate antibiotic treatment and at least one surgery (type 2 R). In cranial (except the mandible) and sternal osteomyelitis, HBO should be started simultaneously with antibiotics and surgical treatment (type 2 R).

New frontiers concern peripheral arteriopathies (early stages), sickle-cell anaemia with chronic leg ulcers, perineal ulcerations and fistula in Crohn's disease, dermatological diseases as epidermolysis bullosa, Hansen's disease, granuloma gangraenescens or pyoderma gangrenosum. At the moment, HBO is not recommended and remains to be evaluated.

Potential benefits and risks of HBO - Oxygen toxicity

Many diseases or syndromes have as a major component a cellular O_2 insufficiency usually locally and HBO represents a technically well-developped approach designed to enhance O_2 supply.

As with any other therapeutic approach, there are potential benefits and risks that have been listed [33]: HBO should increase tissue PO_2 but reactive O_2 species will be generated with potential cellular toxicity; tissue O_2 delivery should be enhanced by increased arterial O_2 and capillary PO_2 but hyperoxic vasoconstriction may reduce blood flow and this tissue delivery of inflammatory cells, nutrient delivery, etc.; growth of certain bacteria is inhibited by high concentrations of O_2, that of others might be enhanced; technically, to provide O_2 at 2 or 3 ATA is straight forward, however the potential for mechanical accidents, O_2 toxicity and this morbidity exists; is HBO cost-effective and ethic since there is a marked resurgence in the number of patients treated with HBO and a lack of sufficient well-controlled clinical trials to determine efficacy?

HBO usually involves no more than 3 atm. of pure oxygen applied for 1 to $1/2$ h at a time. There is no clinical evidence of O_2 toxicity under such conditions, but if cellular damage occurs before clinical toxicity, it is possible that, using HBO, there will be hyperoxic cellular damage. Whether repeated HBO treatment (the rule rather than the exception) induces tolerance to hyperoxic damage or rather produces cumulative damage is not clearly established. Continuous exposures to 2 atm. O_2 is lethel in most animals within 12 to 24h, but intermittent exposure dramatically reduces clinical O_2 toxicity. Vital capacity in humans is not reduced after repetitive 1 to 2h exposures to 2 atm O_2. On the other hand, repeated HBO treatments produce progressive myopia that usually reverses when treatment is complete. Convulsions (CNS toxicity) remains exceptional but clinically in humans, toxic responses to HBO are heterogeneous. The biochemical basis of O_2 toxicity appears to be, initially, the accelerated production of reactive O_2 species caused by the high PO_2. Hydrogen peroxide, superoxide anion and hydroxyl radicals are produced in a dose-dependent manner from most cells (from inflammatory cells, red cells and endothelial cells in particular). The relationship among PO_2, time of exposure, induction of cell damage and induction of tolerance to damage when PO_2 is delivered hyperbarically is under extensive investigation. Recent technical advances have enabled more sophisticated measurements of PO_2 in tissues as well as physiological and pharmacological effects of HBO at the cellular and biochemical levels [34]. This new information has forced reexamination of principles long held basic to HBO effect with regard to the area of HBO and O_2 toxicity and has opened the door to many exciting frontiers in HBO research and therapy. The optimal oxygen dose will be established in the near future for a variety of clinical conditions amenable to HBOT.

Conclusions

Evidence-based hyperbaric oxygen therapy is quite the contrary of a therapy in search of disease: acute and chronic indications for HBOT can be clearly identified. There is no clinical evidence of oxygen toxicity under accepted conditions (no more than 3 ATA, pure oxygen for maximum 1-1^1/$_2$ hours at a time, in a multiplace chamber). However, whether repeated HBOT induces tolerance to hyperoxic damage or rather produces cumulative damage is not yet clearly established.

References

1. Gabb G, Robin ED (1987) Hyperbaric oxygen: a therapy in search of diseases. Chest 92:1074-1082
2. Gyatt G and the Evidence Based Medicine working group (1992) Evidence based medicine. A new approach to teaching the practice of medicine. JAMA 268:2420-2425
3. Wattel F, Mathieu D (1994) Proceedings of the 1st European Consensus Conference on Hyperbaric Medicine, vol. 1. CRAM Nord-Picardie, Lille, p 504
4. Wattel F, Mathieu D (1996) Proceedings of the 2nd Consensus Conference devoted to the treatment of decompression accidents in recreational diving, vol. 1. Faculté de Médecine de Lille, Lille, p 225
5. Marroni A (1996) The Divers Alert Network in Europe: risk evaluation and problem management in a European recreational divers population. In: Oriani G, Marroni A, Wattel F (eds) Handbook on hyperbaric medicine. Springer, Berlin Heidelberg New York, pp 265-267
6. Dutka AJ (1991) Air or gas embolism. In: Camporesi EM, Barker AC (eds) Hyperbaric oxygen therapy: a critical review. Undersea and Hyperbaric Medical Society, Bethesda, pp 1-10
7. Moon RE (1996) Gas embolism. In: Oriani G, Marroni A, Wattel F (eds) Handbook on hyperbaric medicine. Springer, Berlin Heidelberg New York, pp 229-248
8. Mathieu D, Wattel F, Neviere R, Mathieu-Nolf M (1996) Carbon monoxide poisoning: mechanism, clinical presentation and management. In: Oriani G, Marroni A, Wattel F (eds) Handbook on hyperbaric medicine. Springer, Berlin Heidelberg New York, pp 281-296

9. Thom S (1993) Leukocytes in carbon monoxide mediated brain oxidative injury. Toxicol Appl Pharmacol 123:234-247
10. Thom S (1993) Functional inhibition of leukocyte B2 integrins by hyperbaric oxygen in carbon monoxide mediated brain injury in rats. Toxicol Appl Pharmacol 123:248-256
11. Park MK, Muhvich KH, Myers RAM, Mazella L (1994) Effects of hyperbaric oxygen infectious diseases: basic mechanisms. In: Kindwall EP (ed) Hyperbaric medicine practice. Best, Flagstaff, AZ, pp 141-172
12. Hart GB, Strauss MB (1990) Gas gangrene – clostridial myonecrosis – a review. J Hyperbaric Med 5:125-144
13. Bakker DJ, Van der kleij AJ (1996) Clostridial myonecrosis. In: Oriani G, Marroni A, Wattel F (eds) Handbook on hyperbaric medicine. Springer, Berlin Heidelberg New York, pp 362-385
14. Mader JT (1988) Mixed anaerobic and aerobic soft tissue infections. In: Davis JC, Hunt TK (eds) Problem wound: the role of oxygen. Elsevier, New York, pp 153-172
15. Marroni A, Oriani G, Wattel F (1996) Cost-benefit and cost efficiency evaluation of hyperbaric oxygen therapy. In: Oriani G, Marroni A, Wattel F (eds) Handbook on hyperbaric medicine. Springer, Berlin Heidelberg New York, pp 879-886
16. Wattel F, Mathieu D, Neviere R (1996) Les indications de l'oxygénothérapie hyperbare - organisation d'une unité de traitement. Formation des personnels. Bull Acad Nat Med 180: 949-964
17. Wattel F, Ohresser Ph, Mathieu D et al (1986) Perineal gangrene - clinical presentation and management. J Hyperbare Med I:215-221
18. Mathieu D, Neviere R, Chagnon JL, Wattel F (1995) Cervical necrotizing fasciitis - clinical manifestations and management. Clin Infect Dis 21:51-56
19. Bakker DJ, Van der Kleij AJ (1996) Soft tissue infection excluding clostridial myonecrosis: diagnosis and treatment. In: Oriani G, Marroni A, Wattel F (eds) Handbook on hyperbaric medicine. Springer, Berlin Heidelberg New York, pp 343-361
20. Riseman JA, Zamboni WA, Curtis A (1990) Hyperbaric oxygen therapy for necrotizing fasciitis reduces mortality and the need for debridements. Surgery 108:847-850
21. Niniikoski J, Hunt TK (1996) Oxygen and healing wounds: tissue-bone repair enhancement. In: Oriani G, Marroni A, Wattel F (eds) Handbook on hyperbaric medicine. Springer, Berlin Heidelberg New York, pp 485-507
22. Zamboni WA (1994) The microcirculation and ischemia-reperfusion: basic mechanisms of hyperbaric oxygen. In: Kindwall EP (ed) Hyperbaric medicine practice. Best, Flagstaff, AZ, pp 551-564
23. Bouachour G, Cronier P (1996) Hyperbaric oxygen in crush injuries. In: Oriani G, Marroni A, Wattel F (eds) Handbook on hyperbaric medicine. Springer, Berlin Heidelberg New York, pp 428-442
24. Zamboni WA (1996) Applications of hyperbaric oxygen therapy in plastic surgery. In: Oriani G, Marroni A, Wattel F (eds) Handbook on hyperbaric medicine. Springer, Berlin Heidelberg New York, pp 443-483
25. Lind F (1996) HBO therapy in burns and smoke inhalation injury. In: Oriani G, Marroni A, Wattel F (eds) Handbook on hyperbaric medicine. Springer, Berlin Heidelberg New York, pp 509-520
26. Wattel F, Mathieu D (1998) Hyperbaric oxygen in the treatment of post-hanging cerebral anoxia. In: Gullo A (ed) APICE 12. Springer, Berlin Heidelberg New York, pp 459-473
27. Ducasse JL, Cathala B (1996) Brain injuries and HBO. In: G. Oriani, Oriani G, Marroni A, Wattel F (eds) Handbook on hyperbaric medicine. Springer, Berlin Heidelberg New York, pp 404-408
28. Nemiroff PM, Merwin GE, Brant T, Cassisi NJ (1985) Effects of hyperbaric oxygen and irradiation on experimental skin flaps in rats. Otolaryngol Head Neck Surg 93:485-491
29. Mathieu D, Neviere R, Wattel F (1996) Transcutaneous oximetry in hyperbaric medicine. In: Oriani G, Marroni A, Wattel F (eds) Handbook on hyperbaric medicine. Springer, Berlin Heidelberg New York, pp 686-698

30. Van Merkesteyn JPR, Bakker DJ, Kooijman R (1996) Radionecrosis. In: Oriani G, Marroni A, Wattel F (eds) Handbook on hyperbaric medicine. Springer, Berlin Heidelberg New York, pp 387-401
31. Marx RE (1994) Radiation injury to tissue. In: Kindwall EP (ed) Hyperbaric medicine practice. Best, Flagstaff, AZ, pp 448-503
32. Britt M, Calhoun J, Mader JT, Mader JP (1994) The use of hyperbaric oxygen in the treatment of osteomyelitis. In: Kindwall EP (ed) Hyperbaric medicine practice. Best, Flagstaff, AZ, pp 419-427
33. NHLBI Workshop summary (1991) Hyperbaric oxygenation therapy. Am Rev Resp Dis 144: 1414-1421
34. Camporesi EM, Mascia MF, Thom SR (1996) Physiological principles of hyperbaric oxygenation. In: Oriani G, Marroni A, Wattel F (eds) Handbook on hyperbaric medicine. Springer, Berlin Heidelberg New York, pp 35-58

Intrinsically Safe Hyperbaric Centres

R. Scandella

The latest accident that occurred in October 1997 in hyperbaric habitat in Milan was one of the most serious that ever happened since hyperbaric chambers have been used as medical instruments. This fact overbearingly pointed out the importance of considering the risk related to the use of hyperbaric chambers, and consequently, the need to state definite safety levels. Every device or piece of electric or electronic apparatus which is not able to release – even in the case of a breakdown or an accidental damage – a quantity of energy such as to trigger off a combustion or an explosion, is defined, in this specific environment, as "intrinsically safe", although in the presence of extremely inflammable substances.

Applying the same logical principle, it is possible to define as "intrinsically safe" all those hyperbaric centres which, both as for the technical outfit or the set of equipment, and for the organization, management and training of their experts, can consider, control and, if possible, reduce the risks related to hyperbarism. In this way any accident should be avoided or, if that occurs although the necessary precautions, any consequence should be reduced to its minimum, if not avoided. The study of the risks of hyperbarism was divulgated by a great deal of publications, emphasizing the priority of fire-risk: the chances that this could happen are slight, but any consequences could be serious [3-8]. On the other hand, if we consider the mechanism regulating every combustion, we understand that the risk of fire is the most dangerous one, but also the easiest to be under control. In fact, in order to set a combustion it is necessary to have the so-called "combustion triangle", i.e. the simultaneous presence of three factors: the combustible substance, the igniter and the primer [1-3, 6, 8]. On standard conditions of use of the hyperbaric chamber, the combustible substance can be set up by clothing, sheets, sanitary stuffs and internal equipment, but also organic tissues can change, in some hyperoxygenated habitats, from self-estinguishing into combustible. If it is true that all the combustible components can be practically removed or replaced with fireproof materials, it is also true that the subject effecting the hyperbaric therapy must be present. Therefore the combustible substance can be rejected but just partially. Now then it is possible to act on the other components, i.e. the igniter and the primer. Evidently the igniter is made up of O_2, present in the air of compression and necessary for the hyperbaric therapy on the patient; therefore it cannot be totally removed, but it can be kept at levels as much as possible close to the normal ones, eliminating any incidental leak and monitoring the hyperbaric environment so as to maintain the combustibility levels at values as much as possible similar to the normal ones [1, 2, 6, 7, 9, 10]. The primer – a flame, a spark or concentrated heat – is the third basic element enabling combustion. In the ordinary conditions of use of a hyperbaric chamber, pressurized with air, and even in the presence of non-volatile combustible substances, the primer must have a reasonably high energy-level, and it must prime very closely (if not in direct contact) with the combustible substance. A spark induced by an electrostatic discharge is not able to trigger off the combustion of a regular cotton overall unless this is soaked with fatty combustible volatile and easily inflammable substances such as ether, alcohol, fuel, etc.; moreover, unless it is plugged into a hyperoxygenated atmosphere [5-7]. A free flame like that of a match or that of a lighter could certainly be sufficient to trigger off the combustion of the above-mentioned overall or the combustion of a sheet, being very close to them and acting until the ignition temperature is achieved. So it is obvious that the simple removal from a hyperbaric environment of: fatty, inflammable and volatile substances, electrostatic charges, mains supply at a high grade of energy, "free flames" and the excess of "free" oxygen, can drastically reduce fire risks up to very remote chances [1-4]. Therefore, the chance of a fire can successfully be reduced to negligible levels, operating through different intervention lines:

– the kit of equipment
– the operating and procedural organization.

The kit of equipment

The experimental use of hyperbaric chambers in the medical field has been concentrating for a long time on the actuation of the hyperbaric oxygen therapy (HBOT). On that account, not only a larger quantity of O_2 present in the hyperbaric environment – due to a larger existing pressure –, but also and above all the presence of pure O_2 administered to the patient may constitute a risk; in the case of uncontrolled leakage it may produce a further increase of the combustibility of the materials that are exposed to the hyperbaric environment. Recent studies (NFPA 99 Code) proved that an increase of the relative pressure of 1.47 bar (2.5 ATA, an increase of around 150%) raises the speed of combustion of the material (paper) from 1 cm/sec to 1.5 cm/sec in the air containing O_2 at around 21%, with a raise of the speed of 50%; whereas in the case of normobaric pressured combustion but containing O_2 at 100% the speed gets up to 4.5 cm/sec (increase of 350%). At a pressure of 1.47 bar in the presence of O_2 at 30% the speed of combustion gets up to 2 cm/sec (increase of 100%). It is clear that a larger speed of combustion depends greatly on the percentage of O_2 present, and not really on a larger earthed availability of O_2, generated by a larger pressure; in fact increasing the pressure, the earthed availability of both oxygen and nitrogen (the main further component of air) is increased, causing an inhibitory effect on the increased ignitible power of the hyperbaric environment [2].

Starting from these considerations exclusively hyperbaric chambers need to be used: the internal pressuring increase is here obtained by inletting compressed air, conveniently fittered and treated, steadily checking the percentage of O_2 in the hyperbaric environment. Being O_2 indispensable as a basic drug in the hyperbaric therapy, its control must be carried out with maximum efficiency, through consistent timing-distribution and supply systems such as to guarantee that there will be no leak in the equipment and that there will be the lowest level of loss in the zone of contact between the patient and the supply system. Currently it is possible to accept the minimum degree of pollution due to O_2 in a hyperbaric environment (plus 1-2% and no more), but having a set of equipment that permits to point out and to monitor the percentage of O_2 present is fundamental and can avoid O_2 reaching levels such as to increase considerably the speed of combustion. In order to guarantee the higher safety levels possible, a hyperbaric chamber has to be equipped with:

1. a pressurization system with high quality compressed air (rules DIN 3188 or STANAG 1079);

2. current-fed lines with exclusively individual applicated supply units for group therapies;

3. a direct suction system to collect and release outboard O_2 exhaled by the patients. This system should guarantee a ventilatory basic level and an exchange of the internal air;

4. an analysing system of the percentage of O_2, equipped with optical and hearing alarms;

5. a surveying and a recording system of parameters (pressure, temperature, the relative humidity and the percentage of O_2 present);

6. no current-fed electrical system with high energy levels on the inside;

7. a set of equipment such as to prevent the accumulation of electrostatic charges;

8. an automatic device that, in the case of the overcoming of the pre-established alarm threshold, blocks O_2 supplies replacing it with breathable air (% $O_2 > 23$%);

9. an automatic device that, in the case of the overcoming of the pre-established alarm threshold, substitutes the air present in the hyperbaric environment;

10. a fire-fighting plant at air feeding system, suitably carried out and shaped, equipped with devices such as to prevent the use of the hyperbaric chamber in the case of a partial or a total inefficiency;

11. a safety device to prevent the use of the hyperbaric chamber when the division of the emergency transfer is not planned to guarantee a prompt assistance in the same chamber if pressurized [1-3, 5, 10].

These technical features (some of which were already used in particularly sophisticated and advanced centres), emerged while considering the accident that happened in Milan (Italy), October 1997. A specific board of experts was designated by the district of Lombardy in order to define some guidelines for the correct management of a hyperbaric centre from the viewpoint of the maximum safety possible.

Other technical requirements were added just to prevent the arising of risk conditions (for example the inefficiency of the extinguishing system or the wrong use of the oxygen analysing system); these conditions, together with behaviouring mistakes (the non-continuity in the chamber command during all the therapy), and procedural errors (short accuracy while controlling, short information of the users), may contribute to cause an accident with the dramatic consequences we know. There are other risks linked to hyperbarism: any variation in pressure may cause barotrauma or other problems caused by the change in temperature or in the density of the air (sun strokes, respiratory lacks, pneumothorax), or problems depending on the enclosed nature of the environment (claustrophobia, anxiety, non-rapid escaping times) [3]. The technical equipment normally present in a well planned and constructed hyperbaric chamber can hold back to the maximum the chance that the above-mentioned risks may happen (e.g. high precision manometers, pressure gauges, monitoring of the surrounding therapeutical parameters with previously arranged alarms, ergonomic control system, regular shaping of current-fed ducts and tubes, etc...) [3].

The operating and procedural organization

However, technical equipment at its highest level is not sufficient to eliminate completely the intrinsic risk related to the use of any set of machinery, and, in this case, the hyperbaric chamber is not an exception, because the maximum safety guarantees are obtained through the match man/machine. Although sophisticated, the only machine, being a machinery, is exposed to breakdowns or bad running, also if it is checked continually and carefully. So even the operator can make mistakes though his training and executive care; the synergic union of both factors, the human and the technological – supporting and completing one another thanks to a careful reckoning of any mutual weak point –, make possible to guarantee the achievement of the highest efficiency – and operating security – levels, guaranteed by the current state of art. The figures of the operators – both medical and technical – are important above all for the risk that the event may occur; in fact, they have to be rightly informed and trained so as to face, in a lucid and determined manner, any unforeseen event that may happen during the hyperbaric therapy and related to the above-tested risks. First of all a differentiation of the competences of the persons in charge is needed, giving precise responsibility to the medical and to the technical manager; these two figures must act synergically to achieve the aim, i.e. carrying out the technical duty through the use of the hyperbaric chamber at its maximum degree of efficiency and safety. There is no point in telling that it is the medical manager's duty to take all the therapeutical responsibilities and decisions; whereas the technical manager is entrusted with the responsibilities related to the proper management and preservation of the system at the height of its efficiency. It is obvious that the therapeutic decisions will take priority on any other arising problem, if this is not such as to lower, even slightly, the efficiency of the safety systems or to add further sources of risk besides the already estimated ones [1].

If necessary both the persons in charge will have to receive confirmation of the efficiency guarantees of all the hyperbaric system's components and they could check the real need of the therapeutical modalities applied, suspending or interrupting the activity if the distinctive features are lacking. The medical and the technical managers are charged with the definition of the operating procedures of the subjects involved (medical and paramedical staff, technicians, maintenance men), checking at intervals the correct application and the possible updating suggested by practical knowledge. The managers will also have to test the medical, technical and servicing competence of the staff managing the hyperbaric system.

Conclusions

To be "intrinsically safe" a modern hyperbaric centre has to apply the operating and installing modalities so far pointed out; no accident among the possible ones should occur or, if this happens, it should produce the minimum consequences (when nothing at all) thanks to conveniently defined programming, competence and set of equipment.

References

1. Linee guida per la gestione delle camere iperbariche collocate in ambienti sanitari pubblici e privati. Delibera Regione Lombardia n. VI/34873, 27 February 1998
2. – (1996) Hyperbaric facilities. In: Health care facilities. National Fire Protection Association (NFPA code 99)
3. Consensus Conference, Lille, 1994
4. Hamilton RW (1977) Hyperbaric chamber safety - Hyperbaric oxygen therapy. Davis and TK Hunt (eds), UMS 1977
5. US Air Force Manual (1983) Hyperbaric chamber equipment: consolidated equipment list from selected multiplace hyperbaric facilities. Department of the Air Force
6. Youn BA, Gordon D, Moran C, Brown B (1989) Fire in the multiplace hyperbaric chamber. J Hyperbaric Med 4
7. ANSI-ASME (1997) Safety standards for pressure vessel for human occupancy, PVHO. American Society of Mechanical Engineers, New York
8. Sheffled PJ, Desautels DA (1997) Hyperbaric and hypobaric chambers fires: a 73-year analysis. Undersea Hyperbaric Medicine 24(3):153-164
9. SIAARTI (Società Italiana di Anestesia Analgesia Rianimazione e Terapia Intensiva) (1994) Raccomandazioni per l'impiego dell'ossigenoterapia iperbarica
10. SIMSI (Società Italiana di Medicina Subacquea e Iperbarica) (1995) Requisiti minimi organizzativi, strutturali e tecnologici per la terapia iperbarica

LUNG FUNCTION IN THE ICU

Lung Function Monitoring in the ICU: Available Techniques and Future Requirements

B. LACHMANN, S.J.C. VERBRUGGE

Lung function monitoring should provide basic physiological information on gas transport from the air via the lung into the blood and should – depending on the level of care – provide parameters which make a differentiation of the cause of the disturbance in gas exchange possible (Table 1).

Table 1. Monitoring requirements during mechanical ventilation

First level
Arterial oxygen tension (pulse oximetry)
Acid base balance
Airway pressure
Second level
Lung-thorax mechanics (compliance, resistance)
Intra-pulmonary shunt
Cardiac output and haemodynamics
Third level
Oxygen consumption/delivery and carbon dioxide production
Diffusion capacity
Ventilation-perfusion mismatching
Lung water

Arterial oxygenation

The main goal of mechanical ventilation is to overcome or prevent hypoxia, which is the most important and life-threatening parameter during mechanical ventilation. The oxygenation index (PaO_2/FiO_2) measured under standard ventilator settings (e.g. PEEP of 5 cm H_2O, peak pressure of 35 cm H_2O, I/E ratio = 1:1, frequency of 20 breaths per minute), can be used to define the state of impairment of the lung, although a lower than optimal oxygenation index does not differentiate between: 1) ventilation, 2) perfusion, 3) diffusion 4) ventilation/perfusion (V/Q) or 5) perfusion-diffusion problems. At present it is the most reliable and routinely available tool to define the disease state of the lung [1] under standard ventilation conditions.

Lung mechanical parameters

Peak inspiratory pressure at flow constant ventilation is a poor parameter to measure alveolar overstretching as it is influenced by a number of factors independent of alveolar pressure and does not allow to define the state of overinflation and/or openness of different lung areas [2]. To prevent repeated alveolar collapse and reexpansion, it has been suggested that lungs should be ventilated above the lower inflection point of their P-V curve [2, 3]; to prevent overdistension it has been suggested that inspiratory plateau pressures should be reduced below the upper inflection point of the P-V curve, ventilating them in the most compliant part of their P-V curve [2, 3]. Total lung volume and functional residual capacity (FRC) should always be taken into account when interpreting compliance measurements [4], in other words lung compliance measurements which are not normalized for lung volume have only a limited information. That means that the values e.g. from the Murray score also only have very limited information. For a small tiny person a compliance of 40 ml/cm H_2O may be quite normal, whereas for a 2 m tall person it may be a very low value. Thus, if FRC measurements are not possible, one should at least normalize lung compliance values for lean body weight. Furthermore, a normal value for FRC does not differentiate a fully open lung from one with collapsed lung areas in which healthy areas are overinflated. Similarly, as the lower inflection point is the resultant of the P-V curves of different lung parts with a different compliance it may be the resultant of overdistended anterior parts, while posterior lung parts remain collapsed (Fig. 1) and may represent both alveolar recruitment and increases in volume of alveoli that are already open. Thus, considering the quite complicated nature of lung mechanical measurements and the fact that no standardized way of lung volume measurements is possible (functional residual capacity measurements are at this time not routinely available), oxygenation index is at present the best way to define the disease state of the lung.

Morphological measurements

The development of a simple tool for determining regional volumes during ventilation would be a major step forward in the search for safer treatment. Although CT scan may be used for this purpose [5], it is not likely to find its way as a routine applicable tool in clinics because of its price, size and possible hazards. However, electric impedance tomography which has been shown to have the same capabilities as CT scan, but is not limited by its disadvantages, may well find its way as a routine evaluation method in the future [6].

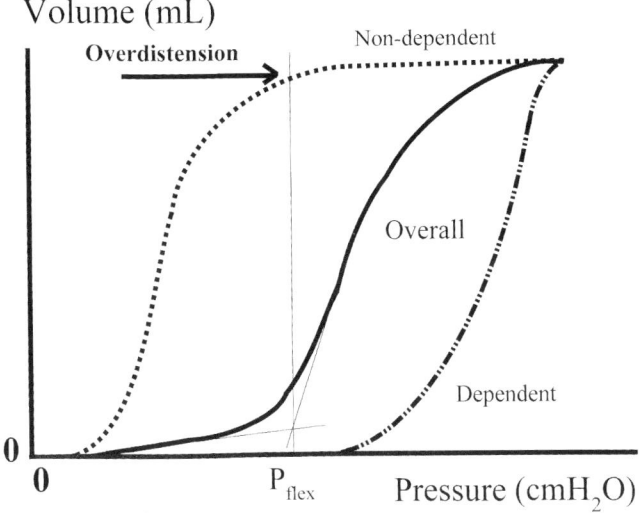

Fig. 1. Because the pressure-volume curve of the whole lung in an ARDS lung is the result of parts which have been affected by the disease process to different extents, the lower inflection point of the pressure-volume curve does not have to represent mass alveolar recruitment, but rather overdistension of non-dependent parts while posterior parts remain collapsed

Biological markers

Finally, numerous biological markers have been identified which may be used to evaluate damage to the alveolo-capillary barrier. These have been recently reviewed elsewhere [7]. For the endothelium, many specific markers are available [7], but at present only increased protein permeability of radio-active tracers from the alveolar lung compartment into the circulation evaluates the epithelial integrity, which is rate-limiting for the transfer of solutes over the alveolo-capillary barrier [7]. A recent preliminary report suggests the use of purines as a specific marker of epithelial injury [8]. The search should continue for highly specific biological markers in the bloodstream, such as are available for other organs, to monitor the metabolic and biological stress inflicted on the lung by our supportive ventilation therapy.

Conclusions

Monitoring of the lung by means of physiological, morphological and biochemical parameters is a prerequisite for an optimal ventilation strategy in the ICU to prevent or to minimize ventilation-induced lung injury. Monitoring techniques should provide us as much as possible with non-invasive continuous analytical data such as FRC measurements or electric impedance tomography or with minimal invasive techniques such as on-line blood gases or continuous monitoring of specific biological markers by means of biosensors. Some of these techniques are already available and some are in the experimental, developmental state. If we learn to use them to make the right therapeutic decisions in our patients, than it may be possible to further reduce the high mortality in the ICU with which we are still confronted.

References

1. Böhm S, Lachmann B (1996) Pressure-control ventilation. Putting a mode into perspective. Int J Intens Care 3:12-27
2. Tremblay NL, Slutsky AS (1996) The role of pressure and volume in ventilation induced lung injury. Appl Cardiopulm Pathophysiol 6:179-190
3. Morris AH, Wallace CJ, Menlove RL et al (1994) Randomized clinical trial of pressure-controlled inverse ratio ventilation and extracorporeal CO_2 removal for adult respiratory distress syndrome. Am J Resp Crit Care Med 149:295-305
4. Radford EP (1964) Static mechanical properties of mammalian lungs. In: Fenn WO, Rahn H (eds) Handbook of physiology. A critical, comprehensive presentation of physiological knowledge and concepts. American Physiological Society, Washington DC
5. Gattinoni L, Pelosi P, Crotti S, Valenza F (1995) Effects of positive end-expiratory pressure on regional distribution of tidal volume and recruitment in adult respiratory distress syndrome. Am J Respir Crit Care Med 151:1807-1814
6. Hahn G, Sipinkova I, Baisch F, Hellige G (1995) Changes in thoracic impedance distribution under different ventilatory conditions. Physiol Meas 16:A161-A173
7. Pittet JF, MacKersie RC, Martin TR, Matthay MA (1997) Biological markers of acute lung injury: Prognostic and pathogenic significance. Am J Resp Crit Care Med 155:1187-1205
8. Verbrugge SJC, de Jong JW, Keijzer E, Lachmann B (1998) Purine in broncho-alveolar lavage fluid as marker of ventilation-induced lung injury. Crit Care Med (in press)

Mechanical Ventilation and Lung Mechanics

B. JONSON

Classical studies by von Neergaard in 1929 and Radford and co-workers in the early 1960's showed in experiments with liquid- and air-filled lungs that surface forces are responsible for a large part of the elastic recoil pressure of the lungs [1, 2]. Concepts which may form the basis for the interpretation of elastic pressure-volume (P_{el}-V) curves in today's intensive care units were laid down. This interpretation is, however, more complex than has previously been understood as will be emphasised in this chapter. The technique for clinical determination of the P_{el}-V curves is another issue that will be discussed.

The elastic pressure-volume curve

A representative P_{el}-V curve recorded in a patient with acute lung injury (ALI) during insufflation following a deep expiration is shown in Fig. 1. The curve comprises three segments. The first segment is flat, which means that compliance initially is very low. This is an indication of collapse of peripheral airways or alveoli during the preceding expiration. The second segment is steeper, compliance is higher. The transition between these two segments is called the lower inflection point (LIP). The second segment linear implies that compliance remains constant. The third segment has a declining slope which means that compliance approaches zero [3-6]. The upper inflection point (UIP) separates the second from the third segment. It has been suggested that the tidal volume, Vt, should be limited to within the linear segment between the LIP and the UIP [6, 7]. Below the LIP repeated collapse and re-opening of lung units could lead to shear forces damaging the lung. Above the LIP the lung might suffer from barotrauma because of over-distension. Below the understanding of the P_{el}-V curve behind this view will be critically analysed.

A lung model

A lung model comprising 100 units with different properties will be analysed so as to mimic the non-homogeneity of the opening pressure of collapsed lung

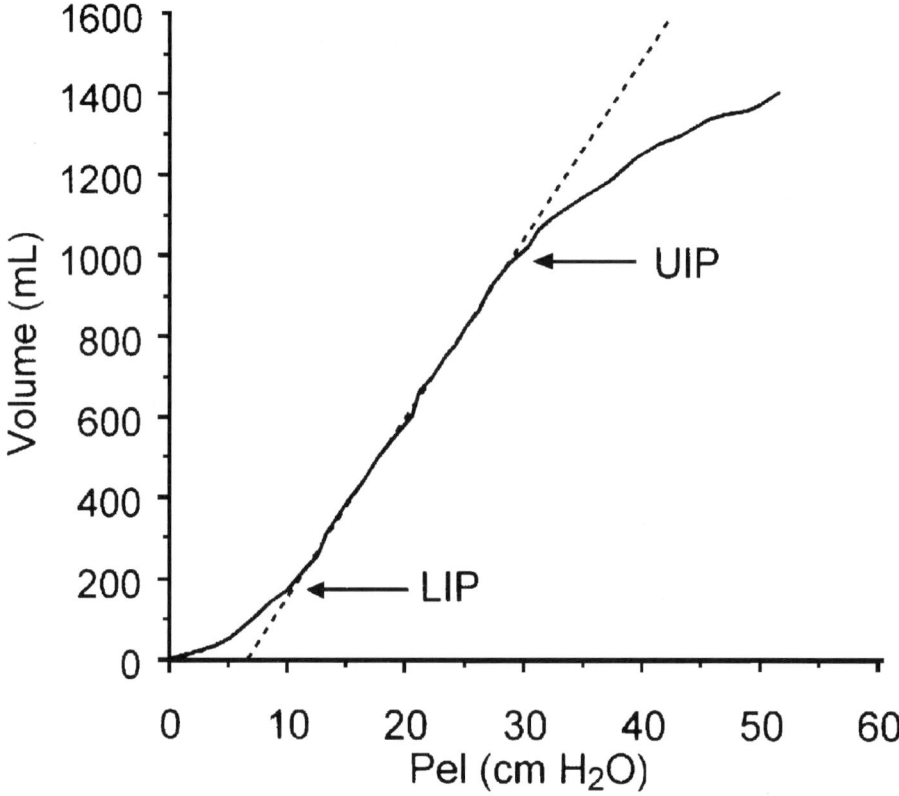

Fig. 1. The elastic pressure-volume (P_{el}-V) curve recorded over an extended volume range from a patient with acute lung injury. The dotted line represents the extrapolation of the linear segment of the P_{el}-V curve

units which is well documented in ALI and in the acute respiratory distress syndrome (ARDS) by Gattinoni et al. [8].

If all the 100 units of the lung model are recruited, the total lung has a compliance of 50 ml/cm H_2O, which is constant up to a P_{el} of 14 cm H_2O (Fig. 2). At pressures above 14 cm H_2O, the compliance falls and approaches zero at a fictive maximum volume of 1500 ml.

Each recruited lung unit has an identical P_{el}-V curve and represents 1% of the volume of the ideal P_{el}-V curve in Fig. 2. To mimic the situation in ARDS it was assumed that a lung unit would collapse or be recruited from the collapsed state at a specific critical pressure in the proximal airway (P_{crit}). The distribution of the critical pressure between the lung units is defined by two parameters: the mean critical pressure (mP_{crit}) and the standard deviation of P_{crit} (sdP_{crit}). The simulated lung model allows a variation of the pressure surrounding a lung unit

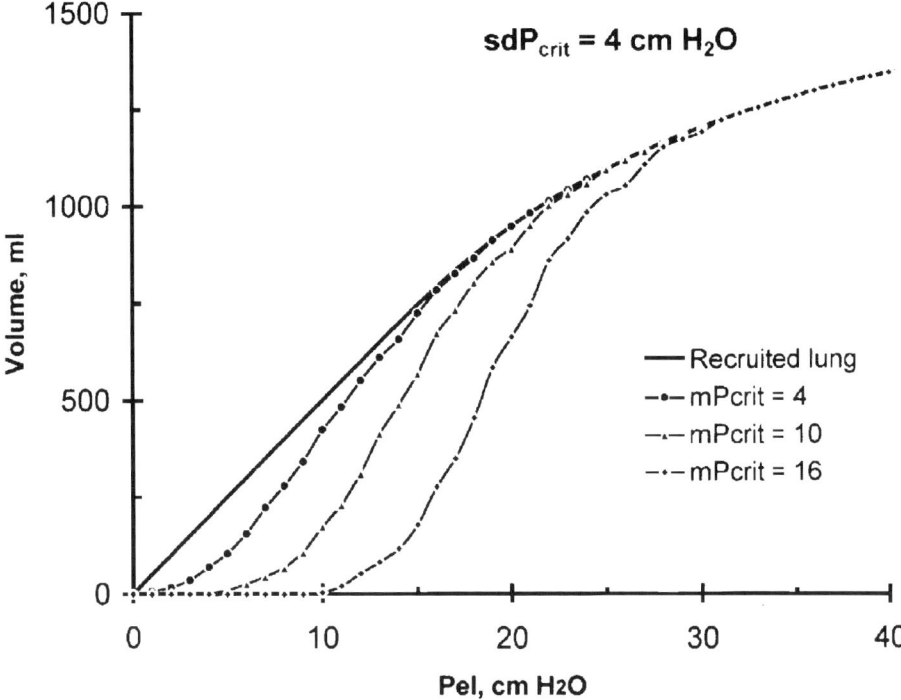

Fig. 2. Elastic pressure-volume (P_{el}-V) curves representing a multi-compartment lung model. The continuous curve shows features of a completely recruited lung. The other curves represent three lungs, with a mean critical opening pressures (mP_{crit}) of 4-16 cm H_2O. All have a standard deviation of mP_{crit} (sdP_{crit}) of 4 cm H_2O. Minor irregularities of the curves reflect a random attribution of P_{crit} of the 100 lung compartments

caused by lung weight, which for simplicity's sake will not be further discussed. During insufflation, when the P_{el}-V curve is recorded a lung unit is considered to "pop" open when the airway pressure reaches the specific value of P_{crit} for the unit. When the unit pops open, the volume increases from zero to the volume of other open units. At airway pressure above its individual P_{crit} a lung unit attains a volume defined by the P_{el}-V curve of open units. This simple model does not incorporate resistive or visco-elastic properties.

When mP_{crit} is allowed to vary between 4 and 16 cm H_2O, at a constant sdP_{crit} of 4 cm H_2O, a LIP is observed at a pressure lower than mP_{crit} (Fig. 2). Above the LIP, a nearly linear segment shows a compliance which is higher than the compliance of the fully recruited lung at similar pressures. The upper inflection point is strongly dependent on the mP_{crit}. Full recruitment occurs at pressures much higher than the LIP, as indicated by the coalescence of P_{el}-V curves with the curve representing the fully recruited lung.

In order to simulate an augmented non-homogeneity of the lung with respect to the critical opening pressure, the sdP_{crit} was varied between 4 and 16 cm H_2O while the mP_{crit} was kept constant at 15 cm H_2O. The LIP, the UIP and the extension of the linear segment and its slope, i.e. the maximum compliance, are all very much depending upon the heterogeneity of the lung expressed as sdP_{crit} (Fig. 3).

What does "compliance" stand for?

By definition compliance is the volume change divided by the pressure change:

$$C = \frac{\Delta V}{\Delta P} \qquad \text{(Eq. 1)}$$

When, during an insufflation lung units get recruited, ΔV consists of two components: 1) ΔV_{dist} represents the distension of open lung units under increasing pressure; 2) ΔV_{recr} represents sudden volume increments when the critical opening pressure of a specific collapsed lung unit is overcome and the unit is recruited. Thus:

$$C = \frac{\Delta V}{\Delta P} = \frac{\Delta V_{dist} + \Delta V_{recr}}{\Delta P} \qquad \text{(Eq. 2)}$$

The more or less abrupt increase in compliance at the LIP (Figg. 2 and 3), indicates the commencement of recruitment of lung units. The second, linear segment with a high compliance reflects that distension and recruitment occur in parallel. In Fig. 2 a low sdP_{crit} implies that lung units open up over a small pressure interval. Then ΔV_{recr} will lead to a particularly high maximum compliance. The UIP indicates the end of the recruitment process. The UIP does not mean that the lung is overdistended. The commonly held opinion that the tidal ventilation should occur within the linear segment of the P_{el}-V curve in order to avoid lung collapse below the LIP and lung overdistension above the UIP appears to be false as the LIP and the UIP reflect the beginning and the end of the recruitment process. When, as in Fig. 3, the sdP_{crit} is varied one may observe that the LIP and the UIP vary depending upon the non-homogeneity of the lung with respect to opening pressures of various lung units.

Is the lung model realistic? Do we need to change our view on the P_{el}-V curve? The form of the P_{el}-V curve of a well recruited lung is well known. The lack of resistive and visco-elastic properties is a limitation of the model. However, these properties are also non-homogeneous, and would further increase the variation of pressure and volume at which different lung units would be recruited. The incorporating of resistive and visco-elastic properties would lead to even

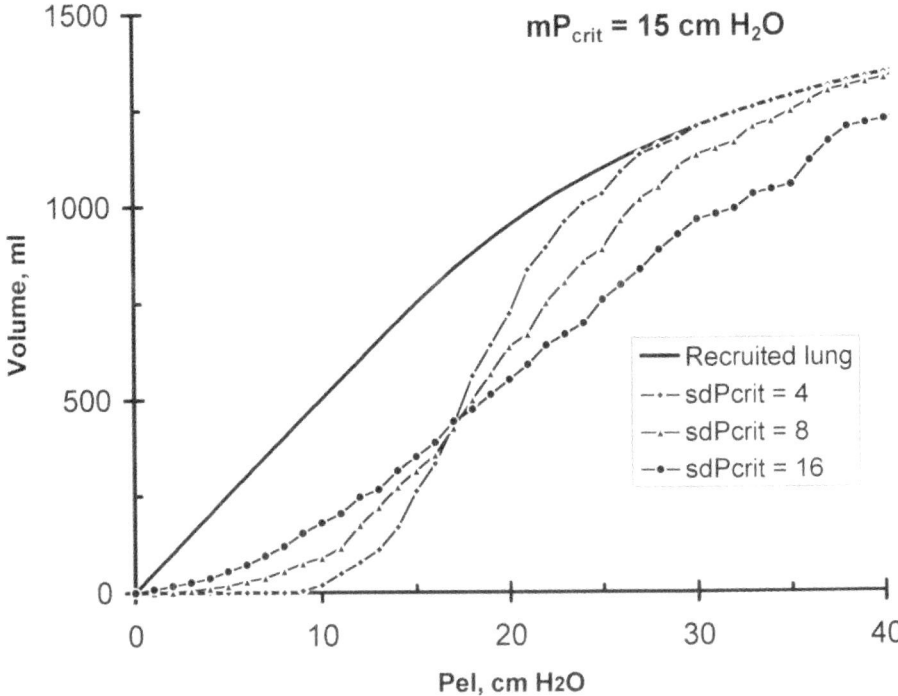

Fig. 3. Three lungs modelled, all with a mP_{crit} of 15 cm H_2O and a sdP_{crit} varying from 4 to 16 cm H_2O. See also Fig. 2

greater deviations from the concept that a linear P_{el}-V segment represents the zone within which collapse/recruitment and overdistension are avoided. Indeed we need to change our perspective on the P_{el}-V curve.

In ALI and ARDS P_{el}-V curves recorded after an expiration to zero end-expiratory pressure, ZEEP, showed a steeper slope (greater compliance) than curves recorded after an expiration to a positive end-expiratory pressure (Fig. 4) [9]. This observation shows that recruitment after a lung collapse during a deep expiration to ZEEP continues far above the LIP. Also data in healthy humans [10] show that a high value of compliance indicates ongoing recruitment in accordance with Eq. 2.

When a collapsed lung is re-expanded in the operating theatre one observes how lung units start to pop open at modest insufflation pressures. Complete lung recruitment takes high distending pressures. Both in health and in ARDS high airway pressures are required to re-inflate condensed lung zones [8, 11]. Accordingly, a model with a wide distribution of opening pressures is realistic. The inhomogeneity between lung compartments modelled in Fig. 3 is warranted.

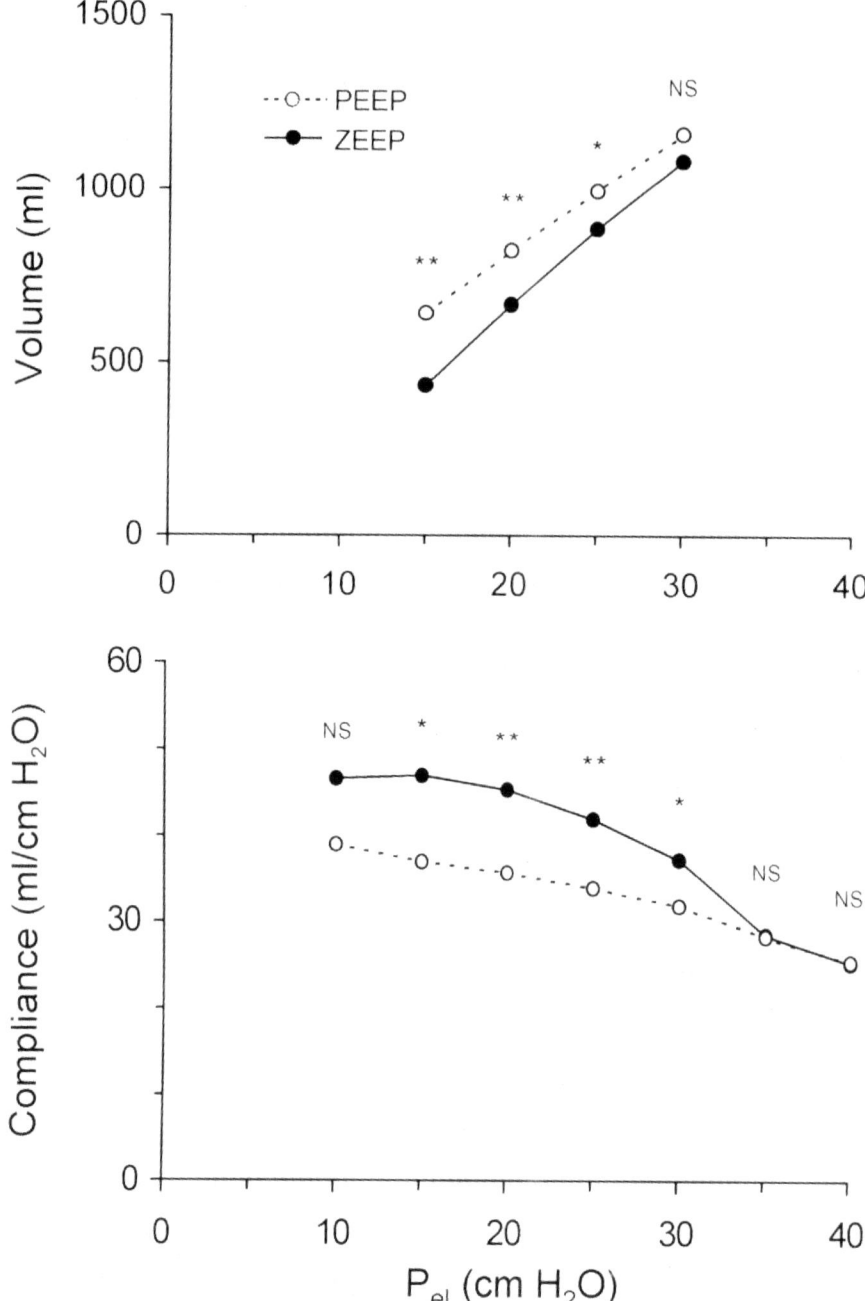

Fig. 4. Mean volume and compliance versus elastic pressure (P_{el}) in 11 patients with ALI/ARDS. The recording was started after either an expiration to zero end-expiratory pressure (ZEEP) or after an expiration at the clinically applied positive end-expiratory pressure (PEEP). NS, non-significant; *, $P < 0.05$; **, $P < 0.01$. Modified from [9]

P_{el}-V curve recording in intensive care

Static P_{el}-V curves. Studies of properly elastic properties of the respiratory system are based upon determination of static elastic P_{el}-V curves. The super-syringe method has been a most valuable method [7, 12]. To avoid problems associated with the method [13, 14] the flow interruption method was developed [15-19]. Computer-control of a commercial ventilator (ServoVentilator 900C, Siemens-Elema AB, Sweden) allows precise control of events preceding and during measurements of the static P_{el}-V curve with high precision and reproducibility [20]. The flow interruption method is based on about 20 interrupted breaths with long pauses and separated by at least two ordinary breaths. The recording of the static P_{el}-V curve takes several minutes.

One may ask whether the static elastic recoil pressure is the most relevant pressure to measure in intensive care. Static pressures exist only under the artificial pauses used for its determination. During inspiration, the dynamic pressure in the lung is the sum of the static elastic and the visco-elastic recoil pressure. To the extent that intrapulmonary pressure is harmful the visco-elastic pressure component can hardly be less dangerous than the static elastic pressure. This implies that dynamic pressure recordings may then be more relevant. This aspect in combination with problems associated with the determination of the static P_{el}-V curve, motivate alternative methods.

Dynamic P_{el}-V curves. Suratt and Owens [21] and Ranieri et al. [22] applied the concept that at constant flow insufflation variations in the rate of pressure change indicate a change in compliance. Servillo et al. used a computer-controlled ventilator for dynamic studies [23]. A prolonged expiration at ZEEP was followed by an insufflation lasting 6 s. The resistive pressure from Y-piece to the trachea and within the patient's airway was subtracted. In ALI and ARDS the dynamic P_{el}-V curves were largely similar to static curves, but showed a clearer decrease in compliance at high airway pressures and a more consistent UIP. The difference was probably due to the visco-elastic pressure which increases fast at high pressures due to the non-linearity of visco-elastic properties [3, 19].

Description of the P_{el}-V curve

The P_{el}-V curve is usually characterised by visual and manual means. Particularly in research a mathematical characterisation of P_{el}-V curves is needed. Venegas et al. [24], who used a symmetrical model based on only four parameters, reported good agreement between their model and data recorded from dogs and humans in health and with ARDS. A model allowing a strictly linear segment between two non-linear segments, which may be asymmetrical, is based upon a non-continuous equation with six parameters [10]. The fit between observed data and the model was excellent at health. This is also the case in ALI/ARDS (Fig. 5).

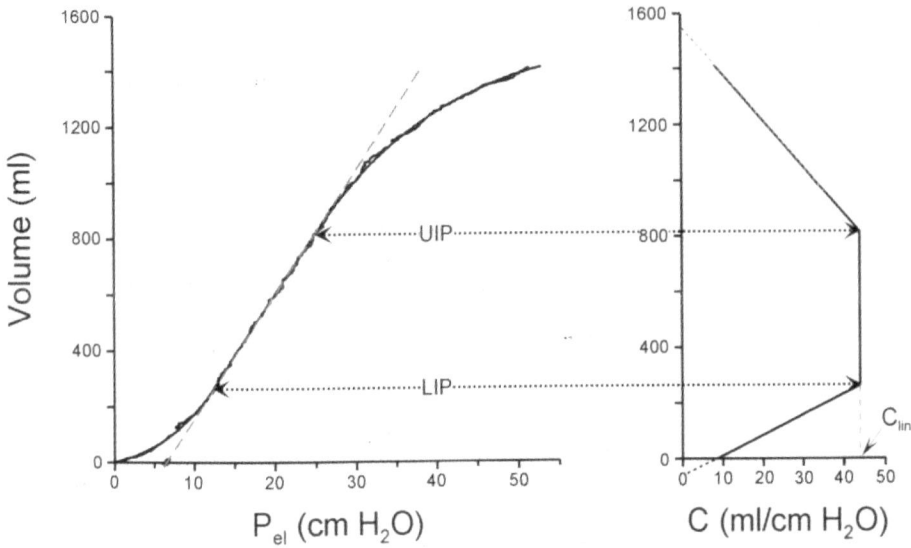

Fig. 5. An elastic pressure-volume (P_{el}-V) curve recorded from a patient with acute lung injury. The smooth curve is calculated according to a six-parameter three-segment model [10]. The linear segment of the P_{el}-V curve is delineated by the lower and upper inflection points (LIP and UIP, respectively). The mathematical model presumes that compliance increases linearly with volume up to the LIP, it then assumes a constant high value, C_{lin}, up to the UIP from which it falls linearly with increasing volume (right panel)

Is the P_{el}-V curve clinically useful?

A large number of reports provide data for or against the clinical value of a "protective ventilation strategy" (PVS). The Pel/V curve has been considered to give important guidelines in ventilator setting [6]. Recently, Amato et al. showed improved results in ARDS patients treated with a PVS [25, 26]. The positive end-expiratory pressure was set to 2 cm H_2O above the LIP, while the tidal ventilation was reduced by allowing moderate degrees of hypercapnic ventilation. It is not easy to estimate which importance the P_{el}-V curve had for the positive outcome. It is, however, promising that this study, which is the first and so far only study in which a PVS has given positive results in a controlled study, used the P_{el}-V curve, for individual titration of the ventilator setting.

Clinically useful techniques for recording and analysis of the P_{el}-V curve are being developed. We understand better the physiological background of the curve. The first positive clinical studies in which the P_{el}-V curve has been used have been presented. After many years of promise, the P_{el}-V curve may at last become an essential tool in improving patient care. However, further studies are needed to finally define the clinical value of the P_{el}-V curve.

References

1. Neergaard KV (1929) Neue Auffassungen über einen Grundbegriff der Atemmechanik: Die Retraktionskraft der Lunge abhängig von der Oberflächenspannung in den Alveolen. Z Ges Exp Med 66:373-394
2. Radford EP Jr (1964) Mechanical properties of mammalian lungs. In: Fenn WO, Rahn H (eds) Handbook of physiology. American Physiological Society, Washington DC, pp 429-449
3. Svantesson C, John J, Taskar V et al (1996) Respiratory mechanics in rabbits ventilated with different tidal volumes. Respir Physiol 106:307-316
4. Paiva M, Yernault JC, Eerdeweghe PV et al (1975) A sigmoid model of the static volume-pressure curve of the human lung. Respir Physiol 23:317-323
5. Svantesson C (1997) Respiratory mechanics during mechanical ventilation in health and in disease [dissertation]. Lund University, Lund
6. Roupie E, Dambrosio M, Servillo G et al (1995) Titration of tidal volume and induced hypercapnia in acute respiratory distress syndrome. Am J Respir Crit Care Med 152:121-128
7. Matamis D, Lemaire F, Harf A et al (1984) Total respiratory pressure-volume curves in the adult respiratory distress syndrome. Chest 86:58-66
8. Gattinoni L, Pelosi P, Crotti S et al (1995) Effects of positive end-expiratory pressure on regional distribution of tidal volume and recruitment in adult respiratory distress syndrome. Am J Respir Crit Care Med 151:1807-1814
9. Richard J-C, Jonson B, Straus C et al (1997) Pressure-volume curves in acute respiratory failure recorded from zero and positive end expiratory pressure. Intensive Care Med 23:S21 (abstract)
10. Svantesson C, Sigurdsson S, Larsson A et al (1998) Effects of recruitment of collapsed lung units on the elastic pressure-volume relationship in anaesthetised healthy adults. Acta Anaesthesiol Scand (in press)
11. Rothen HU, Sporre B, Engberg G et al (1993) Re-expansion of atelectasis during general anaesthesia: a computed tomography study. Br J Anaesth 71:788-795
12. Suter PM, Fairley HB, Isenberg MD (1978) Effect of tidal volume and positive end-expiratory pressure on compliance during mechanical ventilation. Chest 73:158-162
13. Gattinoni L, Mascheroni D, Basilico E et al (1987) Volume/pressure curve of total respiratory system in paralysed patients: artefacts and correction factors. Intensive Care Med 13:19-25
14. Dall'Ava-Santucci J, Armaganidis A, Brunet F et al (1988) Causes of error of respiratory pressure-volume curves in paralyzed subjects. J Appl Physiol 64:42-49
15. Gottfried SB, Rossi A, Higgs BD et al (1985) Noninvasive determination of respiratory system mechanics during mechanical ventilation for acute respiratory failure. Am Rev Respir Dis 131:414-420
16. Bates JH, Baconnier P, Milic-Emili J (1988) A theoretical analysis of interrupter technique for measuring respiratory mechanics. J Appl Physiol 64:2204-2214
17. Levy P, Similowski T, Corbeil C et al (1989) A method for studying the static volume-pressure curves of the respiratory system during mechanical ventilation. J Crit Care 4:83-89
18. Jonson B, Beydon L, Brauer K et al (1993) Mechanics of respiratory system in healthy anesthetized humans with emphasis on viscoelastic properties. J Appl Physiol 75:132-140
19. Beydon L, Svantesson C, Brauer K et al (1996) Respiratory mechanics in patients ventilated for critical lung disease. Eur Respir J 9:262-273
20. Svantesson C, Drefeldt B, Jonson B (1997) The static pressure-volume relationship of the respiratory system determined with a computer-controlled ventilator. Clin Physiol 17:419-430
21. Suratt PM, Owens D (1981) A pulse method of measuring respiratory system compliance in ventilated patients. Chest 80:34-38
22. Ranieri VM, Giuliani R, Fiore T et al (1994) Volume-pressure curve of the respiratory system predicts effects of PEEP in ARDS: "occlusion" versus "constant flow" technique. Am J Respir Crit Care Med 149:19-27
23. Servillo G, Svantesson C, Beydon L et al (1997) Pressure-volume curves in acute respiratory failure. Automated low flow inflation versus occlusion. Am J Respir Crit Care Med 155: 1629-1636

24. Venegas JG, Harris RS, Simon BA (1998) A comprehensive equation for the pulmonary pressure-volume curve. J Appl Physiol 84:389-395
25. Amato MB, Barbas CS, Medeiros DM et al (1995) Beneficial effects of the "open lung approach" with low distending pressures in acute respiratory distress syndrome. A prospective randomized study on mechanical ventilation. Am J Respir Crit Care Med 152:1835-1846
26. Amato MB, Barbas CS, Medeiros DM et al (1998) Effect of a protective-ventilation strategy on mortality in the acute respiratory distress syndrome. N Engl J Med 338:347-354

Pulmonary Gas Exchange in the Intensive Care Unit

R. Naeije

Acute respiratory failure is an acute insufficiency of the gas exchange function of the lungs. Respiratory failure is always associated with abnormal arterial blood gases, in the sense that the gradient between alveolar PO_2 (PAO_2) and arterial PO_2 (PaO_2) ($AaPO_2$) is increased, while $PaCO_2$ is increased, normal or decreased. Respiratory failure therefore is classically defined using arterial blood gases criteria, generally by a PaO_2 lower than 60 mmHg and a $PaCO_2$ higher than 50 mmHg. Accordingly, pulmonary gas exchange in patients admitted to the intensive care unit are evaluated with repetitive arterial blood gas analysis. However, PaO_2 and $PaCO_2$ are determined not only by the gas exchange function of the lungs, but also by extrapulmonary factors including inspired PO_2 (PIO_2) and mixed venous PO_2 (PvO_2) which in turn depends on cardiac output (Q), O_2 extraction, haemoglobin, and P_{50}. Also, the tolerance to abnormal PaO_2 and $PaCO_2$ is largely dependent on the patient's past history and current illness.

In the absence of a diffusion limitation to the alveolo-capillary transfer of O_2 and CO_2, the gas exchange function of the lungs is best described by a distribution of ventilation (VA)/Q relationships. The vast majority of acute respiratory insufficiencies seen in the intensive care unit are accounted for by abnormal distributions VA/Q. The most common causes of severe acute respiratory failure are decompensated chronic obstructive pulmonary disease (COPD) and the adult respiratory distress syndrome (ARDS) [1, 2].

Normal and abnormal VA/Q distributions

In the normal lung, as a consequence of the effects of gravity and of the mechanical properties of the respiratory system, both perfusion and ventilation increase progressively from non dependent to dependent regions, but at a different rate, so that from top to base of an erect lung, VA/Q varies about sixfold (from 3.3 to 0.6). In spite of this rather marked physiological VA/Q inhomogeneity, gas exchange of healthy lungs is very efficient, as indicated by a normally small $AaPO_2$ (less than 10 mmHg).

The distribution of VA/Q can be determined using the multiple inert gas elimination technique. A series of six inert gases (not bound to haemoglobin) dissolved in saline at trace concentrations is slowly infused in a peripheral vein, and after a steady state of elimination by the lung has been achieved, the concentrations are measured in mixed venous and arterial blood and expired gas by gas chromatography. Because the gases have different solubilities, they partition between blood and gas according to the VA/Q ratio of the lung unit. The multiple inert gas elimination technique is complicated, but its results are simple to present as amounts of VA and of Q (both in L/min) distributed to 50 lung compartments of a progressively increasing VA/Q from 0 (the shunt) to 100 (the dead space), passing through an ideal value of 1. A VA/Q distribution recovered in a normal young adult [3] is represented in Fig. 1.

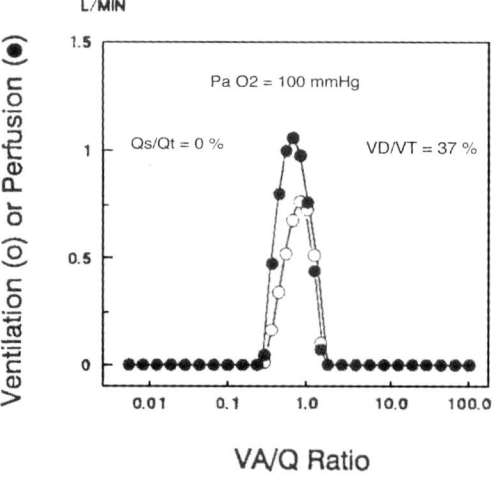

Fig. 1. Distributions of ventilation (VA) and perfusion (Q) as a function of VA/Q in a normal volunteer. Ventilation and perfusion are distributed to one mode centered on lung units with a VA/Q ratio around 1, but ranging from 0.5 to 3.5. (Modified from [3])

VA/Q distributions in COPD are markedly altered, with increased amounts of both ventilation and perfusion distributed to lung units with higher as well as lower than normal VA/Q. Shunt however remains most often normal or minimally increased in these patients. An examplative VA/Q distribution recovered in a patient with an advanced COPD [4] is shown in Fig. 2.

In asthma, VA/Q distributions most often present with a mode of increased perfusion to lung units with a lower than normal VA/Q, and no shunt. Absence of shunt in obstructive lung diseases in general is explained by the efficiency of collateral ventilation in the human species.

In ARDS, most of the severe hypoxaemia characteristic of this disease entity is explained by a shunt. An exemplative case [5] is shown in Fig. 3.

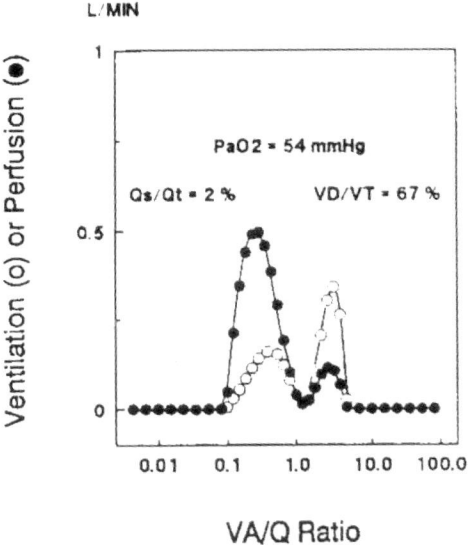

Fig. 2. Distributions of ventilation (VA) and perfusion (Q) as a function of VA/Q in a patient with chronic obstructive pulmonary disease. The distribution is bimodal, with a mode of VA and Q distributed to lung units with lower than normal VA/Q, and a mode of VA and Q distributed to lung units with a higher than normal VA/Q. (Modified from [4])

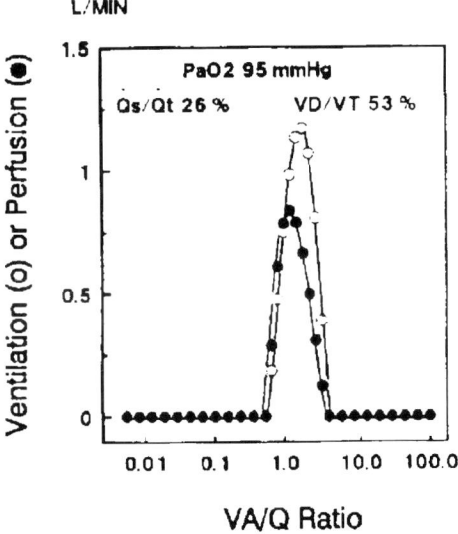

Fig. 3. Distributions of ventilation (VA) and perfusion (Q) as a function of VA/Q in a patient with acute respiratory distress syndrome. Ventilation and perfusion are distributed to a mode centered on lung units with a VA/Q around 1, but there is an additional mode of perfusion to lung units with a VA/Q = 0 (shunt, Q_S/Q_T). (Modified from [5])

Because the multiple inert gas elimination technique rests on the assumption that there is no diffusion limitation for the inert gases, the existence of a diffusion limitation for O_2 can be looked for by comparing measured PaO_2 to PaO_2 predicted from the recovered VA/Q distributions and the mathematical lung model of the method. No significant difference between measured and predicted PaO_2 has been found in studies of pulmonary gas exchange using the multiple inert gas elimination technique in patients with decompensated COPD or ARDS.

Patterns of abnormal arterial blood gases

Various types of respiratory failure are associated with different degrees of hypoxaemia and hypercapnia. Fig. 4 shows an O_2-CO_2 diagram with the line for a respiratory quotient of 0.8. Pure hypoventilation (example: narcotic overdose) moves PO_2 and PCO_2 in the direction indicated by arrow A. Severe VA/Q inequality (example: decompensated COPD) moves PO_2 and PCO_2 along a line such as B. In respiratory failure caused by ARDS, $PaCO_2$ is typically low but hypoxaemia is severe as indicated by arrow C. Oxygen therapy in decompensated COPD raises PaO_2 but also $PaCO_2$ (B to E), mainly because of depression of ventilation. Oxygen therapy in ARDS is associated with little improvement in PaO_2, and does not affect $PaCO_2$ (C to D).

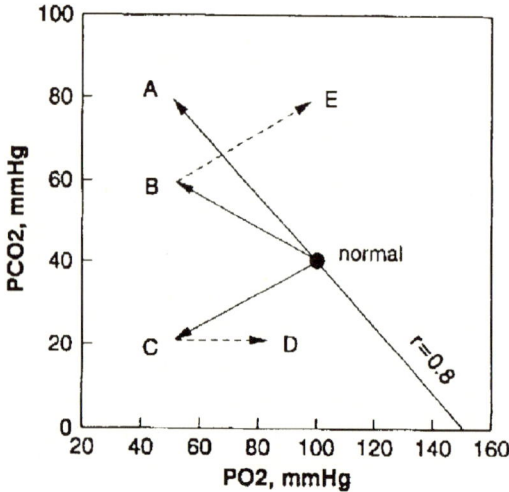

Fig. 4. Patterns of abnormal arterial blood gases. (Modified from [2])

Hypoxaemia in respiratory failure

Four primary pulmonary causes of hypoxaemia are classically recognized:

1. Hypoventilation
2. Diffusion impairment
3. Shunt
4. VA/Q inequality

A fifth cause, reduction of inspired PO_2, such as at high altitude or during breathing of a low O_2 concentration, is seen only in special circumstances.

Hypoventilation

Hypoventilation most often results from extrapulmonary problems. It always causes an increase in $PaCO_2$. There is indeed an inverse relationship between alveolar PCO_2 and ventilation, as can be seen from the alveolar ventilation equation:

$$PACO_2 = VCO_2 \times K/VA$$

where VCO_2 is CO_2 output and K a constant. Thus if VA is halved, $PACO_2$ is doubled. No patient can hypoventilate without hypercapnia.

On the other hand, hypercapnia is necessarily associated with hypoxaemia, as recalled by the alveolar gas equation:

$$PAO_2 = FIO_2 \times (Patm - 47) - PACO_2/R$$

where FIO_2 is the fraction of inspired O_2, 47 the partial pressure of water at 37°C and R the respiratory quotient. Thus if R and $PACO_2$ remain constant, every mmHg rise in PIO_2 will produce a corresponding rise in PAO_2. Hypoxaemia of hypoventilation can be easily corrected with supplemental oxygen.

However, hypoventilation-induced hypoxaemia cannot be severe. For example a doubling of normal $PaCO_2$ to 80 mmHg would reduce PaO_2 to 60 mmHg (the $AaPO_2$ gradient is supposed to remain normal) which, in view of the shape of the oxyhaemoglobin dissociation curve, leads to a decrease in O_2 saturation to 90%.

Causes of hypoventilation are: 1) depression of the respiratory center by drugs (opiates), 2) diseases of the medulla (encephalitis), 3) a spinal injury (high cervical dislocation), 4) anterior horn diseases (poliomyelitis), 5) diseases of the nerves to the respiratory muscles (Guillain-Barré syndrome), 6) diseases of the myoneuronal junction (myasthenia gravis), 7) diseases of the respiratory muscles (progressive muscular dystrophy), 8) thoracic cage abnormalities (crushed chest or extreme obesity) and 9) upper airway obstruction (tracheal stenosis).

Diffusion impairment

A diffusion impairment means that equilibrium does not occur between the PO_2 in the alveolar gas and in the pulmonary capillaries. Normally, under resting conditions, the capillary blood PO_2 almost reaches that of the alveolar gas in about one third of the total contact time of 3/4 sec available in the capillary. There is thus plenty of time in reserve. In fact, recent studies have shown that a diffusion impairment does not account for arterial hypoxaemia at rest even in advanced forms of interstitial lung diseases. Gas exchange in these patients is essentially altered because of an increased perfusion to lung areas with a lower than normal VA/Q. At exercise, however, erythrocyte transit time is reduced along with increased pulmonary blood flow, and a diffusion impairment then may contribute to a substantial part of abnormally increased $AaPO_2$. On the other hand, high altitude decreases the pressure gradient for alveolo-capillary O_2 diffusion, and exercise hypoxaemia develops even in normal subjects mainly because of a diffusion impairment. Exercise and altitude are uncommon features in the intensive care setting, where thus a diffusion impairment can be neglected as possible cause for hypoxaemia.

A common misconception is that hypoxaemia due to a diffusion limitation for O_2 can be measured by the alveolo-capillary transfer of carbon monoxide (DL_{CO}). Carbon monoxide is used to measure the diffusing capacity of the lungs because, when inhaled in low concentration, PCO in the capillaries remains extremely low in relation to its alveolar value. This is due to the very high affinity of CO for haemoglobin, which is about 210 times that of O_2. As a result, in contrast to O_2, there is no perfusion limitation for the alveolo-capillary transfer of CO. Thus the uptake of CO is determined by the diffusion properties of the blood-gas barrier and by the rate of combination of CO with the blood. The diffusion properties of the alveolo-capillary membrane depend on its thickness and area, and therefore DL_{CO} is reduced in interstitial lung diseases, emphysema, and pneumonectomy. The rate of combination of CO with blood is reduced whenever the number of red cells in the capillaries is reduced, and therefore DL_{CO} is decreased in anaemia and in pulmonary embolism. In addition, DL_{CO} is affected by unevenness of distribution of ventilation and perfusion.

Shunt

Shunt means that venous blood reaches the arterial system without passing through ventilated lung areas. The most common shunts are seen in congenital cardiac diseases. Intrapulmonary shunts can be caused by an arterio-venous fistula or (more frequently) by still perfused but completely unventilated lung areas, as seen in ARDS or in cardiogenic pulmonary oedema.

Characteristic of an intrapulmonary shunt is that the hypoxaemia it causes cannot be corrected by supplemental oxygen. This is explained by the shape of the oxyhaemoglobin dissociation curve, as illustrated in Fig. 5.

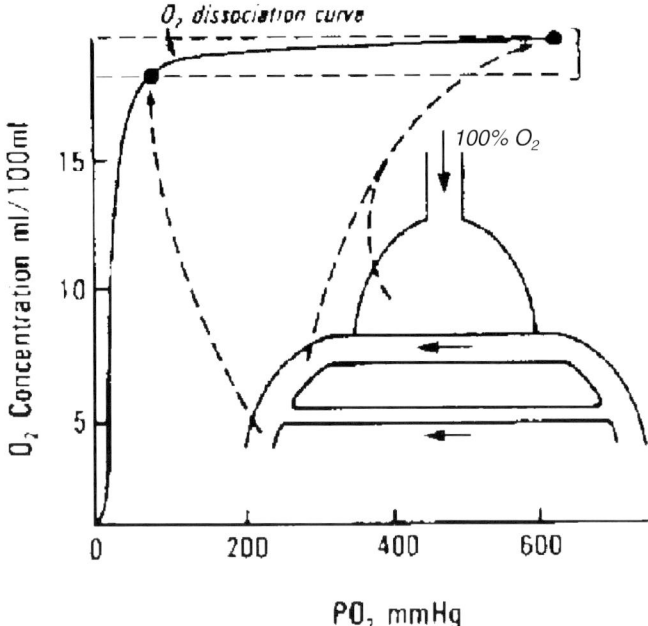

Fig. 5. Oxyhaemoglobin dissociation curve in a patient with a shunt and ventilated with pure oxygen. A small decrease in arterial O_2 content is associated with an important decrease in arterial PO_2. (Modified from [1])

Atelectatic lung areas frequently develop in critically ill patients. Associated shunts, even very small and therefore undetected by a chest X-ray, may be responsible for significant decreases in PaO_2 when the patient is ventilated with or breathes high O_2 concentrations. Small decreases in shunt as seen for example in patients with ARDS treated with inhaled nitric oxide (NO) may for the same reason be associated with sometimes spectacular increases in PaO_2.

The magnitude of a shunt during pure O_2 breathing can be determined from the shunt equation:

$$Qs/Qt = (Cc' - Ca) / (Cc' - Cv)$$

where Qt is pulmonary blood flow, Qs is shunt flow, and Cc', Ca and Cv refer to the O_2 contents of capillary, arterial and mixed venous blood. In this equation, $Cc'O_2$ is calculated from PAO_2 (alveolar gas equation) assuming complete equilibration between alveolar gas and capillary blood.

Shunt does not usually lead to hypercapnia. Shunted CO_2 stimulates the peripheral chemoreceptors which, together with the stimulating effect of hypoxaemia, accounts for the hypocapnia usually seen in these patients. That increased ventilation corrects hypercapnia but not hypoxaemia is explained by the respective shapes of the O_2 and of the CO_2 dissociation curves.

VA/Q inequality

This mechanism of hypoxaemia is ubiquitous. It is typically seen in COPD and in severe asthma, but also accounts for most of the hypoxaemia associated with interstitial lung diseases and pulmonary vascular diseases, including pulmonary embolism.

Characteristic of hypoxaemia caused by an increased perfusion to lung areas with a low VA/Q is that it is easily corrected with small or moderate increases in FIO_2. This observation together with the known hypercapnic effects of O_2 inhalation in decompensated COPD explains why "controlled low-flow O_2" (FIO_2 0.24 to 0.30) is a recommended treatment for such patients.

The severity of VA/Q inequality is evaluated by arterial blood gases determinations. PaO_2 is a good guide, but is best completed by the calculation of the $AaPO_2$ gradient to correct for increased FIO_2 and for the level of PCO_2. If mixed venous blood gases are available (pulmonary artery catheter), a physiologic shunt or venous admixture can be calculated. This is the amount of mixed venous blood which would have to be mixed with "ideal" blood to give the observed PaO_2. Venous admixture is estimated using the shunt equation, with measurements preferably done at a FIO_2 of 0.21.

To evaluate the extent of higher than normal VA/Q, physiological dead space is calculated as:

$$VD/VTphys = (PACO_2 - PECO_2)/PACO_2$$

where $PECO_2$ is mixed expired CO_2.

Effects of mixed venous PO_2 on arterial PO_2

Extrapulmonary haemodynamic events can affect PaO_2 through associated changes in PvO_2. Mixed venous blood oxygenation is dependent on arterial blood oxygenation and on the ratio between O_2 delivery to the tissues (TO_2) and O_2 uptake ($\dot{V}O_2$), as shown by the following arrangement of the Fick equation:

$$CvO_2 = CaO_2 \times (1 - \dot{V}O_2/TO_2)$$

where CvO_2 is mixed venous O_2 content and CaO_2 arterial O_2 content.

Mixed venous PO_2 changes are transmitted to PaO_2 when VA/Q is normal or decreased, as illustrated in Fig. 6. Arterial PO_2 is less sensitive to PvO_2 when VA/Q is increased above normal. Thus profound hypoxaemia, due for example to a shunt and refractory to continuous positive pressure ventilation with high

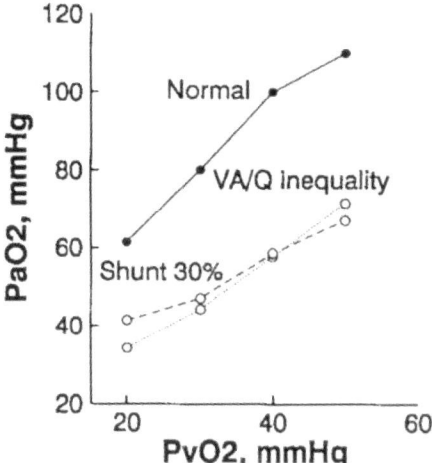

Fig. 6. Effects of mixed venous PO_2 on arterial PO_2. At normal or low ventilation/perfusion ratio (VA/Q), mixed venous PO_2 is transmitted to arterial PO_2 in a close to one-to-one ratio. (Modified from [2])

FIO_2, may be improved by therapeutic interventions aimed at an increase in TO_2 by means of increased cardiac output and/or haematocrit. However, increased cardiac output and associated improved mixed venous oxygenation may also result in a further deterioration in VA/Q matching, probably by an inhibition of hypoxic pulmonary vasoconstriction.

What is required and what is possible for the evaluation of lung function in intensive care

Most problems of abnormal pulmonary gas exchange in the intensive care unit can be resolved with an analysis of expired and blood gases, confronted to sound pathophysiological reasoning. Changes in low VA/Q areas are adequately explored by arterial and mixed venous blood gases. Changes in high VA/Q areas require in addition the measurement of expired PCO_2. Dyspneic patients with advanced emphysema or pulmonary embolism may present with near normal arterial blood gases but with a markedly increased ventilation to lung units with higher than normal VA/Q. Along the same line, ventilated patients with pulmonary embolism, with an excessive PEEP or auto-PEEP, may become hypercapnic because of increased wasted ventilation and inability to increase alveolar ventilation (due for example to a controlled ventilation setting in a deeply sedated or paralyzed patient, or inability to increase VA because of excessive muscle fatigue and/or very high airway resistance).

Any single combination of expired and blood gases is the resultant of a complex interplay between a series of pulmonary and extrapulmonary determinants. These can be qualitatively unravelled by a thorough and careful clinical evaluation, completed with haemodynamic and lung mechanic determinations. For investigational purposes, a quantification of all the pulmonary and extrapulmonary factors of arterial and expired PO_2 and PCO_2 can be done with the multiple inert gas elimination technique.

At present, repeated measurements of blood gases and continuous monitoring of expired PCO_2 and mixed venous O_2 saturation are easily available in most intensive care units. Continuous monitoring of expired PCO_2 and mixed venous O_2 saturation are useful essentially for the automated detection of acute haemodynamic or ventilatory accidents, such as a cardiac arrest or an acutely obstructed tracheal tube. Because of the complex interplay of determinants of the composition of blood gases, it is unlikely that the continuous monitoring of PaO_2, $PaCO_2$, PvO_2, and $PvCO_2$ would contribute to improved or faster diagnosis of altered pulmonary gas exchange. The same can be said about on line diffusion measurements by alveolo-capillary transfer of CO. It would not be difficult by the way to measure a DL_{NO} instead of a DL_{CO} in patients treated with inhaled NO and monitored with fast responder measurement devices. Nitric oxide is indeed at least as diffusible and avid for haemoglobin as CO, but, of course, a DL_{NO} would not be more specific for the diffusing properties of the alveolo-capillary membrane than a DL_{CO}, and would not make diffusion limitation a more frequent cause of hypoxaemia.

It could be theoretically possible to apply the multiple inert gas elimination method using on line or quasi on line mass spectrometry, but there is little perspective of clinical benefit being worth the efforts and expenses.

References

1. JB West (1991) Pulmonary physiology: The essentials. Williams and Wilkins, Baltimore
2. JB West (1985) Pulmonary pathophysiology: The essentials. Williams and Wilkins Baltimore
3. Mélot C, Naeije R, Hallemans R et al (1987) Hypoxic pulmonary vasoconstriction and pulmonary gas exchange in normal man. Respir Physiol 68:11-27
4. Mélot C, Hallemans R, Mols P et al (1984) Deleterious effects of nifedipine on pulmonary gas exchange in chronic obstructive pulmonary disease. Am Rev Respir Dis 130:612-616
5. Mélot C, Lejeune P, Leeman M et al (1989) Prostaglandin E$_1$ in the adult respiratory distress syndrome: benefit for pulmonary hypertension and cost for pulmonary gas exchange. Am Rev Respir Dis 139:106-110

Pulmonary Haemodynamics in the Intensive Care Unit

R. NAEIJE

Steady-flow haemodynamics

Pulmonary vascular pressure measurements throughout the world are made with the Swan-Ganz catheter, which was introduced in 1970 [1]. This catheter is balloon-tipped, which allows placement in the pulmonary artery without fluoroscopic control and measurement successively of right atrial pressure (Pra), right ventricular pressure (Prv), pulmonary artery pressure (Ppa) and occluded Ppa (Ppao). It has two fluid-filled lumens, one for measurement of Ppa and Ppao, and one for the measurement of Pra and injection of saline into the right atrium for the measurement of pulmonary blood flow (Q) by thermodilution. It has a thermistor at the tip for measurement of blood temperature in the pulmonary artery.

It has long been known that fluid-filled catheters lack precision and accuracy for the measurement of instantaneous pressures, because of inadequate frequency response, motion artifacts, errors on zero leveling, and altered signal quality due to debubbling and regular flushing. However, it is generally assumed that fluid-filled catheters provide reliable estimates of mean vascular pressures. On the other hand, a thermodilution pulmonary blood flow necessarily covers several cardiac cycles. Thus, the very use of the Swan Ganz catheter imposes a simplification, which is that the natural pulsatility of the pulmonary circulation is ignored.

In steady-flow haemodynamics, resistance (R) can be calculated as a pressure drop from some upstream point (inflow pressure, Pin) to a downstream point (outflow pressure, Pout) divided by the flow. In smooth walled, thin, nondistensible tubes, with a laminar flow of a Newtonian fluid, Poiseuille's law states that

$$R = (Pin - Pout)/Q = 8.l.\eta/\pi.r^4$$

where l is the length of the tube, η a coefficient of viscosity, and r the radius of the tube. Since the latter is at the fourth power, Pin at a given Q is exquisitively sensitive to small changes in the caliber radius of the tube.

When this approach is transposed to the pulmonary circulation, Pin becomes Ppa, Pout becomes Pla, and the flow becomes Q:

$$PVR = (Ppa - Pla)/Q$$

PVR is sensitive to the flow resistive properties of the pulmonary resistance vessels, which are mainly small arterioles of a diameter approximately between 100 and 250 μm diameter, thus at the periphery of the pulmonary arterial tree. The evaluation of the functional state of the pulmonary resistive vessels is improved when pulmonary vascular pressures are measured at several levels of flow, to generate a multipoint (Ppa-Pla)/Q curve [2]. A passive reference multipoint Ppa/Q curve or (Ppa-Pla)/Q curve can be obtained in clinical practice by an infusion of dobutamine, at doses up to 10 μg/kg/min which probably have no intrinsic effect on pulmonary vascular tone [3].

Left atrial pressure is estimated by Ppao measured downstream to the inflated small balloon at the tip of the pulmonary artery catheter. In most clinical circumstances Ppao gives a valuable estimate of Pla, provided the catheter tip is properly wedged below the level of the left atrium. The pressure measured with the pulmonary artery catheter wedged in a peripheral branch of the pulmonary arterial tree (Ppw) may be higher than Ppao when pulmonary venous resistance is increased [4]. In that circumstance, Ppw overestimates Pla. Pulmonary artery occlusion pressure sometimes is mistaken for pulmonary capillary pressure (Pc). By reference to a pulmonary circulation model consisting in two resistances (arterial and venous) connected by a compliance (capillary), Pc can be estimated by the measurement of the intersection point of the successively rapid and slow pressure decay curves recorded after a rapid occlusion of the pulmonary artery [5].

A typical pulmonary artery occlusion recording to estimate Pc by the extrapolation to 150 ms after the instant of occlusion of a single exponential fitting of the Ppa decay curve with adjustment for Ppao as obtained using an original software designed in our laboratory [6] is shown in Fig. 1. Although this has not been directly investigated, it is likely that determinations of Pc would be improved by the use of a high fidelity micromanometer-tipped Swan Ganz catheter. Such a technical improvement would allow a better detection of the exact instant of occlusion, because of less motion artifacts, and a better definition of the fast initial rapid portion of the Ppa decay curve.

An example of mean Ppa measurements at several levels of mean Q for the definition of the functional state of the resistive pulmonary vessels is presented in Fig. 2, which represents pooled mean Ppa versus Q relationships with Q increased by exercise (full circles) or dobutamine (empty circles) respectively in 11 patients with primary pulmonary hypertension [7]. The calculated regressions are represented by the lines. By reference to the Starling resistor model of the pulmonary circulation [2], the extrapolated pressure intercept of the dobutamine-induced Ppa/Q relationships represents the averaged closing pressure of

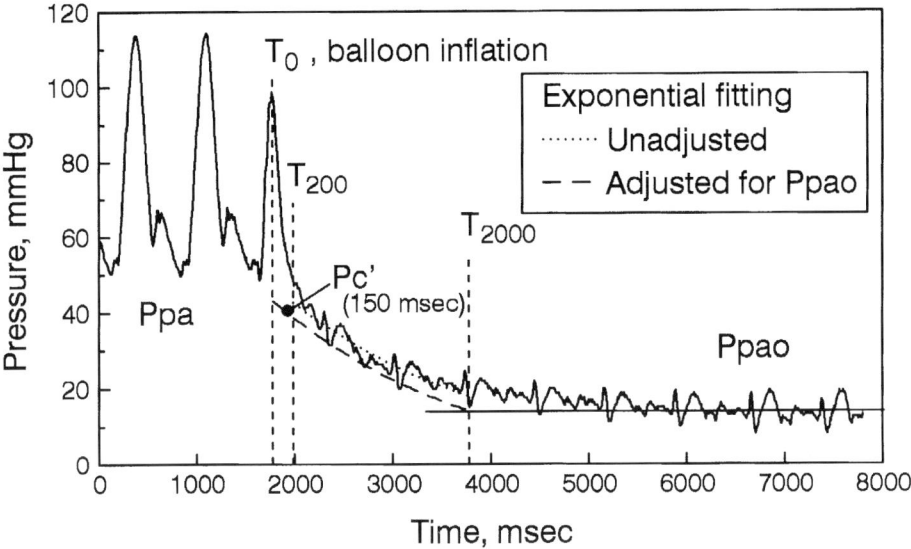

Fig. 1. Estimation of effective pulmonary capillary pressure by the occlusion method in experimental pulmonary hypertension. Modified from [6]

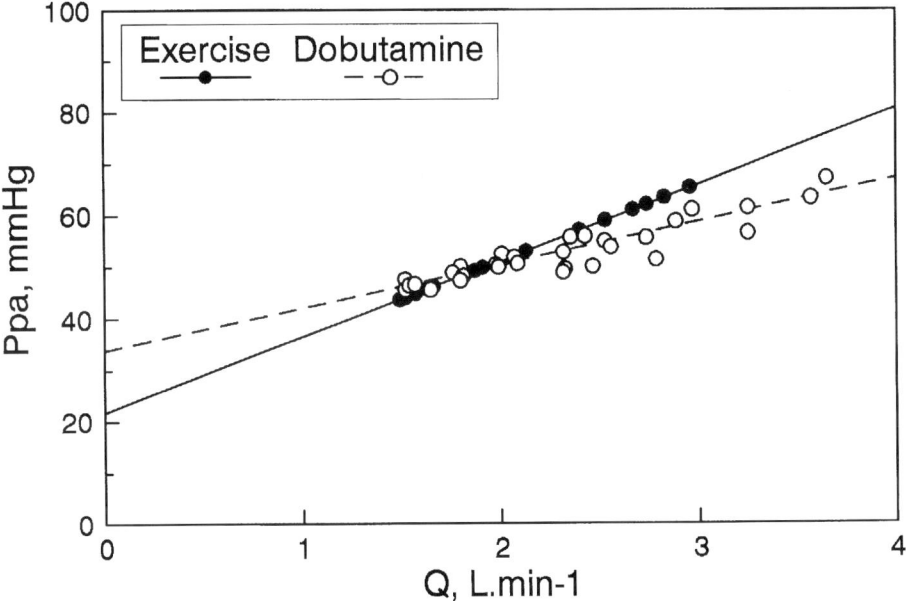

Fig. 2. Pulmonary artery pressure/flow relationships in patients with primary pulmonary hypertension. Modified from [7]

the smallest pulmonary arterioles, and the slope of the dobutamine-induced Ppa/Q plots the incremental upstream arterial resistance. It can be seen that small errors on mean Ppa and mean Q could result in marked changes in estimated closing pressures and incremental resistances.

Since wedging or balloon inflation stop the flow downstream to the Swan Ganz catheter tip, the insufficient frequency response of this fluid-filled catheter poses no problem for measurements of Ppao or Ppw. Estimates of mean Q by thermodilution have been shown to agree very well with mean Q measured by the reference Fick method. Estimates of mean Ppa are probably reasonably accurate and precise, but have to our knowledge not directly been compared to mean Ppa measured by high fidelity micromanometer-tipped catheters in intact animals or in patients. It would be interesting to compare estimates of Pc measured by the arterial occlusion method using high fidelity micromanometer-tipped and fluid-filled Swan Ganz catheters.

Pulsatile flow pulmonary haemodynamics

The first measurement of pulmonary artery and right ventricular pressures was reported by Cournand and coworkers in 1945 [8]. The patient had severe pulmonary hypertension from rheumatic heart disease. As shown in Fig. 3, the right ventricular pressure contour showed a sharp initial upstroke, followed by a short plateau, and a late systolic rise, and the Ppa contour showed a wide pulse pressure and late systolic peaking.

The nowadays easily available echo-Doppler examination of the pulmonary circulation of such a patient would show a pulmonary flow-velocity curve with shortened acceleration time and late or mid-systolic deceleration [2].

The classical reference experiment to explain these pressure and flow wave characteristics and associated consequences for RV function was published in 1980 by Elzinga and coworkers [9], and is illustrated in Fig. 4. These authors connected an isolated cat heart to an artificial pulmonary circulation in which resistance and compliance could be varied independently, and measured Prv, Ppa and Q. An isolated increase in PVR (4 times normal) increased Prv and mean Ppa, and decreased Q. PVR decreased, but there was a small pulse pressure which is not normally seen in severe pulmonary hypertension. A decrease in compliance (1/16 times normal) also increased Prv and decreased Q, but mean Ppa did not increase very much. A combination of increased PVR and decreased compliance typically produced increased Prv, with late systolic peaking, and widened Ppa pulse pressure, and a major decrease in Q.

In a more intact animal model may be more relevant to real critical care clinical situations, Furuno et al. [10] compared the effects of proximal pulmonary artery constriction (corresponding to acute severe pulmonary embolism) and distal pulmonary artery obstruction, by injection of 100 μm beads (corresponding to acute respiratory distress syndrome). Both interventions were titrated

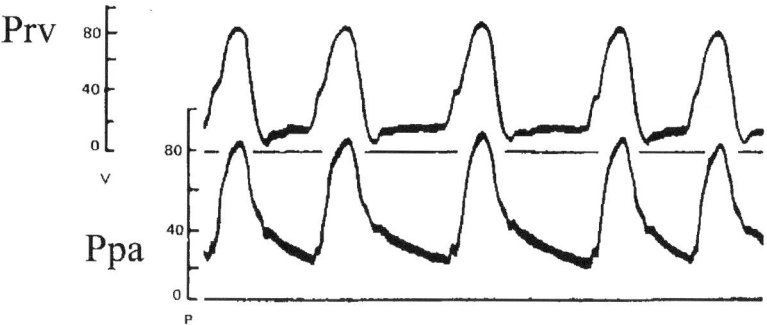

Fig. 3. Pulmonary artery pressure and right ventricular pressure in a patient with pulmonary hypertension secondary to advanced mitral valve disease. Modified from [8]

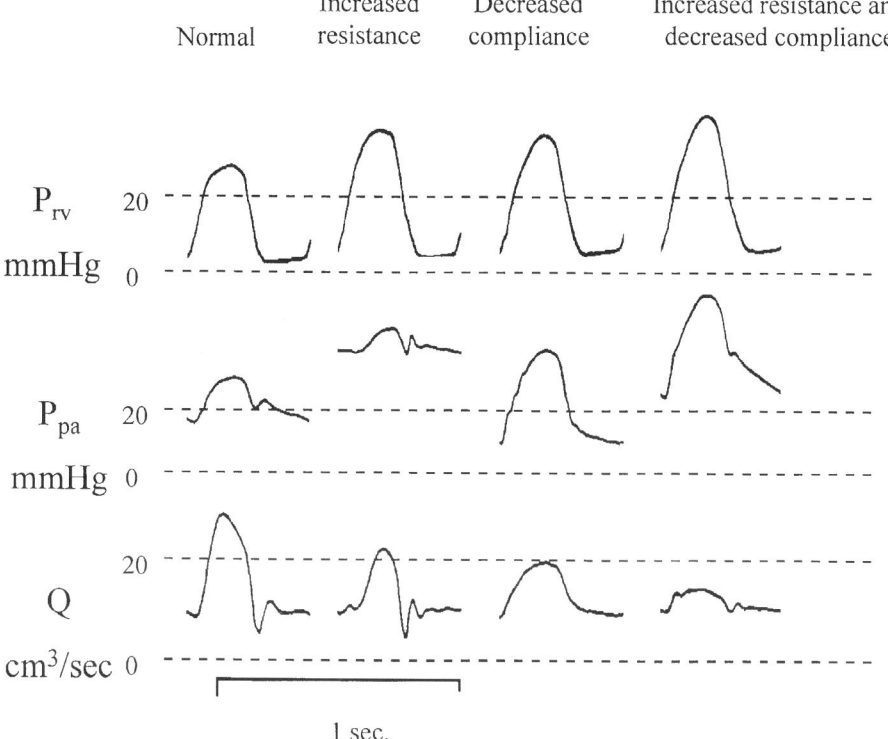

Fig. 4. Effects of resistance and compliance respectively on right ventricular pressure, pulmonary artery pressure, and right ventricular output. Modified from [9]

such as to obtain the same mean Ppa. Flow was maintained constant. Proximal obstruction reproduced typical patterns of increased pulse pressure and late or mid-systolic deceleration of flow, while distal obstruction did not increase pulse pressure and did not produce late systolic flow deceleration. The authors decomposed pressure and flow waves into forward and backward components, and showed very elegantly that the late systolic peaking of pressure and deceleration of flow was mainly due to earlier return of reflected waves. A representative experiment is illustrated in Fig. 5.

In a very recent report, Nakayama and coworkers from Dr Sunagawa's laboratory used pulmonary pressure wave form analysis for the differential diagnosis between thromboembolic and primary pulmonary hypertension (thus proximal versus distal obstruction respectively) [11]. These authors showed that pulse pressure normalized by mean pressure was higher in thromboembolic pulmonary hypertension compared to primary pulmonary hypertension, and was diagnostic in separating the two groups without overlap. Although the authors used the classical fluid-filled Swan Ganz catheter, they recognize that their study should be repeated using high fidelity micromanometer-tipped Swan Ganz catheters.

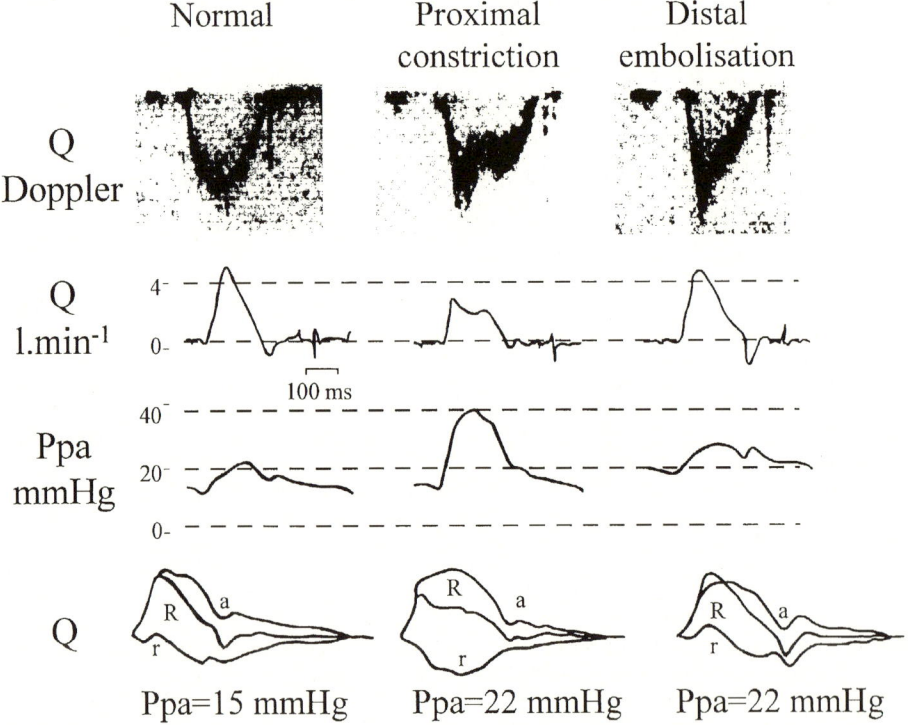

Fig. 5. Effects of proximal versus distal obstruction of pulmonary artery pressure and flow waves. Modified from [10]

Thus resistance is only a part of right ventricular afterload, which is also largely determined by elastance and wave reflection. At least a qualitative idea of the importance of these two determinants can be derived from analysis of pressure and flow wave morphology. A quantification of the respective contributions of resistance, elastance and wave reflection to right ventricular afterload can be obtained by impedance calculations from spectral analysis of pressure and flow waves. In a preliminary study using Ppa measured high fidelity micromanometer-tipped Swan Ganz catheters (manufactured by Ohmeda) and pulmonary artery blood flow velocity evaluated by echo-Doppler, we have been able to show that characteristic impedance (the ratio between proximal pulmonary arterial inertance and compliance) is at least as useful as PVR to predict right ventricular tolerance to moderate pulmonary hypertension in patients with a cardiac transplantation.

High fidelity micromanometer-tipped catheters are becoming increasingly available at a reasonable cost. Surprisingly, no balloon-tipped versions of such catheters have been commercialized until now, and thus their insertion into the pulmonary artery requires special skill and fluoroscopic control. Recent developments have made instantaneous pulmonary blood flow measurements possible by echo-Doppler methods. Instantaneous flow measurement devices incorporated in pulmonary artery catheters are not yet commercially available. Technically, however, pulmonary artery catheters for instantaneous P and Q measurements are feasible and could replace fluid-filled thermodilution catheters soon.

References

1. Swan HJC, Ganz W, Forrester JS et al (1970) Catheterization of the heart in man with use of a flow-directed catheter. N Engl J Med 283:447-451
2. Naeije R (1996) Pulmonary vascular function. In: AJ Peacock (ed) Pulmonary Circulation: A Handbook for Clinicians. Chapman & Hall Medical 2:13-27
3. Naeije R, Lipski A, Abramowicz M et al (1994) Nature of pulmonary hypertension in congestive heart failure. Effects of cardiac transplantation. Am J Respir Crit Care Med 147:881-887
4. Zidulka A, Hakim TS (1985) Wedge pressure in large vs small pulmonary arteries to detect pulmonary venoconstriction. J Appl Physiol 59:1329-1332
5. Cope DK, Grimbert F, Downey JM, Taylor AE (1992) Pulmonary capillary pressure: a review. Crit Care Med 20:1043-1055
6. Mélot C, Vermeulen F, Maggiorini M et al (1997) Site of pulmonary vasodilation by inhaled nitric oxide in microembolic lung injury. Am J Respir Crit Care Med 156:75-85
7. Abdel Kafi S, Mélot C, Vachiéry JL et al (1998) Partitioning of pulmonary vascular resistance in primary pulmonary hypertension. J Am Coll Cardiol 31:1372-1376
8. Cournand A, Bloomfield RA, Lanson HD (1945) Double lumen catheter for intravenous and intracardiac blood sampling and pressure recording. Proc Soc Exp Biol Med 60:73-75
9. Elzinga G, Piene H, de Jong JP (1980) Left and right ventricular pump function and consequences of having two pumps in one heart. Circ Res 46:564-574
10. Furuno Y, Nagamoto Y, Fujita M et al (1991) Reflection as a cause of mid-systolic deceleration of pulmonary flow wave in dogs with acute pulmonary hypertension: comparison of pulmonary artery constriction with pulmonary embolisation. Cardiovasc Res 25:118-124
11. Nakayama Y, Nakanishi N, Sugimachi M et al (1997) Characteristics of pulmonary artery pressure waveform for differential diagnosis of chronic pulmonary thromboembolism and primary pulmonary hypertension. J Am Coll Cardiol 29:1311-1316

PET and Other Nuclear Medicine Techniques

P. WOLLMER

In nuclear medicine, radiolabelled pharmaceuticals are used to study organ and tissue function. There is a large range of nuclear medicine procedures reflecting vital functions, and these techniques are, in principle, well suited for examination of critically ill patients. There are, however, also constraints to the use of nuclear medicine procedures in intensive care. These are due mainly to the use of bulky equipment, the rather long time often required for examinations and the limited repeatability of the tests.

Technical aspects

In conventional nuclear medicine, radiopharmaceuticals are labelled with isotopes emitting single photons. These can be detected with single detector probes over the organ, which record the turnover of the pharmaceutical in the underlying tissue. No information about the distribution of the radiopharmaceutical nor of the function studied is obtained. Detector probes can be made sufficiently small to be used without problems in intensive care units.

The most common equipment in nuclear medicine is the gamma camera. This consists of a large detector which is placed over a part over the body. An image of the distribution of radioactivity is obtained. Dynamic studies of the turnover of the radiopharmaceutical can be made by repeated imaging. A gamma camera is bulky, and for high quality examinations, the patient generally has to be taken out of the intensive care unit. Mobile gamma cameras are available for use bed-side. Several manufacturers work with new detector materials, and there is a possibility that mobile gamma cameras with considerably smaller and lighter detectors will become available in a few years.

With positron emission tomography (PET), radiopharmaceuticals are labelled with positron emitting isotopes. Their decay results in emission of two photons in opposite directions, which are detected by a pair of detectors placed on both sides of the body. There are two unique features of PET. Firstly the use of isotopes of carbon, nitrogen, oxygen and fluorine (used as a hydrogen analogue), virtually any substance can be labelled with no or minimal effect on its biochemical properties. Secondly, PET enables tissue concentration of a labelled substance to be measured quantitatively. Thereby, biological processes such as blood flow, glucose metabolism etc. can be measured quantitatively. In addition, receptor density in various organs can be measured and pharmacokinetics of labelled drugs can be studied at the tissue level.

PET is technically demanding. The short-lived isotopes are produced with a cyclotron, and only fluorine-18 may be transported to any extent. The detector system is bulky, and mobile equipment will not be available in the foreseeable future.

Applications

There are many well established nuclear medicine procedures used in intensive care. These have been recently reviewed by Davis and Fink-Bennett [1, 2]. The rest of this paper will focus on nuclear medicine examinations of the lungs.

Ventilation/perfusion scintigraphy

One of the earliest applications of nuclear medicine to critically ill patients was lung perfusion scintigraphy for the diagnosis of pulmonary embolism. Perfusion scintigraphy is still performed in basically the same way and is now frequently combined with ventilation scintigraphy. This is often performed by inhalation of radiolabelled aerosol, a technique readily applicable to patients on mechanical ventilation. In addition to diagnosis of pulmonary embolism, lung scintigraphy may provide valuable information about airway patency, presence of right-to-left shunts, etc. [3].

Lung water and solute exchange

Nuclear medicine techniques have been used extensively for measurements of lung water. Much of the basic work on indicator dilution techniques was performed using radiolabelled, diffusible and non-diffusible indicators. Non-invasive methods for measurement of regional lung water using radiolabelled indicators and external counting have also been developed. Insight into earlier events in the pathogenesis of high permeability pulmonary oedema is provided by measurement of the leakage of radiolabelled proteins in the pulmonary circulation [4]. This technique entails labelling of a plasma protein (transferrin) and red blood cells with different isotopes. Measurements can be made with probe detectors at bedside.

PET has also been applied to critical lung disease. Techniques have been developed for measurement of regional pulmonary oedema and blood volume. These have been based on measurement of the density of the lung and regional blood volume (labelled red cells) [5, 6] or on the use of radiolabelled water [7]. The technique for measurement of protein leakage in the pulmonary circulation has also been refined using PET. With this technique, very accurate measurements of regional protein leakage can be performed. A clear difference can be demonstrated between hydrostatic and high permeability pulmonary oedema [8]. High leakage is also observed in patients with active pneumonia and active interstitial disease.

Another approach to studies of the integrity of the alveolo-capillary barrier in the lung has been to deliver a tracer – most commonly the small, hydrophilic molecule 99mTc-DTPA – to the alveolus in aerosol form and measure its diffusion into the blood. This is done by simply recording a retention curve over the lungs with a probe detector or a gamma camera and calculating the half-life of the tracer in the lungs. While it was initially assumed that the clearance of the tracer from the lung reflected the properties of the alveolar epithelium [9], it is now clear that the integrity of the surfactant system also affects the clearance [10]. The technique is very sensitive to any derangement of the alveolo-capillary barrier; abnormal clearance is observed not only in lung injury, but also in patients with interstitial lung disease and in normal smokers. The effect of smoking seems to be largely through impaired surfactant function [11]. Clearance of solutes from the lung is also profoundly affected by lung volume [12]. The inability to differentiate between the effects of smoking on the alveolo-capillary barrier and severe lung injury hampers, of course, the use of the technique in clinical practise. Recent studies have shown that the clearance of a larger tracer molecule, albumin, is qualitatively affected in the same way as the clearance of 99mTc-DTPA by smoking, but to a smaller extent [13]. Experimental work has shown that derangement of the surfactant system has considerably smaller effect on the clearance of albumin than is seen in experimental models of lung injury [14]. The use of larger tracer molecules may therefore improve the specificity of studies of the integrity of the alveolo-capillary barrier.

Inflammation of the lung

A new interesting approach to studies of inflammatory conditions in the lung has been developed with PET. The technique is based on measurement of the glucose consumption in the lungs using deoxyglucose labelled with 18F (18FDG). Normal lung tissue has very low glucose consumption. Leukocytes, on the other hand, have very high glucose metabolism, and the uptake of 18FDG in the lung can in many instances be taken to represent the metabolic activity of leukocytes. The technique has been applied to patients with interstitial lung disease [15], bronchiectasis and pneumonia [16]. Of more interest in intensive care are preliminary results obtained in experimental models of abdominal sepsis, showing that increased glucose consumption in the lungs due to infiltrating leukocytes can be demonstrated well before there is any substantial effect on lung function. Measurement of glucose consumption may therefore provide new insight into the development of septic lung injury.

Conclusions

Nuclear medicine contributes greatly to diagnosis and evaluation of seriously ill patients. As for any other diagnostic modality relying on the use of bulky equipment, the full range of nuclear medicine procedures will be difficult to apply in patients under intensive care. While, therefore, the use of nuclear medicine procedures in clinical routine practise may be somewhat limited, nuclear medicine techniques applied in experimental or clinical research will continue to make major contributions to our understanding of pathophysiologic mechanisms in critically ill patients.

References

1. Davis LP, Fink-Bennett D (1994) Nuclear medicine in the acutely ill patient - I. Crit Care Clin 10:365-381
2. Davis LP, Fink-Bennett D (1994) Nuclear medicine in the acutely ill patient - II. Crit Care Clin 10:383-400
3. Juni JE, Alavi A (1991) Lung scanning in the diagnosis of pulmonary embolism: the emperor redressed. Semin Nucl Med 21:281-296
4. Gorin AB, Kohler J, DeNardo G (1980) Noninvasive measurement of pulmonary transvascular protein flux in normal man. J Clin Invest 66:869-877
5. Rhodes CG, Wollmer P, Fazio F et al (1981) Quantitative measurement of regional extravascular lung density using positron emission and transmission tomography. J Comput Assist Tomogr 5:783-791
6. Wollmer P, Rhodes CG, Deanfield J et al (1987) Regional extravascular density of the lung in patients with acute pulmonary edema. J Appl Physiol 63:1890-1895
7. Schuster DP, Marklin GF, Mintun MA (1986) Regional changes in extravascular lung water detected by positron emission tomography. J Appl Physiol 60:1170-1178
8. Kaplan JD, Calandrino FS, Schuster DP (1991) A positron emission tomographic comparison of pulmonary vascular permeability during the adult respiratory distress syndrome and pneumonia. Am Rev Respir Dis 143:150-154
9. Jones JG, Minty BD, Lawler P et al (1980) Increased alveolar epithelial permeability in cigarette smokers. Lancet 1:66-68
10. Wollmer P, Jonson B, Lachmann B (1995) Evaluation of lung permeability in neonatal respiratory distress syndrome and adult respiratory distress syndrome. In: Robertson B, Taeusch HW (eds) Surfactant therapy for lung disease. Marcel Dekker, New York, pp 199-213
11. Schmekel B, Bos JAH, Kahn R et al (1992) Integrity of the alveolo-capillary barrier and alveolar surfactant system in smokers. Thorax 47:603-608

12. Taskar V, Wollmer P, Evander E et al (1996) Effect of detergent combined with large tidal volume ventilation on alveolocapillary permeability. Clin Physiol 16:103-114

13. Nilsson K, Evander E, Wollmer P (1997) Pulmonary clearance of [^{99m}Tc]DTPA and [^{99m}Tc] albumin in smokers. Clin Physiol 17:183-192

14. Nilsson K, Wollmer P (1992) Pulmonary clearance of ^{99m}Tc-DTPA and ^{99m}Tc-albumin in rabbits with surfactant dysfunction and lung injury. Clin Physiol 12:587-594

15. Brudin LH, Valind SO, Rhodes CG et al (1994) Fluorine-18 deoxyglucose uptake in sarcoidosis measured with positron emission tomography. Eur J Nucl Med 4:297-305

16. Jones HA, Sriskandan S, Peters AM et al (1997) Dissociation of neutrophil emigration and metabolic activity in lobar pneumonia and bronchiectasis. Eur Respir J 10:795-803

Lung Function Monitoring: Data Provided by CT Scan

I. Ravagnan, L. Brazzi, L. Gattinoni

In the last 10 years the role of computed tomography (CT) in the clinical evaluation of thoracic diseases has rapidly gained popularity becoming one of the most important research and diagnostic tool. In particular, CT played a major role in improving our knowledge in the physiopathology of the Acute Respiratory Distress Syndrome (ARDS) and in evaluating the impact of the different approaches commonly used to therapeutically treat the syndrome.

In this brief review we will focus on:

1. the lung structure and function relationship in baseline conditions and at different stages of the ARDS evolution;
2. the modifications introduced applying therapeutical manouvres such as Positive End-Expiratory Pressure (PEEP), mechanical ventilation and prone positioning to ARDS lungs.

The quantitative analysis of the CT scan

The quantitative analysis of the CT scan relies on the analysis of "CT numbers", which roughly define the density (i.e. mass/volume) of each voxel composing the image [1]. When a given voxel (dimension 1.5 mm * 1.5 mm * 9 mm) is composed by gas, the CT number, in Hounsfield Units (H), is – 1000 H; when it is composed by water (or blood, or lung tissue) is equal to 0 H. Knowing the density and the total lung volume (computed by CT scan image) or the gas volume (by helium dilution technique) it is possible to compute both in the entire lung, or in a given lung region: 1) the amount of gas; 2) the amount of "tissue"; 3) the gas/tissue ratio. Moreover, knowing either the lung density at different lung levels (by CT scan) or the lung height and assuming that pressures are transmitted throughout the lung parenchyma as in a fluid (i.e. pressure at a given height is equal to density times height), it is possible to estimate, at a given lung height, the hydrostatic superimposed pressure at that height. Finally, taking CT scan at different intrathoracic pressure or in different position it is possible to estimate the "lung recruitment" defined as the amount of gasless tissue which regains inflation.

Lung morphology at different stages of ARDS

The CT scan clearly shows that the densities in ARDS lung, at least in the early phase, are primarily distributed in the dependent lung regions. This dishomogeneity of the lung lesions distribution, with a sparing of the non dependent regions, led us initially [2] to model the ARDS lung as composed by three compartments: one "healthy" (non dependent), one "recruitable" and one "consolidated". The difference between recruitable and consolidated compartment was inferred studying the ARDS lung at different PEEP levels. Some patients, in fact, had spectacular clearing of densities increasing pressure (recruitment), while others showed only increased inflation of the regions already inflated, with unmodified densities distribution (consolidation). Using the quantitative approach described above, we found that the lung weight, during ARDS, was two-three fold than normal and that the amount of excess tissue mass (likely oedema) was positively correlated with the shunt fraction and the dead space [3]. More interestingly, a positive correlation was found between the excess tissue mass and the pulmonary artery pressure (1 mmHg of pulmonary artery pressure was associated with 14% increase of the original lung weight). From these early studies, however, the most important finding was that the lung compliance was not related to the amount of "diseased" lung tissue but, rather, to the amount of residual inflated lung: the smaller the lung, the lower the compliance [2]. This led to the concept of "baby lung" which emphasized that the functioning part of the ARDS lung has the dimension of the lung of a five or six year old baby [4].

Initially, we hypothesized the lung oedema as distributed according to gravity. Later on, analyzing quantitatively the different lung regions dividing the lung in 10 levels from sternum to vertebra, we realized that the excess tissue mass, in each lung level, was approximately the same (twofold normal) being the lung oedema distribution clearly not gravity dependent [5]. The pulmonary parenchyma seems, hence, homogeneously affected by the disease. The densities are mainly located in the dependent lung regions due to the fact that the increased lung weight, due to oedema accumulation, progressively compresses the lung regions along the vertical axis and the gas is gradually squeezed out from the dependent regions, with development of compression atelectasis.

It has been reported that, with time, the lung structure and function changes markedly [6]. The application of CT scan in ARDS gave us the opportunity to investigate in a more specific and detailed way the changes in lung morphology occurring *in vivo* with time: the most important finding is the presence of cysts and emphysema-like lesions prevalently in the dependent lung regions. In late ARDS these enphysema-like lesions are associated with an increased incidence of pneumothorax as well as an increase in dead space and arterial $PaCO_2$. Moreover, in late ARDS the development of lung fibrosis reduces the transmission of hydrostatic forces with a consequent decrease in the occurrence of atelectasis in the dependent part of the lung.

Response to PEEP

Having in mind the model described above, we tested the hypothesis that lung collapse is due to the hydrostatic superimposed pressure and that PEEP is effective in counteracting this forces [7]. Ten ARDS patients were studied at several PEEP levels, from 0 to 20 cm H_2O. This allow to construct, at each lung level, a gas/tissue ratio-pressure curve. Three different kind of curves were obtained: 1) straight lines, which suggested the presence of open pulmonary units inflating according to their own compliance; 2) biphasic curves, which presented an inflection point (Pflex) suggesting the presence of collapsed units which are recruited only when a critical pressure is reached; 3) not significant gas/tissue ratio-pressure curves in which the gas/tissue ratios did not increase with pressure at any point, suggesting the presence of consolidated pulmonary units. As expected, we evidenced that the non dependent lung regions were characterized by straight line while the frequency of biphasic response increased along the sterno-vertebral axis with a progressive increase in the measured inflection point pressure (i.e. the more dependent the level, the higher the inflection point pressure). These data, hence, supported the hypothesis that compression is the main cause of alveolar collapse in the dependent part of the lung and that PEEP acts as a counterforce, keeping the pulmonary units with lower inflection point pressure open. Two potential clinical implications may be inferred from these findings: 1) optimal PEEP does not exist since counteracting the hydrostatic forces in the most dependent lung regions causes hyperexpansion of the upper lung units which do not need any pressure; 2) for the same lung density (i.e. relative amount of oedema), the distance from sternum to vertebra is important to be considered since cause superimposed pressure in the dependent lung regions to be different in amount and, hence, the PEEP to apply to counteract this force to be accordingly chosen.

Response to prone positioning

The hydrostatic forces, which cause the compression atelectasis in the dorsal regions of the lung while in supine position, change their directions when the patients are turned prone. According to the model previously described we can expect that, in prone position, the dorsal regions are reinflated, while the ventral ones collapse. The results obtained when studying, with the CT scan, the modification observed when changing patients position from supine to prone fit the hypothesized model since, even if the total density of the lung does not change, we found a density redistribution from dorsal to ventral pulmonary regions [8]. The response to PEEP and the body positioning seems hence to share a common mechanism which is to counteract, in different ways, the superimposed pressure which causes compression atelectasis in the more dependent lung regions.

Effect of mechanical ventilation

It is widely reported in literature [9] that mechanical ventilation with high peak airway pressure and lung overdistension are contributing factors for iatrogenic lung injury during ARDS treatment. To evaluate the distribution of ventilation and the regional changes in lung volume associated with the use of mechanical ventilation at different PEEP level, we recently evaluated 8 ARDS patients treated with volume controlled mechanical ventilation at different PEEP level from 0 to 20 cm H_2O [10]. We found that, at 0 cm H_2O PEEP in supine position, ventilation was mainly distributed in the upper part of the lung. Increasing PEEP, the distribution of the inspired tidal volume becomes progressively more homogeneous with a decrease of compliance in the upper part of the lung, no change in the middle part and an increase in the lower part. It is well known that respiratory system compliance depend either on the intrisic elasticity of the pulmonary units (i.e. specific compliance) or on the number of ventilable alveolar units. Since the specific compliance, in ARDS, it has been reported as quite normal in each lung regions [7, 11], the observed modification in compliance, and hence in ventilation distribution, has to be attributed mainly to a modification in the number of ventilable alveolar units. The analysis of the recruitment distribution, as possible by means of CT scan, confirmed the hypothesis: in the upper levels, in fact, where the superimposed pressure is low and atelectatic regions are few, the recruitment is negligible and the compliance minimally affected. On the contrary, in the middle and lowest levels, where the superimposed pressure is higher causing atelectasis to be present, application of PEEP may cause recruitment with a consequent increase in regional compliance.

Conclusions

Data reported above, support the hypothesis that the introduction of thoracic CT scan deeply influenced our knowledge of lung physiopathology during ARDS. A number of previously established concepts on physiopathology and on the mechanisms of action of different therapeutic manouvres such as PEEP and body position changes have been recently challenged. It is nowadays diffusely accepted that the use of CT scan may be extremely useful in titrating the "optimal" ventilatory strategy at different stage of ARDS. However, due to the fact that some authors found that CT scan seems inadequate for optimizing mechanical ventilation being expensive and hardly repeatible in everyday clinical practice [12], its role in routine clinical management of ARDS has still to be defined.

References

1. Gattinoni L, Pesenti A, Torresin A (1986) Adult respiratory distress syndrome profiles by computed tomography. J Thorac Imag 3:25-30
2. Gattinoni L, Pesenti A, Avalli L et al (1987) Pressure-volume curve of total respiratory system in acute respiratory failure. Am Rev Respir Dis 36:730-736
3. Gattinoni L, Pesenti A, Bombino M et al (1988) Relationship between lung computed tomographic density, gas exchange and PEEP in acute respiratory failure. Anesthesiology 69: 824-832
4. Gattinoni L, Pesenti A (1987) ARDS: the non homogeneous lung; fact and hypothesis. Intens Crit Care Digest 6:1-4
5. Pelosi P, D'Andrea L, Vitale G et al (1994) Vertical gradient of regional lung inflation in adult respiratory distress syndrome. Am J Respir Crit Care Med 149:8-13
6. Gattinoni L, Bombino M, Pelosi P et al (1994) Lung structure and function in different stages of severe adult respiratory distress syndrome. JAMA 271:1772-1779
7. Gattinoni L, D'Andrea L, Pelosi P et al (1993) Regional effect and mechanism of positive end-expiratory pressure in early adult respiratory distress syndrome. JAMA 269:2122-2127
8. Gattinoni L, Pelosi P, Vitale G et al (1991) Body position changes redistribute lung computed tomographic density in patients with acute respiratory failure. Anesthesiology 74:15-23
9. Manning HL (1994) Peak airway pressure: why the fuss. Chest 105:242-247
10. Gattinoni L, Pelosi P, Crotti S, Valenza F (1995) Effects of PEEP on regional distribution of tidal volume and recruitment in patients with adult respiratory distress syndrome. Am J Respir Crit Care Med 151:1807-1814
11. Pelosi P, Cereda M, Foti G et al (1995) Alterations of lung and chest wall mechanics in patients with acute lung injury: effects of positive end-expiratory pressure. Am J Respir Crit Care Med 152:531-537
12. Brunet F, Jeanbourquin D, Monchi M et al (1995) Should mechanical ventilation be optimized to blood gases, lung mechanics or thoracic CT scan? Am J Respir Crit Care Med 152:524-530

Bedside Replacement of Computed Tomography by Electrical Impedance Tomography

P.W.A. Kunst, S.H. Böhm, B. Lachmann

In the adult respiratory distress syndrome (ARDS) mechanical ventilation is used to maintain adequate oxygenation, but mechanical ventilation can be hazardous to the lung itself. Different ventilation approaches have been developed to open the lung and to reduce the risk of any trauma to the alveoli during mechanical ventilation [1, 2]. However, in the vertical gradient from anterior to posterior lung density increases, indicating an increase in collapse of alveoli in this gradient due to pulmonary oedema, loss of surfactant and alveolar damage [3]. With increasing pulmonary oedema the differences in the vertical gradient are even more pronounced. The increase in lung weight due to pulmonary edema causes collapse of alveoli at the posterior site of the lungs owing to gravitational forces. Knowing whether and in what region alveoli are collapsed or open might help in the adjustment of mechanical ventilation and/or might give insight in the severity of pulmonary oedema. Therefore, regional information about the division of functional lung volume is needed. CT-scanning of the lung has already been proven useful for the assessment of the regional information [3], but is impractical at the intensive care unit (ICU) since it can not be used at the bedside. With a recent non-invasive bedside method, called Electrical Impedance Tomography (EIT), regional information about the division of functional lung volume can also be obtained. EIT registers changes in impedance due to lung volume changes in a 2-D image plane [4, 5]. In this abstract we will briefly describe the basics of EIT and some experimental results.

Basics

Electrical impedance tomography

In this study EIT measurements were performed using the Sheffield Applied Potential Tomograph (DAS-01P Portable Data Acquisition System, Mark I, IBEES, Sheffield, England), which has been described previously [6, 7]. Briefly, EIT is a technique that produces 2-D images of changes in electrical impedance by means of 16 standard ECG electrodes that are placed around the object measured. An alternating current (50 kHz, 5 mA peak-peak) is injected between a pair of adjacent electrodes and the remaining electrodes are used to measure impedance. When all pairs of adjacent electrodes have been used as injecting electrodes, one data collection cycle is completed. In order to minimise artefacts, in the present study 10 data collection cycles were averaged to obtain one image or frame. During the entire measurement a sequence of frames at 1.13 second intervals was recorded. The Sheffield Tomograph generates different images to a reference set. Therefore, only physiological processes that cause changes in impedance can be imaged. In the thorax, major changes in impedance occur due to the inspiration and expiration of air [6, 7]. Therefore, in the sequence of images, the change in impedance due to the inflation of air can be visualized and studied. After defining a region of interest in the 2-D image, the impedance changes occurring over time are plotted in a curve and numerical values are obtained. Since the reconstruction algorithm of the EIT is based on differences in impedance, the average impedance change has no unit and is expressed as an arbitrary unit (AU). In the results mentioned here we analyzed the curves of the whole image containing 788 pixels, and those of the anterior half (394 pixels) and the posterior half (394 pixels) separately. From the obtained curves the maximal difference in impedance between inspiration and expiration was calculated. This difference was called ventilation-induced impedance change.

Results

Measurement of different lung regions

In ARDS an increasing lung density exists in the vertical gradient from anterior to posterior when the patient is in the supine position, as Gattinoni et al. showed by using CT-scan [3]. Therefore, alveoli in the anterior part are mostly filled with air whereas alveoli in the posterior part are frequently collapsed. As EIT can distinguish the anterior from the posterior part, these differences may well become visible by using this technique.

In a recent study, in which animals underwent lung lavages in order to create ARDS, differences in ventilation-induced impedance changes (oscillating signal) of the anterior part of the lung occurred after lung lavage in comparison with the posterior part (Fig. 1). As can be seen, the ventilation-induced impedance changes of the anterior part remained the same after lung lavage (i.e. the sudden impedance decrease), whereas those of the posterior part decreased after both lavages.

As mentioned differences in lung density should exist in the vertical gradient from anterior to posterior. In Fig. 2 regional pressure impedance curves were constructed using EIT in an experimental setting (pressure was measured simultaneously with the EIT-measurements at the end of the tube. Afterwards the time-axis was converted into a pressure-axis). The EIT image was divided into 4 regions and for each region a pressure-impedance curve was plotted.

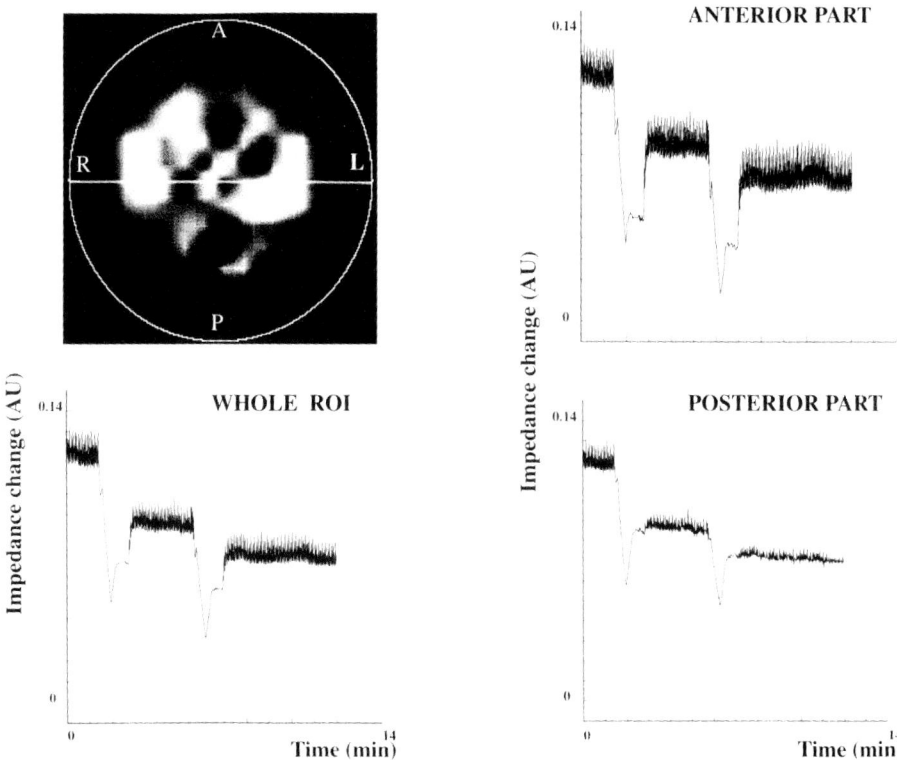

Fig. 1. *Left*: EIT-image divided into an anterior and a posterior part (upper image). Lower graph: impedance changes measured over the whole image plotted as a function of time. *Right*: Impedance changes of the anterior part (upper graph) and the posterior part (lower graph). The deep decrease is due to the lavage

Looking at the inflation limb (the lower limb) from region 1 to 3 the pressure to induce a sudden impedance remains the same. From region 4 to 5 this pressure increases. Also the plateau of the inflation limb is easily reached in the upper parts of the lungs, whereas in the posterior parts no plateau is reached. These results indicate the potential for measurement of recruitment by EIT in the vertical gradient, as was already possible with CT [3]. Although these preliminary results in the ARDS patients underline the findings that EIT might be a tool to help to establish the optimal ventilator settings for an ICU patient, a lot of research has to be performed to indicate the use of EIT for this application at the ICU.

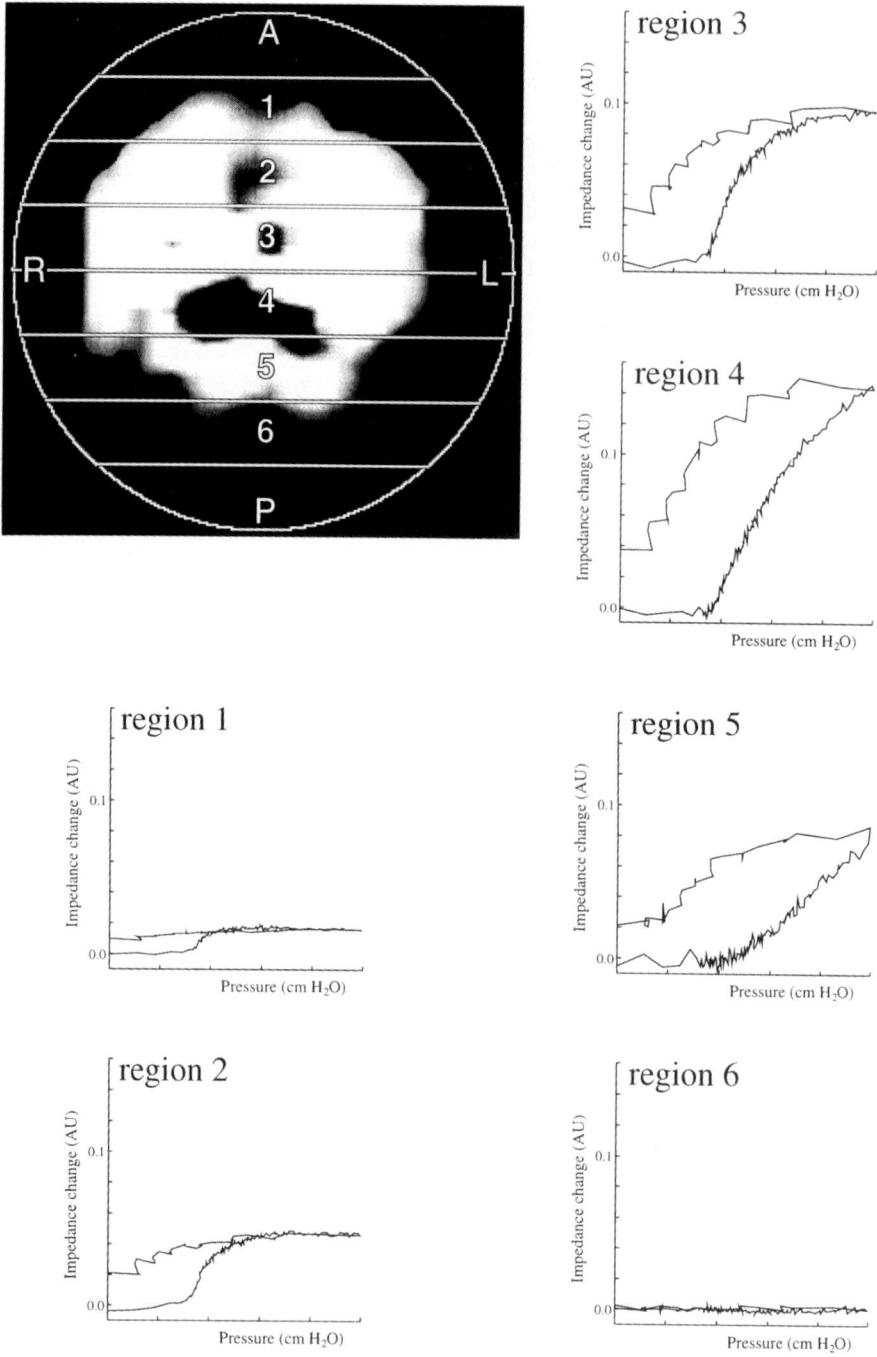

Fig. 2. Regional differences in impedance pressure curves

References

1. Sjöstrand UH, Lichtwark-Aschoff M, Nielsen JB et al (1995) Different ventilatory approaches to keep the lung open. Intensive Care Med 21:310-318
2. Amato MBP, Barbas CSV, Medeiros DM et al (1995) Beneficial effect of the "Open lung approach" with low distending pressures in acute respiratory distress syndrome. Am J Respir Crit Care Med 152:1835-1846
3. Gattinoni L, Pelosi P, Crotti S, Valenza F (1995) Effects of positive end-expiratory pressure on regional distribution of tidal volume and recruitment in adult respiratory distress syndrome. Am J Respir Crit Care Med 151:1807-1814
4. Harris ND, Suggett AJ, Barber DC, Brown BH (1987) Applications of applied potential tomography (APT) in respiratory medicine. Clin Phys Physiol Meas 8[Suppl A]:155-165
5. Hahn G, Sipinkova I, Baisch F, Hellige G (1995) Changes in thoracic impedance distribution under different ventilatory conditions. Physiol Meas 16:A161-A173
6. Smith RWM, Freeston IL, Brown BH (1995) A real time electrical impedance tomography system for clinical use - Design and preliminary results. IEEE Trans Biomed Eng 40(2):133-139
7. Brown BH, Barber DC (1988) Possibilities and problems of real-time imaging of tissue resistivity. Clin Phys Physiol Meas 9[Suppl A]:121-125

VENTILATORY PERFUSION MISMATCH IN ARDS

Volume Distribution and Ventilatory Modes in Patients with Acute Respiratory Distress Syndrome

C. Chopin, M.C. Chambrin

Since the first publication by Gattinoni et al., who used high resolution CT scans, it is well documented that acute respiratory distress syndrome (ARDS) is a heterogeneous lung disease [1]. Morphological examination of the lung shows structural alterations depending on the stage of this disease [2]. In the acute exudative stage an increased permeability of the alveolar barrier is responsible for a widespread interstitial oedema. As the disease progresses, interstitial fluid containing fibrin escapes toward the alveolar space, generating alveolar oedema, hyaline membrane; leukocytes accumulation occurs. Interstitial and alveolar oedema are predominantly distributed in the dependent area of the lung which are the dorsal regions for patients in supine position. Measured at this early stage, lung compliance (C_L) and end expiratory lung volume (EELV) are low, airway resistance (Raw) is normal or slightly high. Application of moderate positive end expiratory pressure (PEEP) is sufficient to recruit a large amount of non functional alveoli. This recruitment phenomenon is responsible for a decrease in the intrapulmonary shunt along with PaO_2, EELV and C_L increase [3]. The subacute proliferative stage is characterized by type II pneumocyte hyperplasia and fibroblast colonization. At this stage main features are a decrease in C_L and EELV and an increase in airway resistance [4, 5]. Application of PEEP and positive inspiratory pressure (PIP), even at high level, is not able to recruit the consolidated parts of the lung. However, high level of PIP is responsible for overdistension of the remaining normally aerated pulmonary units submitted to very high transpulmonary pressure gradient which therefore receive the main part of the tidal volume. Then mechanical ventilation induces, by itself, additional acute lung injury definitively compromising the prognosis [6, 7]. Few days later, interstitial and intraalveolar fibrosis may occur.

In summary, ARDS is a heterogeneous lung disease characterized by lung units with great differences in compliance and resistance and consequently with huge differences in regional time constant ($\tau = RC$). A recent American-European consensus conference has recommended for ventilatory support in patients with ARDS [8]:

– to ensure appropriate oxygen delivery with sufficient CO_2 removal,
– to ensure the most complete recruitment at the lesser mean airway pressure (MAP) by adding PEEP and by extending the inspiratory time fraction (TI),

– to maintain the recruited alveoli opened throughout most of the tidal range, while avoiding overdistension of normal remaining areas, mechanical ventilation related lung injury, and haemodynamic depression.

The consensus committee did not recommend any peculiar mode of ventilation, but underlined the need for future research on the influence of breathing pattern and gas flow delivery on ventilation perfusion matching in ARDS.

Briefly, current ventilatory modes are divided in two main classes: flow preset ventilation (FPV) and pressure preset ventilation (PPV). A review of the technical aspect of PPV was published by Blanch et al. [9, 10]. When FPV is time cycled, the mode is termed flow controlled (V'C). When PPV is time cycled, the mode is termed pressure controlled (PC).

In mechanical ventilation the respiratory cycle is divided in three phases: time of insufflation (Ti), end inspiratory pause (EIP) and expiratory time (TE). By convention TI is the sum of Ti and EIP. The inspiratory to expiratory time ratio (TI/TE) is termed inverse when TI is longer than TE.

Because there is a good rationale for inverse ratio ventilation (IRV) in ARDS, this paper will mainly focus on the influence of extending TI on gas volume distribution. Hypotheses and conclusions will be based on the results obtained from a mathematical model and from clinical and experimental studies.

The model

To investigate the consequence of applying either a constant pressure or a linear flow to a heterogeneous two-compartmental lung model, we used the model proposed by Bates et al. [11]. To illustrate the behavior of the system as it could be observed on flow and pressure waveforms at airway opening at patient's bedside, a common resistance representing upper airway and endotracheal tube was added. To solve the equations governing the model, its representation was considered as an analogous electrical circuit (Fig. 1). In such a model, the charge $[Q(t)]$, the intensity $[I(t) = \delta Q(t)$, which is the derivative of the charge with respect to time] and the tension $[U(t)]$ respectively correspond to volume $[V(t)]$, flow $[\delta V(t)]$ and pressure $[P(t)]$. The applied source could be either a current generator or a tension generator. R_0 is the resistance of the endotracheal tube and trachea, C_1 and C_2 are the compliances of the two compartments and R_1 and R_2 the corresponding airway resistances. PEEP is represented by a constant tension applied to the system. Total compliance (static compliance) is equal to the sum of the compliances of the two compartments: $C_T = C_1 + C_2$. Elastance (E) is the inverse of compliance: $E = 1/C$. Total resistance is a function of both the resistances and the compliances.

In such a model the following equations are always valid at each phase of the respiratory cycle (inspiration, EIP or expiration):

$$\text{Ptrach}(t) = R_1\, \delta V_1(t) + E_1\, V_1(t) = R_2\, \delta V_2(t) + E_2\, V_2(t) \qquad \text{(eq. 1)}$$

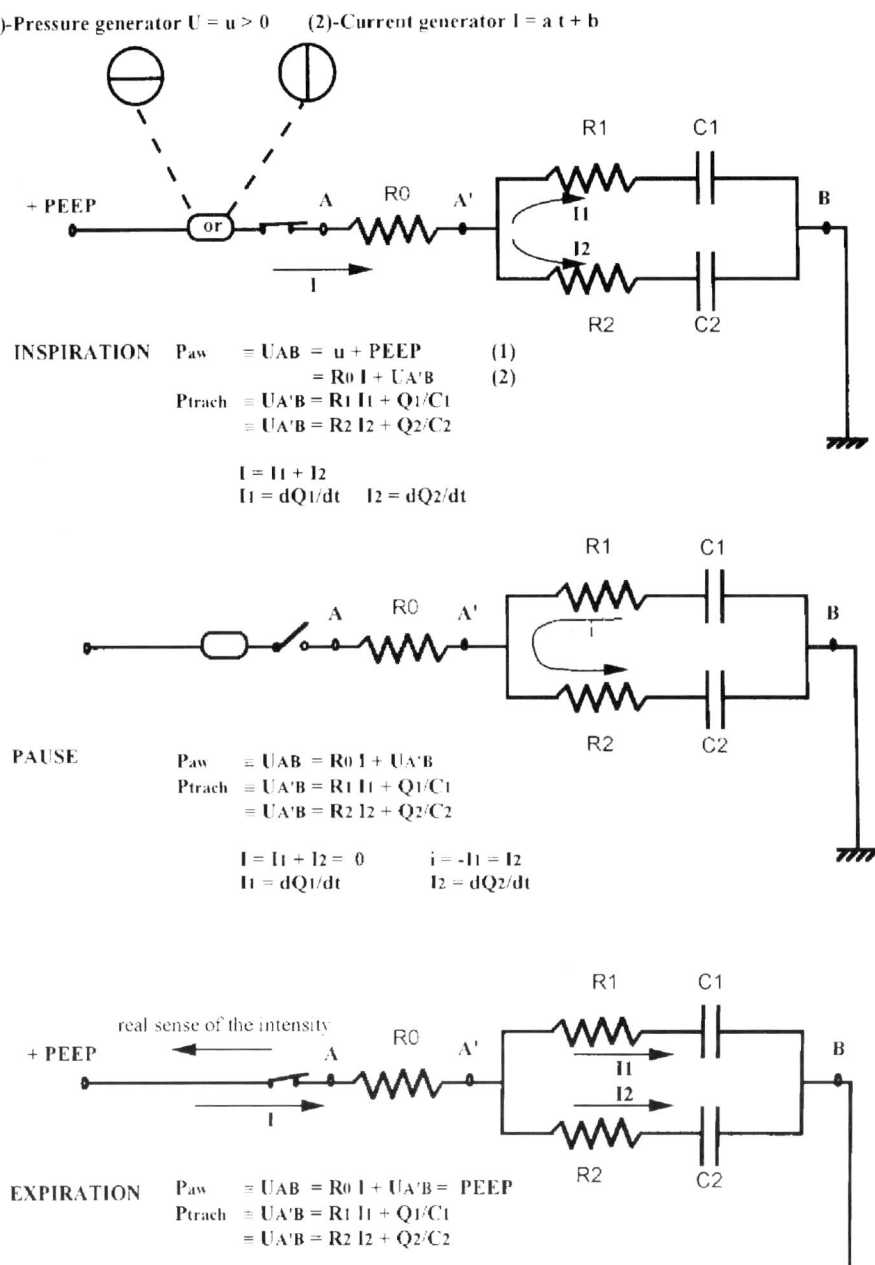

(1)-Pressure generator U = u > 0   (2)-Current generator I = a t + b

INSPIRATION P_{aw} = U_{AB} = u + PEEP   (1)
                       = R_0 I + $U_{A'B}$ (2)
         P_{trach} = $U_{A'B}$ = R_1 I_1 + Q_1/C_1
                = $U_{A'B}$ = R_2 I_2 + Q_2/C_2

         I = I_1 + I_2
         I_1 = dQ_1/dt I_2 = dQ_2/dt

PAUSE P_{aw} = U_{AB} = R_0 I + $U_{A'B}$
         P_{trach} = $U_{A'B}$ = R_1 I_1 + Q_1/C_1
                = $U_{A'B}$ = R_2 I_2 + Q_2/C_2

         I = I_1 + I_2 = 0   i = $-I_1$ = I_2
         I_1 = dQ_1/dt I_2 = dQ_2/dt

real sense of the intensity

EXPIRATION P_{aw} = U_{AB} = R_0 I + $U_{A'B}$ = PEEP
         P_{trach} = $U_{A'B}$ = R_1 I_1 + Q_1/C_1
                = $U_{A'B}$ = R_2 I_2 + Q_2/C_2

         I = I_1 + I_2
         I_1 = dQ_1/dt I_2 = dQ_2/dt

Fig. 1. Representation of the model according to an electrical circuit. The equations governing each phase are given. Their equivalent in a mechanical model are given in the text. For expiration, the same conventions related to the directions of intensities are used and the resolution produces, of course, negative values for all these intensities

where $\delta V(t)$ is the derivative function of $V(t)$ with respect to t. $V(t)$ is the volume and $\delta V(t)$ is the flow.

We can define the value of the resistive and elastic pressures as follows:

$$\begin{array}{ll} \mathrm{Pres}_1(t) = R_1\, \delta V_1(t) & \mathrm{Pres}_2(t) = R_2\, \delta V_2(t) \\ \mathrm{Pel}_1(t) = E_1\, V_1(t) & \mathrm{Pel}_2(t) = E_2\, V_2(t) \end{array}$$

and

$$\mathrm{Paw}(t) = R_0\, \delta V(t) + \mathrm{Ptrach}(t) \qquad\qquad \text{(eq. 2)}$$

$$V(t) = V_1(t) + V_2(t) \qquad\qquad \text{(eq. 3)}$$

Inspiration

Whatever the applied command is, the equations describing the model during inspiration are:

$$\delta V(t) = \delta V_1(t) + \delta V_2(t) \qquad\qquad \text{(eq. 4)}$$

initial conditions   at $t = 0$, $V_1(0) = Q_1$ and $V_2(0) = Q_2$

For the first inspiration, it was postulated that inspiration started from the elastic equilibrium volume (define as zero volume), so $Q_1 = Q_2 = 0$. For the following cycles, the remaining volume was taken into account when it exists.

With *linear applied flow* $[\delta V(t)]$ the equations describing the model during inspiration are:

$$\delta V(t) = at + b \qquad\qquad \text{(eq. 5)}$$

Integrating equation 5 we obtain $V(t) = 1/2at^2 + bt + K$. At $t = 0$, $V(0) = Q_1 + Q_2 = K$, then

$$V(t) = 1/2at^2 + bt + Q_1 + Q_2 \qquad\qquad \text{(eq. 6)}$$

Combination of equations 1, 3, 4, 5 and 6 leads to the following differential equation:

$$R_1\, \delta V_1(t) + E_1\, V_1(t) - R_2\, (at + b - \delta V_1(t)) - E_2\, (1/2at^2 + bt + Q_1 + Q_2\, \delta V_1(t)) = 0$$

The general solution for this equation is:

$$V_1(t) = aK_1 t^2 + K_1't + K_1'' + K_1'''\, e^{-t/\tau} \text{ with } \tau = R_1 + R_2 / E_1 + E_2$$

In a same way, we have:

$$V_2(t) = aK_2 t^2 + K_2't + K_2'' + K_2'''\, e^{-t/\tau}$$

If the flow is constant, a is equal to zero, so the term in t^2 disappears. When t increases, the term with exponential disappears and volume evolves linearly.

If the flow is accelerating or decelerating, a is respectively positive or negative and the evolution of the volume is strongly dependent on the term in t^2.

With *constant applied pressure* (u), the equations describing the model during inspiration are:

$$R_1 \, \delta V_1(t) + E_1 \, V_1(t) = u + \text{PEEP} - R_0 \, (\delta V_1(t)) + \delta V_2(t)) \qquad \text{(eq. 7)}$$

whose derivative is

$$R_1 \, \delta^2 V_1(t) + E_1 \, \delta V_1(t) = - R_0 \, (\delta^2 V_1(t) + \delta^2 V_2(t)) \qquad \text{(eq. 7bis)}$$

In the same way, we have:

$$R_2 \, \delta V_2(t) + E_2 \, V_2(t) = u + \text{PEEP} - R_0 \, (\delta V_1(t)) + \delta V_2(t)) \qquad \text{(eq. 8)}$$

whose derivative is

$$R_2 \, \delta^2 V_2(t) + E_2 \, \delta V_2(t)) = - R_0 \, (\delta^2 V_1(t)) + \delta^2 V_2(t)) \qquad \text{(eq. 8bis)}$$

By extracting $\delta V_2(t)$ from eq. 7 and $\delta^2 V_2(t)$ from eq. 7bis, replacing by their values in eq. 8bis and rearranging, we obtain the following differential equation:

$$(R_0(R_1 + R_2) + R_2 R_1) \, \delta^2 V_1(t) + (R_0(E_1 + E_2) + E_2 R_1 + E_1 R_2) \, \delta V_1(t)$$
$$+ E_1 E_2 V_1(t) - E_2(u + \text{PEEP}) = 0$$

for which the general solution is:

$$V_1(t) = (u + \text{PEEP} + K_1 \, e^{-\beta t} + K_1{}' \, e^{-\mu t}) \, / \, E_1$$

In a same way, we have:

$$V_2(t) = (u + \text{PEEP} + K_2 \, e^{-\beta t} + K_2{}' \, e^{-\mu t}) \, / \, E_2$$

If time is long enough, the exponential terms are near zero, and the repartition only depends on each compartment elastance.

End inspiratory pause

When an end inspiratory pause is set, a volume is transferred from one compartment to the other to equalize the pressures in the two compartments. To solve the problem we hypothesize that the flow will be positive from *compartment 1* to *compartment 2* (the inverse hypothesis leads to the same results). This is expressed by:

$$\delta V(t) = \delta V_2(t) = - \delta V_1(t) \qquad \text{(eq. 9)}$$

and

$$\delta^2 V(t) = \delta^2 V_2(t) = - \delta^2 V_1(t) \qquad \text{(eq. 10)}$$

By deriving eq. 1 we obtain:

$$R_1 \delta^2 V_1(t) + E_1 \delta V_1(t) = R_2 \delta^2 V_2(t) + E_2 \delta V_2(t) \qquad \text{(eq. 11)}$$

By combining equation 9, 10 and 11, we obtain:

$$(R_1 + R_2) \delta^2 V_1(t) + (E_1 + E_2) \delta V_1(t) = 0 \qquad \text{(eq. 12)}$$

The solution for this equation is:

$$V_1(t) = (E_1 Q_1 - E_2 Q_2) / (E_1 + E_2) e^{-\alpha t} + (Q_1 + Q_2) E_2 / (E_1 + E_2)$$

with

$$\alpha = (E_1 + E_2) / (R_1 + R_2)$$

In the same way:

$$V_2(t) = (E_1 Q_1 - E_2 Q_2) / (E_1 + E_2) e^{-\alpha t} + (Q_1 + Q_2) E_1 / (E_1 + E_2)$$

When EIP is long enough, the final repartition only depends on the distribution of the elastances.

Expiration

At the end of inspiration, when breathing is purely passive, the applied pressure returns immediately to PEEP and the volume decreases in an exponential manner during the subsequent expiration.

The equations describing the model during passive expiration are:

$$R_1 \delta V_1(t) + E_1 V_1(t) = PEEP - R_0 (\delta V_1(t)) + \delta V_2(t)) \qquad \text{(eq. 13)}$$

whose derivative is

$$R_1 \delta^2 V_1(t) + E_1 \delta V_1(t) = - R_0 (\delta^2 V_1(t) + \delta^2 V_2(t)) \qquad \text{(eq. 13bis)}$$

and

$$R_2 \delta V_2(t) + E_2 V_2(t) = PEEP - R_0 (\delta V_1(t)) + \delta V_2(t)) \qquad \text{(eq. 14)}$$

whose derivative is

$$R_2 \, \delta^2 V_2(t) + E_2 \, \delta V_2(t) = - R_0 \, (\delta^2 V_1(t) + \delta^2 V_2(t)) \qquad \text{(eq. 14bis)}$$

By extracting $\delta V_2(t)$ from eq. 13 and $\delta^2 V_2(t)$ from eq. 13bis, replacing by their values in eq. 14bis and rearranging, we obtain the following differential equation:

$$(R_0(R_1 + R_2) + R_2 R_1) \, \delta^2 V_1(t) + (R_0(E_1 + E_2) + E_2 R_1 + E_1 R_2) \, \delta V_1(t))$$
$$+ E_1 E_2 V_1(t) - E_2 PEEP = 0$$

The general solution for this equation is:

$$V_1(t) = (PEEP + K_1 \, e^{-\beta t} + K_1' \, e^{-\mu t}) \, / \, E_1$$

In a same way, we have:

$$V_2(t) = (PEEP + K_2 \, e^{-\beta t} + K_2' \, e^{-\mu t}) \, / \, E_2$$

At sufficiently long time (when expiration is complete), the two exponential terms disappear and volume depends only on the level of PEEP and elastance of each compartment.

Limitations of the model

Some limitations of the model have to be pointed out. In clinical practice, the ventilators usually do not deliver a perfect constant pressure. Airway resistances are normally higher during expiration than during inspiration because of the flow turbulence created by the abrupt decrease in pression in the cross-sectional area at the tip of the endotracheal tube [12]. In the model, RI and RE are considered identical. The respiratory system is represented as a collection of compliant and resistive elements with constant individual characteristics at a given flow.

Despite these limitations, this model is relevant enough to produce useful insight in the behavior of patient's respiratory system when PFV or PPV modes are applied.

To illustrate this behavior we have defined 3 models whose characteristics have been chosen in order to have a "normal" compartment (*compartment 1*) and a "pathological" compartment (*compartment 2*). In ARDS, the "pathological" compartment (increased resistance (in cm $H_2O/L/s$) and decreased compliance (in $L/cm \, H_2O$) is supposed to have the longer time constant, but this remains questionable. For this reason, we have defined three models with different repartition of time constants, but identical total compliance ($C_T = C_1 + C_2$) (Table 1).

Table 1. Characteristics of the mechanical models

Model	R_1	C_1	τ_1	R_2	C_2	τ_2
M1 ($\tau_1 < \tau_2$)	8	0.040	0.32	32	0.020	0.64
M2 ($\tau_1 = \tau_2$)	6	0.040	0.24	12	0.020	0.24
M3 ($\tau_1 > \tau_2$)	8	0.050	0.40	24	0.010	0.24

Resistances (R) are expressed in cm $H_2O/L/s$, compliances (C) in L/cm H_2O and time constants (τ) in seconds. Compartment 1 represents "normal" lung and compartment 2 "pathological" lung

Inverse ratio ventilation in ARDS

The concept of IRV was proposed thirty years ago, based on the experience in neonates with hyaline membrane disease [13]. In adults, IRV has also been proposed on the basis of improved gas exchange with reduction of the peak airway pressure [14, 15]. The rationale for implementation of IRV in adults has extensively been described in a review by Marcy and Marini [16]. The main argument to use IRV is that heterogeneous lung injury in ARDS causes a wide variation in regional τ, from very high (slow lung units) to very low (fast lung units) values. The slow lung units require longer TI to be fully inflated. As a result, IRV should improve gas exchanges and ventilation to perfusion matching (VA/Q). IRV can be administered both in FPV – this mode is termed flow controlled inverse ratio ventilation (V'CIR) – and in PPV – this mode is termed pressure controlled inverse ratio ventilation (PCIR). In PCIR, IRV is only applied by increasing TI. In V'CIR, IRV is applied by either EIP or a slow constant or decelerating flow. Whatever the IRV mode, as TE decreases, a positive value of the static recoil pressure of the respiratory system occurs when the inspiration starts before complete return to the previous EELV. This pressure is termed auto or intrinsic PEEP (PEEPi). We successively focus on the effects related with the lengthening of TI, use of V'CIR versus PCIR, and shortening of TE.

For the same inverse TI/TE ratio, lengthening of TI may be obtained either by setting an EIP or by using a low inspiratory flow.

When constant flow ventilation is applied on the model at different values (Table 2), the volume distribution is dependent on the elastance and time constant of each compartment.

When the time constants of the two compartments are equal, the inspiratory flow level has no influence on the volume distribution which depends only on the ratio of elastances of the compartments. In model M2 ($C_1 = 0.040$ and $C_2 = 0.020$), the volume in compartment 1 would be twice the volume of compartment 2.

When the time constants are different, as flow decreases, the volume decreases into the compartment with smaller time constant. Inversely, as flow decreases, the volume increases into the compartment with longer time constant.

Table 2. Results on the models when applying different flow patterns

Waveform $at + b$	Constant $a=0, b=1.4$			Constant $a=0, b=0.7$			Constant $a=0, b=0.46$			Constant $a=0, b=0.35$			Accelerating $a=1.4, b=0$			Decelerating $a=-1.4, b=1.4$			Decelerating $a=-0.35, b=0.70$		
Ti	0.5			1.0			1.5			2.0			1.0			1.0			2.0		
Model type	M1 ($\tau_1 < \tau_2$)	M2 ($\tau_1 = \tau_2$)	M3 ($\tau_1 > \tau_2$)	M1 ($\tau_1 < \tau_2$)	M2	M3 ($\tau_1 > \tau_2$)	M1 ($\tau_1 < \tau_2$)	M2	M3 ($\tau_1 > \tau_2$)	M1 ($\tau_1 < \tau_2$)	M2	M3 ($\tau_1 > \tau_2$)	M1 ($\tau_1 < \tau_2$)	M2	M3 ($\tau_1 > \tau_2$)	M1 ($\tau_1 < \tau_2$)	M2	M3 ($\tau_1 > \tau_2$)	M1 ($\tau_1 < \tau_2$)	M2	M3 ($\tau_1 > \tau_2$)
V_1 (Ti)	527	466	557	509		568	498		573	491		575	521		560	496		576	478		581
V_2 (Ti)	173	233	143	191		132	202		127	209		124	179		140	204		124	221		119
Δ(V(Ti))	**354**	**233**	**414**	**318**		**436**	**296**		**446**	**282**		**451**	**342**		**420**	**292**		**452**	**257**		**462**
Pel_1 (Ti)	13.2	11.7	11.1	12.7		11.4	12.4		11.5	12.3		11.5	13		11.2	12.4		11.5	11.9		11.6
Pel_2 (Ti)	8.6	11.7	14.3	9.6		13.2	10.1		12.7	10.5		12.4	8.9		13.9	10.2		12.4	11.1		11.0
ΔPel (Ti)	**4.5**	**0**	**-3.2**	**3.2**		**-1.8**	**2.3**		**-1.2**	**1.8**		**-0.9**	**4.1**		**-2.7**	**2.2**		**-0.9**	**0.9**		**-0.2**
$Pres_1$ (Ti)	8	5.6	9.2	3.8	2.8	4.7	2.5	1.9	3.1	1.8	1.4	2.3	8.1	5.6	9	-0.4	0	0.2	-0.1	0	0.1
$Pres_2$ (Ti)	12.6	5.6	6	7	2.8	2.8	4.8	1.9	1.9	3.6	1.4	1.4	12.2	5.6	6.3	1.7	0	-0.6	0.7	0	-0.2
Ptrach (Ti)	21.2	17.3	20.3	16.6	14	16	14.9	13	14.6	14.1	13.1	13.8	21.1	17	20.3	11.9	11.7	11.7	11.8	11.7	11.7
Paw (Ti)	25.4	21.5	24.5	18.7	16	18.1	16.4	15	15.9	15.2	14.1	14.9	25.4	21	24.5	11.9	11.7	11.7	11.8	11.7	11.7
Paw, mean	19.3	15.6	18.6	12.7	11	12.2	10.4	9	10.1	9.3	8.3	9	10.7	8.8	10.3	14.7	12.7	14.2	11.3	10.2	11

Evolution of the parameters of mechanical ventilation at different flow patterns for a given tidal volume set to 0.7 L and with $Q_1 = Q_2 = 0$, $R_0 = 3$, PEP = 0. The difference Δ is always computed by value of *compartment 1* minus value of *compartment 2*

In model M1, the time constant of the "normal lung" (compartment 1) is smaller than the time constant of the "pathological" one (compartment 2). Then, as flow decreases, the volume into compartment 1 decreases and the volume in compartment 2 increases. This is a favorable effect for the "pathological" compartment. The difference of volume between the two compartments decreases when flow decreases. Conversely, in model M3, time constant of the "normal lung" (compartment 1) is longer than the time constant of the "pathological" one (compartment 2). So, as flow decreases, volume in compartment 1 increases and volume in compartment 2 decreases. There is a deleterious effect for the "pathological" compartment. The difference of volume between the two compartments increases when flow decreases.

For different flow patterns (constant, accelerating or decelerating), the volume distribution is also a function of the elastance and time constant of each compartment (Table 2).

When the time constants are equal, flow pattern makes no difference.

When the time constants are different, as flow waveform is modified from an accelerating form to a decelerating form, the volume decreases in the compartment with smaller time constant. Conversely, the volume increases in the compartment with longer time constant. In model M1, the time constant of the "normal lung" (compartment 1) is smaller than the time constant of the "pathological" one (compartment 2). So, when moving from an accelerating form to a decelerating one, there is a decrease of the volume in compartment 1 and an increase of the volume in compartment 2. There is a favorable effect for the "pathologic" compartment. The difference of volume between the two compartments decreases when the flow waveform goes from an accelerating pattern to a decelerating pattern. Conversely, in model M3, the time constant of the "normal" lung (compartment 1) is longer than the time constant of the "pathological" one (compartment 2). So, there is a deleterious effect for the "pathologic" compartment. The difference of volume between the two compartments increases when the flow waveform goes from an accelerating pattern to a decelerating pattern.

During EIP, the volume redistribution is again a function of the time constant of each compartment (Table 3).

When the time constants are equal there is no influence of EIP.

When the time constants are different, the compartment with the longest time constant will be filled with gas coming from the compartment with the smallest time constant.

In model M1, the time constant of the "normal " lung (compartment 1) is smaller than the time constant of the "pathological" one (compartment 2). So, when applying a pause there is a favorable effect for the "pathological" compartment. EIP must be long enough to allow the volume repartition according to elastances. Conversely, in model M3, there is a deleterious effect for the "pathological" compartment. EIP is not suitable, if the objective is to increase the aeration of the "pathological" area.

Table 3. Results on the models when applying EIP

Flow waveform $(at+)b$	Constant $a = 0$, $b = 0.7$			Constant $a = 0$, $b = 0.7$		
Ti	1.0			1.0		
Tp	0.5			1.0		
Model type	M1 $\tau_1<\tau_2$	M2 $\tau_1=\tau_2$	M3 $\tau_1>\tau_2$	M1 $\tau_1<\tau_2$	M2 $\tau_1=\tau_2$	M3 $\tau_1>\tau_2$
$V_1(Ti)$	509	466	568	509	466	568
$V_2(Ti)$	191	233	132	191	233	132
$V_1(Ti)$ - $V_2(Ti)$	**318**	**233**	**436**	**318**	**233**	**436**
$V_1(Tp)$	483	466	581	473	466	583
$V_2(Tp)$	217	233	119	227	233	117
$V_1(Tp)$ - $V_2(Tp)$	**266**	**233**	**462**	**246**	**233**	**466**
$Pel_1(Ti)$ - $Pel_2(Ti)$	3.1	0	−1.8	3.2	0	−1.82
$Pel_1(Tp)$ - $Pel_2(Tp)$	1.2	0	−0.3	0.5	0	0
$Pres_1(Tp)$	−0.2	0	0.1	−0.1	0	0
$Pres_2(Tp)$	0.99	0	−0.2	0.4	0	0
$Ptrach(Tp)$	11.83	11.67	11.69	11.73	11.67	11.67
$Paw(Tp)$	11.83	11.67	11.69	11.73	11.67	11.67

Evolution of the parameters of mechanical ventilation during a pause for a given tidal volume set to 0.7 l, after an insufflation at constant flow for Ti = 1 second

To summarize, when applying on a heterogeneous lung with similar time constants, square waveform inspiratory flow only results in a compliance-dependency, flow-independency volume distribution. When time constants are different, a low flow and/or decelerating pattern and/or EIP profits to the slower compartment.

In experimental previous studies on animal models of acute lung injury, alteration of TI/TE without EIP produced no significant change in haemodynamic, oxygenation or ventilation parameters when MAP [17] or total PEEP (PEEPtot) [18] were kept constant. Moreover, when shunt and dead space effects, measured by inert gas elimination technique were compared in patients with ARDS submitted to V'C PEEP [TI/Ttot 0,24] vs V'CIR [TI/Ttot 0,72] at similar level of PEEPtot, distribution of VA/Q ratios was identical [19]. In patients with ARDS, V'C with decelerating flow resulted in a decrease in PaO_2 and MAP, and an increase in PIP when compared to V'C with square flow wave form, at similar level of VT, RR, TI/TE and PEEP. There was no difference in VD/VT haemodynamic parameters [20]. Similar results were obtained in a pig model of ARDS by Markström et al. [21].

Considering the results of these studies, it remains to be established whether these small differences are sufficient to warrant clinical and therapeutic considerations in the choice of inspiratory flow pattern in V'CIR.

Few papers have compared effect of IRV with and without EIP. Pillet et al. [22] studied the effect of various TI/Ttot ratio without end-expiratory pause

(EIP) on VA/Q mismatching in subjects with slight lung impairment submitted to V'C with square flow wave form. Ti was increased from 20 to 67% of Ttot. In the absence of EIP, lowering flow leads to change in volume distribution with a reduction in ventilation distribution. There was a shift in ventilation distribution toward low VA/Q compartments with recruitment of slower units. The authors concluded "that omission of EIP has detrimental effects on VA/Q and that the shorter the time of insufflation the worse the effect was".

Flow-preset controlled versus pressure-preset controlled IRV

In adults critical care, the V'C has been the most commonly and extensively mode used for the last decades. In the early nineties, the attention was drawn on the frequency of mechanical ventilation induced lung injuries including pneumothorax, interstitial emphysema, systemic gas embolism, bronchodysplasia and lung inflammatory response [23, 24]. Many experimental studies underlined the detrimental role of excessive tidal volume and alveolar pressure [6, 7] and most clinicians recognized PC mode of ventilation as standard practice in the ventilatory management of ARDS [25]. Indeed PC mode strictly controls the alveolar pressure, thereby avoiding barometric injury and it is speculated that the rapid initial flow rate will open and fill the alveoli quicker and maintain them longer inflated therefore improving gas exchange [26].

When PC is applied to the model (Table 4), it can be seen that the lungs are filled according to their time constant and elastance. This point stresses the importance in the choice of TI when using pressure controlled ventilation, the slow lung unit requiring a long time to be fully inflated.

For example, in model 1, to be fully inflated, the "pathological" compartment 2 requires a TI > 2.5 s.

If we compared the results of the models at TI = 2 s of all the different modalities of ventilation that are used in ARDS patients (Table 5), it could be concluded that, in these models, for a given tidal volume, there are little differences between constant flow + EIP, decelerating flow and constant pressure. Insufflating with low constant flow will produce lower MAP. In term of volume distribution, the best result for model M1 is to use constant flow + EIP, for model M3, it is to use low constant flow. But, to be sure to avoid overdistension of the "normal" lung, it is better to use PC.

The first studies comparing V'CIR and PCIR were performed in patients with ARDS demonstrating a poor response to conventional V'C with a worsening hypoxaemia and respiratory function. The authors underlined that PC mode improved the outcome when compared with predictive mortality rate of severe ARDS [27-29]. Muñoz et al. [30] were the first to compare PC with V'C with a decelerating inspiratory flow pattern in a small group of patients with ARF of various etiologies including COPD. This study failed to demonstrate any impor-

Table 4. Results on the models when applying PPV

TI	0.5			1.0			1.5			2.0			2.5		
Model type	M1	M2	M3	M1	M2	M3	M1	M2	M3	M1	M2	M3	M1	M2	M3
V_1 (TI)	301	325	335	404	424	480	441	454	541	456	463	566	462	465	576
τ_1	0.32	0.24	0.40	0.32	0.24	0.4	0.32	0.24	0.4	0.32	0.24	0.4	0.32	0.24	0.40
% V_{1theo}	66	70	57	86	91	82	94	97	93	98	99	97	99	100	99
V_2 (TI)	102	162	83	163	212	105	197	227	112	215	231	115	223	233	116
τ_2	0.64	0.24	0.24	0.64	0.24	0.24	0.64	0.24	0.24	0.64	0.24	0.24	0.64	0.24	0.24
% V_{2theo}	44	70	70	70	91	90	85	97	96	92	99	98	96	100	99
Pel_1 (TI)	7.5	8.1	6.7	10.1	10.6	9.6	11	11.3	18.8	11.4	11.6	11.3	11.5	11.6	11.5
Pel_2 (TI)	5.1	8.1	8.3	8.1	10.6	10.5	9.8	11.3	11.2	10.7	11.6	11.5	11.2	11.6	11.6
$Pres_1$ (TI)	2.7	2	3.4	1	0.6	1.5	0.3	0.2	0.6	0.1	0.1	0.2	0.1	0	0.1
$Pres_2$ (TI)	5.1	2	1.8	2.9	0.6	0.5	1.5	0.2	0.2	0.8	0.1	0.1	0.4	0	0
Ptrach (TI)	10.2	11.1	10.1	11	11.2	11	11.4	11.5	11.4	11.5	11.6	11.6	11.6	11.6	11.6
V (TI)	403	487	418	567	636	585	638	681	653	671	694	681	685	698	692
% V_{theo}	57	69	58	81	91	83	91	97	93	96	99	97	98	100	99

The level of pressure has been computed in order to assure the same tidal volume (0;7 l) as in flow controlled ventilation. As in the model $C_T = 0.060$ l/cm H_2O, the level of pressure must be set to 0.7/0.06 = 11.67 cm H_2O.

If the time of insufflation TI is long enough, the volume would be distributed according to the compliance of each compartment. The rate of filling of each compartment will depend on its own time constant.

We have reported the value of the volume at TI as the percentage of its theoretical final value, as % V_{theo}

Table 5. Comparison of the different modalities of ventilation at t = 2 s for models M1 and M3

| | M1 at t = 2 s | | | |
	$\tau_1 < \tau_2$			
Mode	Low constant flow	Constant flow + EIP	Decelerating flow	Constant pressure
% V_{1theo} (TI)	105	101	102	97.7
% V_{2theo} (TI)	89.5	97	94.7	92
% V_{theo} (TI)	100	100	100	95.8
Paw, mean	9.3	12.2	11.3	11.7

| | M3 at t = 2 s | | | |
	$\tau_1 > \tau_2$			
Mode	Low constant flow	Constant flow + EIP	Decelerating flow	Constant pressure
% V_{1theo} (TI)	98.5	100	99.6	97
% V_{2theo} (TI)	106	100	102	98.5
% V_{theo} (TI)	100	100	100	97.3
Paw, mean	9	11.9	11	11.7

The results are expressed in percentage of their theoretical value obtained for a TI long enough in PC to fill each compartment according to their elastance. A value greater than 100 represents an overdistension. *Compartment 1* is the "normal" lung, *compartment 2* is the "pathological" lung

tant difference between the two modes of ventilation and the authors concluded that they "do not believe that PC contributes any uniqueness to the theory or practice of mechanical ventilation".

In ARDS patients, Mercat et al. have reported the results of two protocols comparing PC (TI/TE = 1/2) vs PCIR (TI/TE = 2/1) [31] and V'C (TI/TE = 1/2) with a constant inspiratory flow pattern vs PCIR (TI/TE = 2/1) [32], at similar frequency, VT, and PEEPtot. The authors concluded that PC, neither with IR nor without IR, brings any benefit compared with V'C.

In the above mentioned study, Ludwigs et al. [18] have compared in a pig model of ARDS induced by infusion of physiologic saline VCPEEP (I/E ratio = 1/2), VCIR (I/E ratio = 4/1) and PCIR (I/E = ratio 4/1). In comparison to VCPEEP, PCIR resulted in reduced PIP, increased MAP and similar functional residual capacity (FRC). Oxygen delivery and VDphys/VT were significantly lower with PCIR.

In an experimental study using a pig model of oleic acid lung injury [33], V'C and PCIR were randomly applied at constant PEEPtot level and compared in terms of gas exchange, haemodynamics, lung mechanics. Interestingly in this study recruitment of lung tissues, regional lung density and distribution of inspiratory gas were assessed by computed tomography [34]. The authors did not found any significant difference between V'CPEEP and PCIR but a slight decrease in cardiac output, a decrease in peak airway pressure and an increase in MAP.

In summary, up to date no clinical studies have convincingly demonstrated the superiority of neither PC vs V'C nor PCIR versus V'CIR under similar PEEP,tot. This feature probably indicates that the effect of PEEPi and shortened expiration are more important and clinically relevant than alteration of the inspiratory phase, raising the question of compared effect of PEEPi and PEEPe.

PEEPe versus PEEPi

Expiration is "clinically" complete when TE is at least equal to 3 expiration time constants of the respiratory system. IRV produces PEEPi when the inspiration starts before complete return to the previous EELV. PEEPi would occur and increase when lengthening TI, increasing RR or VT. The occurrence rate of PEEPi is high in mechanically ventilated patients with ARF [34, 35]. PEEPi induces an increase in mean alveolar pressure which is occulted and not associated with an equivalent increase in MAP. The trapped air volume cannot be predicted unless the changes of EELV are monitored by thoracic impedance pletysmography [36]. The dynamic hyperinflation has adverse effects on cardiocirculatory system which are similar to PEEPe at identical level.

Using a four chambers model with each chamber having a different time constant from 0.05 s to 0.74 s, Kacmarek et al. [37] showed that when

PEEPe is applied to the local model, local PEEP were all equal to applied PEEPe, whereas during PEEPi local PEEP were dramatically heterogeneous. Similarly local EELVs were more heterogeneously distributed with PEEPi than with PEEPe.

The results obtained with our models are presented in Fig. 2. Local variations of PEEPi may occur depending on the regional time constants. The longer time constant of lung unit, the higher the local PEEPi [38]. By contrast PEEPe is homogeneously distributed within the lung, with an increase in regional EEVs which depends on units elastance.

In summary, from clinical and experimental studies, we can conclude that IRV at a TI/TE ratio that results in PEEPi, does not significantly improve gas exchange and VA/Q mismatching in ARDS patients whatever the mode of ventilation is, when the same level of MAP or PEEPtot is used. These results are somewhat conflicting with theoretical considerations pleading in favor of IRV with decelerating flow and PCIR as regards of volume distribution. This contradiction may be explained by that a redistribution phenomenon does not imply a favorable effect on VA/Q mismatch. Low TI, EIP and PEEPi, together tend to favor slow compartment and the best effect may only be expected if slow compartment and poorly aerated areas are merged. When the fast compartment is represented by the poorly aerated area, the volume redistribution will only lead to underventilation of the pathological area and overdistension of the remaining normal lung. The same problem may occur with PEEPi: when occurring in the poorly aerated part of the lung, recruitment may be responsible for a decrease in intrapulmonary shunt, by contrast when occurring in the near normal part of the lung, PEEPi may be responsible for an overdistension with increase in VA/Q mismatching and deleterious haemodynamic effects as alveolar pressure exceeds capillary pressure.

Another point that must be discussed is whether beneficial effects of IRV may be delayed. Interestingly, in a study from Rappaport [39], two groups of patients with ARDS were randomized to be submitted to either PC or V'C. At 72 h, in patients treated with PC mode, there was a trend toward a more rapid normalization of $PaCO_2$, a more rapid increase in PaO_2/FiO_2 ratio and in compliance. These patients required fewer days of mechanical ventilation. The reason why PC modes could have delayed beneficial effects is somewhat unclear. During this study, the need for sedation was clinically assessed by the physician. Because the physical principle of PC allows a better adaptation of the patients to the ventilator and to breath spontaneously, fewer patients were probably sedated or paralyzed in PC. It must be noted, that in almost all of the previously mentioned studies, the patients were heavily sedated, sometimes even paralyzed to allow acute measurement of mechanics and gas exchange. In a very elegant study, Putensen et al. have compared biphasic positive airway pressure ventilation (BIPAP - Evita Dräger, Germany) with and without spontaneous breathing in a dog model of acute lung injury [40]. In the control group, animals were paralyzed and in the treated group, they were allowed to breath spontaneously. Af-

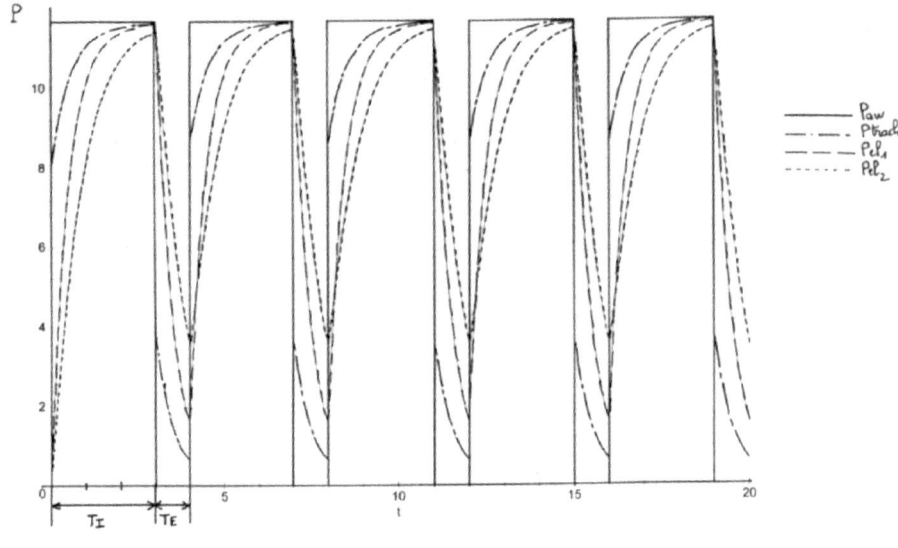

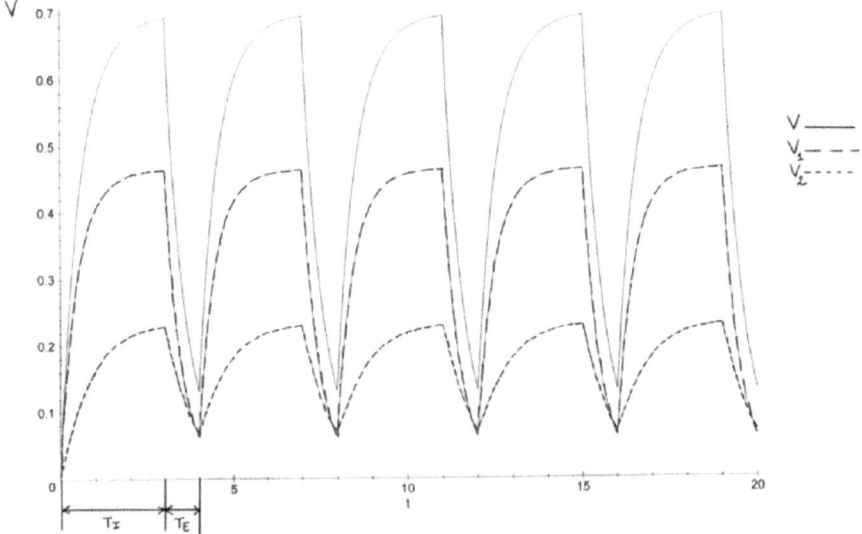

Fig. 2. Example of PCIRV applied to model M1 ($\tau_1 < \tau_2$). In the model, at airway opening, their is no evidence of PEEPi. PEEPi appears in the two compartments, but it is higher in the compartment with the higher time constant ($Pel_2 > Pel_1$). In this specific case, PEEPi could be considered as beneficial allowing a better aeration of the "pathological" compartment

ter 40 min of equilibration on each ventilatory modes, they found that, in the spontaneous breathing group, PaO_2 increased from 61 to 78 mmHg, cardiac output from 4.2 to 4.6 L/min, intrapulmonary shunt and VD/VT decreased respectively of 17% and 6%. Spontaneous breathing accounted only for a 10% increase of minute ventilation. The authors concluded that uncoupling of spontaneous and mechanical breaths during PPV could have substantial beneficial effects on VA/Q mismatching in ARDS patients, perhaps because spontaneous ventilation is mostly directed to well-perfused, dependent lung regions during diaphragmatic contraction.

This beneficial effect of "permissive" spontaneous ventilation added to PPV in mechanical ventilation of ARDS, deserves further clinical investigations.

References

1. Gattinoni L, Pesenti A, Torresini A (1986) Adult respiratory distress syndrome profiles by computed tomography. J Thorac Imag 1:25-30
2. Schlag G, Redl H (1988) The morphology of the adult respiratory distress syndrome. In: Kox W, Bihari D (eds) Shock and the adult respiratory distress syndrome. Springer, Berlin, pp 21-31
3. Suter PM, Fairley HB, Isemberg MD (1978) Effect of tidal volume and positive end expiratory pressure on compliance during mechanical ventilation. Chest 73:158-162
4. Wright P, Bernard G (1989) The role of airflow resistance in patient with the adult respiratory distress syndrome. Am Rev Respir Dis 139:1169-1174
5. Pesenti A, Pelosi P, Rossi N et al (1991) The effects of positive end expiratory pressure on respiratory resistance in patients with adult respiratory distress syndrome and in normal anesthetized subjects. Am Rev Respir Dis 144:101-107
6. Dreyfuss D, Basset G, Soler P et al (1985) Intermittent positive hyperventilation with high inflation pressure produces pulmonary microvascular injury in rats. Am Rev Respir Dis 132: 380-384
7. Dreyfuss D, Saumon G (1993) Role of tidal volume, FRC and end expiratory volume in the development of pulmonary edema following mechanical ventilation. Am Rev Respir Dis 148: 1194-1203
8. Artigas A, Bernard GR, Carlet J et al and the Consensus Committee (1998) The American-European consensus conference on ARDS. Part 2. Ventilatory, pharmacologic, supportive therapy, study design strategies and issues related to recovery and remodeling. Intensive Care Med 24:3 785-398
9. Blanch PB, Jones M, Layon AJ, Camner N (1993) Pressure preset ventilation. Part 1: physiologic and mechanical consideration. Chest 104:590-599
10. Blanch PB, Jones M, Layon AJ, Camner N (1993) Pressure preset ventilation. Part 2: Mechanics and safety. Chest 104:904-912
11. Bates JHT, Rossi A, Milic-Emili J (1985) Analysis of the behavior of the respiratory system with constant inspiratory flow. J Appl Physiol 58:1840-1848
12. Chang HK, Mortola JP (1981) Fluid dynamic factors in tracheal pressure measurement. J Appl Physiol 51:218-225
13. Reynolds E (1971) Effect of alterations in mechanical ventilator settings on pulmonary gas exchange in hyaline membrane disease. Arch Dis Child 46:152-159
14. Cole ACG, Weller SF, Sykes MK (1984) Inverse ratio ventilation compared with PEEP in adult respiratory distress syndrome. Intensive Care Med 10:227-232

15. Gurevitch MJ, Van Dyke J, Young ES, Jackson K (1986) Improved oxygenation and lower peak airway pressure in severe adult respiratory distress syndrome: treatment with inverse ratio ventilation. Chest 89:211-213
16. Marcy WT, Marini JJ (1991) Inverse ratio ventilation, rationale for implementation. Chest 100:494-504
17. Mang H, Kacmareck RM, Ritz R et al (1995) Cardiorespiratory effects of volume and pressure controlled ventilation at various I/E ratios in an acute lung injury model. Am J Respir Crit Care Med 151:731-736
18. Ludwigs U, Klingstedt C, Baehrendtz S, Hedenstierna G (1997) A comparison of pressure and volume-controlled ventilation at different inspiratory to expiratory ratio. Acta Anaesthesiol Scand 41:71-77
19. Zavala E, Ferrer M, Polese G et al (1998) Effect of inverse ratio ventilation on gas exchange in acute respiratory distress syndrome. Anesthesiology 88:35-42
20. Davis K, Branson RD, Campbell RS, Porembka DT (1996) Comparison of volume control and pressure control ventilation: is flow wave form the difference? J Trauma 41:808-814
21. Markström AM, Lichtwarck-Aschoff M, Svensson BA et al (1996) Ventilation with constant versus decelerating inspiratory flow in experimentally induced acute respiratory failure. Anesthesiology 84:882-889
22. Pillet O, Choukroun ML, Castaing Y (1993) Effects of inspiratory flow rate alteration on gas exchange during mechanical ventilation in normal lungs. Chest 103:1161-1165
23. Gammon RB, Shin MS, Groves RH et al (1995) Clinical risk factors for pulmonary barotrauma: a multivariate analysis. Am J Respir Crit Care Med 152:1235-1240
24. Rouby JJ, Lherm T, De Lasalle ME et al (1993) Histological aspect of pulmonary barotrauma in critically ill patients with acute respiratory failure. Intensive Care Med 19:383-389
25. MacIntyre NR (1993) Clinically available new strategies for mechanical ventilatory support. Chest 104:560-565
26. Abraham E, Yoshihara G (1989) Cardiorespiratory effect of pressure controlled ventilation in severe respiratory failure. Chest 96:1356-1359
27. Tharratt RS, Allen RP, Albertson TE (1988) Pressure controlled inverse ratio ventilation in severe adult respiratory failure. Chest 94:755-762
28. Sassoon CSH (1991) Positive pressure ventilation: alternate modes. Chest 100:494-604
29. Lachmann B, Schairer W, Armbrusters S et al (1989) Improved arterial oxygenation and CO_2 elimination following changes from generated PEEP ventilation with inspiratory/expiratory ratio of 1/2 to pressure generated ventilation with I/E of 4/1 in patients with severe ARDS. Adv Exp Med Biol 248:779-786
30. Muñoz J, Guerrero JE, Escalante J et al (1993) Pressure controlled ventilation versus controlled mechanical ventilation with decelerating flow. Crit Care Med 21:1143-1148
31. Mercat A, Graïni L, Teboul JL et al (1993) Cardiorespiratory effects of pressure controlled ventilation with and without inverse ratio in the adult respiratory distress syndrome. Chest 104:871-875
32. Mercat A, Titiriga M, Anguel N et al (1997) Inverse ratio ventilation (I/E = 2/1) in acute respiratory distress syndrome. A six-hour controlled study. Am J Respir Crit Care Med 155: 1637-1642
33. Ludwigs U, Klingstedt C, Baehrendtz S et al (1994) A functional and morphologic analysis of pressure-controlled ventilation in oleic acid lung injury. Chest 106:925-931
34. Brown DG, Pierson DJ (1986) Auto-PEEP in mechanically ventilated patients: A study of incidence, severity and detection. Respir Care 31:1069-1074
35. Patel H, Yang KL (1995) Variability of positive end-expiratory pressure in patient receiving mechanical ventilation. Crit Care Med 23:1074-1079
36. Hoffman RA, Ershowsky P, Krieger BP (1989) Determination of auto-PEEP during spontaneous and controlled ventilation by monitoring changes in end expiratory thoracic gas volume. Chest 96:613-616

37. Kacmarek RM, Kirmse M, Nishimura N et al (1995) The effects of applied vs auto-PEEP on local lung unit pressure and volume in a four-unit lung model. Chest 108:1073-1979
38. Pepe PE, Marini JJ (1982) Occult end expiratory pressure in mechanically ventilated patients with airflow obstruction. Am J Respir Dis 126:166-170
39. Rappaport SH, Shpiner R, Yoshiara G et al (1994) Randomized prospective trial of pressure-limited versus volume-controlled ventilation in severe respiratory failure. Crit Care Med 22:22-32
40. Putensen C, Räsänen J, Lopez FA (1994) Ventilation-perfusion distribution during mechanical ventilation with surimposed spontaneous breathing in canine lung injury. Am J Respir Care Med 150:101-108

Problems Associated with Clinical Determination of Pulmonary Shunting

H.M. LOHBRUNNER, K.J. FALKE

A disturbance of pulmonary gas exchange results in hypoxaemia and hypercarbia. Given a stable cardiac output and a known FiO_2, it is possible to explain changes in arterial PO_2 and PCO_2 by mismatch of alveolar ventilation to pulmonary perfusion or disturbance of the distribution of the alveolar ventilation to perfusion ratio ($\dot{V}_A/\dot{Q}$). The normal healthy lung consists of more than 300 million alveoli which all receive the same inspiratory gas and mixed venous blood. Nevertheless the composition of intraalveolar and endcapillary partial pressures of O_2, CO_2 and N_2 differ between various areas of the lung because the partial pressures in the alveoli (P_A) depend upon the $\dot{V}_A/\dot{Q}$.

Three main causes lead to an increased alveolar-arterial oxygen difference ($AaDO_2$):

$\dot{V}_A/\dot{Q}$ mismatching (lung areas with low $\dot{V}_A/\dot{Q}$ resulting in a $\dot{Q}\bar{v}a/\dot{Q}_T$ effect) and the physiological or "true" right-to-left shunt ($\dot{Q}_S/\dot{Q}_T$) in compartments with $\dot{V}_A/\dot{Q} = 0$ and diffusion impairment.

Abbreviations

$\dot{Q}$	blood flow
P	partial pressure
Pa	arterial partial pressure
P_A	alveolar partial pressure
P_U	partial pressure of the gas in the arterialized blood of the underventilated compartment
Pi	partial pressure of the gas in the "ideal" compartment
$P\bar{v}$	partial pressure of the gas in the mixed venous blood
CaO_2	arterial oxygen content
$C\bar{v}O_2$	mixed venous oxygen content
CcO_2	capillary oxygen content
$\dot{Q}_U$	blood flow of the underventilated compartment
$\dot{Q}\bar{v}a/\dot{Q}_U$	venous admixture of the underventilated compartment
$\dot{V}_A/\dot{Q}$	ratio of alveolar ventilation and perfusion
$\dot{V}i/\dot{Q}i$	$\dot{V}_A/\dot{Q}$ ratio of the "ideal" compartment
$\dot{V}_U/\dot{Q}_U$	$\dot{V}_A/\dot{Q}$ ratio of the underventilated compartment
$\dot{Q}\bar{v}a/\dot{Q}_T$	venous admixture including $\dot{Q}_S/\dot{Q}_T$, low $\dot{V}_A/\dot{Q}$ (and diffusion impairment)
$\dot{Q}_S/\dot{Q}_T$	"true" right-to-left shunt ($\dot{V}_A/\dot{Q} = 0$)
SO_2	oxygen saturation of haemoglobin

The role of diffusion impairment in producing hypoxaemia appears to be quite small in most ICU patients with respiratory diseases [1, 2]. Consequently, in order to explore an increased $AaDO_2$, it is necessary to differentiate between the effect of $\dot{V}_A/\dot{Q}$ mismatching from $\dot{Q}_S/\dot{Q}_T$.

Estimation of $\dot{Q}\overline{v}a/\dot{Q}_T$ - venous admixture at $FiO_2 < 1.0$

In 1949, Riley and Cournand [3] developed a three-compartment model of the lung for quantification of $\dot{V}_A/\dot{Q}$ mismatch causing $AaDO_2$:

a) "ideal" compartment with normal ventilation and perfusion $\Rightarrow \dot{V}_A/\dot{Q} \approx 1$;

b) normal ventilation, no perfusion $\Rightarrow \dot{V}_A/\dot{Q} = \infty \Rightarrow V_D/V_T$ physiologic dead space (Appendix 1);

c) no ventilation, normal perfusion $\Rightarrow \dot{V}_A/\dot{Q} = 0 \Rightarrow$ physiological "true" shunt $\dot{Q}_S/\dot{Q}_T$;

plus

   venous admixture produced by areas of low $\dot{V}_A/\dot{Q}$ between $0 - 0.1$ (Appendix 2).

In 1942, Berggren [4] derived:

$$\dot{Q}\overline{v}a/\dot{Q}_T = (CcO_2 - CaO_2) / (CcO_2 - C\overline{v}O_2) \text{ (compare Fig. 1)}$$

Under clinical conditions, however, measurement of capillary oxygen content (CcO_2) is impossible without analysis of P_AO_2 by a mass spectrograph. Thus an estimation under consideration of FiO_2 is necessary [5]: $P_AO_2 = FiO_2$ x $(P_{baro} - P_{H_2O}) - PaCO_2$.

With $CcO_2 = (Hb \times SO_2 \times 1.39) + (P_AO_2 \times 0.0031)$ $\dot{Q}\overline{v}a/\dot{Q}_T$ can be calculated. Furthermore, met- and CO-haemoglobin must directly be measured because the haemoglobin is not completely saturated with oxygen [6]. Finally, determination of $\dot{Q}\overline{v}a/\dot{Q}_T$ at $FiO_2 < 1.0$ does not permit differentiation between true shunt $\dot{Q}_S/\dot{Q}_T$ and areas of low $\dot{V}_A/\dot{Q}$ (compare again Fig. 1).

Determination of physiological shunt at FiO_2 1.0

The most usual clinical method of differentiating $\dot{Q}_S/\dot{Q}_T$ from $\dot{Q}\overline{v}a/\dot{Q}$ – first described by Berggren [4] – is the ventilation with FiO_2 1.0. After 10-20 minutes of breathing 100% oxygen until all alveolar N_2 has been washed out, alveolar gas consists only of O_2, CO_2 and H_2O vapore:

$$P_AO_2 = P_{baro} - P_{H_2O} - P_ACO_2$$

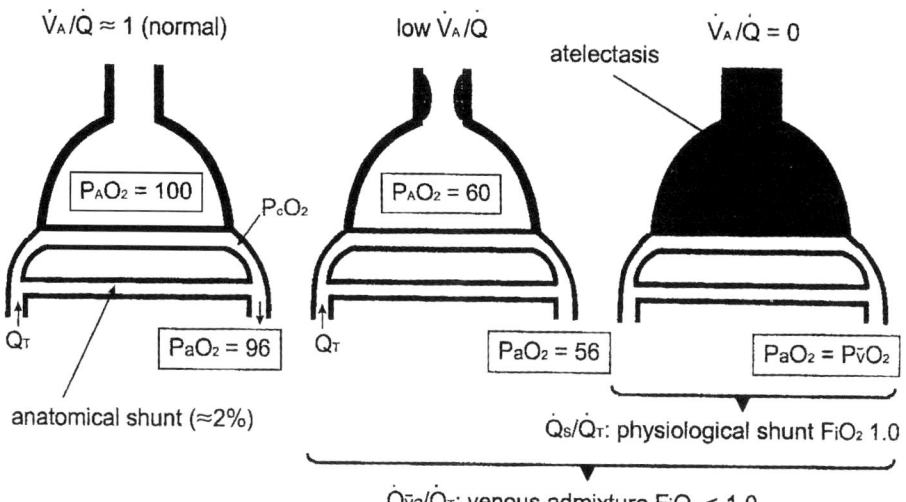

Fig. 1. The components of pulmonary venous admixture

The assumption, however, is necessary that P_ACO_2 is equal to $PaCO_2$, which is clinically easy to measure. With high tensions of alveolar oxygen, equilibration between gas phase and capillary blood is (again assumed) complete:

$$CcO_2 = (Hb \times SO_2 \times 1.39) + (P_AO_2 \times 0.0031)$$

Now $\dot{Q}_S/\dot{Q}_T$ can be calculated as:

$$\dot{Q}_S/\dot{Q}_T = (CcO_2 - CaO_2) / (CcO_2 - C\overline{v}O_2)$$

provided 100% O_2 has been breathed for sufficient time to remove N_2 from areas of low $\dot{V}_A/\dot{Q}$. Thus by differentiating $\dot{Q}\overline{v}a/\dot{Q}_T$ and $\dot{Q}_S/\dot{Q}_T$ at $FiO_2 < 1.0$ and $FiO_2 = 1.0$ an estimation of venous admixture by areas of low $\dot{V}_A/\dot{Q}$ is possible.

If the shunt – expressed by this equation – produces relevant desaturation of arterial blood, CaO_2 must be determined as well as $C\overline{v}O_2$ in analogy to the above mentioned equation for the calculation of CcO_2.

The 100% oxygen method yields conflicting results [7-12]. Alterations can be explained by:

a) collapse of alveolar units in areas of low $\dot{V}_A/\dot{Q}$ if inspiratory ventilation is lower than gas absorption. Formation of atelectasis increases $\dot{Q}_S/\dot{Q}_T$ [8, 13];

b) ventilation with 100% oxygen ameliorates the hypoxical pulmonary vasoconstriction in non-ventilated areas. The effect of this phenomenon on $\dot{Q}_S/\dot{Q}_T$ is not definitively explained [14].

The overestimation of $\dot{Q}_S/\dot{Q}_T$ by the oxygen method compared with inert gas retention results from an incomplete washout of nitrogen affecting mostly low $\dot{V}_A/\dot{Q}$ areas [15].

Sulfur hexafluoride retention

The determination of sulfur hexafluoride retention (SF_6; gas partition coefficient $\lambda = 6 \times 10^{-3}$ ml ml^{-1} 760 mmHg^{-1}) is a simple method, based on accepted physiological principles, to differentiate between true shunt and $\dot{V}_A/\dot{Q}$ maldistribution at maintenance FiO_2, without any disturbances of the patients pathophysiology. SF_6 is a commonly used inert gas in respiratory physiology. By infusing the gas into the venous circulation it is possible to create the following equation for a considered homogeneous compartment of the lung [2, 16]:

$$\frac{Pa}{P\bar{v}} = \frac{\lambda}{\lambda + \dot{V}_A/\dot{Q}}$$

"Underventilation" $(_U)$ of any lung compartment will contribute to a venous admixture effect of the whole lung. Now it is possible to consider the blood returning from underventilated compartments as two separated components:

1. one component with Pa = Pi of the "ideal" lung, with "ideal" $\dot{V}_A/\dot{Q} = \dot{V}i/\dot{Q}i$
2. the other component in which Pa = $P\bar{v}$.

Farhi and Yokoyama [17] have shown that the venous admixture of the underventilated compartment can be calculated as:

$$\frac{\dot{Q}\bar{v}a}{\dot{Q}_U} = \frac{P_U - Pi}{P\bar{v} - Pi} = \frac{\dot{V}i/\dot{Q}i - \dot{V}_U/\dot{Q}_U}{\dot{V}i/\dot{Q}i} \times \frac{1}{\lambda \times (\lambda + \dot{V}_U/\dot{Q}_U)}$$

For a given $\dot{V}_U/\dot{Q}_U$ and using a gas like SF_6 with a very low value of λ the $\dot{Q}\bar{v}a/\dot{Q}$ of the compartment considered homogeneously is as low as the factor λ. Any compartment with a $\dot{V}_A/\dot{Q}$ ratio ≥ 0.05 does not contribute significantly to the overall $\dot{Q}\bar{v}a/\dot{Q}(SF_6)$. Hence, even if 50% of $\dot{Q}$ flows through compartments with a $\dot{V}_A/\dot{Q}$ ratio = 0.05, the overall lung $\dot{Q}\bar{v}a/\dot{Q}(SF_6)$ will only be 0.05 [15]. On the other hand, when blood perfuses alveoli with a $\dot{V}_A/\dot{Q}$ ratio = 0, their contribution to $\dot{Q}_S/\dot{Q}_T$ will be the same for gases of any λ. If the ventilation is truly 0, SF_6 cannot leave the capillaries. Than $\dot{Q}\bar{v}a/\dot{Q}(SF_6)$ measures only $\dot{Q}_S/\dot{Q}_T$, and is just marginally affected by $\dot{V}_A/\dot{Q}$ mismatch ($\dot{Q}\bar{v}a/\dot{Q}(SF_6) \approx \dot{Q}_S/\dot{Q}_T(SF_6)$). Because of the extremely low partial pressure of SF_6 (PSF_6) the measure of $\dot{Q}_S/\dot{Q}_T(SF_6)$ can be reduced to:

$$\dot{Q}S/\dot{Q}T(SF_6) = \frac{Pa - Pi}{P\bar{v} - Pi} \approx \frac{Pa}{P\bar{v}} = \text{Retention of } SF_6$$

Thus measurement of SF_6 retention permits the differentiation of $\dot{Q}\bar{v}a/\dot{Q}$ effect of O_2:

1. "true" shunt $\dot{Q}_S/\dot{Q}_T \approx \dot{Q}_S/\dot{Q}_T(SF_6)$ with $\dot{V}_A/\dot{Q} \approx 0$
2. $\dot{V}_A/\dot{Q}$ mismatch, indicated by $\dot{Q}\bar{v}a/\dot{Q}(O_2) - \dot{Q}_S/\dot{Q}_T(SF_6)$

Multiple inert gas elimination technique

The multiple inert gas analysis is technically very complex and has never reached widespread clinical use [15], but it is still the most powerful investigational tool and the gold standard for analyzing $\dot{V}_A/\dot{Q}$ distributions. The method is based on the law of mass maintenance for six inert gases: SF_6, ethane, cyclopropane, halothane, ether and acetone which represent a widespread range of λ (0.005 SF_6 – 300 acetone) [18]. After continuous intravenous infusion and under steady-state conditions partial pressures of the inert gases in mixed expired gas, arterial blood and mixed venous blood will be measured by gas chromatography. After calculation of retention R = $Pa/P\bar{v}$ and excretion E = $P_{exp}/P\bar{v}$ and determination of individual solubility the description of continuous ventilation-perfusion distributions over the whole range of $\dot{V}_A/\dot{Q}$ ratios is possible in a lung model with 50 compartments. An increased retention of gases with low solubility indicates the presence of areas with low $\dot{V}_A/\dot{Q}$. A decreased excretion of gases with high λ represents regions with high $\dot{V}_A/\dot{Q}$ ratios [17-20].

What are the problems under clinical circumstances?

The differentiation of the relative amount of hypoxaemia due to $\dot{Q}_S/\dot{Q}_T$ from the amount due to $\dot{V}_A/\dot{Q}$ mismatch is important for treatment and understanding of impaired gas exchange during respiratory failure.

Total intrapulmonary shunting can be devided into two main components:

1. constant or anatomical shunt caused by bronchial, pleural, Thebesian veins and arteriovenous communications ($\approx 2\%$ of cardiac output);
2. variable or capillary shunt caused by atelectasis, $\dot{V}_A/\dot{Q}$ mismatch and diffusion impairment.

When air is breathed, the total venous admixture provides an estimation of the amount of blood which has to be shunted past the lung in order to produce a combined effect of $\dot{V}_A/\dot{Q}$ mismatch and true right-to-left shunt. This estimation is theoretically only applicable, if all the shunted blood has the same composition and all alveoli contain the same "ideal" gas. Anatomical shunting will be ignored, and also it is assumed that all shunted blood is mixed venous. Furthermore, it will be assumed that alveolar and end-capillary oxygen tensions are equal. These assumptions and the necessity of five measurements with individual faults lead to inaccuracy and unreliable data. Differentiation of $\dot{Q}_S/\dot{Q}_T$ from $\dot{Q}\overline{v}a/\dot{Q}_T$ at FiO_2 1.0 – which eliminates the "ideal" alveolar gas problem – is limited by formation of atelectasis and amelioration of hypoxical pulmonary vasoconstriction. Provided that limitations of these analyses are understood, the methods allow a useful clinical estimation of the failure of the lung to oxygenate the mixed venous blood. In pulmonary diseases with a high amount of $\dot{Q}_S/\dot{Q}_T$ – for example severe ARDS – venous admixture and 100% method overestimate the intrapulmonary shunt. This effect is mainly caused by an incomplete washout of N_2 affecting low $\dot{V}_A/\dot{Q}$ areas [15].

The intrinsic features of SF_6 make this inert gas an ideal tool for the determination of $\dot{Q}_S/\dot{Q}_T$. Due to its very low solubility in blood $\dot{Q}\overline{v}a/\dot{Q}_T$ of SF_6 is the best estimation of physiological shunt, also in diseases with abnormal high $\dot{Q}_S/\dot{Q}_T$, under extracorporeal circulation or for investigation of the influence of FiO_2 on the effect of nitric oxide (NO) on intrapulmonary shunt. MIGET offers hardly the most information about the true shunt and $\dot{V}_A/\dot{Q}$ distributions, but is much more complex than SF_6 retention method alone. The effects of any selected therapy on pulmonary gas exchange – for example different modes of mechanical ventilation modifying the $\dot{V}_A/\dot{Q}$ mismatch – could relatively easily and satisfactory be tested with a combination of SF_6 retention, venous admixture and 100% O_2 breathing method.

Today there are several different models available for quantifying the ventilation perfusion mismatch. Measurement of PO_2 and PCO_2 in blood and expired gas permits an estimation of $\dot{V}_A/\dot{Q}$ and physiological dead space. Usually, this suffices enough for clinical practice. The inert gas elimination technique allows determination of nearly continuous ventilation-perfusion distributions over the whole range of $\dot{V}_A/\dot{Q}$ ratios, but is technically more than complex and thus will remain a tool for scientific investigations. The use of SF_6 retention to identify the true shunt at maintenance FiO_2 is suggested feasible for clinical use because absolute gas calibration or data of absolute gas partial pressures are not required [15].

Conclusion

The determination of intrapulmonary shunting ($\dot{Q}_S/\dot{Q}_T$) is of great interest in applying and evaluating different therapeutic approaches in critically ill patients. Investigation of the ventilation and perfusion mismatch ($\dot{V}_A/\dot{Q}$) helps to explain frequent respiratory problems which result in hypoxaemia and hypercarbia. Different methods are available for evaluating $\dot{V}_A/\dot{Q}$ mismatching.

Analysis of PO_2 and PCO_2 in arterial and mixed venous blood and mixed expired gas, calculation of the physiologic dead space (V_D/V_T) and venous admixture ($\dot{Q}\overline{v}a/\dot{Q}_T$) makes estimation of the degree of present mismatching possible. These data allow a quantitative analysis according to a three compartment model of the lung [21]. The necessity, however, to make an assumption of the capillary oxygen content (CcO_2) by inspiratory oxygen fraction (FiO_2) < 1.0 leads to an overestimation of alveolar PO_2 (P_AO_2) and to inaccuracy.

Estimation of $\dot{Q}_S/\dot{Q}_T$ at FiO_2 1.0 alters the lung conditions *per se* by vasodilatation, formation of absorption atelectasis, and amelioration of hypoxic pulmonary vasoconstriction (HPV). Therefore the method appears unsatisfactory for the shunt determination in patients with distinct HPV.

The multiple inert gas elimination technique (MIGET) permits nearly continuous precise description of ventilation-perfusion distributions over the whole range of $\dot{V}_A/\dot{Q}$ ratios. This technique has contributed to explain the pathophysiology in most of pulmonary diseases. Its application, however, is more than complex and the validity of the results depends on stable haemodynamics for a long lasting period of investigation [21].

The use of sulfur hexafluoride (SF_6) retention is an easier way to identify the true shunt ($\dot{V}_A/\dot{Q} < 0.05$) at maintenance FiO_2. $\dot{Q}_S/\dot{Q}_T$ estimation is given by the ratio $PaSF_6/P\bar{v}SF_6$. This method is suggested as appropriate for clinical use [15].

Appendix

1. Enghoff [22] calculated V_D/V_T:

$$V_D/V_T = (PaCO_2 - P_{exp}CO_2) / PaCO_2$$

This equation is a simplification of the Bohr-equation [23] because P_ACO_2 will be replaced by $PaCO_2$.

Dead space is the amount of inspiratory gas which is added to the "ideal" alveolar gas, and yields expiratory gas mixture. If P_ACO_2 is supposed to be identical with $PaCO_2$, calculation of V_D/V_T is not influenced by CO_2-retention in areas of low $\dot{V}_A/\dot{Q}$.

Total ventilation V_T is the sum of alveolar ventilation and ventilation of the dead space:

$$V_T = V_A + V_D$$

Only ventilated areas of the lung can excrete CO_2:

$$VCO_2 = V_A \times F_ACO_2 = V_T \times F_{exp}CO_2$$

After exchange of FCO_2 with PCO_2 and the assumption that $P_AO_2 = PaO_2$ results:

$$V_D/V_T = (PaCO_2 - P_{exp}CO_2) / PaCO_2$$

2. Cardiac output $\dot{Q}_T$ is the sum of $\dot{Q}_{shunt}$ ($\dot{Q}_S$) and $\dot{Q}_{lung\ capillary}$ ($\dot{Q}c$):

$$\dot{Q}_T = \dot{Q}_S + \dot{Q}c \text{ (compare with Fig. 1)}$$

If $\dot{Q}_T \times CaO_2 = \dot{Q}_S \times C\bar{v}O_2 + \dot{Q}c \times CcO_2$ follows:

$$\dot{Q}_S/\dot{Q}_T = (CcO_2 - CaO_2) / (CcO_2 - C\bar{v}O_2) = \dot{Q}\bar{v}a/\dot{Q}_T \text{ in the "ideal" compartment with } \dot{V}_A/\dot{Q} \approx 1$$

If PaO_2 is > 150 mmHg and haemoglobin is completely saturated with oxygen, $\dot{Q}_S/\dot{Q}_T$ can be calculated also as:

$$\frac{\dot{Q}_S}{\dot{Q}_T} = \frac{AaDO_2 \times 0.0031}{AaDO_2 \times 0.031 + (CaO_2 - C\bar{v}O_2)}$$

and $AaDO_2^{1.0}$ as:

$$AaDO_2^{1.0} = (P_{baro} - PaCO_2 - P_{H_2O}) - PaO_2$$

The application, however, of this equation in patients suffering from lung diseases with high $\dot{Q}_S/\dot{Q}_T$, for example in severe Adult Respiratory Distress Syndrome (ARDS), is not allowed. These patients *per se* do not have completely oxygen-saturated haemoglobin or a PaO_2 > 150 mmHg.

References

1. Dantzker DR, Brook CJ, Dehart P et al (1979) Ventilation-perfusion distributions in the adult respiratory distress syndrome. Am Rev Respir Dis 120:1039-1052
2. West JB, Wagner PD (1998) Pulmonary gas exchange. Am J Respir Crit Care Med 157: S82-S87
3. Riley RL, Cournand A (1949) "Ideal" alveolar air and the analysis of ventilation-perfusion relationships in the lung. J Appl Physiol 1:825
4. Berggren S (1942) The oxygen deficit of arterial blood caused by non-ventilating parts of the lung. Acta Physiol Scand [Suppl II]:1
5. Martin L (1986) Abbreviating the alveolar gas equation: an argument for simplicity. Resp Care 31:40
6. Cane RD, Shapiro BA, Harrison RA et al (1980) Minimizing errors in intrapulmonary shunt calculations. Crit Care Med 8:294-297
7. Carlon GC, Howland WS, Turnbull AD et al (1980) Pulmonary venous admixture during mechanical ventilation with varying FIO_2 and PEEP. Crit Care Med 8:616-619
8. Dantzker DR, Wagner PD, West JB (1974) Proceedings: Instability of poorly ventilated lung units during oxygen breathing. J Physiol Lond 242:72P
9. Quan SF, Kronberg GM, Schlobohm RM et al (1980) Changes in venous admixture with alterations of inspired oxygen concentration. Anesthesiology 52:477-482
10. Shapiro AR, Virgilio RW, Peters RM (1977) Interpretation of alveolar-arterial oxygen tension difference. Surg Gynecol Obstet 144:547-552
11. Shapiro BA, Cane RD, Harrison RA et al (1980) Changes in intrapulmonary shunting with administration of 100 percent oxygen. Chest 77:138-141
12. Suter PM, Fairley HB, Schlobohm RM (1975) Shunt, lung volume and perfusion during short periods of ventilation with oxygen. Anesthesiology 43:617-627
13. Wagner PD, Laravuso RB, Uhl RR et al (1974) Distributions of ventilation-perfusion ratios in acute respiratory failure. Chest 65[Suppl]:32S-35S
14. Lampron N, Lemaire F, Teisseire B et al (1985) Mechanical ventilation with 100% oxygen does not increase intrapulmonary shunt in patients with severe bacterial pneumonia. Am Rev Respir Dis 131:409-413
15. Pesenti A, Latini R, Riboni A et al (1982) Simple estimate of the true right to left shunt (Qs/Qt) at maintenance FIO_2 by sulphur hexafluoride retention. Intensive Care Med 8: 283-286
16. Fahri LE (1967) Elimination of inert gases by the lung. Respir Physiol 3:1
17. Fahri LE, Yokoyama T (1967) Effects of ventilation perfusion inequality on elimination of inert gases. Respir Physiol 3:12

18. Wagner PD, Saltzman HA, West JB (1974) Measurement of continuous distributions of venti-
    lation-perfusion ratios: theory. J Appl Physiol 36:588-599
19. Evans JW, Wagner PD, West JB (1974) Conditions for reduction of pulmonary gas transfer by
    ventilation-perfusion inequality. J Appl Physiol 36:533-537
20. Wagner PD, Naumann PF, Laravuso RB (1974) Simultaneous measurement of eight foreign
    gases in blood by gas chromatography. J Appl Physiol 36:600-605
21. Radermacher P, Cinotti L, Falke KJ (1988) Grundlagen der methodischen Erfassung von Ven-
    tilations-Perfusions-Verteilungsstörungen. Anaesthesist 37:36-42
22. Enghoff H (1937) Volumen inefficax. Bemerkungen zur Frage des schädlichen Raumes. Up-
    sala Laekareforen Foerh 44:191
23. Bohr C (1891) Über die Lungenatmung. Scand Arch Physiol 2:236

Pulmonary Hypertension

J.O.C. Auler Jr, M.J.C. Carmona

Acute respiratory distress syndrome (ARDS) presents a combination of nonspecific alveolar damage and extensive pulmonary vascular disease [1]. Noncardiogenic pulmonary oedema, hypoxaemia, decreased lung compliance, increased pulmonary artery pressures, and the requirement for mechanical ventilation are important signs of this syndrome [2]. Pulmonary artery hypertension and increased pulmonary vascular resistance have been identified as markers of the severity of ARDS and are related to vascular thrombosis [3] and pulmonary vasoconstriction.

The normal pulmonary circulation

Haemoglobin is normally oxygenated to nearly full capacity and the blood is cleansed of much particular matter and bacteria during the passage of blood cells through the lungs. Generally, the pulmonary vascular bed offers remarkably little resistance to flow. Pulmonary hypertension results from reductions in the caliber of the pulmonary vessels and/or increases in pulmonary blood flow [4, 5].

The normal pulmonary artery pressure has a peak systolic value of 18 to 25 mmHg, an end-diastolic value of 6 to 10 mmHg and a mean value ranging from 12 to 16 mmHg, in a person living at sea level. Definite pulmonary hypertension is present when pulmonary artery systolic and mean pressure exceed 30 and 20 mmHg, respectively. The normal mean pulmonary venous pressure is 6 to 10 mmHg; therefore, the normal arteriovenous pressure difference, moves the entire cardiac output from 2 to 10 mmHg. This small pressure gradient is all the more remarkable when one considers that to move the same amount of blood per minute through the systemic vascular bed, a pressure differencial of approximately 90 mmHg (systemic arterial mean pressure minus right atrial mean pressure) is required.

Thus, the normal pulmonary vascular bed offers less than one-tenth the resistance to flow offered by the systemic bed. Vascular resistance is generally quantified, by analogy to Ohm's law, as the ratio of drop in pressure (ΔP in mm

Hg) to mean flow (Q in liters/min). The ratio is commonly multiplied by 79.9 to express the results in dynes.s.cm^{-5}. The calculated pulmonary vascular resistance in normal adults is 67 ± 23 dynes.s.cm^{-5} or 1 Wood unit.

Vascular resistance reflects a composite of variables that includes, but is not limited to, the cross-sectional area of small muscular arteries and arterioles. Other determinants are blood viscosity, the total mass of lung tissue (i.e., resistance is higher in infants and children than in adults), proximal vascular obstruction (e.g., pulmonary coarctation, pulmonary embolism, peripheral pulmonary stenosis), and extramural compression of vessels (perivascular oedema).

Because the pulmonary vascular bed contains considerable elastic tissue, the cross-sectional area of the bed varies directly with transmural pressure and flow. Therefore, pulmonary vascular resistance decreases passively with increases in flow. This fall in resistance results in part from the increase in the radius of distensible vessels secondary to increased flow. From a consideration of the Poiseuille relationship – in which $R = \Delta P/Q = 8 \, \eta l/\pi r^4$, where R = resistance, ΔP = pressure drop, Q = flow, η = viscosity of fluid, and l and r = length and radius of the vessel, respectively – it is apparent that resistance can be effectively influenced by even small changes in the radius of the vessel. Recruitment of additional vascular channels also contributes to the fall in resistance that characterizes increased flow through the pulmonary circuit. This phenomenon is particularly prominent in the upright position, where vessels in the upper parts of the lungs are in a partially collapsed state owing to low hydrostatic pressure.

The reduction in resistance in a distensible vascular bed that occurs with increased flow has been offered as the explanation for the absence of pulmonary hypertension in many patients with large left-to-right intracardiac shunts, particularly atrial septal defects. However, it must be pointed out that increased distensibility of pulmonary vessels in such situations has developed over years and that this principle is not necessarily applicable to acute increase in pulmonary blood flow. In this regard, the results of studies with unilateral occlusion of a pulmonary artery using a balloon catheter are relevant. Acute increases in flow in the supine position were associated with increase in ΔP, so that vascular resistance of the lung (the slope of the line relating ΔP to flow) remained unchanged. In the upright position, however, blood vessels in the upper part of the lung are usually in a partially or fully collapsed state and with an increase in flow, these vessels may expand, thereby reducing vascular resistance.

Pulmonary hypertension

Pulmonary hypertension results from reductions in the caliber of the pulmonary vessels and/or increases in pulmonary blood flow. Unlike the systemic blood vessels, where the response to hypoxaemia is vasodilation, the pulmonary vessels respond with vasoconstriction [5-7]. This occurs in small arteries and arterioles (less than 200 μm in diameter) when the alveolar PO_2 decreases to less than 60 mmHg [8, 9]. The exact mechanism governing this response is unclear, and there are at least two proposed pathways: a direct effect on the vascular smooth muscle and an indirect effect causing release of vasoactive substances from the pulmonary parenchyma [10]. Although both adrenergic and cholinergic fibers are found in the lung and may be of importance in reflex responses in the foetus, they apparently play a minor role if any in the adult response to hypoxia. Pulmonary vasoconstriction may represent a self-regulatory mechanism for adjusting capillary perfusion to alveolar ventilation.

It is well established that acute hypoxia elicits pulmonary vasoconstriction, and it is general agreement that this response is part of a self regulatory mechanism for adjusting capillary perfusion to alveolar ventilation. There appears to be an age dependency and a considerable species variability in the magnitude of this vasoconstrictor response, which is quite intense in cattle, intermediate in humans and the pig, and comparatively mild in dogs and sheep; hypoxic vasoconstriction is more profound in the infant or young mammal than in the adult. Variability exists within a given species as well, and there is strong evidence for a genetic determination of individual reactivity to hypoxia in animals.

The mechanism of the acute pulmonary vasoconstriction that occurs in response to hypoxia is uncertain. There is some evidence that hypoxia-induced local release of histamine may play an important role with pulmonary vasoconstriction secondary to stimulation of pulmonary vascular H_1-receptors. There has been considerable speculation about the role of vascular endothelium as a mediator of hypoxis-induced pulmonary vasoconstriction. This is based on recent findings concerning the role of vascular endothelium in the regulation of vascular smooth muscle contraction and relaxation. Balanced release of endothelial-derived relaxing factor (EDRF) and of the vasoconstrictor peptide endothelin by endothelial cells plays a critical role in the regulation of tone in systemic vascular resistance vessels and may be of considerable importance in the pulmonary circulation as well.

Considerable evidence suggests a role for increased Ca^{++} entry into vascular smooth muscle mediating hypoxic pulmonary vasoconstriction. The concentration of Ca^{++} in the vicinity of the contractile machinery represents a balance between the inflow and outflow across the cell membrane. Although most of the evidence favors an influx of Ca^{++} from extracellular fluid, the relative contribution of differential mobilization from intracellular stores is unsettled. The mechanism responsible for intracellular mobilization of Ca^{++} is also unclear.

Changes in alveolar oxygenation affect the oxygenation of blood in small pulmonary arteries and arterioles by direct gaseous diffusion from the alveoli, respiratory bronchioles, and alveolar ducts in the pulmonary arterioles, even though the latter are "upstream" in relation to the alveoli. This fact, taken together with evidence for a reduction in pulmonary arterial blood volume during hypoxia, supports the view that small pulmonary arteries and arterioles are the main sites of vasoconstriction and increased resistance during hypoxia. Although alveolar oxygen tension is a major physiological determinant of pulmonary arteriolar tone, a reduction in the oxygen tension in the mixed venous blood flowing through the small pulmonary arteries and arterioles may also lead to pulmonary arterial vasoconstriction. Acidaemia appears to potentiate the effects of hypoxaemia, whereas alkalosis may be protective.

Pulmonary hypertension in ARDS

Pulmonary arterial hypertension and increased pulmonary vascular resistance have been identified as markers of the severity of ARDS and are related to vascular thrombosis [4] and pulmonary vasoconstriction.

Possible causes of the increased resistance include vasoconstriction, vascular obstruction by endothelial cell oedema, microembolism, or thrombosis, and destruction of the microvasculature. There are numerous studies of obstructive and structural factors in pulmonary hypertension, but direct evidence for pulmonary vasoconstriction is scarce [11-13].

Studies of experimental lung injury suggest evidence for involvement of pulmonary vasoconstriction in the pathogenesis of ARDS. For example, intravenous endotoxin elicits acute pulmonary hypertension in many mammals mainly due to the release of constrictor substances, rather than to direct vascular effects of endotoxin or to mechanical obstruction by leukocyte or platelet aggregation [14]. Although numerous vasoactive agents (e.g., histamine, serotonin, cathecholamines, angiotensin, kinins, and arachidonic acid metabolites) are apparently released after intravenous endotoxin, it appears that only the latter are important in the pulmonary constriction. Thus whereas endotoxin-induced pulmonary vasoconstriction was not blocked by antagonists of histamine, serotonin, and α-adrenergic receptors, it was reduced by inhibitors of ciclooxygenase [15].

Acute respiratory distress syndrome presents a combination of nonspecific alveolar damage and extensive pulmonary vascular disease [1]. Noncardiogenic pulmonary oedema, intrapulmonary shunting, hypoxaemia, decreased lung compliance, increased pulmonary artery pressures, and the requirement for mechanical ventilation are important signs of this syndrome [2]. In addition, many factors can act to promote the pulmonary hypertension observed in ARDS, such as associated pathologies, the presence of mediators, the use of positive end expiratory pressure, and the use of hypercapnia, permissive or not.

The effects of acute hypercapnia on pulmonary and systemic circulation have been extensively evaluated experimentally. Haemodynamically, acute hypercapnia causes pulmonary vasoconstriction and pulmonary hypertension through an increase in both cardiac output and pulmonary vascular resistance [16-19].

Most of this effect is likely mediated by the release of endogenous catecholamines [20-22].

The lungs, in addition to functioning as a blood acid-base balance by excreting carbon dioxide, help to maintain an optimal blood pH. A direct effect of carbon dioxide on the pulmonary vasculature is controversial, some authors report pulmonary vasodilation and others pulmonary vasoconstriction [18, 19, 23].

The presumptively beneficial strategy of "optimally recruiting" as much lung as possible is therefore highly questionable and alternative modes of mechanical ventilation, all based on a reduction in tidal volume, have been proposed to limit lung barotrauma [24].

The control of pulmonary hypertension in ARDS

In the absence of definitive therapy for ARDS, management involves supportive care using mechanical ventilation increased inspired oxygen concentrations and positive end-expiratory pressure (PEEP). Since hypoxaemia in ARDS is primarily a result of alveolar collapse, which results in intrapulmonary shunting, patients may remain hypoxemic despite such a therapy. The treatment of hypoxaemia and alveolar collapse are the principal ways to control pulmonary hypertension.

Oxygen therapy is central to the management of different situations associated with alveolar hypoxia. Along with the harmful systemic effects associated with oxygen arterial content deprivation, modification in the haemodynamics of the pulmonary circulation is also important. Arterioles in the pulmonary vascular bed seem morphologically common; however, these vessels are the most responsive system of any organ, in addition to being responsible for changes in oxygen levels. During alveolar hypoxia there is a probable detriment in NO synthesis or activity, and hypoxic vasoconstriction may result from a reduced NO dilating effect. As observed in acute hypoxia, during chronic pulmonary hypertension experimental data has shown a reduced response of the endothelium-dependent relaxation factor. A possible mechanism to explain the impairment of L-arginine-NO pathway during chronic hypoxia could arise from modified NO synthase or guanylate cyclase function [25, 26]. Oxygen plays an important role in pulmonary vascular tone and NO is continuously released in the pulmonary circulation and is associated with endothelium-dependent vasodilation. Therefore, some points involving NO still remain open to discussion. First, the contribution of continuous NO to low pulmonary vascular tone remains to be totally clarified. The second point involves acute and chronic hypoxia, NO and hypoxic pulmonary vasoconstriction. One could speculate that hypoxaemia exerts an inhibitory effect on NO synthesis, thus enhancing the vasoconstriction and shunting blood from collapsed areas to ventilated ones. The contrary view is that oxygen deprivation increases NO production and the vasoconstrictive reflex could be attenuated. In this way NO could be acting in favor of the ventilation-perfusion matching mechanism. Considering these points, the basis of the treatment of pulmonary hypertension secondary to acute or chronic alveolar hypoxia should be reviewed. More needs to be learned about the cellular and molecular adaptation to hypoxia in man, but the future may soon bring novel approaches to the treatment of patients with chronic obstructive lung disease and secondary pulmonary hypertension, as well as those with respiratory failure [27]. Oxygen may be an effective vasodilator, mainly when hypertension is due to hypoxic stimulation of the precapillary arteriolar vasculature.

Selective reduction of pulmonary vascular resistance continues to be a therapeutic goal for the treatment of pulmonary hypertension, and this reduction is based on the belief that pulmonary vasoconstriction is an important component of pulmonary hypertension. The ultimate response to vasodilator therapy is reduction of pulmonary artery pressure with a rise in cardiac output. The successful pharmacological manipulation of pulmonary vascular control is influenced by such factors as lack of specificity and systemic effects, as well as the choice between a wide variety of drugs that have been employed in the treatment of pulmonary hypertension.

Lung tissue is particularly active in the synthesis, metabolism, and release of a number of prostaglandins, some of which may play a role in the regulation of pulmonary vascular resistance. Prostaglandins I_2 and E are active pulmonary vasodilators, whereas $F_2\alpha$ and A_2 are pulmonary vasoconstrictors. Prostacyclin (PGI_2) is a powerful vasodilator that also inhibits platelet aggregation through activation of adenylate cyclase. Its metabolic half-life in the bloodstream is less than one circulation time with its metabolite 6-keto-prostaglandin $F_1\alpha$ having little biological activity. A variety of drugs with diverse mechanisms of action are reported to encourage prostacyclin production and include calcium channel blockers, angiotensin-converting enzyme inhibitors, diuretics, and nitrates. Physiologically, prostacyclin is a local hormone rather than a circulating one. The release of prostacyclin by endothelial cells causes relaxation of the underlying vascular smooth vessel and prevents platelet aggregation within the bloodstream. Because the biological actions of prostacyclin are the opposite from those of thromboxane, the balance between these two peptides appears to control the local environment within the vascular bed.

The biological action of nitric oxide (EDRF) is quite similar to that of prostacyclin in that it relaxes vascular smooth muscle and potentially inhibits the aggregation and adhesions of platelets by raising platelet levels of cyclic GMP. The observation that activation of the same receptors or a change in membrane confirmation induced by shear stress leads to the release of both nitric oxide and prostacyclin suggests that these substances act in unison as a common mechanism that defends the vascular endothelium.

In contrast to septic shock with overproduction of NO, pulmonary hypertension in patients with acute lung injury, with chronic obstructive lung disease, and in newborns with primary pulmonary hypertension may be associated with a relative or absolute lack of endogenous NO production within the pulmonary vasculature.

In humans, NO is produced by the upper respiratory airway, as demonstrated by Kobzig et al. using immunocytochemical and histochemical methods. In volunteers and patients, Gerlach et coll. measured NO concentrations in different parts of the upper airway. The highest concentrations were in the nose (0.649 ± 0.109 ppm), whereas in intubated patients the NO concentration was < 0.01 ppm. This suggests that the nasopharynx synthetized NO is normally inhaled and reabsorbed by the lower respiratory tract. Here, it may take part in the physiological regulation of the ventilation-perfusion ratio.

Intravenously infused vasodilators have been used to reduce pulmonary hypertension, but due to their general vasodilator effects on the systemic and pulmonary circulation they may also decrease mean systemic arterial pressure and impair pulmonary gas exchange by increasing perfusion to unventilated lung areas. Based on the properties of the agent, inhalation of gaseous NO may induce selective pulmonary vasodilation. As a gas, it reaches the pulmonary blood vessels from the abluminal surface adjacent to the ventilated airways. Thereby, in contrast to intravenous vasodilators, inhaled NO may increase perfusion of ventilated lung regions.

Administration of NO has been found to reduce pulmonary hypertension in a patient with severe acute respiratory distress syndrome [28]. If NO is inhaled, 50-80% of the inhaled NO is reabsorbed. NO freely diffuses from the alveoli into the surrounding lung tissue and nearby blood vessels. In blood, NO becomes inactivated within seconds by binding to haemoglobin, since NO has a high affinity to the haemoglobin molecule. Nitrosul-haemoglobin (NOHb) is produced and in the presence of oxygen, oxidized into methaemoglobin from which ferrous Hb is rapidly regenerated by methaemoglobin reductase in red blood cells with nitrate as a by product. The metabolism of the inhaled NO after its conversion to nitrate is identical to that of the nitrate taken up via foodstuffs. Most of the nitrate is excreted by the kidneys in urine.

The use of inhaled nitric oxide is still experimental, however it has been increasingly used during mechanical ventilation to treat pulmonary hypertension and hypoxaemia related to ARDS [29-31].

In patients with ARDS, low doses of NO reverse the increased pulmonary resistance induced by permissive hypercapnia, and significantly improve the oxygenation [24]. According to this study, nitric oxide could be an effective combination with hypoventilation during mechanical ventilation in severe ARDS cases. In ARDS, NO can improve transpulmonary vascular mechanics without intrinsic right ventricular change when permissive hypercapnia is used [32].

During the early phases of ARDS, the main determinant of the decrease in pulmonary vascular resistance induced by inhaled NO is the basal level of pulmonary vascular resistance index (PVRI). The greater the baseline PVRI, the greater the inhaled NO-induced decrease in PVRI [33, 34]. In the absence of a previous constriction of the pulmonary vessels, no decrease in PVRI is observed. Nitric oxide induced decrease in PVRI varies from 0 to 50%.

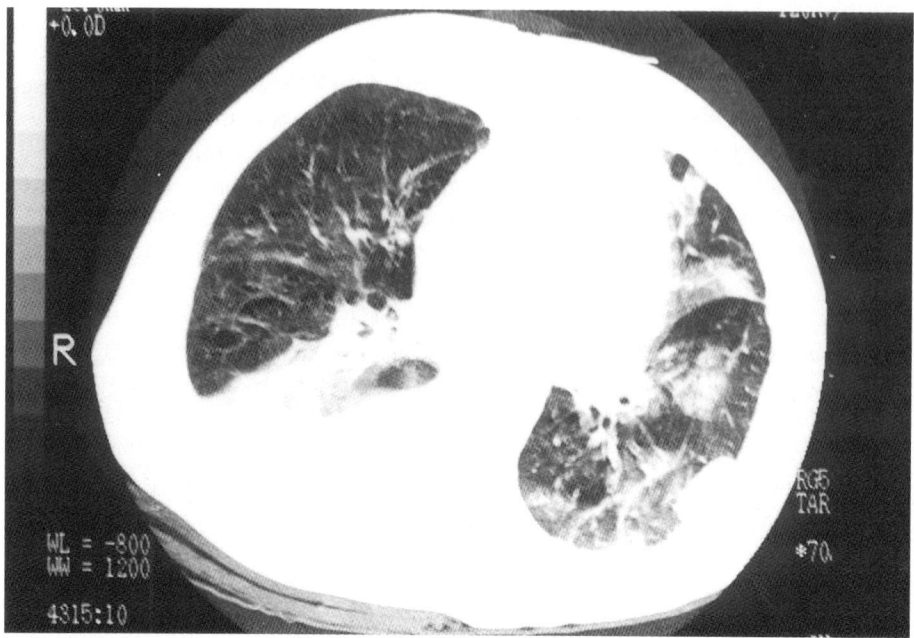

Fig. 1. Thoracic CT scan of a patient with acute respiratory failure after cardiac surgery

The increased PVRI observed in acute respiratory failure, which in the initial phases is mainly related to the constrictor effect of circulatory inflammatory mediators such as thromboxane A_2, platelet activating factor or endothelin, becomes partly fixed, at a later stage due to irreversible mechanisms such as microthrombosis or an increase in vascular thickness secondary to smooth muscle proliferation [35, 36].

The so-called "NO-responders" are patients with an increase in PVRI related to vasoconstriction. "NO non-responders" are either patients with normal pulmonary vascular tone or patients with an increase in PVRI mainly related to thrombosis or to anatomical remodeling of the pulmonary vessels. The correlation between the basal level of PVRI and the NO-induced decrease in PVRI observed during early stages of ARDS has also been documented in pulmonary hypertension complicating cardiac surgery [37]. In septic ARDS, inhaled NO seems to be effective only in a subgroup of patients characterized by increased right ventricular ejection fraction accompanied by higher cardiac index, oxygen delivery and oxygen extraction ratio [38].

However, the presence of gravitational gradients of pulmonary perfusion is useful for understanding the heterogeneity of pulmonary blood flow, a considerable amount of recent studies demonstrate that gravitation is not very important [39, 40].

The outcome of ARDS complicating cardiopulmonary bypass has changed little in recent years. Some predictors for ARDS in cardiac surgery are intra and postoperative intervention score, the total volume of blood pumped bypass and age [41, 42]. These risk factors should alert the clinician to the possibility of severe postoperative pulmonary complications. In patients undergoing cardiac surgery, many factors can change pulmonary function during the perioperative period [43, 44], and atelectasis is probably the major cause of hypoxaemia after cardiopulmonary bypass. In thoracic CT scan of patients with acute respiratory failure after cardiac surgery, we can see many different densities in the lung (Fig. 1). An increment in transpulmonary pressure by PEEP may not necessarily improve ventilation-perfusion relationship, because high alveolar pressure may induce a spatial perfusion distribution and an expansion of open lung tissue. However, the ventilation-perfusion alterations, the cardiac disease and PEEP contribute to pulmonary hypertension. In ARDS the severe disturbances of ventilation-perfusion and secondary hypertension allow NO to show its effects and, therefore, show an improvement in oxygenation, but in patients undergoing cardiac surgery and with pulmonary hypertension without ARDS, no improvement in oxygenation is observed with nitric oxide inhalation [45].

Aside from pharmacological therapy, a general approach to the control of acute pulmonary hypertension includes sedation, adequate ventilation, and acid-base equilibrium, since hypoxia, agitation and acidosis may induce and exacerbate pulmonary arterial reactivity.

References

1. Ashbaugh D, Bigelow D, Petty T et al (1967) Acute respiratory distress in adults. Lancet 2:319
2. Fowler AA, Hamman RF, Zerbe GO et al (1985) Adult respiratory distress syndrome: prognosis after onset. Am Rev Resp Dis 132:472
3. Malik AB (1990) Pulmonary microembolism and lung vascular injury. Eur Respir J 3:499s
4. Stuart R, Braunwald E, Grossman W (1997) Pulmonary hypertension. In: Braunwald E (ed) Heart disease, 5th edn, p 780
5. Zapol WM, Rimar S, Gillis N et al (1994) Nitric oxide and the lung. Am J Respir Crit Care Med 149:1375-1380
6. Sylvester JT, Gottlieb JE, Rock P et al (1986) Acute hypoxic responses. In: Bergofsky EH (ed) Abnormal pulmonary circulation, p 127
7. Auler Jr JOC, Ruiz Neto PP (1997) Treatment of pulmonary hypertension. In: Coriat P (ed) Clinical cardiovascular medicine in anaesthesia, p 213
8. Fishman AP, Fritts HW, Cournand A (1960) Effects of acute hypoxia and exercise on the pulmonary circulation. Circulation 22:204
9. Bergofsky EH, Haas F, Porcelli R (1968) Determinations of the sensitive vascular sites from which hypoxia and hypercapnia elicit rises in pulmonary artery pressure. Fed Proc 27:1420
10. Fishman AP (1976) Hypoxia on the pulmonary circulation: how and where it acts. Circ Res 38:221
11. Zapol WM, Kobayaki K, Snider MT et al (1977) Vascular obstruction causes pulmonary hypertension in severe acute respiratory syndrome. Chest 71:306

12. Snow RL, Davies P, Pontoppidan H et al (1982) Pulmonary vascular lesions of the adult respiratory distress syndrome. Am Rev Respir Dis 126:887
13. Tomashefski JF Jr, Davies P, Boggis C et al (1983) The pulmonary vascular lesions of the adult respiratory distress syndrome. Am J Pathol 112:112
14. Casey LC, Fletcher JR, Zmudka MI et al (1982) Prevention of endotoxin-induced pulmonary hypertension in primates by the use of a selective thromboxane synthetase inhibitor, OXY 1581. J Pharmacol Exp Ther 222:441
15. Paratt JR, Sturgess RM (1977) The possible roles of histamine, 5-hydroxytryptamine and prostaglandin F2alfa as mediators of the acute pulmonary effects of endotoxin. Br J Pharmacol 23:273
16. Linde LM, Simmons DH, Lewis N (1963) Pulmonary hemodynamics in respiratory acidosis in dogs. Am J Physiol 205:1008
17. Horwitz LD, Bishop VS, Stone HL (1968) Effects of hypercapnia on the cardiovascular system of conscious dogs. J Appl Physiol 25:346
18. Noble WH, Kay JC, Fisher JÁ (1981) The effect of PCO_2 on hypoxic pulmonary vasoconstriction. Can Anaesth Soc J 28:422
19. Weil P, Salisbury PF, State D (1957) Physiological factors influencing pulmonary artery pressure during separate perfusion of the systemic and pulmonary circulations in the dog. Am J Physiol 191:453
20. Frumin MJ, Epstein RM, Cohen G (1959) Apneic oxygenation in man. Anesthesiology 20:789
21. Sechzer PH, Egbert LD, Linde HW et al (1960) Effect of CO_2 inhalation on arterial pressure, ECG and plasma catecholamines and 17-OH corticosteroids in normal man. J Appl Physiol 15:454
22. Noble O, Folwle NO, Westcott RN et al (1951) The effect of norepinephrine upon pulmonary arteriolar resistance in man. J Clin Invest 30:517
23. Baudouin SV, Evans TW (1993) Action of carbon dioxide on hypoxic pulmonary vasoconstriction in the rat lung: Evidence against specific endothelium-derived relaxing factor-mediated vasodilation. Crit Care Med 21:740
24. Puybasset L, Stewart T, Rouby JJ et al (1994) Inhaled nitric oxide reverses the increase in pulmonary vascular resistance induced by permissive hypercapnia in patients with acute respiratory distress syndrome. Anesthesiology 80:1254
25. Eddahib S, Adnot S, Carville C et al (1992) L-arginine restores endothelium-dependent relaxation in pulmonary circulation of chronically hypoxic rats. Am J Physiol 72:194
26. Dinh-Xuan AT, Higgenbottam TW, Clelland CA et al (1991) Impairment of endothelium-dependent pulmonary artery relaxation in chronic obstructive lung disease. N Engl J Med 324:1539
27. Higgenbottam T, Cremona G (1993) Acute and chronic hypoxic pulmonary hypertension. Eur Respir J 8:1207
28. Falke K, Rossaint R, Pison U et al (1991) Inhaled nitric oxide selectively reduces pulmonary hypertension in severe ARDS and improves gas exchange as well as right heart ejection fraction: a case report. Am Rev Respir Dis 143:A248
29. Rossaint R, Gerlach H, Schmidt-Ruhnke H et al (1995) Efficacy of inhaled nitric oxide in patients with sever ARDS. Chest 107:1107
30. Geralch H, Pappert D, Lewandowski K et al (1993) Long-term inhalation with evaluated low doses of nitric oxide for selective improvement of oxygenation in patients with adult respiratory distress syndrome. Intensive Care Med 19:443
31. Gerlach H, Rossaint R, Pappert D et al (1993) Time course and dose-response of nitric oxide inhalation for systemic oxygenation and pulmonary hypertension in patients with adult respiratory distress syndrome. Eur J Clin Invest 23:499
32. Cheifetz IM (1996) Nitric oxide improves transpulmonary vascular mechanics but does not change intrinsic right ventricular contractility in an acute respiratory distress syndrome model with permissive hypercapnia. Crit Care Med 24:1554

33. Bigatelo LM, Hurford WE, Kacmarek RM et al (1994) Prolonged inhalation of low concentrations of nitric oxide in patients with severe adult respiratory distress syndrome. Anesthesiology 80:761

34. Puybasset L, Rouby JJ, Mourgeon E et al (1995) Factors influencing cardiopulmonary effects of inhaled nitric oxide in acute respiratory failure. Am J Resp Crit Care Med 152:318

35. Langleben D, Demarchie M, Laporta D et al (1993) Endothelin-1 in acute lung injury and the adult respiratory distress syndrome. Am Rev Respir Dis 148:1646

36. Zapol WM, Snider MT, Rie MA (1985) Pulmonary circulation during adult respiratory distress syndrome. In: Zapol WM, Falke KJ (eds) Acute respiratory failure. Dekker, New York, p 209

37. Rich FR, Murph GD, Roos CM et al (1993) Inhaled nitric oxide: Selective pulmonary vasodilation in cardiac surgical patients. Anesthesiology 78:1028

38. Krafft P, Fridrich P, Fitzgeral RD et al (1996) Effectiveness of nitric oxide inhalation in septic ARDS. Chest 109:486

39. Melsom MN, Flatebo T, Kramer-Johansen J et al (1995) Both gravity and non-gravity dependent factors determine regional blood flow within the goat lung. Acta Physiol Scand 153:343

40. Walther SM, Domino KB, Glenny RW et al (1997) Pulmonary blood flow distribution has a hilar-to peripheral gradient in awake, prone sheep. J Appl Physiol 82:678

41. Messent M, Sullivan K, Keogh BF et al (1992) Adult respiratory distress syndrome following cardiopulmonary bypass: incidence and prediction. Anaesthesia 47:267

42. Matthay MA, Wiener-Kronish JP (1989) Respiratory management after cardiac surgery. Chest 95:424

43. Auler Jr JOC, Carmona MJC, Bocchi EA et al (1996) Low doses of inhaled nitric oxide in heart transplant recipients. J Heart Lung Transplant 15:443

44. Hachenberg T, Tenling A, Nystrom SO et al (1994) Ventilation-perfusion inequality in patients undergoing cardiac surgery. Anesthesiology 80:509

45. Carmona MJC, Auler Jr JOC (1998) Effects of inhaled nitric oxide on respiratory system mechanics, hemodynamics, and gas exchange after cardiac surgery. J Cardiothorac Vasc Anesth 12:157

LUNG DYSFUNCTION
AND VENTILATORY MANAGEMENT

Pathophysiology of Unresolving ARDS: The Role of the Host Defense Response

G.U. Meduri

Acute respiratory distress syndrome (ARDS) describes the clinical syndrome associated with the morphologic lesion termed *diffuse alveolar damage* (DAD). At presentation, early ARDS manifests with acute and diffuse injury to the endothelial and epithelial linings of the terminal respiratory units and causes increased vascular permeability with protein-rich exudative oedema. In nonsurvivors of ARDS, DAD rapidly advances through three histological phases (exudative, fibroproliferative, and fibrotic) with different clinico-physiological features. The objective of this review is to describe systematically the pathophysiology of unresolving ARDS relating to mechanisms of its development, structural alterations induced in the lung, and functional consequences of these morphologic changes.

Most ARDS patients (85-95%) survive the initial, direct or indirect, insult that precipitated acute respiratory failure and progress into the *reparative stage*, where outcome varies (Table 1) from complete recovery (group 3) to rapid death due to accelerated pulmonary fibrosis (group 5) [1]. In patients who recover, the permeability defect and gas exchange abnormalities do improve (adaptive response) [2]. Conversely, ineffective repair is manifestsed by progression of fibroproliferation, inability to improve lung function (groups 4 and 5), and unfavorable outcome (maladaptive response) [3]. Most nonsurvivors die after a prolonged period of ventilatory support (group 4) and invariably develop fever, systemic inflammatory response syndrome (SIRS), clinical manifestations of sepsis [4], and multiple organ dysfunction syndrome (MODS) [5] antemortem.

Tissue homeostasis and the host defense response

Tissue consists of organized groups of cells attached to an extracellular matrix (ECM) and is surrounded by a network of blood vessels. The ECM occupies a significant proportion of the volume of any tissue and is indispensable for its structural integrity [6]. Tissue steady state, or homeostasis, is maintained by coordinating cell growth and proliferation with the production and turnover of ECM [7]. Cells achieve a remarkable coordination by constant signaling to themselves (autocrine activity) and each other (paracrine activity) by means of

Table 1. Clinical classification of ARDS

Clinical group	1	2	3	4	5
Source of injury controlled	No	Yes	Yes	Yes	Yes
Percentage of patients %	5-15	10	20-40	40-60	5-10
Average duration of ARF days	≤ 3	≤ 7	7-28	7-28	≤ 7
Evolution	Rapidly fatal	Rapid recovery	Slow improvement	Slow deterioration	Rapidly fatal
Survival	No	Yes	Yes	No	No
Causes of death	MODS	–	–	10-40% pulmonary 60-90% MODS	Pulmonary
Histological findings	Exudative phase of ALI	–	Fibroproliferation *	55% extensive fibrosis 69% pneumonia **	Severe fibrosis

ARF, acute respiratory failure; MODS, multiple organ dysfunction syndrome; ALI, acute lung injury

*   Data obtained from open-lung biopsy [73, 128, 79]
** Data obtained from autopsy series [5, 72, 74, 119, 122, 130, 174]

(Modified from [3])

polypeptides called cytokines (also known as growth factors). Cell-cell and cell-matrix interactions, through cytokine networking, are essential not only for maintaining homeostasis but also for providing a rapid defense (stress) response against intrinsic or extrinsic disturbing (infectious and noninfectious) forces.

The host defense response (HDR) to insults is similar regardless of the tissue involved and consists of an interactive network of simultaneously activated pathways that act in synergy to increase the host's chance of survival. Among this complex cascade of integrated pathways, five aspects of the HDR (Table 2) are important for understanding the clinical development and evolution of ARDS: inflammation, coagulation (intravascular clotting and extravascular fibrin deposition), modulation of the immune response, tissue repair, and activation of the hypothalamic-pituitary-adrenal (HPA) axis with production of glucocorticoids. Sympathetic system release of cathecholamines and hepatic production of acute-phase reactants are an integral part of the HDR and are under the influence of glucocorticoids. The host defense response is essentially a protective response of tissues, which serves to destroy, dilute, or wall off injurious agents [8] and to repair any consequent tissue damage. Repair consists of replacing injured tissue by regenerating native parenchymal cells and filling defects with fibroblastic tissue. Three aspects of the HDR – inflammation, coagulation, and tissue repair – can be analyzed separately to explain the histological and physiological changes occurring at the tissue level in unresolving ARDS.

Table 2. Components of the host defense response

Inflammation
    Vasodilation and stasis
    Increased expression of adhesion molecules
    Increased permeability of the microvasculature with exudative oedema
    Leukocyte extravasation *
    Release of leukocyte products potentially causing tissue damage
Coagulation
    Activation of coagulation
    Inhibition of fibrinolysis
    Intravascular clotting
    Extravascular fibrin deposition
Modulation of the immune response
    Fever and induction of heat-shock proteins
    Release of neutrophils from the bone marrow
    Priming of phagocytic cells
    T-cell proliferation
    Antibody production
    Downregulation
Tissue repair
    Angiogenesis
    Epithelial growth
    Fibroblast migration and proliferation
    Deposition of extracellular matrix and remodeling
    Activation of the hypothalamic-pituitary-adrenal axis
    Release of ACTH with cortisol production
    ACTH and cortisol modulation of the sympathetic nervous system
    Cortisol modulation of acute-phase protein production by the liver **

*   Initially polymorphonuclear cells and later monocytes
** Elevated levels of circulating glucocorticoids synergize with IL-6 in inducing hepatic synthesis and secretion of acute-phase reactants such as fibrinogen, protease inhibitors, complement C3, ceruloplasmin, haptoglobin, and C-reactive protein

Cellular responses in HDR are regulated by a complex interaction among cytokines with final local and systemic effects not directly induced by the initiating insult. In this regard, cytokines have concentration-dependent biologic effects [9]. At low concentration, they regulate homeostasis, and at progressively higher concentrations, they mediate proportionally stronger local and then systemic responses. Among a broad spectrum of proximal mediators, cytokines of the interleukin-1 (IL-1) and tumor necrosis factor (TNF) family appear uniquely important in initiating all key aspects of the HDR (for a review, see references 10 and 11). TNF-α and IL-1β stimulate their own and each other's secretion, and both promote the release of IL-6 (NF-IL6 is the transcription factor responsible for IL-6 gene activation after IL-1 stimulation). The term "inflammatory cytokines" (as they are commonly known) is restrictive, because their action extends well beyond this essential pathway of the HDR to include (among others) activation of coagulation [12], fibroproliferation [13], and HPA axis [14, 15]. The cell most commonly associated with initiating the HDR cascade is the tissue macrophage or the blood monocyte [10]. Once released, TNF-α and IL-1β act on epithelial cells, stromal cells (fibroblasts and endothelial), the ECM, and recruited circulating cells (neutrophils, platelets, lymphocytes) to cause second-ary waves of cytokine release, with amplification of the HDR [10]. Generation of inflammatory cytokines is normally strongly controlled by a number of homeostatic regulatory mechanisms, including shedding of specific cytokine re-ceptors on host cells, synthesis of endogenously generated cytokine antagonists, synthesis of antiinflammatory cytokines, downregulation, and activation of the HPA axis with production of glucocorticoids (GC) [11].

The host defense response in ARDS

ARDS is characterized by acute onset of diffuse and severe HDR of the lung parenchyma to a direct or indirect insult that disrupts the alveolocapillary mem-brane with loss of compartmentalization [16]. The magnitude of the initial HDR appears to be a major determinant of the progression and outcome in ARDS. Our group recently reported that on day 1 of mechanical ventilation (MV) non-survivors of ARDS had significantly ($p < 0.0001$) higher plasma (Fig. 1) and bronchoalveolar lavage (BAL) TNF-α, IL-1β, IL-2, IL- 4, IL-6, and IL-8 levels than survivors had [17, 18]. Although cytokine levels may not reflect activity, these findings are similar to those reported by others and agree with studies in-dicating that the evolution of ARDS is determined by the extent of initial pul-monary HDR in the form of alveolar denudation, basement membrane destruc-tion, vascular permeability, and quantity of intraalveolar exudate [19-22].

Of significant importance, during the progression of ARDS, we have found nonsurvivors to have persistent and marked elevation of plasma and BAL in-flammatory cytokine levels over time, while survivors had a rapid reduction in inflammatory cytokine levels [17, 18]. Other groups have also reported that non-survivors of ARDS or sepsis had persistent elevation of inflammatory cytokines (Table 3) or other components of the HDR (i.e., PLA$_2$, leukotrines, and comple-ment) over time [23-27]. This finding is important to understanding why treat-ment modalities of limited duration may be ineffective in ARDS. It is well ac-cepted that during ARDS the HDR is not limited to the lung [28]. In patients with unresolving ARDS, disruption of alveolocapillary membranes [29] causes release of cytokines into the systemic circulation and contributes to the develop-ment and/or maintenance of SIRS and MODS [16, 30]. Strong correlation among TNF-α, IL-1β, IL-6, and IL-8 at the onset of ARDS and over time is consistent with a broad and integrated HDR [17].

Overall, a strong line of evidence supports the view that an overaggressive and protracted HDR, rather than the etiologic condition precipitating respiratory failure, is the major factor influencing outcome in ARDS [4]. In agreement with this statement are the findings that ARDS patients may not improve despite ap-propriate treatment of the precipitating disease, while mortality is decreased

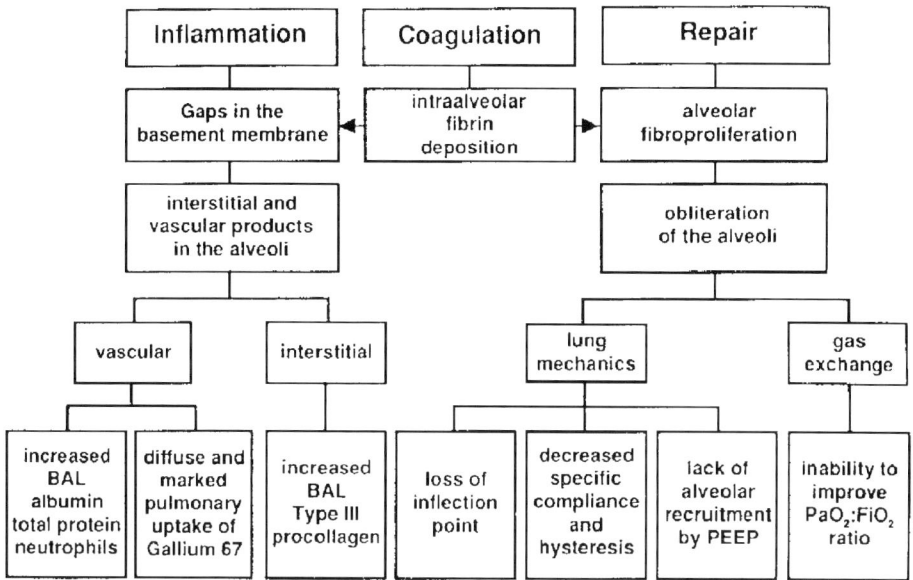

Fig. 1. Alveolar epithelial changes in unresolving ARDS. (Modified from [29])

when the HDR is adequately suppressed by sustained glucocorticoid administration (discussed later) [31]. In the absence of inhibitory signals, the continued exaggerated production of HDR mediators prevents effective restoration of lung anatomy and function (maladaptive response) by sustaining ongoing injury, coagulation, and fibroproliferation (the three act in synergy). Histology of lung tissue obtained by open-lung biopsy in patients with unresolving ARDS (8 to 22 days into ARDS) showed new injury to previously spared endothelial and epithelial surfaces to occur in conjunction with an amplified reparative (coagulation and fibroproliferation with deposition of extracellular matrix) process over previously damaged areas [29]. Persistent endothelial and epithelial injury protracts vascular permeability in the lung and systemically. Intravascular coagulation decreases available pulmonary vascular bed, while intraalveolar fibrin deposition promotes cell-matrix organization by fibroproliferation [32]. Most clinical and physiological derangements observed in unresolving ARDS are attributable to unrestrained coagulation and fibroproliferation and are discussed below.

Coagulation

During ARDS, normal intraalveolar fibrinolytic activity (urokinase-like plasminogen activators produced by alveolar macrophages) and endothelium anticlotting activity (heparin-like molecules, thrombomodulin) are severely compro-

Table 3. Host defense response and progression of ARDS

Variables at day 3-7 of ARDS	Survivors	Nonsurvivors	References
Clinical manifestations of inflammation			
Body temperature	↓	↑	[88]
Mean arterial blood pressure	↑	−↓	[45, 88, 89]
Laboratory manifestations of inflammation			
Blood inflammatory cytokine levels	↓	↑	[17, 24, 30, 121]
BAL inflammatory cytokine levels	↓	↑	[18, 122]
Blood phospholipase A_2 levels	↓	↑	[23, 24]
Complement activation	↓	NA	[26, 121]
Laboratory manifestations of pulmonary endothelial permeability			
BAL neutrophil percentage	↓	−↑	[26, 90, 93, 98, 99, 122]
BAL albumin and protein concentration	↓	−↑	[18, 90, 93]
Increased gallium-67 pulmonary uptake	↓	−	[102, 107]
Clinical manifestations of systemic endothelial permeability			
Positive fluid balance	↓	↑	[88, 89]
Laboratory manifestations of coagulation			
Platelet count	↓	↑	[43, 45, 121]
BAL antifibrinolytic activity	↓	−↑	[36, 123]
Physiological and radiographic manifestations of fibroproliferation			
$PaO_2:FiO_2$	↑	−↓	[18, 36, 45, 81, 85-91, 121]
PEEP requirements	↓	−↑	[45, 89, 121]
Static compliance	↑	↓	[81, 86]
Dead space ratio	↓	↑	[81, 113]
Pulmonary artery pressure	↓	−↑	[45, 81, 89]
Alveolar infiltration	↓	↑	[29, 85, 87, 121]
Laboratory manifestations of fibroproliferation			
BAL procollagen-III	↓	↑	[124, 125]
Serum procollagen-III	↓	↑	[75-77, 124, 125]

Variables on day 3-7 of ARDS in comparison to day 1
−, no change; ↑, increased; ↓, decreased; NA, not available

mised and lead to accelerated vascular and extravascular fibrin deposition [33-35]. In patients with ARDS, BAL increases procoagulant activity due to tissue factor associated with factor VII [36, 37] and concomitant depression of fibrinolytic activity attributable to increased levels of both plasminogen activator inhibitor-1 (PAI-1) and antiplasmin [36, 38, 39]. In humans [36, 40], similar to experimental models [41], derangements of intraalveolar fibrin turnover occur early (1-3 days) and persist for ≥ 14 days. Depressed BAL fibrinolytic activity at day 7 of ARDS correlates with poor outcome [36]. Despite a depression in fibrinolytic activity, BAL fibrinogen degradation products (FDP) are markedly increased and remain elevated over time and correlate significantly with BAL total protein concentration and number of neutrophils [40]. Patients with ARDS also have marked and prolonged systemic procoagulant activity and rapid exhaustion of the fibrinolytic system [42]. Virtually all ARDS patients have increased circulating FDP levels [43]. Disseminated intravascular coagulation (DIC) is a frequent finding in ARDS and carries a higher mortality rate [44]. Even in patients without DIC, a reduction in circulating platelets of at least 50% of the initial values is frequently seen during the course of ARDS, and nonsurvivors have a greater degree of thrombocytopenia than survivors do [45]. Thrombocytopenia is not due to decreased platelet production, but to decreased platelet survival (one third of normal) because of increased pulmonary sequestration [46].

Patients with early ARDS as well as patients with late unresolving ARDS show diffuse pulmonary sequestration of intravenously administered radiolabeled fibrinogen [47]. Pathways for increased fibrinogen uptake include: 1) increased microvascular permeability with exudation of fibrinogen into pulmonary interstitial and intraalveolar oedema, 2) intravascular and extravascular fibrin formation, and 3) fibrinogen binding to injured endothelial cells [47]. Recovery from lung injury is associated with normalization of radiolabeled fibrinogen uptake [47]. Cytokines TNF-α, IL-1β, and IL-6 alter the surface of the endothelium from an anticoagulant into a procoagulant moiety, due to downregulation of thrombomodulin and the expression of tissue factor, and are able to enhance the synthesis of PAI-1 [48-50].

Pulmonary thromboemboli are a frequent histological finding in patients with unresolving ARDS subjected to open-lung biopsy [29] and are found on postmortem exam in 95% of ARDS nonsurvivors [51, 52]. Macrothrombi (in arteries greater than 1 mm diameter) are found by postmortem angiography in 86% of patients and are more prevalent in patients who died in the early phase of ARDS [52]. Microthrombi are as prevalent as macrothrombi but tend to be distributed throughout all phases of ARDS. In one study, filling defects at angiography correlated with the severity of ARDS, the degree of pulmonary hypertension, and the presence of DIC [51]. Unfortunately, anticoagulant treatment does not improve outcome in ARDS [51], and this has applied to any treatment directed at one single facet of the complex host response. Ischemic or avascular necrosis, particularly in the subpleural regions, is a common feature of unresolving ARDS (see *barotrauma*) [29, 51].

Fibrin deposition also influences the course of tissue injury and repair. Thrombin, fibrin, and its degradation products (FDP) play an important role in amplifying inflammation by promoting neutrophil chemotaxis and adhesiveness and by directly causing increased endothelial permeability [35, 53, 54, 55]. Thrombin is also a potent inducer of platelet degranulation with additional release of HDR mediators. Coagulation and fibrinolysis are also interactive with the kallikrein-kinin system with release of bradykinin. Bradykinin increases vascular permeability and stimulates collagen production by fibroblasts [56].

Animal studies have demonstrated that intraalveolar fibrin deposition is typical of DAD, even when injury resolves without fibrosis, indicating that fibrin deposition of limited duration is essential for effective lung repair [57]. In the presence of a protracted HDR, however, persistent intraalveolar fibrin deposition contributes to airspace organization and fibrosis [33, 57, 58, 59]. *In vitro* data demonstrate that fibrin forms a matrix on which fibroblasts may aggregate and secrete collagen [60]. In addition, thrombin binds to thrombin receptors on fibroblasts and promotes their proliferation [61].

Fibroproliferation

Fibroproliferation is a stereotypical reparative response to injury. In ARDS, pulmonary fibroproliferation manifests with the accumulation of myofibroblasts and their connective tissue products in the airspaces, interstitium, respiratory bronchioles, and walls of the intraacinar microvessels [52, 62]. Pulmonary fibroproliferation is a diffuse process, as indicated by the findings of chest computed tomography [29], gross inspection at surgery, microscopic analysis of biopsies from different lobes [63], and bilateral BAL findings [18]. At microscopy, however, regional heterogeneity exists, and focal areas of normal parenchyma are occasionally found [64, 65]. Unhalted fibroproliferation results in extensive fibrotic remodeling of the lung parenchyma. Macroscopically, the lung shows irregular zones of diffuse scarring with formation of numerous microcystic reorganized airspaces measuring between 1 and 2 mm, most prominent in the subpleural zones [29].

Pulmonary fibroproliferation in ARDS shares a common pathogenetic mechanism with other fibroproliferative diseases, where degree and duration of the HDR dictate the ultimate reparative outcome [66]. In this "linear" concept of tissue response to injury, mediators of the HDR sustain the fibrotic process [67]. Fibrosis ensues when the HDR is intense and prolonged, leading to released profibrotic moieties and trophic factors for mesenchymal cells. Experimental work indicates that severity of acute lung injury determines the intensity of chronic inflammation and fibrosis [68]. We have also found that patients with higher plasma IL-6 on days 1-3 of ARDS are more likely to develop accelerated fibroproliferation unresponsive to GC rescue treatment [31].

Morphometric analysis of lung tissue in late ARDS has shown that intraalveolar fibroproliferation predominates over interstitial fibroproliferation [62]. The histological sequence leading to intraalveolar fibroproliferation has been clearly characterized [62]. Epithelial injury provides focal discontinuities (gaps) in the alveolar basement membrane (BM) resulting in direct communication of interstitial cells and matrix elements with the alveolar airspaces [29, 69]. Activated myofibroblasts from the interstitium migrate into the alveoli in response to chemotactic signals and attach to the luminal surface of the damaged BM [62,

69]. Myofibroblasts, once they have migrated into the alveoli, proliferate and become active in collagen production [69], transforming the initially fibrinous intraalveolar exudate into myxoid connective tissue matrix and eventually into dense acellular fibrous tissue. TNF-α and IL-1β, among other HDR mediators, stimulate chemotaxis and are important modulators of fibroblast proliferation and collagen deposition [1, 70, 71].

Morphometric studies in nonsurvivors of ARDS have shown intraalveolar (and, to a lesser degree, interstitial) fibroproliferation to occur within 7 days of the onset of ARDS and to have a rapid increase in the second and third week of respiratory failure [62]. The rate of progression varies [64, 72, 73]. Newly produced matrix stains intensely for cell-associated fibronectin and type 3 procollagen [69]. Type III collagen (newly formed, flexible, and more susceptible to digestion by collagenase) predominates in the intermediate proliferative phase, while type I collagen (composed of thick fibrils, more resistant to digestion) is the major collagen present in the late fibrotic phase. In nonsurvivors, the collagen content of the lung is increased 2- to 3-fold after 2 weeks of ARDS, and it parallels the development of fibrosis [74]. Patients with ARDS dying after 7 days of respiratory failure have, in contrast to survivors, persistent elevation in the BAL and serum of extracellular matrix components (procollagen III), indicating ongoing fibrogenesis (Table 3) [22, 75, 76, 77]. Patients with a procollagen III level greater than 1.75 U/ml in BAL on day 7 had a 72% mortality rate compared with a 20% mortality rate for patients with a procollagen III level less than 1.75 U/ml [22]. BAL procollagen III levels correlate with histological evidence of intraalveolar fibrosis [78]. Finding fibrosis at open-lung biopsy or transbronchial biopsy is a poor prognostic factor [79, 80].

The patterns of fibrous reorganization of the lung in ARDS have been described [19]. Intraalveolar fibroblastic aggregation is continuous with a similar process in the terminal bronchioles, respiratory bronchioles, alveolar ducts, and the interstitium [72]. The bronchiolar intraluminal (bud-like) fibrosis found in patients with fibroproliferation [73] is similar to that described in interstitial lung disorders [59]. The coexistence of unaffected bronchioles surrounded by parenchymal interstitial and alveolar space fibrosis indicates that lung injury induces patchy bronchial epithelial and basement membrane damage. In our experience, intraluminal fibrosis at open-lung biopsy in patients with unresolving ARDS predicts reversibility of fibroproliferation with GC rescue treatment [73], similar to the response seen in patients with bronchiolitis obliterans organizing pneumonia [32].

Of significance, we and others have described microscopic and ultrastructural evidence of ongoing epithelial and endothelial injury in patients with advanced fibroproliferation [29, 52, 64, 73]. Despite the high turnover rate and ability of endothelial cells to repair themselves, acute endothelial injury is more pronounced in the proliferative phase than in the exudative phase of ARDS [52, 64], consistent with a continuous injury process. Fibrocellular intimal proliferation, the sequela of endothelial injury, involves predominantly the small arteries, but also the veins and lymphatics. Absence of arteriolar subintimal fibroproliferation at open-lung biopsy in patients with unresolving ARDS predicts reversibility of fibroproliferation with GC rescue treatment [73].

Pathophysiology of unresolving ARDS

Morphological changes at epithelial and endothelial levels, caused by recurrent injury, ongoing coagulation, and amplified fibroproliferation, can explain the physiological and laboratory findings seen in patients with unresolving ARDS.

Gas exchange and lung mechanics. As shown in Fig. 1, gaps in the alveolar BM in unresolving ARDS [29], allow communication between the alveoli and the interstitium for entrance of vascular and interstitial components into the airspaces. Myofibroblasts migrate, proliferate, and produce collagen. Progressive fibroproliferation leads to obliteration of the respiratory units, changing their mechanical properties (loss of inflection point in the pressure-volume [P-V] curve and lack of recruitability by positive end-expiratory pressure [PEEP]), increasing dead space ventilation (VD/VT), and further compromising gas exchange. [81-84]. A concomitant reduction in capillary volume and thickening of the alveolar septa additionally contribute to reducing gas transfer and increasing VD/VT [64]. In several studies (Table 3), the PaO_2: FiO_2 ratio, although similar at the onset of ARDS, clearly separated by day 3-7 survivors (increased) from nonsurvivors (decreased or no change) [18, 36, 45, 81, 85-91]. In one report, mortality rate in patients with and without improvement in lung function by day 7 of ARDS was 43% and 97%, respectively [87].

Pulmonary vascular permeability. As shown in Fig. 2, endothelial injury [29] in unresolving ARDS favors the passage of vascular products in the alveoli. Among the many cells and substances that exude in the airspaces, the following have been the subject of clinical investigations: albumin, proteins, neutrophils, and ^{67}Ga.

BAL albumin and total protein are markers of pulmonary endothelial permeability in ARDS [92]. At the onset of ARDS, we have found BAL albumin and total protein levels to be similar in survivors and nonsurvivors. In agreement with others [90, 93], we have found in survivors, in contrast to nonsurvivors, a progressive decline in BAL albumin and total protein levels over time, suggesting effective repair of the alveolar-endothelial surface. We have also identified a consistent correlation between BAL albumin and total protein levels and BAL TNF-α, IL-1β, IL-6, and IL-8 levels [18].

BAL neutrophilia ($\geq$ 70%) is invariably found in early ARDS [93-95]. The percentage of BAL neutrophils parallels BAL protein [20, 90] and albumin [18] concentration and correlates with the severity in gas exchange [93]. We and others have identified a positive correlation between total neutrophil count and

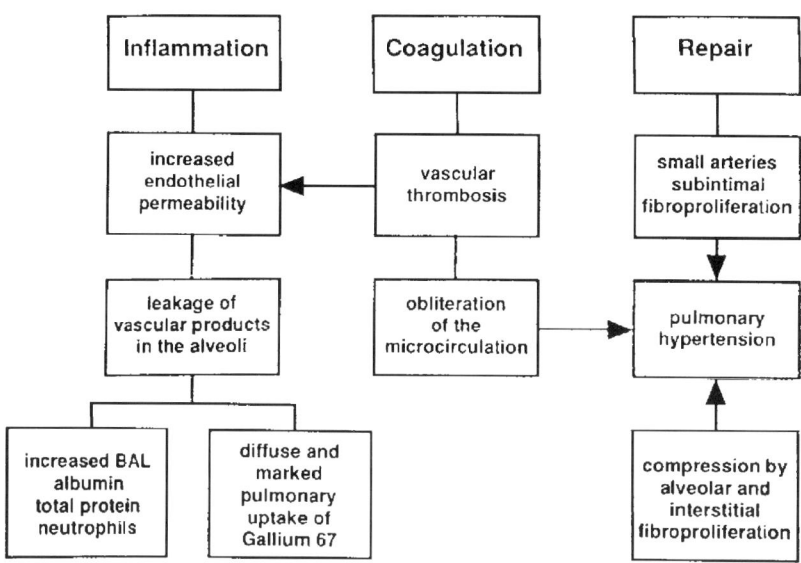

Fig. 2. Pulmonary endothelial changes in unresolving ARDS. (Modified from [29])

BAL TNF-α, IL-1β, and IL-8 levels [18, 96, 97]. Persistent elevation of neutrophils in the BAL by days 7 and 14 of ARDS is associated with poor outcome [98, 99]. Resolution of ARDS, on the contrary, is associated with a dramatic fall in neutrophils and increased number of macrophages [98].

The origin of neutrophils recovered by BAL in unresolving ARDS requires clarification. In patients with unresolving ARDS subjected to both bronchoscopy and open-lung biopsy an average of 14 days into respiratory failure, we have found a significant discrepancy between marked BAL neutrophilia (60% of recovered cells) and an almost complete absence of neutrophils in the airways, alveoli, and interstitium at histology [73]. It has been recognized that the alveolocapillary membrane is permeable to fluids and that in normal patients 39% of the aspirated BAL fluid originates from the circulation [100]. In conditions associated with disruption of vascular and epithelial integrity, such as unresolving ARDS, the circulatory component of BAL effluent becomes more significant, and cells such as neutrophils and erythrocytes are aspirated into the alveoli when negative pressure is applied during suction [100]. Therefore, BAL neutrophilia in unresolving ARDS is a marker of endothelial permeability [20, 73, 90], not a reflection of "neutrophilic alveolitis", and it is unlikely that neutrophils play a major role in the progression of unresolving of ARDS.

[67]Ga uptake in the lung is an additional marker of endothelial permeability [101]. The mechanism of ^{67}Ga uptake was recently reviewed [102]. In the lung, ^{67}Ga concentration is normally low. Diffuse ^{67}Ga uptake has been used as a sen-

sitive but nonspecific test to identify patients with active pulmonary inflammation who may respond to GC treatment. Five reports (total of 44 patients) have described marked and diffuse uptake of ^{67}Ga in the lung of patients with unresolving ARDS and who subsequently responded to GC rescue treatment [73, 103-106]. Diffuse and marked pulmonary uptake of ^{67}Ga in unresolving ARDS correlates with BAL neutrophilia [102]. Decreased pulmonary ^{67}Ga uptake correlates with improvement in gas exchange [107]. The diagnostic role of ^{67}Ga scintigraphy in ARDS was reported [102].

Pulmonary hypertension. While in early ARDS the pulmonary vasculature is available for dilation and/or recruitment, vascular changes in unresolving ARDS are less responsive to vasodilator treatment [108]. In these patients, vascular obstruction from thrombosis, subintimal fibroproliferation of the small arteries, and compression from alveolar and interstitial expansion significantly reduces the capacity of the pulmonary microcirculation (Fig. 2) [64] and subjects the patent vascular bed to abnormally high flow, stimulating medial hypertrophy of the muscular and partially muscular arteries [109]. These changes are similar to those seen in pulmonary hypertension of thromboembolic origin [109], and they worsen with progression of fibroproliferation [45, 81, 89]. In early ARDS, there is a marked elevation in circulating levels of endothelin-1, a mediator of vascular remodeling and pulmonary hypertension [110]. With the progression of ARDS, endothelin-1 levels drop to normal values in patients improving lung function but remain elevated in patients who worsen [110]. Persistent elevation or worsening pulmonary artery pressure is a poor prognostic sign [45, 81, 89]. In the final stages of ARDS, the mean pulmonary artery pressure can exceed 40 mmHg due to a 4-fold elevation of vascular resistance [108].

Barotrauma. In unresolving ARDS, vascular obstruction with subpleural tissue necrosis and endoluminal fibrosis with intraparenchymal pseudocyst formation contribute to alveolar rupture. Barotrauma may manifest as intraparenchymal and subpleural pneumatoceles, large compliant air collections or bullae, pulmonary interstitial emphysema, pneumomediastinum, pneumothorax, subcutaneous emphysema, and rarely pneumoperitoneum [111]. Barotrauma in ARDS is related to the severity of lung dysfunction and is associated with a higher mortality [112-114]. An increase in the alveolar-arterial pressure gradient, from either hyperinflation and/or reduced blood flow, causes disruption at the common border between the alveolar base and the vascular sheath [109, 115]. Partial obliteration (endoluminal fibrosis) of terminal airways leads to cyst formation by valvular mechanism and by compensatory dilatation of neighboring bronchioles [114]. Tissue necrosis distal to pulmonary artery thrombi [51] is prominent in the subpleural regions where insufficient collateral blood flow makes lung tissue particularly susceptible to ischaemia [116]. At angiography, a "picket-fence" appearance is seen, caused by dilated subpleural arteries bridging regions of oligaemia and necrosis distal to the thrombotic arterial occlusion [116]. With progressive fibroproliferation, preferential ventilation to these hypoperfused peripheral areas may occur, contributing to the development of barotrauma [116].

References

1. Snyder LS, Hertz MI, Harmon KR et al (1990) Failure of lung repair following acute lung injury: Regulation of the fibroproliferative response. Chest 98:733-738
2. Calandrino Jr FS, Anderson DJ, Mintun MA et al (1988) Pulmonary vascular permeability during the adult respiratory distress syndrome: A positron emission tomographic study. Am Rev Respir Dis 138:421-428
3. Meduri GU (1993) Late ARDS. New Horiz 1:563-577
4. Headley AS, Tolley E, Meduri GU (1997) Infections and the inflammatory response in acute respiratory distress syndrome. Chest 111:1306-1321
5. Bell RC, Coalson JJ, Smith JD et al (1983) Multiple organ system failure and infection in adult respiratory distress syndrome. Ann Intern Med 99:293-298
6. Raghow R (1994) The role of extracellular matrix in postinflammatory wound healing and fibrosis. FASEB J 8:823-831
7. Border WA, Noble NA (1994) Transforming growth factor β in tissue fibrosis. N Engl J Med 331:1286-1292
8. Gallin JK, Goldstein IM, Snyderman R (eds) (1988) Overview. In: Inflammation: Basic principles and clinical correlates. Raven, New York, pp 1-3
9. Cerami A (1992) Inflammatory cytokines. Clin Immunol Immunopathol 62:S3-S10
10. Baumann H, Gauldie J (1994) The acute phase response. Immunol Today 15:74-80
11. Heumann D, Glauser MP (1994) Pathogenesis of sepsis. Sci Med 1:28-37
12. Van Der Poll T, Buller HR, Cate HT et al (1990) Activation of coagulation after administration of tumor necrosis factor to normal subjects. N Engl J Med 322:1622-1627
13. Elias JA, Freundlich B, Kern JA et al (1990) Cytokine networks in the regulation of inflammation and fibrosis in the lung. Chest 97:1439-1445
14. Perlstein RS, Whitnall MH, Abrams JS et al (1993) Synergistic roles of interleukin-6, interleukin-1, and tumor necrosis factor in the adrenocorticotropin response to bacterial lipopolysaccharide in vivo. Endocrinology 132:946-952
15. Hermus ARMM, Sweep CGJ (1990) Cytokines and the hypothalamic-pituitary-adrenal axis. J Steroid Biochem Molec Biol 37:867-871
16. Tutor JD, Mason CM, Dobard E et al (1994) Loss of compartmentalization of alveolar tumor necrosis factor after lung injury. Am J Respir Crit Care Med 149:1107-1111
17. Meduri GU, Headley S, Kohler G et al (1995) Persistent elevation of inflammatory cytokines predicts a poor outcome in ARDS. Plasma IL-1β and IL-6 are consistent and efficient predictors of outcome over time. Chest 107:1062-1073
18. Meduri GU, Kohler G, Headley S et al (1995) Inflammatory cytokines in the BAL of patients with ARDS. Persistent elevation over time predicts poor outcome. Chest 108:1303-1314
19. Burkhardt A (1989) Alveolitis and collapse in the pathogenesis of pulmonary fibrosis. Am Rev Respir Dis 140:513-524
20. Harris TR, Bernard GR, Brigham KL et al (1990) Lung microvascular transport properties measured by multiple indicator dilution methods in patients with adult respiratory distress syndrome. Am Rev Respir Dis 141:272-280
21. Kawamura M, Yamasawa F, Ishizaka A et al (1994) Serum concentration of 7S collagen and prognosis in patients with the adult respiratory distress syndrome. Thorax 49(2):144-146
22. Clark JG, Milberg JA, Steinberg KP et al (1995) Type III procollagen peptide in the adult respiratory distress syndrome. Association of increased peptide levels in bronchoalveolar lavage fluid with increased risk for death. Ann Intern Med 122:17-23
23. Vadas P, Pruzanski W, Stefanski E et al (1988) Concordance of endogenous cortisol and phospholipase A_2 levels in gram-negative septic shock: A prospective study. J Lab Clin Med 111:584-590
24. Romaschin AD, DeMajo WC, Winton T et al (1992) Systemic phospholipase A_2 and cachectin levels in adult respiratory distress syndrome and multiple-organ failure. Clin Biochem 25:55-60

25. Bernard GR, Korley V, Chee P et al (1991) Persistent generation of peptide leukotrienes in patients with the adult respiratory distress syndrome. Am Rev Respir Dis 144:263-267
26. Robbins RA, Russ WD, Rasmussen JK et al (1987) Activation of the complement system in the adult respiratory distress syndrome. Am Rev Respir Dis 135:651-658
27. Dofferhoff ASM, De Jong HJ, Bom VJJ et al (1992) Complement activation and the production of inflammatory mediators during the treatment of severe sepsis in humans. Scand J Infect Dis 24:197-204
28. Crouser ED, Dorinsky PM (1994) Gastrointestinal tract dysfunction in critical illness: Pathophysiology and interaction with acute lung injury in adult respiratory distress syndrome/multiple organ dysfunction syndrome. New Horiz 2:476-487
29. Meduri GU, ElTorky M, Winer-Muram HT (1995) The fibroproliferative phase of late adult respiratory distress syndrome. Semin Respir Infect 10:154-175
30. Roumen RMH, Hendriks T, van der Ven-Jongekrijg J et al (1993) Cytokine patterns in patients after major vascular surgery, hemorrhagic shock, and severe blunt trauma. Relation with subsequent adult respiratory distress syndrome and multiple organ failure. Ann Surg 218(6):769-776
31. Meduri GU, Headley S, Tolley E et al (1995) Plasma and BAL cytokine response to corticosteroid rescue treatment in late ARDS. Chest 108:1315-1325
32. Cordier J-F, Peyrol S, Loire R (1994) Bronchiolitis obliterans organizing pneumonia as a model of inflammatory lung disease. In: Epler GR (ed) Diseases of the bronchioles. Raven, New York, pp 313-345
33. Idell S (1994) Extravascular coagulation and fibrin deposition in acute lung injury. New Horizons 2:566-574
34. Bone RC (1992) Modulators of cogulation: A critical appraisal of their role in sepsis. Arch Intern Med 151:1381-1389
35. Hasegawa N, Husari AW, Hart WT et al (1994) Role of the coagulation system in ARDS. Chest 105:268-277
36. Idell S, Koenig KB, Fair DS et al (1991) Serial abnormalities of fibrin turnover in evolving adult respiratory distress syndrome. Am J Physiol 261:L240-L248
37. Gunther A, Nix F, Heinemann S et al (1995) Alteration of procoagulant and fibrinolytic properties in acute inflammatory and chronic interstitial lung disease. Am J Resp Crit Care Med 151:A77
38. Bertozzi P, Astedt B, Zenzius L et al (1990) Depressed bronchoalveolar urokinase activity in patients with adult respiratory distress syndrome. N Engl J Med 322:890-897
39. Moalli R, Doyle JM, Tahhan HR et al (1989) Fibrinolysis in critically ill patients. Am Rev Respir Dis 140:287-293
40. Fuchs-Buder T, de Moerloose P, Ricou B et al (1996) Time course of procoagulant activity and D dimer in bronchoalveolar fluid of patients at risk for or with acute respiratory distress syndrome. Am J Respir Crit Care Med 153:163-167
41. Idell S, James KK, Gillies C et al (1989) Abnormalities of pathways of fibrin turnover in lung lavage of rats with oleic acid and bleomycin-induced lung injury support alveolar fibrin deposition. Am J Pathol 135:387-399
42. Kirschstein W, Heene DL (1985) Fibrinolysis inhibition in acute respiratory distress syndrome. Scand J Clin Lab Invest 45:87-94
43. Carvalho AC (1985) Blood alterations during ARDS. In: Zapol WM, Falke KJ (eds) Acute respiratory failure. Marcel Dekker, New York, pp 303-346
44. Bone RC, Francis PB, Pierce AK (1976) Intravascular coagulation associated with the adult respiratory distress syndrome. Am J Med 61:585-589
45. Bone RC, Balk R, Slotman G et al (1992) Adult respiratory distress syndrome. Sequence and importance of development of multiple organ failure. Chest 101:320-326
46. Schneider RC, Zapol WM, Carvalho AC (1980) Platelet consumption and sequestration in severe acute respiratory failure. Am Rev Respir Dis 122:445-451
47. Quinn DA, Carvalho AC, Geller E et al (1987) ^{99m}Tc-fibrinogen scanning in adult respiratory distress syndrome. Am Rev Respir Dis 135:100-106

48. Nawroth PP, Stern DW (1986) Modulation of endothelial cell hemostatic properties by tumor necrosis factor. J Exp Med 163:740-745
49. de Boer JP, Creasy AA, Chang A et al (1993) Activation patterns of coagulation and fibrinolysis in baboons following infusion with lethal or sublethal dose of Escherichia coli. Circ Shock 39:59-67
50. Taylor FB (1994) The inflammatory-coagulant axis in the host response to Gram-negative sepsis: Regulatory roles of proteins and inhibitors of tissue factor. New Horiz 2:555-565
51. Greene R, Zapol WM, Snider MT et al (1981) Early bedside detection of pulmonary vascular occlusion during acute respiratory failure. Am Rev Respir Dis 124:593-601
52. Tomaseski JF, Davies P, Boggis C et al (1983) The pulmonary vascular lesions of the adult respiratory distress syndrome. Am J Pathol 112:112-126
53. Malik AB (1990) Pulmonary microembolism and lung vascular injury. Eur Respir J 3: 499S-506S
54. Neuhof H, Seeger W, Wolf HRD (1986) Generation of mediators by limited proteolysis during blood coagulation and fibrinolysis: Its pathogenetic role in the adult respiratory distress syndrome (ARDS). Resuscitation 14:23-32
55. Leavell KJ, Peterson MW, Gross TJ (1996) The role of fibrin degradation products in neutrophil recruitment to the lung. Am J Respir Cell Mol Biol 14:53-60
56. Schapira M, Gardaz JP, Py P et al (1985) Prekallikrein activation in the adult respiratory distress syndrome. Bull Eur Physiopathol Respir 21:237-247
57. McDonald JA (1990) The yin and yang of fibrin in the airways. N Engl J Med 322:929-931
58. Kuhn C III, Boldt J, King TE et al (1989) An immuno-histochemical study of architectural remodeling and connective tissue synthesis in pulmonary fibrosis. Am Rev Respir Dis 140:1693-1703
59. Basset F, Ferrans VJ, Soler P et al (1986) Intraluminal fibrosis in interstitial lung disorders. Am J Pathol 122:443-461
60. Colvin RB, Gardner PI, Roblin RO et al (1979) Cell surface fibrinogen-fibrin receptors on cultured human fibroblasts. Lab Invest 41:464-473
61. Cherington PV, Pardee AB (1980) Synergistic effects of epidermal growth factor and thrombin on the growth stimulation of diploid chinese hamster fibroblasts. J Cell Physiol 105: 25-32
62. Fukuda Y, Ishizaki M, Masuda Y et al (1987) The role of intraalveolar fibrosis in the process of pulmonary structural remodeling in patients with diffuse alveolar damage. Am J Pathol 126:171-182
63. Lamy M, Fallat RL, Koeniger E et al (1976) Pathologic features and mechanisms of hypoxemia in adult respiratory distress syndrome. Am Rev Respir Dis 114:267-284
64. Bachofen M, Weibel ER (1977) Alterations of the gas exchange apparatus in adult respiratory insufficiency associated with septicemia. Am Rev Respir Dis 116:589-615
65. Zapol WM, Snider MT, Rie M (1992) Pulmonary circulation in adult respiratory distress syndrome. In: Artigas A, Lemaire F, Suter PM (eds) Adult respiratory distress syndrome. Churchill Livingstone, Singapore, pp 259-278
66. Kovacs EJ, Dipietro LA (1994) Fibrogenic cytokines and connective tissue production. FASEB J 8:854-861
67. Bitterman PB, Henke CA (1991) Fibroproliferative disorders. Chest 99:81S-84S
68. Shen AS, Haslett DC, Feldsien C et al (1988) The intensity of chronic lung inflammation and fibrosis after bleomycin is directly related to the severity of acute injury. Am Rev Respir Dis 137:564-571
69. Kuhn C III, Boldt J, King Jr TE et al (1989) An immunohistochemical study of architectural remodeling and connective tissue synthesis in pulmonary fibrosis. Am Rev Respir Dis 140:1693-1703
70. King RJ, Jones MB, Minoo P (1989) Regulation of lung cell proliferation by polypeptide growth factors. Am J Physiol 257:L23-L38

71. Postlethwaite AE, Seyer JM (1990) Stimulation of fibroblast chemotaxis by human recombinant tumor necrosis factor α (TNF-α) and a synthetic TNF-α 31-68 peptide. J Exp Med 172:1749-1756

72. Collins JF, Smith JD, Coalson JJ et al (1984) Variability in lung collagen amounts after prolonged support of acute respiratory failure. Chest 85(5):641-646

73. Meduri GU, Chinn AJ, Leeper KV et al (1994) Corticosteroid rescue treatment of progressive fibroproliferation in late ARDS. Patterns of response and predictors of outcome. Chest 105:1516-1527

74. Zapol WM, Trelstad RL, Coffey JW et al (1979) Pulmonary fibrosis in severe acute respiratory failure. Am Rev Respir Dis 119:547-554

75. Entzian P, Huckstadt A, Kreipe H et al (1990) Determination of serum concentrations of type III procollagen peptide in mechanically ventilated patients. Pronounced augmented concentrations in the adult respiratory distress syndrome. Am Rev Respir Dis 1420:1079-1082

76. Kropf J, Grobe E, Knoch M et al (1991) The prognostic value of extracellular matrix component concentrations in serum during treatment of adult respiratory distress syndrome with extracorporeal CO_2 removal. Eur J Clin Chem Clin Biochem 29:805-812

77. Waydhas C, Nast-Kolb D, Trupka A et al (1993) Increased serum concentrations of procollagen type III peptide in severely injured patients: An indicator of fibrosing activity? Crit Care Med 210:240-247

78. Farjanel J, Hartmann DJ, Guidet B et al (1993) Four markers of collagen metabolism as possible indicators of disease in the adult respiratory distress syndrome. Am Rev Respir Dis 147(5):1091-1099

79. Angus DC, Linde-Zwirble W, Sirio CA et al (1995) Understanding post-discharge mortality after prolonged mechanical ventilation. Crit Care Med 23:A55

80. Martin C, Papazian L, Payan MJ et al (1995) Pulmonary fibrosis correlates with outcome in established ARDS. Usefulness and safety of the transbronchial lung biopsy in mechanically ventilated patients. Chest 107:196-200

81. Shimada Y, Yoshiya I, Tanaka K et al (1979) Evaluation of the progress and prognosis of adult respiratory distress syndrome: Simple respiratory physiologic measurement. Chest 76:180-186

82. Matamis D, Lemaire F, Harf A et al (1984) Total respiratory pressure-volume curves in the adult respiratory distress syndrome. Chest 86:58-66

83. Klose R, Osswald PM (1981) Effects of PEEP on pulmonary mechanics and oxygen transport in the late stages of acute pulmonary failure. Intensive Care Med 7:165-170

84. De Latorre FF (1992) Study of gas exchange as a prognostic factor in adult respiratory distress syndrome. In: Artigas A, Lemaire F, Suter PM (eds) Adult respiratory distress syndrome. Churchill Livingstone, Singapore, pp 371-378

85. Heffner JE, Zamora CA (1990) Clinical predictors of prolonged translaryngeal intubation in patients with the adult respiratory distress syndrome. Chest 97:447-452

86. Maunder RJ, Kubilis PS, Anardi DM et al (1989) Determinants of survival in the adult respiratory distress syndrome (ARDS). Am Rev Respir Dis A220

87. Bernard GR, Luce JM, Sprung CL et al (1987) High-dose corticosteroids in patients with the adult respiratory distress syndrome. N Engl J Med 317:1565-1570

88. Simmons RS, Berdine GG, Seidenfeld JJ et al (1994) Fluid balance and the adult respiratory distress syndrome. Am Rev Respir Dis 135:924-929

89. Sloane PJ, Gee MH, Gottlieb JE et al (1992) A multicenter registry of patients with acute respiratory distress syndrome. Am Rev Respir Dis 146:419-426

90. Sinclair DG, Braude S, Haslam PL et al (1994) Pulmonary endothelial permeability in patients with severe lung injury. Chest 106:535-539

91. Heffner JE, Brown LK, Barbieri CA et al (1995) Prospective validation of an acute respiratory distress syndrome predictive score. Am J Respir Crit Care Med 152:1518-1526

92. Holter JF, Weiland JE, Pacht ER et al (1986) Protein permeability in the adult respiratory distress syndrome. Loss of selectivity of the alveolar epithelium. J Clin Invest 78:1513-1522 (abstract)

93. Weiland JE, Davis WB, Holter JF et al (1986) Lung neutrophils in the adult respiratory distress syndrome. Clinical and pathophysiologic significance. Am Rev Respir Dis 133: 218-225

94. Fowler AA, Hamman RF, Zerbe GO et al (1985) Adult respiratory distress syndrome: Prognosis after onset. Am Rev Respir Dis 132:472-478

95. Martin TR, Pistorese BP, Hudson LD et al (1991) The function of lung and blood neutrophils in patients with the adult respiratory distress syndrome. Implications for the pathogenesis of lung infections. Am Rev Respir Dis 144:254-262

96. Jorens PG, VanDamme J, DeBacker W et al (1992) Interleukin 8 (IL-8) in the bronchoalveolar lavage fluid from patients with the adult respiratory distress syndrome (ARDS) and patients at risk for ARDS. Cytokine 4(6):592-597

97. Miller EJ, Cohen AB, Magao S et al (1992) Elevated levels of NAP-1/interleukin-8 are present in the airspaces of patients with the adult respiratory distress syndrome and are associated with increased mortality. Am Rev Respir Dis 146:427-432

98. Steimberg KP, Milberg JA, Martin TR et al (1994) Evolution of bronchoalveolar lavage cell population in the adult respiratory distress syndrome. Am J Respir Crit Care Med 150: 113-122

99. Gunther K, Baughman RP, Rashkin M et al (1993) Bronchoalveolar lavage results in patients with sepsis-induced adult respiratory distress syndrome: Evaluation of mortality and inflammatory response. Am Rev Respir Dis 147:A346

100. Kelly CA, Fenwick JD, Corris PA et al (1988) Fluid dynamics during bronchoalveolar lavage. Am Rev Respir Dis 138:81-84

101. Bégin R, Canton A, Drapeau G et al (1983) Pulmonary uptake of gallium-67 in asbestos-exposed humans and sheep. Am Rev Respir Dis 127:623-630

102. Meduri GU, Belenchia JM, Massey JD et al (1996) ^{67}Ga scintigraphy in diagnosing sources of fever in ventilated patients. Intensive Care Med 22:395-403

103. Meduri GU, Belenchia JM, Estes RJ et al (1991) Fibroproliferative phase of ARDS. Clinical findings and effects of corticosteroids. Chest 100:943-952

104. Hooper RG, Kearl RA (1990) Established ARDS treated with a sustained course of adrenocortical steroids. Chest 97:138-143

105. Hooper RG, Kearl RA (1996) Established adult respiratory distress syndrome successfully treated with corticosteroids. South Med J 89:359-364

106. Passamonte PM, Martinez AJ, Singh A (1984) Pulmonary gallium concentration in the adult respiratory distress syndrome. Chest 85:828-830

107. Baughman RP, Thorpe JE, Staneck J et al (1987) Use of the protected specimen brush in patients with endotracheal or tracheostomy tubes. Chest 91:233-235

108. Zapol WM, Snider MT (1977) Pulmonary hypertension in severe acute respiratory failure. N Engl J Med 296:476-480

109. Snow RL, Davies P, Pontoppidan H et al (1982) Pulmonary vascular remodeling in adult respiratory distress syndrome. Am Rev Respir Dis 126:887-892

110. Langleben D, Demarchie M, Laporta D et al (1993) Endothelin-1 in acute lung injury and the adult respiratory distress syndrome. Am Rev Respir Dis 148:1646-1650

111. Unger JM, England DM, Bogust GA (1989) Interstitial emphysema in adults: Recognition and prognostic implications. J Thorac Imaging 4:86-94

112. Woodring JH (1985) Pulmonary interstitial emphysema in the adult respiratory distress syndrome. Crit Care Med 13:786-791

113. Gattinoni L, Bombino M, Pelosi P et al (1994) Lung structure and function in different stages of severe adult respiratory distress syndrome. JAMA 271:1722-1779

114. Rouby JJ, Lherm T, de Lassale EM et al (1993) Histologic aspects of pulmonary barotrauma in critically ill patients with acute respiratory failure. Intensive Care Med 19:383-389

115. Macklin MT, Macklin CC (1944) Malignant interstitial emphysema of the lungs and mediastinum as an important occult complication in many respiratory diseases and other conditions: An interpretation of the clinical literature in light of laboratory experiments. Medicine (Baltimore) 23:281-358

116. Tomasheski Jr JR (1990) Pulmonary pathology of the adult respiratory distress syndrome. Clin Chest Med 11:593-619
117. Ashbaugh DG, Maier RV (1985) Idiopathic pulmonary fibrosis in adult respiratory distress syndrome. Diagnosis and treatment. Arch Surg 120:530-535
118. Andrews CP, Coalson JJ, Smith JD et al (1981) Diagnosis of nosocomial bacterial pneumonia in acute, diffuse lung injury. Chest 80:254-258
119. Ashbaugh DG, Petty TL (1972) Sepsis complicating the acute respiratory distress syndrome. Surgery 135:865-869
120. Pratt PC, Vollmer RT, Shelburne JD et al (1979) Pulmonary morphology in a multihospital collaborative extracorporeal membrane oxygenation project. Am J Pathol 95:191-214
121. Groeneveld ABJ, Raijmakers PGHM, Hack CE et al (1995) Interleukin 8-related neutrophil elastase and the severity of the adult respiratory distress syndrome. Cytokine 7:746-752
122. Baughman RP, Gunther KL, Rashkin MC et al (1996) Changes in the inflammatory response of the lung during acute respiratory distress syndrome: Prognostic indicators. Am J Resp Crit Care Med 154:76-81
123. Gando S, Nakanishi Y, Tedo I (1995) Cytokines and plasminogen activator inhibitor-1 in posttrauma disseminated intravascular coagulation: Relationship to multiple organ dysfunction syndrome. Crit Care Med 23:1835-1842
124. Lotz M, Guerne PA (1991) Interleukin-6 induces the synthesis of tissue inhibitor of metalloproteinases-1/erythroid potentiating activity (TIMP-1/EPA). J Biol Chem 266(4):2017-2020
125. Meduri GU, Tolley E, Chinn A et al (1998) Procollagen type I and III aminoterminal propeptide levels during ARDS and in response to methylprednisolone treatment. Am J Resp Crit Care Med (in press)

Pathophysiology of Ventilator-Associated Pneumonia

N. Fábregas, A. Torres

Ventilator-associated pneumonia (VAP) is a frequent complication of mechanical ventilation with an incidence that ranges between 9% and 70% [1-4]. VAP seems to be particularly frequent in patients with acute respiratory distress syndrome (ARDS) in whom several local and systemic factors apparently predispose its development [5]. Crude mortality rates of VAP varies from 25% to 50% [6-7], while mortality directly attributable is 27% [8]. Clinical and radiological parameters are not very specific to diagnose VAP [9]. Among several prognostic factors, both inappropriate and prior antibiotic therapy have a particular importance and they indirectly highlight the need for a correct clinical and microbiological diagnosis of pneumonia [3, 7, 10-12]. Most of our knowledge about VAP comes from clinical and or microbiological studies that have been published in the last decade. However, the histology of VAP has been only known in recent years mainly through immediate post-mortem studies that have been performed to validate techniques used to elicit microbial diagnosis of pneumonia in mechanically ventilated patients [13-24]. These studies have extensively investigated the lungs of patients mechanically ventilated for several days and along with experimental models of pneumonia [25-27] have allowed to describe the peculiar histological and microbiological characteristics and interactions of human VAP. From this information important clinical implications have been concluded.

Histological definition of ventilator-associated pneumonia

The histological presence of VAP has classically been accepted [13, 15, 17] as the presence of foci of consolidation with intense leukocyte accumulation in bronchioles and adjacent alveoli. This definition is very simplistic since it does not take into account severity and distribution of lesions. Rouby and co-workers [16], studying whole lungs in patients after mechanical ventilation, could define four different stages of severity and/or extension of VAP as follows: 1) bronchiolitis or "early infection" characterised by intense proliferation of polymorphonuclear leukocytes (PMNL) localised within the lumen of bronchioles and associated with purulent mucus plugs and bronchiolar wall alterations; 2) focal bronchopneumonia: scattered neutrophilic infiltrates localised to terminal bronchioles and surrounding alveoli; 3) confluent bronchopneumonia: defined as the extension of these elementary lesions to several adjacent lobes; and, 4) lung abscess: which is defined as the confluent bronchopneumonia associated with tissue necrosis and disruption of normal lung architecture.

Other histological descriptions of VAP have been recently published, partially modifying initial definitions of VAP. These published studies used modifications of the classification described by Johanson et al. [25] in a baboon model of VAP. Chastre and colleagues [18], examining lungs of patients who have been mechanically ventilated, defined three grades of severity: 1) mild bronchopneumonia: presence of scattered neutrophilic infiltrates localised to terminal bronchioles and some surrounding alveoli. According to these authors, lesions may be non-specific of pneumonia when severe pulmonary underlying disease, such as acute respiratory distress syndrome (ARDS) or extensive chronic obstructive lung disease coexist; 2) moderate bronchopneumonia: defined when the extension of the inflammatory process caused grossly evident confluence of infiltrates between adjacent lobules and when purulent mucus plugs were present in bronchioles; 3) severe bronchopneumonia: considered when there was extensive confluence of inflammation and this was occasionally associated with tissue necrosis. Marquette et al. [19] in a post-mortem study in mechanically ventilated patients considers VAP when there is consolidation at the level of secondary lobules with intense accumulation of PMNL, fibrinous exudate, and cellular debris within alveolar spaces, whether or not the lesions were centred on terminal or respiratory bronchioles. In this study, lesions of pneumonia were defined as confluent if the areas of consolidation extended to several adjacent secondary lobules. Lung abscess was defined when the lesions of pneumonia were associated with tissue necrosis and destruction of the surrounding lung architecture.

In a post-mortem study with bilateral multiple biopsy sampling [21] and according to modified classification from Blackmon [28], we described four evolution stages of pneumonia: 1) early phase (0-2 days of evolution) which shows the presence of capillary congestion with increased number of PMNL at this level, the alveolar spaces usually showed a fibrinous exudate (Fig. 1); 2) intermediate phase [3-4 days of evolution) characterised by presence of fibrin, few erythrocytes and several PMNL within the alveoli; 3) advanced phase [5-7 days of evolution) showing PMNL filling up most of the alveoli and macrophages incorporating cellular debris in the cytoplasm; 4) resolution phase (> 7 days of evolution) when the inflammatory exudate is eliminated due to phagocytic activity of mononuclear cells. We have also defined two degrees of severity in relation to the lung extension of the lesion: mild and severe. Another recent classification from Corley et al. [29] included the following: 1) early stage pneumonia characterised by the accumulation of neutrophils within small bronchi. At this stage, bacteria are not easy to find; 2) progression to neutrophilic inflammation with or without necrosis. It is occasionally possible to identify bacteria in asso-

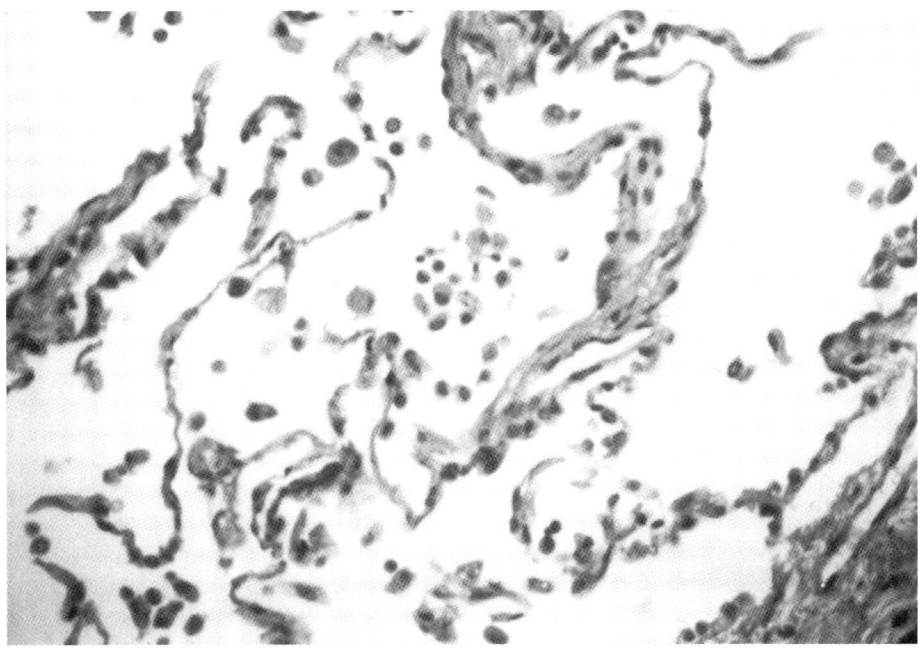

Fig. 1. Early phase of pneumonia: accumulation of polymorphonuclear leukocytes within the capillaries. Hematoxylin & Eosin (x 200)

ciation with neutrophils in the lumens of small bronchi, and 3) late stage of resolving or organising pneumonia. This classification is very similar to ours [21].

Human and experimental post-mortem histological and microbiological studies on VAP

Chastre and colleagues [13] were the first to develop a post-mortem human model upon critically ill patients. In the immediate post-mortem period (within 30 min) they performed a left thoracotomy, under surgical aseptic conditions, and obtained six superficial small specimens from the anterior segment of the left lower lobe for culture. In addition a 1 cm^3 specimen was obtained for histological analysis. They found a good association between histologic and bacteriologic findings (quantitative cultures). Similar results were obtained by Gaussorgues and co-workers [15]. Rouby and colleagues [14] performed a more extensive approach and analysed histologically two small lung specimens obtained from an area of consolidation of the lower lobe. Another small specimen was cut from the same area and bacteriologically examined. Then the entire lung was surgically removed and a complete lung autopsy was done. They were the first in describing that pneumonia in ventilated patients is a multifocal process disseminated within each pulmonary lobe. These foci of pneumonia were predominantly distributed to lower lobes and in dependent zones of the lung. The histologic lesions of bronchopneumonia were always located within large zones of altered lung parenchyma. They demonstrated that a single lung specimen will miss the histological pneumonia in around 30% of cases. The latter finding must be taken into account when interpreting the results of earlier studies which limited histological examination to a single sample. The same group performed another post-mortem study [16] analysing extensively a whole lung from 83 deceased critically ill patients. Five to 10 slices per lung segment were obtained and examined using the histologic classification alluded to above. They reconfirmed the multifocal nature of VAP and described the frequent association of VAP with bronchiolitis.

In 1995 Chastre et al. [18] published the results of a post-mortem study analysing two large specimens from each anterior segment of the left lower lobe and upper lobe obtained in 20 patients who had not suffered prior episodes of pneumonia and were free of recent antibiotic changes. Interestingly in that study the histologic grade of severity of the two matched segments was discordant in 7 out of 19 patients (36%) in whom the two segments were analysed. Marquette et al. [19] studied the histological characteristics of the entire fixed lungs and they confirmed the findings of the previous studies. Pneumonia was found in 50% of the dependent segments and in 37% of the non dependent segments. One of the major characteristics of the lesions was their typically scattered pattern of distribution within normal or damaged lung parenchyma. Only 14 of 83 examined lobes (16,8%) had all of their segments involved by the infectious process. The scattering of the lesions was even more prominent at the segmental level, where the infectious alveolar damage ranged from limited foci of pneumonia to large areas of confluent pneumonia. A distinctive finding in several cases was the absence of pneumonia from the peripheral lung samples, while more central areas of the same segment displayed typical foci.

Our group studied single bilateral post-mortem biopsies in mechanically ventilated patients who died with prior antibiotic treatment [17]. We obtained, from the lower lobe of each lung, one specimen for histological analysis and one for bacteriologic quantitative cultures. In this study we observed a poor relationship between histologic and microbiologic results, perhaps due to the administration of prior antibiotic treatment in all patients. In other words quantitative cultures of lung samples could not easily discriminate the presence or absence of histological pneumonia. This prompted us to perform a subsequent study [21] including patients with and without antibiotic treatment (48 hours at least free of antibiotic treatment). Several specimens from each lobe of the two lungs were aseptically obtained (average of 16 samples per patient). Applying the evolution classification of VAP described above, we confirmed the disseminated multifocal heterogeneous pattern of VAP predominantly involving lower lobes. Interestingly, we observed that all the phases alluded above coexisted in the same patient and in the same lung exhibiting a pleomorphic histological pattern. Overall intermediate phase (Fig. 2) and advanced phase (Fig. 3) were the most common stages of pneumonia observed in this study. As in other studies non-specific alveolar damage and bronchiolitis were also frequent findings.

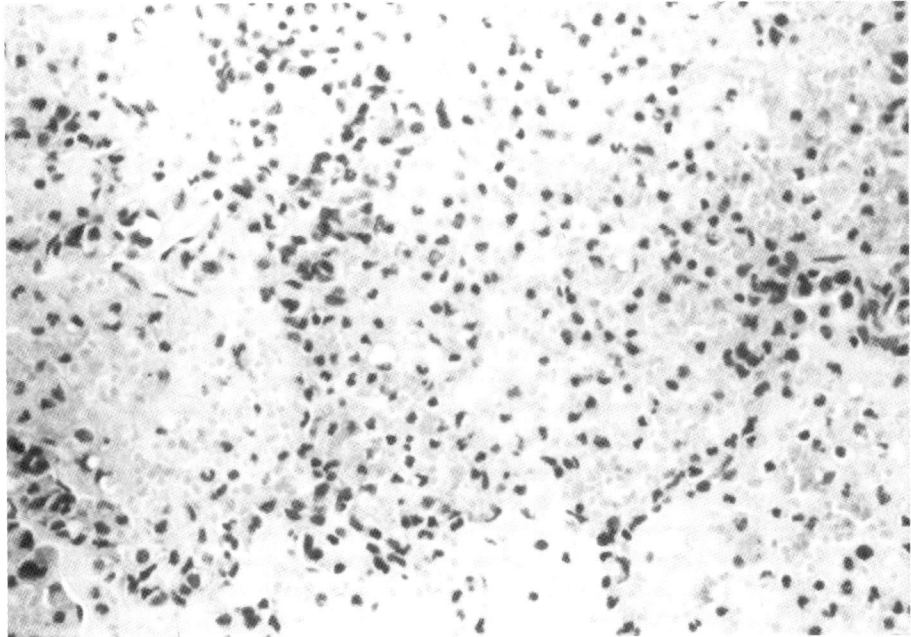

Fig. 2. Intermediate phase of pneumonia: polymorphonuclear leukocytes, fibrin and a few erythrocytes in the alveolar lumina. Hematoxylin & Eosin (x 200)

Papazian and co-workers [20] analysed one entire lung of 38 patients, histologic classification was performed according to Johanson and co-workers [25]. They found no sign of bronchopneumonia in 20 cases. Conversely, in the remaining 18 cases they confirmed bronchopneumonia histologically. There was no relationship between the results of the various cultures and the pathology results. Bronchiolitis was noted in 8 patients, out of whom 5 had concomitant histologic signs of pneumonia. The remaining 3 patients had negative lung cultures. Additional histologic findings were fibrosis in 9 cases and diffuse alveolar damage in 7 cases. These authors examined the significance of the isolation of *Candida* spp. in their samples. Despite frequent lung colonisation by *Candida*, only 2 patients exhibited histologic signs of *Candida* pneumonia. Lung tissue cultures were positive for *Candida albicans* in these 2 patients. This agrees with

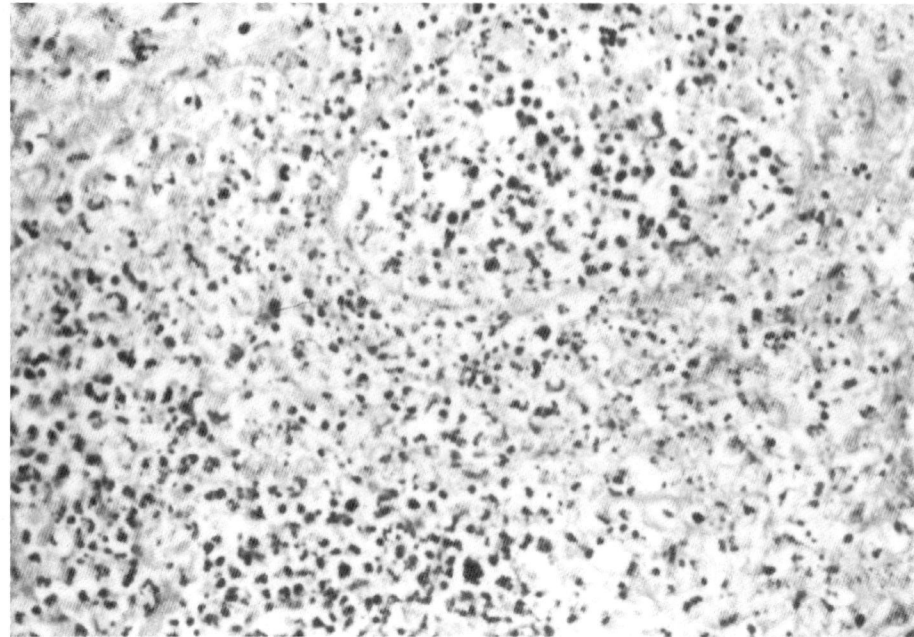

Fig. 3. Advanced phase of pneumonia: polymorphonuclear leukocytes and macrophages filling the alveolar lumina. Hematoxylin & Eosin (x 200)

the results of El-Ebiary's et al. study [30] who found that the incidence of *Candida* pneumonia was 8%. Nevertheless, in this study, the incidence of *Candida* isolation from pulmonary biopsies in critically ill mechanically ventilated non-neutropenic patients who die is high (40%), indicating that *Candida* is a frequent colonising agent in very critically ill patients.

In order to avoid confounding factors such as antibiotic presence or lung injury described in other studies, Marquette et al. [26] induced pneumonia in pigs free from antibiotics and previous concomitant lung disease secondary to tracheobronchial stenosis. They found that the histologic lesions of pneumonia, as well as the lung bacterial burden were unequally distributed within the lungs and even within the lung segments. Moreover, specimens showing histologic evidence of pneumonia had significantly higher bacterial burden than specimens with bronchial infections and specimens with neither bronchial nor lung infection. However, the authors could not define a clear threshold for quantitative cultures to discriminate the presence or absence of pneumonia. This study providing experimental insights into the relationship between microbiologic and histologic features in bacterial pneumonia confirms previous findings in humans. However, a prior study from Johanson et al. in baboons [25] could find acceptable correlation between lobar bacterial index (sum in log scale of different species isolated) and the degree of histological pneumonia severity.

In humans, with one exception [18], there is now compelling evidence that quantitative biopsy cultures cannot reliably discriminate between patients with and without evidence of histological pneumonia. The use of a specific threshold to define the presence of pneumonia does not take into account the fact that lung infection occurs along a bacteriologic continuum. Thus, when pneumonia begins or if infectious bronchiolitis is present, the diagnostic threshold may not be met. The same case occurs when prior antibiotic has been given. Another explanation for low qualitative lung cultures in presence of histological pneumonia is the normal functioning of antibacterial lung defences which clear lung bacterial burden. On the other hand the specificity of lung cultures is low with a high rate of false-positive cultures. In post-mortem studies false-positive lung cultures (without pneumonia) may be due to bacterial colonisation, and bronchiolitis. It has been suggested that closely to death, in critically ill patients, the lung could suffer from massive bacterial colonisation which could explain the frequent presence of bacteria in distal airways without histological pneumonia [30]. From all these findings it is clear, due to the poor relationship between quantitative lung cultures and histological examination, that quantitative lung biopsy cultures alone cannot be used to validate in vivo diagnostic techniques used to microbiologically investigate VAP.

Clinical implications of histological and microbiological findings in post-mortem VAP studies

The histological findings of human post-mortem studies have the following clinical implications: 1) initial phases of VAP that probably need to be treated with antibiotics cannot be detected at portable chest X-ray [31]; 2) since VAP is a multifocal process the techniques that explore broad lung regions such as bronchoalveolar lavage are clearly preferred to those that only explore a segment (protected specimen brush) [32, 33]; 3) blind diagnostic methods that can sample lung dependent zones are probably as accurate as visually guided methods [34-36].

The microbiological findings have the following clinical implications: 1) as mentioned above, quantitative post-mortem lung cultures cannot be used as gold standard to validate microbiological diagnostic techniques; 2) when interpreting quantitative bacteriology at the bedside, the clinician should weight a number of factors that can modify bronchial and alveolar bacterial burden: presumed stage of bronchopneumonia, administration of antibiotics, technique of distal sampling, natural host bacterial defences, duration of mechanical ventilation and presence of acute lung injury. The microbiological complexity of VAP does not support the concept of a standard threshold for the diagnosis of pneumonia [37, 38]. Thus, treatment algorithms based upon definite thresholds of quantitative cultures may lead to undertreat patients. Since early and adequate initial antibiotic treatment is one of the major factors related with prognosis of VAP, the strict execution of treatment based upon quantitative thresholds without clinical judgement may be hazardous to patients.

References

1. Fagon JY, Chastre J, Hance AJ et al (1988) Detection of nosocomial lung infection in ventilated patients: use of a protected specimen brush and quantitative culture techniques in 147 patients. Am Rev Respir Dis 138:110-116
2. Joshi N, Localio R, Hamory BH (1992) A predictive risk index for nosocomial pneumonia in the intensive care unit. Am J Med 93:135-142
3. Kollef MH (1993) Ventilator-associated pneumonia. A multivariate analysis. JAMA 270: 1965-1970
4. Andrews CP, Coalson JJ, Smith JD, Johanson WG (1981). Diagnosis of nosocomial pneumonia in acute diffuse lung injury. Chest 80:254-258
5. Torres A, Aznar R, Gatell JM et al (1990) Incidence, risk, and prognosis factors of nosocomial pneumonia in mechanically ventilated patients. Am Rev Respir Dis 2:523-552
6. Craven DE, Kunches LM, Kilinsky V et al (1986) Risk factors for pneumonia and fatality in patients receiving continuous mechanical ventilation. Am Rev Respir Dis 133:792-796
7. Celis R, Torres A, Gatell JM et al (1988) Nosocomial pneumonia. A multivariate analysis of risk and prognosis. Chest 93:318-324
8. Fagon JY, Chastre J, Hance AJ et al (1993) Nosocomial pneumonia in ventilated patients: A cohort study evaluating attributable mortality and hospital stay. Am J Med 94:281-288
9. Wunderink RG, Woldenberg LS, Zeiss J et al (1992) The radiologic diagnosis of autopsy-proven ventilator-associated pneumonia. Chest 101:458-463
10. Meduri GU, Johanson WG (1992) International consensus conference: Clinical investigation of ventilator-associated pneumonia. Chest 102:551S-588S
11. Fagon JY, Chastre J, Hance AJ et al (1993) Evaluation of clinical judgement in the identification and treatment of nosocomial pneumonia in ventilated patients. Chest 103:547-553
12. Rello J, Ausina V, Ricart M et al (1993) Impact of previous antimicrobial therapy on the etiology and outcome of ventilator-associated pneumonia. Chest 104:1230-1235
13. Chastre J, Viau F, Brun P et al (1984) Prospective evaluation of the protected catheter brush for the diagnosis of pulmonary infections in ventilated patients. Am Rev Respir Dis 130: 924-93911
14. Rouby JJ, Rossignon MD, Nicolas MH et al (1989) A prospective study of protected bronchoalveolar lavage in the diagnosis of nosocomial pneumonia. Anesthesiology 71:679-685
15. Gaussorgues P, Piperno D, Bachmann P et al (1989) Comparison of nonbronchoscopic alveolar lavage to open lung biopsy for the bacteriologic diagnosis of pulmonary infections in mechanically ventilated patients. Intensive Care Med 15:98-102
16. Rouby JJ, Martin de Lassale EM, Poete P et al (1992) Nosocomial bronchopneumonia in the critically ill. Am Rev Respir Dis 146:1059-1066
17. Torres A, El-Ebiary M, Padro L et al (1994) Validation of different techniques for the diagnosis of ventilator-associated pneumonia. Comparison with immediate post-mortem pulmonary biopsy. Am J Crit Care Med 149:324-331
18. Chastre J, Fagon JY, Bornet-Lecso M et al (1995) Evaluation of bronchoscopic techniques for the diagnosis of nosocomial pneumonia. Am J Respir Crit Care Med 152:231-240
19. CH Marquette, MC Copin, F Wallet et al (1995) Diagnostic tests for pneumonia in ventilated patients: prospective evaluation of diagnostic accuracy using histology as a diagnostic gold standard. Am J Respir Crit Care Med 151:1878-1888

20. Papazian L, Thomas P, Garbe L et al (1995) Bronchoscopic or blind sampling techniques for the diagnosis of ventilator associated pneumonia. Am J Respir Crit Care Med 152:1982-1991
21. Fábregas N, Torres A, El-Ebiary M et al (1996) Histopathologic and microbiologic aspects of ventilator-associated pneumonia. Anesthesiology 84:757-759
22. Solé-Violán J, Rodriguez de Castro F, Rey A et al (1996) Comparison of bronchoscopic diagnostic techniques with histological findings in brain dead donors without suspected pneumonia. Thorax 51:929-931
23. Papazian L, Autillo-Touatti A, Thomas P et al (1997) Diagnosis of ventilator-associated pneumonia. An evaluation of direct examination and presence of intracellular organisms. Anesthesiology 87:268-276
24. Kirtland SH, Corley DE, Winterbauer RH et al (1997) The diagnosis of ventilator-associated pneumonia. A comparison of histologic, microbiologic and clinical criteria. Chest 112: 445-457
25. Johanson WG, Seidenfeld J, Gomez P et al. (1988) Bacteriologic diagnosis of nosocomial pneumonia following prolonged mechanical ventilation. Am Rev Respir Dis 137: 259-264
26. CH Marquette, Wallet F, Copin MC et al (1996) Relationship between microbiologic and histologic features in bacterial pneumonia. Am J Respir Crit Care Med 154:1784-1787
27. Wermert D, Marquette CH, Copin MC et al (1998) Influence of pulmonary bacteriology and histology in the yield of diagnostic procedures in ventilator acquired pneumonia. Am J Respir Crit Care Med (in press)
28. Blackmon JA (1994) Bacterial infection. In: Dail DH, Hammar SP (eds) Pulmonary pathology. Springer, Berlin Heidelberg New York, pp 255-330
29. Corley DE, Steven HK, Winterbauer RH et al (1997) Reproducibility of the histologic diagnosis of pneumonia among a panel of four pathologists. Analysis of a gold standard. Chest 112:458-465
30. El-Ebiary M, Torres A, Fàbregas N et al (1997) Significance of the isolation of Candida species from respiratory samples in critically ill, non-neutropenic patients. An immediate post-mortem histologic study. Am J Crit Care Med 156:583-590
31. Rouby JJ (1996) Nosocomial infection in the critically ill: The lung as a target organ. Anesthesiology 84:757-759
32. Rouby JJ (1996) Histology and microbiology of ventilator-associated pneumonia. Semin Respir Infect 11:54-61
33. A'Court CD, Garrard CS (1995) Nosocomial pneumonia in the ICU. New perspectives on current controversies. In: Vincent JL (ed) Yearbook of intensive care and emergency medicine vol. 99. Springer, Berlin Heidelberg New York, pp 726-747
34. Rodriguez de Castro F, Sole J, Elcuaz R et al (1994) Quantitative cultures of protected brush specimens and bronchoalveolar lavage in ventilated patients without suspected pneumonia. Am J Respir Crit Care Med 149:320-323
35. Pham LA, Brun-Bruisson C, Legrand P et al (1991) Diagnosis of nosocomial pneumonia in mechanically ventilated patients. Comparison of a plugged telescoping catheter with protected specimen brush. Am J Respir Dis 143:1055-1061
36. El-Ebiary M, Torres A, Gonzalez J et al (1993) Quantitative cultures of endotracheal aspirates for the diagnosis of ventilator-associated pneumonia. Am Rev Respir Dis 148:1552-1557
37. Pugin J, Auchenthaler R, Mili N et al (1991) Diagnosis of ventilator-associated pneumonia by bacteriologic analysis of bronchoscopic and non bronchoscopic "blind" bronchoalveolar lavage fluid. Am Rev Respir Dis 143:1121-1129
38. American Thoracic Society (1995) Hospital-acquired pneumonia in adults. Diagnosis, assessment of severity, initial antimicrobial therapy, and preventative strategies. A consensus statement. Am J Respir Crit Care Med 153:1711-1725

How to Diagnose Ventilator Associated Pneumonia

M. LANGER

Ventilator associated pneumonia (VAP) is a frequent infectious complication in ICU [1] and contributes to increase mortality in the ICU patients [2].

Diagnosis of VAP is difficult and remains controversial in spite of innumerable investigations. On several points, however, the consensus is nearly universal:

– Abnormal findings at the physical examination as well as clinical data (fever, abnormal respiratory secretions, evidence of inflammation in the laboratory tests, worsening of gas exchange) may be important but have a very low diagnostic specificity. These data are part of the daily clinical evaluation of the ventilated patient and abnormalities or changes should alert the intensivist and trigger further investigations [3].

– Radiological examinations of the lungs are usually performed as portable postero-anterior radiograph. Although their wide spread use, their diagnostic accuracy is rather low [4]. This is particularly true if the single examination is considered and many diagnostic protocols of VAP request in fact "a new and persistent infiltrate" as a valid diagnostic element. Newer techniques as CT scan of the lungs increase certainly the sensitivity but are obviously unable to increase the specificity. Only particular radiological findings as a lung abscess or empyema, very rare events in patients with VAP, allow a definite radiological diagnosis.

– Bacterial isolation from respiratory secretions is an important step in the diagnosis of VAP [5]. Pneumonia in the ventilated patient is in fact mainly a bacterial disease and most of the time the so called "nosocomial" bacteria are involved. Compared to the most frequent pathogens of the community acquired pneumonia (CAP), the "VAP pathogens", as *P. aeruginosa*, *MRSA*, *Acinetobacter* and other Gram negative microorganisms, can be easily cultured from a respiratory specimen. Microbiological analysis of respiratory secretion in patients with suspected VAP is recommended in order to define the pathogen(s) and to assess the in vitro susceptibility. The recovery of bacteria, however, doesn't per se allow to distinguish between a simple bacterial presence in the tracheo-bronchial tree (colonization), a localized infection (tracheitis/bronchitis) and a bacterial infection of the lung parenchyma. A concomitant and concordant positive blood culture increases of course the positive diagnostic value.

It is easy to understand that the area of consensus on the diagnosis of VAP is not large enough to solve the everyday problems and big efforts have been made to define diagnostic tools able to identify VAP with more specificity without loosing too much sensitivity.

The aim of the research in this field was therefore to assess the diagnostic value of more sophisticated microbiological assessments in patients with suspected VAP able to avoid contamination by the flora from the upper respiratory tract and assessments able to distinguish, via the quantification of bacteria present in the specimen, between colonization and infection.

In order to understand the discussion and to make the best choice for a single patient it is important to know exactly the characteristics of the different sample methods and the interpretation of the quantitative culture results.

Tracheal aspirate (TA)

It is the easiest, cheapest and most widely used sampling technique in the intubated patient. It is known to have a high sensitivity [1, 6-8] and negative standard culture results virtually exclude pneumonia due to the common aerobic pathogens, but of course not if the infection is due to *Legionella pneumophila*, *Mycoplasma pneumoniae*, *Chlamydia pneumoniae*, mycobacteria, *Pneumocystis carinii*, anaerobes or viruses. The specificity is much lower (a positive result doesn't always identify a patient with bacterial pneumonia) because of the frequent contamination of the trachea with saliva from the upper airways and because of the inability of the positive test to differentiate between tracheitis/bronchitis and pneumonia. Some recent investigations [6-8] show that unprotected tracheal aspirates are not so bad in diagnosing pneumonia and that their specificity can be improved by adopting a quantitative analysis with a cut off point $\geq 10^5$ or 10^6 cfu/ml. A very recent study [9] compared quantitative results from TA to diagnoses of pneumonia confirmed by PSB ($\geq 10^3$ cfu/ml) plus > 5% of BAL cells containing intracellular bacteria on direct examination. As expected, the sensitivity of this diagnostic procedure decreased from 90%, considering a cut off value $\geq 10^3$ cfu/ml, to 21% for a threshold $\geq 10^7$ cfu/ml. Conversely the specificity increased from 26% to 92%. Repeated analyses can be easily performed and reasonably increase the diagnostic accuracy.

Protected specimen brush (PSB)

It is mostly performed through a bronchoscope utilizing a protected brush [10] but also as blind sampling [11] with a double lumen catheter. In bronchoscopy the sampling area is selected based on the location of the new or progressive infiltrate on the chest radiograph or the segment visualized as having purulent secretion. Purulent secretions should be sampled at a subsegmental level. If purulent secretions are not evidenced, the brush should be advanced peripherally until it is not visualized, being careful not to wedge it into a peripheral position. Wedging may minimize sampling area and increase the risk for bleeding and pneumothorax [10].

Because of the antibacterial properties of lidocaine, bronchoscopy should be performed in general anaesthesia whenever possible. Inadequate sampling and previous antimicrobial therapy are the most frequent causes of false negative results and may contribute a relatively low sensitivity sometimes reported. Concerning the cut off point of the quantitative analysis, there is a wide agreement on $\geq 10^3$ cfu/ml in patients without antibiotic treatment. The microbiological analysis of the sample must be performed within a short time (15 minutes to maximal of 2 h) and the small sample volume may be an important limit of this method and makes direct examination (Gram stain) difficult and not sensitive.

Broncho-alveolar lavage (BAL)

It was first introduced to diagnose pneumonia in the immunocompromised patients [12] and is now used in many modifications as unprotected or protected sampling method through a wedged bronchoscope or also "blind", with a catheter directly introduced through the tracheal tube [10, 13, 14]. The most evident characteristic of BAL, compared to PSB, is the ability of this technique to investigate a much larger sampling area (about 1 million alveoli) if the lavage is properly done and a lavage fluid of 60-240 ml of sterile saline is injected in serial aliquot portions [10]. The dilution of alveolar secretions is 10-100 fold which makes the interpretation of results and cut off points (10^4-10^5 cfu/ml) more difficult to interpret than in PSB. Recently started or modified antibiotic treatment may significantly change the results as happens also for other sample techniques [15].

Direct cytologic and microbiologic examination of BAL fluid [16] may contribute to an appropriate and quick diagnosis of pneumonia (number of phagocytic cells with intracelluar bacteria) and rough microbiological diagnosis by Gram staining.

Unprotected BAL has of course a risk of contamination from upper airways or the bronchial tree. Suction through the working channel of the fibroscope should therefore be avoided before performing BAL and the first aspirated aliquot should not be submitted for quantitative analysis.

BAL is a relatively safe technique but in patients with respiratory failure and pneumonia acute worsening of PaO_2 and haemodynamics have been observed. [17]. A more recent modification of the usual BAL technique as the miniBAL [18] has probably a similar diagnostic accuracy.

Well defined indications [19] to approach suspected pulmonary infection with BAL are respiratory infections in the immunocompromised patient (*Pneu-*

mocystis carinii, *cytomegalovirus*, *mycobacterium tuberculosis* and *atypical mycobacteria* and also *Legionella pneumophila* by direct fluorescent antibody examination).

Sensitivity and specificity are established comparing test results with the true diagnosis but in the case of VAP the true diagnosis is difficult to assess. A "gold standard", a reliable reference method in diagnosing VAP is very difficult to obtain and the results are controversial.

Few studies compared diagnostic results from quantitative microbiological analysis with the histology and the bacterial burden of lung tissue in immediate postmortem findings of ventilated ICU-patients with suspected ventilator associated pneumonia [20-23]. This is probably the best available approach in humans, even if a dying patient might behave differently from a critically ill patient, as far as response to bacterial invasion is concerned. Selection of the study population seems therefore a crucial step and different characteristics of included patients may explain some different findings. This becomes very evident in comparing the findings from the most recent studies [22, 23]. Fabregas et al. [23] found a poor correspondence between bacterial burden of the lung tissue and the histologic grade of lung infection. The lungs of their patients were characterized by multifocal and polymicrobial processes and showed different evolution stages at the same time. Most of the included patients, however, had been admitted to ICU because of pneumonia and died without resolution of the infection.

J. Chastre et al. [22] studied 20 dying patients, who had either never developed pneumonia or developed it only during the terminal phase of their disease, just before death. These patients either were not treated with antibiotics for this episode or treatment was unchanged from several days. The aim of the selection was clearly to investigate a condition as close as possible to a first episode of suspected, ventilator associated pneumonia.

The study of Chastre et al. [22] shows very well the usefulness of quantitative microbiological analysis of specimens obtained by broncoalveolar lavage (BAL) and protected specimen brush (PSB) to diagnose pneumonia, as proven by histology and quantitative microbiology of lung tissue. Quantitative bacteriological results of specimens retrieved by BAL and PSB are in good agreement with histology and lung segment cultures. Also the correlation between BAL and PSB was very good with sensitivity and specificity of both methods ranging from 80 to 90%.

Conclusions

The available evidence tells us that adopting one of the "invasive" techniques and performing quantitative bacteriology we have a higher probability to make a correct diagnosis of VAP and probably we can avoid some useless treatment.

Tracheal aspirates, if combined with quantitative analysis, seem today an acceptable alternative but the lower specificity due to the proximal unprotected sampling must lead to a higher prescription rate of antimicrobials.

Both sampling methods must be combined with blood cultures which can always be drawn before starting antibiotics.

The advantage of the more complex invasive approach with quantitative microbiology has not yet been proved in terms of better outcome of patients [24] and a more sophisticated sampling technique should probably not delay significantly the start of an empiric treatment in high risk patient [25, 26].

References

1. Vincent JL, Bihari DJ, Suter PM et al for the EPIC International Advisory Committee (1995) Prevalence of nosocomial infection in intensive care units in Europe. Results of the European Prevalence of Infection in Intensive Care (EPIC) Study. JAMA 274:639-644
2. Fagon JY (1997) Influence of pneumonia on the mortality of the critically ill. Curr Op Crit Care 3:56-64
3. O'Grady NP, Barie PS, Bartlett J et al (1998) Practice parameters for evaluating new fever in critically ill adult patients. Crit Care Med 26:392-408
4. Winer Muram HT, Rubin SA, Ellis JV et al (1993) Pneumonia and ARDS in patients receiving mechanical ventilation: diagnostic accuracy of chest radiography. Radiology 188:479-485
5. Baselski VS, Wunderink RG (1994) Bronchoscopic diagnosis of pneumonia. Clin Microbiol Rev 7:533-558
6. Chevret S, Hemmer M, Carlet J et al and the European Cooperative Group on Nosocomial Pneumonia (1993) Incidence and risk factors of pneumonia acquired in intensive care units. Results from a multicenter prospective study on 996 patients. Intensive Care Med 19:256-264
7. Baselski VS, El-Torky M, Coalson JJ, Griffin JP (1992) The standardization of criteria for processing and interpreting laboratory specimens in patients with suspected ventilator-associated pneumonia. Chest 102:571S-579S
8. Marquette CH, Georges H, Wallet F et al (1993) Diagnostic efficiency of endotracheal aspirates with quantitative bacterial cultures in intubated patients with suspected pneumonia. Comparison with the protected specimen brush. Am Rev Respir Dis 148:138-144
9. Jourdain B, Novara A, Joly-Guillou et al (1995) Role of quantitative cultures of endotracheal aspirates in the diagnosis of nosocomial pneumonia. Am J Respir Crit Care Med 152:241-246
10. Meduri GU, Chastre J (1992) The standardization of bronchoscopic techniques for ventilator associated pneumonia. Chest 102:557S-564S
11. Pham LH, Brun Buisson C, Legrand P et al (1991) Diagnosis of nosocomial pneumonia in mechanically ventilated patients. Comparison of a plugged telescoping catheter with the protected specimen brush. Am Rev Respir Dis 143:1055-1061
12. Kahn FW, Jones JM (1987) Diagnosing bacterial respiratory infection by bronchoalveolar lavage. J Infect Dis 155:862-869
13. Pugin J, Auckenthaler R, Mili N et al (1991) Diagnosis of ventilator associated pneumonia by bacteriologic analysis of bronchoscopic and nonbronchoscopic "blind" bronchoalveolar lavage fluid. Am Rev Respir Dis 143:1121-1129
14. Meduri GU, Beals DH, Maijub AG, Baselsky V (1991) Protected bronchoalveolar lavage. A new bronchoscopic technique to retrive uncontaminated distal airway secretions. Am Rev Respir Dis 143:855-864
15. Souweine B, Veber B, Bedos JP et al (1998) Diagnostic accuracy of protected specimen brush and bronchoalveolar lavage in nosocomial pneumonia: impact of previous antimicrobial treatments. Crit Care Med 26:236-243

16. Chastre J, Fagon JY, Soler P et al (1989) Quantification of BAL cells containing intracellular bacteria rapidly identifies ventilated patients with nosocomial pneumonia. Chest 95: S190-S192
17. Pugin J, Suter PM (1992) Diagnostic bronchoalveolar lavage in patients with pneumonia produces sepsis like effect. Intensive Care Med 18:6-10
18. Kollef MH, Bock KR, Richards RD et al (1995) The safety and diagnostic accuracy of mini-bronchoalveolar lavage in patients with suspected ventilator-associated pneumonia. Ann Intern Med 122:743-748
19. Shelhamer JH, Gill VJ, Quinn TC et al (1996) The laboratory evaluation of opportunistic pulmonary infections. Ann Intern Med 124:585-599
20. Rouby JJ, Martin De Lassale E, Poete E et al (1992) Nosocomial bronchopneumonia in the critically ill. Histologic and bacteriologic aspects. Am Rev Respir Dis 146:1059-1066
21. Torres A, El-Ebiary M, Padr L et al (1994) Validation of different techniques for the diagnosis of ventilator-associated pneumonia. Comparison with immediate postmortem pulmonary biopsy. Am Rev Respir Crit Care Med 149:324-331
22. Chastre J, Fagon JY, Bornet-Lecso M et al (1995) Evaluation of bronchoscopic technique for the diagnosis of nosocomial pneumonia. Am J Respir Crit Care Med 152:231-240
23. Fabregas N, Torres A, El-Ebiary M et al (1996) Histopathologic and microbiologic aspects of ventilator-associated pneumonia. Anesthesiology 84:760-771
24. Niederman MS (1998) Bronchoscopy for ventilator associated pneumonia: show me the money (outcome benefit)! Crit Care Med 26:198-199
25. Kollef MH, Ward S (1998) The influence of mini-Bal cultures on patient outcomes. Chest 113:412-420
26. American Thoracic Society (1994) Hospital acquired pneumonia in adults: diagnosis, assessment of severity, initial antimicrobial therapy, and preventive strategy: a consensus statement. Am J Respir Crit Care Med 153:1711-1725

Can Hygienic Measures Prevent Pneumonia?

M.L. Moro

Available evidence on pneumonia associated with cross-infection

Several sources of infection for pneumonia, both endogenous and exogenous, have been implicated in ventilated patients. Colonized or contaminated hands and/or gloves, inadequately disinfected/sterilized devices, and contaminated water/solutions have all been found to be associated with the contamination of respiratory equipment and subsequent aspiration or inhalation of bacteria into the lower respiratory tract [1]. Most of the available evidence has come from outbreak investigations.

Transmission through hands. Pathogens causing nosocomial pneumonia, such as Gram-negative bacilli and *Staphylococcus aureus*, are ubiquitous in intensive care units (ICU). The health care workers' hands frequently become contaminated or transiently colonized with these microorganisms, which can then be transmitted to patients. Procedures such as tracheal suctioning and manipulation of ventilator circuit or endotracheal tubes increase the opportunity for cross-contamination [6]. Carriage of microorganisms on hands was implicated in more than 40 nosocomial outbreaks before 1978 [7], and it continues to be reported as the major source of infection in recent ICU outbreaks [8-10].

Contaminated respiratory and anaesthetic equipment. Several reports of outbreaks, published between 1965 and 1980, have incriminated respiratory and anaesthetic equipment as infection sources in ventilator-associated pneumonias (VAP), mostly caused by Gram-negative bacteria. In an extensive review of this topic, Hovig [2] reported at least 12 outbreaks traced to contamination of humidifier systems, and several other outbreaks due to contamination of the humidifier and expiratory tubing, of resuscitation equipment, of the catheter for tracheal suction, and to inhalation of contaminated aerosol in incubators and humidification tents, and in unheated room humidifiers. With the introduction of an appropriate decontamination protocol for respiratory devices and of sterile heated cascade humidifiers, the risk of transmission of bacteria was greatly reduced. Today, the mechanical ventilator is perceived as an "uncommon source of microorganisms that cause VAP" [3], and the only remaining concerns are the condensate in ventilator circuits and contaminated medication nebulizers. Nevertheless, outbreaks due to failure of decontamination of respiratory circuits or to in-use contamination have been recently reported, demonstrating that though this infection source has been greatly reduced, it has not been eliminated [4, 5].

Proportion of endemic pneumonias attributable to cross-infections

The above described outbreaks have proved that contaminated respiratory devices and the hands of health care workers can cause hospital-acquired pneumonias. However, the risk for endemic pneumonias attributable to non-adherence to the recommended standard for preventing cross-infections is unknown and only indirect evidence is available.

The huge variability existing in the ventilator-associated pneumonia rates among the same type of ICUs [11], for example, suggests that the observed differences cannot be explained exclusively on the basis of the severity of patients or the accuracy in detecting pneumonias. The measures adopted for preventing cross-infections, as well as other infection control measures, certainly have an impact on the incidence of pneumonia, yet the proportion of pneumonias attributable to these mechanisms still need to be determined.

According to Van Saene [12], the infections acquired while staying in the ICU (secondary endogenous or exogenous infections) represent, on average, only half of all infections in ICU patients, though this proportion greatly varies with the type of ICU. No estimate was provided in the paper on the proportion of pneumonias acquired within the ICU.

Effectiveness of handwashing and barrier precautions

Handwashing. All of the available guidelines recommend handwashing as the single most important measure for preventing the spread of infection in hospital [6]. This recommendation is based on the demonstrated association between hand colonization and hospital outbreaks, and on the fact that adequate handwashing is an effective way of removing transient bacteria from the hands. However, few studies have addressed the issue of handwashing and the reduction of endemic infections [13-15]. Moreover, the results of these studies are difficult to interpret due to the potential influence of several factors on handwashing efficacy in removing bacteria, such as compliance rates achieved, microbial agent used, duration of its use, and the technique employed. Simmons [14], for example, found no reduction in infection rates, whereas Conly [15] found a significant reduction. However, in the former study, the average handwashing compliance rate achieved after the intervention was 30% and the program did not target health care personnel other than nurses; in the latter study, all of the ICU personnel were involved and high rates of compliance were achieved (73% and 81% before and after patient's contact).

Several studies have found that routine hand antisepsis is superior to hand-washing with bland soap in ICU settings, indirectly pointing out that effective reduction of hand contamination has an impact on nosocomial infection rates [16-18]. Thus it seems that handwashing, when adequately carried out, could have a significant, but difficult to quantify, effect in reducing infection rates or, as concluded by Bryan [13] in a critical review of 18 handwashing studies, "hand washing can add incremental value to infection-control strategies in acute care settings". The problem is that compliance with handwashing is very difficult to achieve, as extensively demonstrated by all the studies in this field [19]. Moreover, when it is achieved, it is not maintained in the long-term [15].

Barrier measures (gloves and gowns). Given the low compliance with hand-washing, the routine use of gloves has been advocated to help prevent cross-contamination in ICUs. Klein [20] demonstrated that glove and gown precautions were effective in reducing nosocomial infection with bacteria and Candida in vulnerable children who were exposed to numerous invasive devices and required prolonged mechanical ventilatory support in the ICU. Routine gloving and gowning was also associated with a decreased incidence of nosocomial respiratory syncytial virus [21]. However, nosocomial pathogens can colonize gloves, and outbreaks have been traced to gloves not changed between patients' contacts [6]. Moreover, it has been shown that it may not be prudent to wash and reuse gloves between patients [22]. The use of gowns as an added barrier has been recommended to help control the spread of resistant microorganisms within hospitals. However, in one ICU study, gowns were found to provide no benefits beyond that afforded by gloves in controlling the spread of endemic vancomycin-resistant enterococci [23].

Effectiveness of comprehensive intervention programs

Recent quality improvement studies have shown the benefit of VAP prevention programs, aimed at reducing VAP incidence by modifying known extrinsic risk factors (rigorous hand-washing techniques, autoaspiration precautions, ventilator circuit maintenance) [24, 25]. These studies have reported a significant reduction in the VAP incidence, from 7/1000 to 3/1000 patients and from 26/1000 to 21/1000 ventilator-days. As concluded by Cook [26], "such multimodal prevention strategies informed by studies of modifiable risk factors for ICU-acquired pneumonia are potentially fruitful directions for future health service research programs".

References

1. Craven DE, Steger KA (1989) Nosocomial pneumonia in the intubated patients. New concepts on pathogenesis and prevention. Infect Dis Clin North Am 3(4):843-867
2. Hovig B (1981) Lower respiratory tract infections associated with respiratory therapy and anaesthesia equipment. J Hosp Infect 2:301-305
3. Mayhall CG (1997) Nosocomial pneumonia. Diagnosis and prevention. Infect Dis Clin North Am 11(2):427-457
4. Cefai C, Richards J, Gould FK et al (1990) An outbreak of Acinetobacter respiratory tract infection resulting from incomplete disinfection of ventilatory equipment. J Hosp Infect 15: 177-182
5. Hartstein AI, Rashad AL, Liebler JM et al (1988) Multiple intensive care unit outbreak of Acinetobacter calcoaceticus subspecies anitratus respiratory tract infection and colonization associated with contaminated, reusable ventilatory circuits and resuscitation bag. Am J Med 85:624-631
6. Centers for Disease Control (1994) Guidelines for prevention of nosocomial pneumonia. Resp Care 39(12):1191-1236
7. Maki D (1978) Control of colonization and transmission of pathogenic bacteria in hospital. Ann Intern Med 89:33-46
8. Chang HJ, Miller HL, Watkins N et al (1998) An epidemic of Malassezia pachydermatis in an intensive care nursery associated with colonization of health care workers' pet dogs. N Engl J Med 338(11):706-711
9. Struelens MJ, Carlier E, Maes N et al (1993) Nosocomial colonization and infection with multiresistant Acinetobacter baumanii: outbreak delineation using DNA macrorestriction analysis and PCR-fingerprinting. J Hosp Infect 25(1):15-32
10. Villarino ME, Stevens LE, Schable B et al (1992) Risk factors for epidemic Xanthomonas maltophilia infection/colonization in intensive care unit patients. Infect Control Hosp Epidemiol 13(4):201-206
11. CDC. National Nosocomial Infection Surveillance (NNIS) Report, data summary from October 1986-April 1997, Issued May 1997. Available on the CDC-Hospital Infection Program (HIP) web site: http://www.cdc.gov/ncidod/hip/hip.htm
12. Van Saene HKF, Damjanovic V, Murray AE, De La Cal MA (1996) How to classify infections in intensive care units - the carrier state, a criterion whose time has come? J Hosp Infect 33:1-12
13. Bryan JL, Cohran J, Larson EL (1995) Hand washing: a ritual revisited. Crit Care Nurs Clin North Am 7(4):617-625
14. Simmons B, Bruyant J, Neiman K et al (1990) The role of handwashing in prevention of endemic intensive care unit infections. Infect Control Hosp Epidemiol 11:589-594
15. Conly JM, Hill S, Ross J et al (1989) Handwashing practices in an intensive care unit: the effects of an educational program and its relationship to infection rates. Am J Infect Control 17: 330-339
16. Doebbeling BN, Stanley GL, Sheetz CT et al (1992) Comparative efficacy of alternative hand-washing agents in reducing nosocomial infections in intensive care units. N Engl J Med 327:88-93
17. Maki DG (1989) The use of antiseptics for handwashing by medical personnel. J Chemother 1[Suppl 1]:3-11
18. Massanari RM, Hierholzer WJ Jr (1984) A crossover comparison of antiseptic soaps on nosocomial infection rates in intensive care units. Am J Infect Control 12:247-248
19. Fridkin SK, Sharon F, Welbel, Weibstein RA (1997) Magnitude and prevention of nosocomial infections in the intensive care unit. Infect Dis Clin North Am 11(2):479-496
20. Klein B, Perloff WH, Maki DG (1989) Reduction of nosocomial infection during pediatric intensive care by protective isolation. N Engl J Med 320:1714-1721

21. Leclaire JM, Freeman J, Sullivan BF et al (1987) Prevention of nosocomial respiratory syncytial virus infections through compliance with glove and gown isolation precautions. N Engl J Med 317:329-334
22. Doebbeling BM, Pfaller MA, Houston AK et al (1988) Removal of nosocomial pathogens from the contaminated glove. Implications for reuse and handwashing. Ann Intern Med 109: 394-398
23. Slaughter S, Hayden MK, Nathan C et al (1996) A comparison of the effect of universal use of glove and gowns with that of glove use alone on acquisition of vancomycin-resistant enterococci in a medical intensive care unit. Ann Intern Med 125:448-456
24. Kelleghan SI, Salemi C, Padilla S et al (1993) An effective continuous quality improvement approach to the prevention of ventilator-associated pneumonia. Am J Infect Control 21: 322-330
25. Joiner GA, Salisbury D, Bollin GE (1996) Utilizing quality assurance as a tool for reducing the risk of nosocomial ventilator-associated pneumonia. Am J Med Qual 11:100-103
26. Cook D, Kollet MH (1998) Risk factors for ICU-acquired pneumonia. JAMA 279:1605-1606

Ventilatory Support in Different Stages of Lung Dysfunction

L. Brazzi, I. Ravagnan, L. Gattinoni

Adult respiratory distress syndrome (ARDS) is usually caused by disorders that cause intra-alveolar fluid accumulation resulting in severe ventilation-perfusion mismatch and hypoxaemia. In normal subjects, this kind of fluid accumulation is not present since the forces inducing fluid movement in and out of the intravascular space are almost in balance and also the small amount of fluid trasudation into the perivascular space (500 ml/day) is rapidly cleared by lymphatic drainage. Excluding the hypothesis of an imbalance between the forces justifying the fluids movements, the pathophysiologic mechanism behind ARDS is difficult to be understood even if the duration of the syndrome seems to play an important role. In this paper we will discuss: 1) the pathophysiology of ARDS; 2) the lung structure and function at different stages of the evolution of ARDS; 3) the possible physiopathologic and clinical implications of the observed differences.

Pathophysiology

The early phase of ARDS, classically termed as the exudative phase, is characterized by endothelial injury consisting of cellular swelling, denudation of type I epithelial cells, hyaline membrane formation, fibrin deposition and interstitial neutrophilic infiltrates. These changes are usually associated with a diffuse pulmonary vasoconstriction, the presence of microthromboemboli and interstitial oedema, which, all together, cause the pulmonary vascular pressure to increase. Clinically, this early phase is characterized by a thoracic X-ray showing diffuse, symmetric, bilateral disorder involving the lung parenchyma. It usually lasts for 3 to 7 days and is associated with markedly impaired oxygenation.

The second or proliferative stage is characterized by the organization of the alveolar and interstitial infiltrate: this includes fibroblast proliferation and type II cell hyperplasia. The lung vasculature is characterized by vascular intimal hyperplasia often associated with increased muscolarization of arterial walls. From the clinical point of view, the second phase of the syndrome is usually characterized by a progression from a simple hypoxic respiratory failure to hypercapnia mainly due to the fact that the workload of the respiratory muscles starts to exceed their capacity to sustain ventilation.

Three to 4 weeks after the onset, the patient enters the fibrotic phase characterized by extensive replacement of connective tissue by collagen. This period is clinically characterized by diffuse interstitial infiltrates and ventilator dependence secondary to high ventilatory dependence and dead space fraction.

Lung structure and function at different stages of ARDS

To evaluate the clinical consequences of time on lung structure and function during ARDS, in 1994 we studied, retrospectively, a group of patients who have been referred to our center to be treated with extracorporeal respiratory support [1]. Eighty-four patients (41 males and 43 females) with a mean age of 31.1 ± 14.4 years entered the study and had their ARDS duration estimated as the period of time spent between the day of intubation and the day of connection to extracorporeal support. According to such an interval, the patients were arbitrarily divided into three groups: 1) early ARDS (ARDS duration up to 1 week); 2) intermediate ARDS (ARDS duration between 1 and 2 weeks); and 3) late ARDS (ARDS duration longer than 2 weeks). The early ARDS group consisted of 37 patients, the intermediate ARDS group consisted of 24 patients and the late ARDS group consisted of 23 patients. We found that even if PaO_2 (66 ± 24, 73 ± 29 and 78 ± 42 mmHg, respectively; $p = 0.34$) and FiO_2 were similar in the three groups (86 ± 14, 83 ± 17 and 81 ± 19%, respectively; $p = 0.45$), the venous admixture was significantly lower in late ARDS (51 ± 13, 47 ± 12 and 42 ± 11, respectively; $p = 0.02$), despite a significantly lower level of PEEP (14 ± 4, 12 ± 4 and 9 ± 5 cm H_2O, respectively; $p = 0.002$). Moreover, we found that the PEEP level of the individual patients were significantly correlated with ARDS duration [PEEP = (17.4-0.44) * days of ARDS; $r = 0.67$, $p < 0.05$] while at comparable minute ventilation, both $PaCO_2$ (48.5 ± 10.6, 56.5 ± 24.4 and 61.8 ± 19.4 mmHg, respectively; $p = 0.03$) and dead space fraction (73 ± 9, 78 ± 10 and 79 ± 7%, respectively; $p = 0.04$) were significantly higher in late ARDS. Among the 84 patients, 41 (48.8%) had pneumothorax, defined as the presence of one or more thoracic tubes for pneumothorax drainage on the day of connection to the extracorporeal support: their incidence was significantly higher in late ARDS (87% of the patients) compared with early and intermediate ARDS (30% and 46% respectively; $p < 0.01$). Overall, we did not find any difference in the number or type of organ dysfunctions among the early, intermediate and late ARDS groups while the survival rate was lower in the late ARDS group (35%) compared with the intermediate ARDS group (50%) and early ARDS group (51%), even if the difference did not reach the level of statistical significance. Sixteen patients among the 84 included in the study underwent thoracic tomographic (CT) scan: nine were in the early ARDS group, two were in the intermediate ARDS group and five in the late ARDS group. Three slices of the CT scan at apex, hilum and base were taken at end expiration with the PEEP in clinical use. Each CT slice was divided into four quadrants and lung density was scored arbitrarily [1]. Bullae were defined as an emphysematous space larger than 1 cm in diameter in the distended state [2]. We found that the total CT scan density score per lung was similar in the three groups (21.1 ± 5.8, 19.8 ± 2.4 and 18.2 ± 6.6, respectively; $p = $ ns) with the densities prevalent at the hilum and basal sections. The number of bullae per lung was significantly increased in the late and intermediate ARDS groups compared with the early ARDS group (8.4 ± 4.1, 4.3 ± 5.3 and 1.9 ± 3.9, respectively; $p < 0.01$) and was significantly correlated with ARDS duration (bullae/lung = $[-0.07 + 0.91]$ * days of ARDS; $r = 0.74$; $p < 0.01$). The number of bullae was significantly higher at the hilum and basal sections compared with the apex ($p < 0.01$) and they were significantly higher in the dependent part of the lung ($p < 0.01$).

Physiopathologic and clinical implications

The data reported above seem to support the hypothesis that the lung structure and function change markedly with time, and that mechanical ventilation could contribute to the observed modifications. More in detail, in early ARDS, the severe oedema causes compression atelectasis in the dependent lung regions [3]: the lungs are reduced in size (baby lung) but still normal being the parenchyma just oedematous. The fraction of pulmonary flow to the atelectatic regions is lost to gas exchange (true shunt) and the ventilation-perfusion ratio maldistribution is, at this stage, negligible [4]. PEEP is, at this stage, effective since it acts as a counterforce, preventing the compression atelectasis [5, 6], while normocapnia is easily maintained at the price of high ventilation. With time, the lung structure changes: oedema is partially reabsorbed, the fibrous processes start developing while "broncopulmonary dysplasia" [7], "bronchiolectasis" [8] and bullae progressively characterize the pulmonary parenchyma. In the course of this process, the atelectatic areas progressively reduce their entity causing the air spaces open to gas exchange to increase and the global oxygenation to improve. The presence of fibrous structure [5] progressively reduces the transmission of the hydrostatic forces throughout the lung parenchyma and PEEP progressively looses its efficacy. Hypoxaemia could still be present even if it is no longer attributable to pulmonary shunt only, but ventilation-perfusion diffusion impairment and oxygen diffusion impairment [9] start to play a major role. As regards the carbon dioxide retention observed in late ARDS this is mainly due to the presence of the bullae above described, which causes the dead space of the lung to increase and the alveolar ventilation to decrease even if the vessel obliteration which characterizes the disease progression [10, 11] could contribute to the phenomenon.

The finding that the observed bullae were mainly distributed in the dependent lung, especially in intermediate and late ARDS, deserves some comments.

In fact, if the respiratory treatment alone would be the factor leading to their formation, we would expect a significant distributions of the lesions in the non dependent lung, as it is more exposed to barotrauma [3, 6, 12]. Our findings suggest that factors other than mechanical ventilation alone may cause the formation of bullae. One hypothesis is that, in the early stages of ARDS, the infection processes and ischemic necrosis are prevalent in the dependent collapsed lung; when the oedema is reabsorbed and the gas may reach the dependent lung regions, the gas pressure in the infected necrotic regions may cause the bullae formation: up to now, no study, to our knowledge, has clinically tested this hypothesis.

Conclusions

The acute respiratory distress syndrome is thought to be a uniform expression of a diffuse inflammatory reaction of the pulmonary parenchyma to a variety of underlying diseases. The possible differences in lung dysfunction among early, intermediate and late ARDS and ARDS resulting from pulmonary and extrapulmonary disease [13] have never been considered as major factors in designing the therapeutic approach to be applied to patients. A number of observations seems now to suggest that a different therapeutical effect could be expected according to the type and the stage of the disease. Care should hence be taken not only to the duration of the disease but to its etiology (pulmonary vs. extrapulmonary) as well as looking for the best therapeutical approach to be clinically used to treat the ARDS patients.

References

1. Gattinoni L, Bombino M, Pelosi P et al (1994) Lung structure and function in different stages of severe adult respiratory distress syndrome. JAMA 271:1772-1779
2. Sanders C (1991) The radiographic diagnosis of emphysema. Radiol Clin North Am 29: 1019-1030
3. Gattinoni L, Pesenti A, Bombino M et al (1988) Relationship between lung computed tomographic density, gas exchange and PEEP in adult respiratory failure. Anesthesiology 69: 824-832
4. Dantzker DR, Brook LJ, Dehart P et al (1979) Ventilation perfusion distributions in the ARDS. Am Rev Respir Dis 120:1039-1052
5. Gattinoni L, D'Andrea L, Pelosi P et al (1993) Regional effects and mechanism of positive end-expiratory pressure in early adult respiratory distress syndrome. JAMA 269:2122-2127
6. Gattinoni L, Pelosi P, Vitale G et al (1991) Body position changes redistribute lung computed tomographic density in patients with acute respiratory failure. Anesthesiology 74:15-23
7. Churg A, Golden J, Fligiel S et al (1983) Bronchopulmonary dysplasia in the adult. Am Rev Respir Dis 127:117-120
8. Slavin G, Nunn JF, Crow J et al (1982) Bronchiolectasis: a complication of artificial ventilation. BMJ 28:931-934

9. Lemaire F, Harf A, Teisseire BP (1985) Oxygen exchange across the acutely injured lung. In: Zapol WM, Falke K (eds) Acute respiratory failure. Marcel Dekker, New York, pp 521-552
10. Tomashefski JF Jr, Davies P, Boggis C et al (1983) The pulmonary vascular lesions of the adult respiratory distress syndrome. Am J Pathol 112:112-126
11. Snow RL, Davies P, Pontoppidan P et al (1982) Pulmonary vascular remodelling in adult respiratory distress syndrome. Am Rev Respir Dis 126:887-892
12. Maunder RJ, Shuman WP, McHugh JW et al (1986) Preservation of normal lung regions in the adult respiratory distress syndrome: analysis by computed tomography. JAMA 255: 2463-2465
13. Gattinoni L, Pelosi P, Suter PM et al (1998) Acute respiratory distress syndrome caused by pulmonary and extrapulmonary disease. Am J Respir Crit Care Med 157 (in press)

Strategies to Minimize Alveolar Stretch Injury During Mechanical Ventilation

N.R. MacIntyre

The concept of stretch injury during mechanical ventilation

The potential for positive pressure breaths to injure the lungs has long been appreciated. The best known form of injury occurs when positive pressure breaths grossly overinflate the lungs and result in pneumothorax, pneumomediastinum, subcutaneous emphysema, and other forms of "volutrauma" or "barotrauma" [1-4]. The mechanism for this type of injury is thought to be actual alveolar rupture into the perivascular space with subsequent dissection of air into the mediastinum, pleura and other locations [3-5]. The risk for alveolar overdistension and rupture becomes clinically significant when transalveolar pressures exceeds the normal maximum and approach 50-60 cm H_2O (Fig. 1).

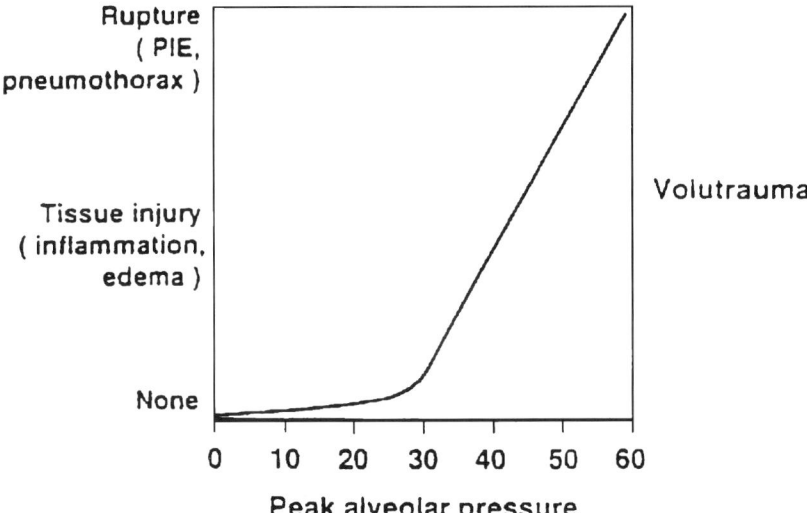

Fig. 1. Lung "stretch" injury (volutrauma) as a function of peak transalveolar pressure. The risk for stretch injury probably begins to rise when transalveolar pressure exceeds the normal maximum of 30-40 cm H_2O. Lung injury is initially characterized by alveolar-capillary inflammation. At higher transalveolar pressure, lung injury is manifest by alveolar rupture producing pulmonary interstitial emphysema (PIE) and other forms of extraalveolar air

In recent years there has been increasing data showing that alveolar distension resulting from transpulmonary pressures only marginally above the normal
maximal voluntary transpulmonary pressure of 30-40 cm H_2O may also be associated with lung injury [6-19]. This injury, however, does not involve alveolar
rupture but rather is characterized by a tissue injury involving the alveolar capillary interface. The presumed mechanism is that alveolar "stretch" beyond its
normal maximum disrupts the alveolar capillary membrane. This causes
parenchymal inflammation, capillary fracture [20], increased vascular permeability, abnormal accumulation of lung water, abnormal surfactant function [21],
alveolar flooding, atelectasis, radiographic infiltrates, and hypoxaemia from
shunt. Of note is that this injury may be most pronounced in previously healthy
lung units. This is because diffuse lung injury is often quite heterogenous (i.e.
certain lung units are severely injured and atelectatic while other units remain
relatively normal) [22, 23], and thus positive pressure ventilation delivered to the
airway may only minimally inflate abnormal units but may grossly overdistend
and consequently injure the healthier units. Conventional mechanical ventilation
goals to aggressively recruit and ventilate abnormal lung units with distending
pressures in excess of 30-40 cm H_2O, therefore, may run the risk of overdistending (stretching) and injuring the remaining healthier units.

Most of the evidence for this stretch injury comes from animal studies (Table
1). From these studies, it appears that *maximal* stretch is the key component of
injury although increasing *duration* and *frequency* of stretch may further increase injury [9, 17, 18]. The role of positive end expiratory pressure (PEEP) in
the development of stretch injury is more complex [6, 19, 24-26]. On one hand,
if PEEP elevates FRC primarily by distending already patent alveoli, further increases in PEEP for a given tidal volume will increase maximal (end inspiratory)
stretch. On the other hand, PEEP may increase FRC through recruitment of collapsed alveoli. This may affect stretch injury differently because alveolar collapse during expiration requires that the next positive pressure breath must "snap
open" that alveolar unit before gas can be delivered [24, 25]. This repetitive collapse and snapping open appears to potentiate the potential injury from positive
pressure breathing. Indeed, a number of animal studies have shown that providing enough expiratory pressure to prevent collapse (i.e. maintain alveolar recruitment) significantly reduces the potential for alveolar injury from a variety
of lung injuries [6, 19, 24-26]. Moreover, studies listed in Table 1 show that this
is also true in lung injuries resulting from overdistension. Additional support for
this concept comes from animal work during high frequency oscillatory ventilation where recruitment of a certain baseline lung volume reduced histologic abnormalities in injured lungs [29]. There is much less human data on this subject
but neonates on extracorporeal systems (ECMO) have been shown to have their
need for ECMO shortened if expiratory pressure was provided [30]. All of these
data taken together would suggest that, although PEEP can increase maximal
end inspiratory alveolar distension (and thus *increase* the potential for stretch injury), it also appears that a certain minimal PEEP to prevent collapse may *decrease* the stretch injury.

Table 1. Animal models of stretch injury

| Author | Model | Lung distension pressures (cm H$_2$O) | | Relative lung | |
		Ppeak	PEEP	Pmean	injury (1-4 + compared to normal)
Webb [6]	rats	14	0	3.6	1+
		30	0	6.7	2.5+
		45	0	9.7	3.5+
		30	10	14.2	2+
		45	10	17.8	3+
Parker [14, 16]	dogs	60	0		2+
		50	0		1.5+
		40	0		1+
		30	0		0
		15	0		0
Tsuno [17]	sheep	15	4		1+
		30	4 (rate = 4)		2+
		30	4 (rate = 15)		3+
Kolobow [9]	sheep	20	7		1+
		50	7 (rate = 3)		3+
		50	7 (rate = 12)		4+
Tsuno [18]	pigs	18	4		0
		40	4		1.5
Dreyfuss [19]	rats	8	0		0
		15	0		0
		45	0		3+
		22	10		0
		45	10		1.5+
		37	15		1+

Since pathologic findings related to stretch injury are very similar to those observed in acute lung injury (ALI) and acute respiratory distress syndrome (ARDS), it may be that lung injury from overdistension may exacerbate or prevent resolution from ARDS. Recovery from respiratory failure and survival might therefore be better if ventilation strategies are used that avoided or reduced excessive stretching forces applied to the lung. Indeed, this is the conclusion of an uncontrolled trial of low stretch ventilation [27] as well as a recent preliminary clinical trial [28]. It is also the reason that a number of recent consensus groups have recommended avoidance of high ventilation pressures to reduce stretch induced lung injury (see below) [1].

Measuring alveolar distension and setting ventilator targets

Measuring and monitoring alveolar volume is difficult to do clinically. Instead, approaches that assess pressures or pressure-volume relationship can be taken to indirectly assess the risk of stretch injury and guide strategies to manage it.

The simplest approach is to use the so called airway "plateau" pressure. This is the airway pressure at end inspiration under "no flow" conditions and, as such, is the alveolar pressure at end inspiration. Assuming that chest wall and extrapulmonary pressures are low (i.e. patient is not dys-synchronous, chest wall has normal compliance, and abdominal pressures are small), this is a reasonable reflection of maximal transalveolar pressure and can be used to estimate the distension of lung units of varying compliance. As a simple rule, many consensus groups recommend keeping plateau pressures below 30-40 cm H_2O in order to keep normally compliant units from exceeding their normal maximal volume [1].

A more sophisticated approach that assesses both alveolar overdistension as well as recruitment is the use of a static pressure-volume (P-V) plot (Fig. 2) [31-33]. Properly done, this plot can be used to detect both a lower and an upper "inflection" point (Pflex) which represent clear changes in the lung's pressure-volume relationship. The lower inflection point (lower Pflex) has been argued as a level above which PEEP should be set to use to avoid collapse injury (see

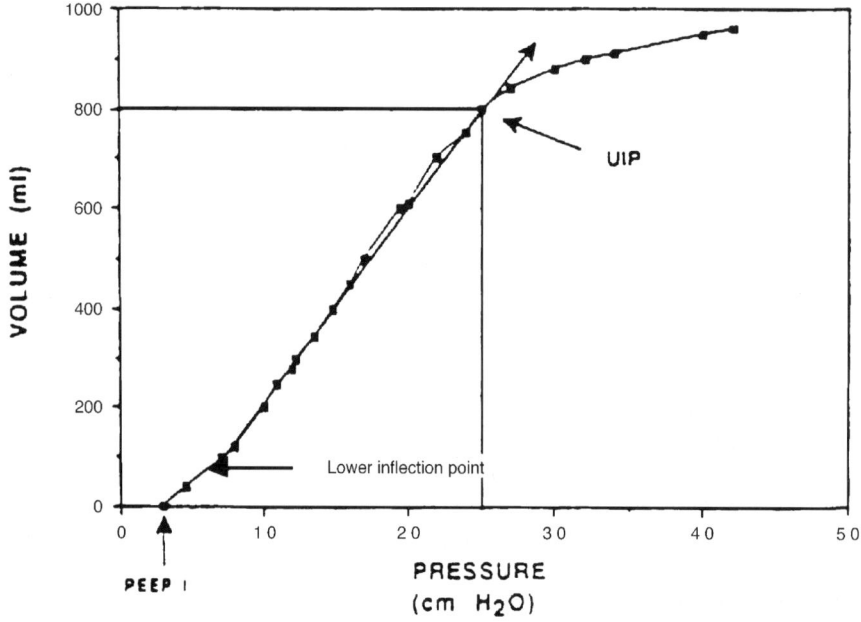

Fig. 2. Static pressure-volume plot in a patient with ARDS. In this example, 3 cm H_2O intrinsic PEEP (PEEPi) is present. Lower and upper inflection points can be appreciated from this plot. These are often taken as points representing minimal recruitment pressures (lower inflection point) and overdistending pressures (upper inflection point). The ideal ventilatory pattern using these measurements would be a PEEP just above the lower inflection point and a tidal volume - PEEP combination that kept maximal pressures below the upper inflection point (From: Rouple E, Dambrosio M, Servillo G et al (1995) Titration of tidal volume and induced hypercapnia in acute respiratory distress syndrome. Am J Resp Crit Care Med 152:121-128. With permission)

above). At the other end of the curve, the upper inflection point (upper Pflex) has been argued as a level above which additional volume/pressure changes are associated with overdistension. Plotting a static P-V relationship, however, is a cumbersome procedure requiring multiple breaths of varying size and often requires patient sedation or paralysis. It is thus not a practical clinical procedure. A more promising clinically applicable approach has been proposed that utilizes a constant flow mechanical breath at varying levels of PEEP to identify minimal recruitment PEEP and overdistension volumes [32].

Practical ways to assess proper mechanical PEEP and tidal volume are clearly needed. In the absence of P-V plots, one approach would be to utilize gas exchange parameters. For instance, clinical studies have demonstrated that the lower Pflex is generally in the range of 5-15 cm H_2O in ARDS patients requiring $FiO_2 > 0.40$ [28, 31-33]. Thus, providing a minimal PEEP of 10-15 cm H_2O in these types of patients would probably provide an appropriate level from a mechanical perspective. An alternative approach would be to recognize that the P-V relationship between the lower Pflex and the upper Pflex reflects the best lung compliance [34]. Thus, optimizing this parameter may be a reasonable surrogate for plotting the two inflection points. With this approach, a tidal breath approaching maximal normal distension (i.e. 25-30 cm H_2O) and a PEEP of 15 cm H_2O might be used to initially recruit all recruitable alveoli. A lower PEEP setting that remained above the lower Pflex might then be determined by measuring the best compliance as one progressively lowered PEEP to a minimum of 5 cm H_2O.

Strategies to minimize alveolar overdistension

Reducing alveolar overdistension during mechanical ventilation can be accomplished by either keeping baseline pressure and volume to a minimum or by keeping tidal pressures and volume distension to a minimum. Tradeoffs, however, are required (Table 2):

1. Minimizing PEEP. Since PEEP is the baseline pressure, it determines baseline alveolar volume (FRC). Minimizing PEEP, however, requires tradeoffs. On the one hand, as noted above, a certain level of PEEP to prevent alveolar collapse may be needed to reduce lung injury. Moreover, alveoli that do not collapse provide better gas exchange and thus a lower FiO_2 requirement. On the other hand, providing high levels of PEEP in an attempt to "normalize" PaO_2 may be counterproductive if it results in alveolar overdistension. As noted above, appropriate PEEP is probably in the 5-15 cm H_2O range and mechanical considerations may be the best guide to setting the minimally required PEEP.

   Because a mechanically determined level of PEEP may not give maximal values for PaO_2, this strategy may require a higher FiO_2. In addition, arterial haemoglobin saturations lower than usual may be tolerated (e.g. 85-88%) if

Table 2. Tradeoffs when minimizing PEEP and VT

Minimizing PEEP:
    Advantage
        lower baseline volume and pressure to reduce overdistension with the applied tidal breath
    Tradeoffs
        higher FiO_2, lower SaO_2, and loss of protection from alveolar collapse related injury if
        PEEP too low
Minimizing VT:
    Advantage - lower tidal volume and pressure to prevent overdistension
    Tradeoffs - higher PCO_2, lower pH, lower SaO_2

oxygen delivery can be maintained with other methods (i.e. improving cardiac output and/or increasing haemoglobin concentration) [1]. Prolonging the inspiratory time can also be used as an alternative to additional PEEP when mechanical recruitment seems optimal but oxygenation is not. A longer inspiratory time has two effects. First, there is a longer mixing period and exposure of capillaries to gas filled alveoli. This alone may serve to reduce the alveolar-arterial oxygen difference [35]. A second effect is the prevention of complete lung emptying because of consequently shorter expiratory times. This is the phenomenon of air trapping and produces "intrinsic PEEP" [36]. It is well known that the development of intrinsic PEEP functions much like applied PEEP in its effects on functional residual capacity and lung volumes [37]. Alveolar overdistension can thus again become a problem when air trapping and intrinsic PEEP develop. Using longer inspiratory times must therefore be done with caution and with careful monitoring of air trapping.

2. Minimizing tidal volume. The second component of alveolar distension is tidal distension. Historically, delivered tidal volumes were often recommended to be as high as 15-20 ml/kg. This, however, was a reflection of practice in anaesthesia before the development of PEEP when large tidal volumes were required to overcome atelectasis. Lowering tidal volumes to 6-8 ml/kg will clearly reduce alveolar pressures and alveolar distension [27, 28, 37]. Alveolar ventilation can be maintained up to a point by increasing the respiratory frequency. Ultimately, however, rapid rates cannot compensate for the loss of tidal volume. Under these circumstances, alveolar ventilation will fall, arterial PCO_2 will rise and arterial pH will fall [1, 27, 28, 38, 39]. This hypercapnia is often referred to as "permissive hypercapnia" and pHs with this strategy have been reported to fall below 7.0. The effects of normoxic hypercapnia under those circumstances are only beginning to be understood. In general, however, humans seem to tolerate an arterial pH of 7.15 and PCO_2 of 80 torr quite well [38]. The rate at which the $PaCO_2$ is allowed to should probably be slow (e.g. 10 torr/hr) so as to permit intracellular pH to adjust [38].

Caution shall be used in permitting respiratory acidosis in patients with intracranial mass effects, recent myocardial infarcts, pulmonary hypertension and possibly gastrointestinal bleeding [38-40]. Respiratory acidosis may also contribute to dyspnea and agitation in critically ill patients and this may require heavy sedation or paralysis [38]. In the animal model with acute lung injury, pulmonary shunt was higher when ventilation was achieved with smaller tidal volumes [41]. Thus smaller tidal volumes may require an increased level of PEEP and/or FIO_2 to maintain acceptable levels of arterial oxygenation. As noted previously, a low tidal volume strategy has been reported to show lower mortality when compared to historical controls matched for physiologic scores [27]. More compelling is a recent preliminary report of a controlled trial using both small tidal volume and PEEP set above the lower Pflex demonstrating favorable trends in favor of the lung protection strategy [28].

Conclusions

The concept of stretch injury has considerable data to support it. Indeed, it stands to reason that lung units "designed" to have transalveolar pressures of 30-40 cm H_2O at maximal volume would be subject to injury when distended beyond that. "Lung protection" ventilatory strategies using lower baseline and tidal pressure applications involve tradeoffs.

Lower baseline distension with PEEP must be balanced against higher FiO_2 requirements, lower SaO_2 values and the possibility that a certain degree of alveolar recruitment with PEEP may be necessary to reduce ventilator related lung injury. Similarly, low tidal breath distension and "permissive" hypercapnia must be balanced against the potential consequences of respiratory acidosis. Improved outcome is suggested by both uncontrolled early controlled trials using "lung protective" strategies. However, carefully done randomized controlled studies are needed to fully assess the role of these approaches.

References

1. ACCP Consensus Group (1993) Mechanical ventilation. Chest 104:1833-1859
2. American Association for Respiratory Care (1992) Consensus on essentials of mechanical ventilation. Resp Care 37:1000-1009
3. Samuelson WM, Fulkerson WF (1991) Barotrauma in mechanical ventilation. Prob Resp Care 4:52-67
4. Steier M, Ching N, Roberts E et al (1974) Pneumothorax complicating continuous ventilatory support. J Thorac Cardiovasc Surg 67:17-23
5. Macklin M, Macklin C (1950) Malignant interstitial emphysema of the lungs and mediastinum as an important occult complication in many respiratory diseases and other conditions. Medicine (Baltimore) 23:281-358
6. Webb HH, Tierney DF (1974) Experimental pulmonary edema due to intermittent positive pressure ventilation with high inflation pressure. Protection by positive end-expiratory pressure. Am Rev Resp Dis 199:556-565
7. Corbridge TC, Wood LD, Crawford GP et al (1990) Adverse effects of large tidal volume and low PEEP in canine acid aspiration. Am Rev Resp Dis 142:311-315
8. Hernandez LA, Coker PJ, May S et al (1990) Mechanical ventilation increases microvascular permeability in oleic acid injured lungs. J Appl Physiol 69:2057-2061
9. Kolobow T, Moretti MP, Fumagalli R et al (1987) Severe impairment in lung function induced by high peak airway pressure during mechanical ventilation. Am Rev Resp Dis 135:312-315
10. Mascheroni D, Kolobow T, Fumagalli R et al (1988) Acute respiratory failure following pharmacologically induced hyperventilation: an experimental animal study. Intensive Care Med 15:8-14
11. Dreyfuss D, Soler P, Basset G, Saumon G (1988) High inflation pressure pulmonary edema. Am Rev Resp Dis 137:1159-1164
12. Dreyfuss D, Basset G, Soler P, Saumon G (1985) Intermittent positive-pressure hyperventilation with high inflation pressures produces pulmonary microvascular injury in rats. Am Rev Resp Dis 132:880-884
13. Bowton DL, Kong DL (1989) High tidal volume ventilation produces increased lung water in oleic acid injured rabbit lungs. Crit Care Med 17:908-911
14. Parker JC Townsley MI, Rippe B et al (1984) Increased microvascular permeability in dog lungs due to high peak airway pressures. J Appl Physiol 57:18091816
15. Parker JC, Hernandez LA, Peevy KJ (1993) Mechanisms of ventilator-induced lung injury. Crit Care Med 21:131-143
16. Parker JC, Hernandez LA, Longenecker GL et al (1990) Lung edema caused by high peak inspiratory pressures in dogs. Am Rev Resp Dis 142:321-328
17. Tsuno K, Prato P, Kolobow T (1990) Acute lung injury from mechanical ventilation at moderately high airway pressures. J Appl Physiol 69:956-961
18. Tsuno K, Miura K, Takeya M et al (1991) Histopathologic pulmonary changes from mechanical ventilation at high peak airway pressures. Am Rev Resp Dis 143:1115-1120
19. Dreyfuss D, Saumon G (1993) The role of tidal volume, FRC and end inspiratory volume in the development of pulmonary edema following mechanical ventilation. Am J Resp Crit Care Med 148:1194-1203
20. Fu Z, Costello ML, Tsukimoto K et al (1992) High lung volume increases stress failure in pulmonary capillaries. J Appl Physiol 73:123-133
21. Wyszogrodski I, Kyei-Aboagye K, Taeusch HW, Avery ME (1975) Surfactant inactivation by hyperventilation: conservation by end expiratory pressure. J Appl Physiol 38:461-466
22. Gattinoni L, Pesenti A, Avalli L et al (1987) Pressure-volume curve of total respiratory system in acute respiratory failure: computed tomographic scan study. Am Rev Resp Dis 136:730-736
23. Gattinoni L, Pelosi P, Crotti S, Valenza F (1995) Effects of positive end expiratory pressure on regional distribution of tidal volume and recruitment in adult respiratory distress syndrome. Am J Resp Crit Care Med 151:1807-1814

24. Sandhar BK, Niblett DJ, Argiras EP et al (1988) Effect of positive end expiratory pressure on hyaline membrane formation in a rabbit model of the neonatal respiratory distress syndrome. Intensive Care Med 14:538-546

25. Muscedere JG, Mullen JB, Gan K, Slutsky AS (1994) Tidal ventilation at low airway pressure can augment lung injury. Am J Resp Crit Care Med 149:1327-1334

26. Ranieri VM, Eissa NT, Corbeil C et al (1991) Effects of positive end expiratory pressure on alveolar recruitment and gas exchange in patients with the adult respiratory distress syndrome. Am Rev Resp Dis 144:544-551

27. Hickling KG, Walsh J, Henderson S, Jackson R (1994) Low mortality rate in adult respiratory distress syndrome using low-volume, pressure-limited ventilation with permissive hypercapnia: a prospective study. Crit Care Med 22:1568-1578

28. Amato MBP, Barbas CSV, Medeiros DM et al (1993) Beneficial effects of the "open lung approach" with low distending pressures in ARDS. Am J Resp Crit Care Med 147: (abstract)

29. Bond DM, McAloon J, Froese AB (1994) Substantial inflations improve respiratory compliance during high frequency oscillatory ventilation but not during large tidal volume positive pressure ventilation in rabbits. Crit Care Med 22:1269-1277

30. Kezzler M, Ryckman FC, McDonald JV et al (1992) A prospective randomized study of high vs low PEEP during ECMO. J Pediatr 120:107-113

31. Rouple E, Dambrosio M, Servillo G et al (1995) Titration of tidal volume and induced hypercapnia in acute respiratory distress syndrome. Am J Resp Crit Care Med 152:121-128

32. Ranieri VM, Giuliani R, Fiore T et al (1994) Volume pressure curve of the respiratory system predicts effects of PEEP in ARDS: occlusion vs constant flow technique. Am J Resp Crit Care Med 149:19-27

33. Putensen C, Bain M, Hormann C (1993) Selecting ventilator settings according to the variables derived from the quasi static pressure volume relationship in patients with acute lung injury. Anesth Analg 77:436-447

34. Suter PM, Fairley HB, Isenberg MD (1975) Optimic end expiratory pressure in patients with acute pulmonary failure. N Engl J Med 292:284-289

35. Armstrong BW, MacIntyre NR (1995) Pressure-controlled, inverse ratio ventilation that avoid air trapping in the adult respiratory syndrome. Crit Care Med 23:279-285

36. MacIntyre NR (1991) Intrinsic positive end expiratory pressure. Prob Resp Care 4:44-51

37. Darioli R and Perret C (1984) Mechanical controlled hypoventilation in status asthmaticus. Am Rev Resp Dis 129:385-387

38. Fiehl F, Perret C (1994) Permissive hypercapnia - how permissive should we be? Am J Resp Crit Care Med 150:1722-1737

39. Tuxen DV (1994) Permissive hypercapnic ventilation. Am J Resp Crit Care Med 150:870-874

40. Simon RJ, Mawilmada S, Ivatury RR (1984) Hypercapnia: is there a cause for concern? J Trauma 74-81

41. Hedley-Whyte J, Laver MB, Bendixen HH (1964) Effect of changes in tidal ventilation on physiologic shunting. Am J Physiol 206:891-897

Modes of Ventilation and Weaning Strategies

C. Putensen, F. Stüber, H. Wrigge

The traditional mechanically ventilatory management of patients with acute lung injury has been based on the perception of a uniformly distributed lung damage. Conventionally, full ventilatory support has been provided with large tidal volumes of 10 to 15 ml/kg, low ventilatory frequencies of 10 to 15 breaths/min, and PEEP levels that allowed adequate arterial oxygenation without using toxic inspiratory oxygen fractions (FiO$_2$) = 0.5 [1]. Discontinuation of mechanical ventilation has been determined mainly by the clinical and often subjective judgment of a well trained physician and was accomplished with T-tube trials ("sink or swim" technique). Downs et al. [2] in 1973 introduced intermittent mandatory ventilation (IMV), that allows unsupported spontaneous breathing to occur between mechanically delivered tidal volumes. Although introduced as a weaning technique [2, 3], IMV rapidly became a standard technique for primary mechanical ventilatory support in most intensive care units [4]. This occurred despite a debate regarding the usefulness of IMV, because clinical experience demonstrated that an adjustable ventilatory support was advantageous. However, controlled mechanical ventilation and IMV represent different levels of ventilatory support administered by using the same technique.

Evolution of pathophysiologic knowledge and technology has resulted in a variety of new modalities and techniques designed to augment alveolar ventilation, decrease the work of breathing, improve the matching between ventilation and perfusion ($\dot{V}_A/\dot{Q}$), and thereby the oxygenation of the arterial blood. However, new ventilatory support modalities are only likely to result in a significant clinical improvement if the method to effect changes in lung volume or the interfacing of mechanical and spontaneous ventilation differs from previous techniques [5, 6]. The following discussion will attempt to clarify the principles of new ventilatory support modalities and their expected and observed physiological effects.

Full ventilatory support

Intermittent positive pressure mechanical ventilation is still widely used to support adequately alveolar ventilation in patients with neuromuscular inability, decreased drive to breath, after severe trauma or major operative procedures in many intensive care units.

Techniques

Volume controlled mechanical ventilation (VCV) delivers periodically a preset tidal volume at a constant inspiratory flow. Following mechanical insufflation an end-inspiratory non flow period (an inflation hold) can generally be adjusted. Insufflation is terminated when a preset time has elapsed and expiration occurs passively under the action of the elastic recoil of the respiratory system. Resulting airway pressures are mainly the result of the mechanics of the respiratory system. Hence, VCV takes over the total work of ventilation. Although the tidal volume is preset during VCV, a deterioration in lung mechanics may cause a significant reduction of the tidal volume delivered to the patient because of an increase of the compressible gas volume trapped in the ventilator circuit.

Pressure controlled mechanical ventilation (PCV) switches periodically between to preset airway pressure levels [1]. The typical decelerating inspiratory flow pattern with an initial peak followed by a gradual decrease is determined by the reduction of the pressure difference between airway opening and the alveoli. Because changes in respiratory mechanics may considerably affect tidal volume, careful monitoring of tidal and minute ventilation has to be recommended during PCV.

Inverse ratio ventilation (IRV) extends the inspiration time while reducing the expiration time and may cause an intrinsic PEEP (PEEPi) which has been suggested to improve alveolar recruitment in patients with acute respiratory distress syndrome (ARDS) [7-9]. In addition, holding a high but not overdistending airway pressure level has been suggested to contribute to alveolar recruitment and better distribution of ventilation to lung units with different time constants [7-9].

Numerous investigations compared IRV with a conventional VCV in patients with acute lung injury and observed lower peak airway pressures, reduction in dead space, and improved arterial oxygenation [7-10]. However, no change has been found in arterial oxygenation when total PEEP was kept constant between the tested ventilatory modalities [10]. Recent observations in patients with ARDS suggest that increasing inspiration time even in the absence of PEEPi may improve arterial oxygenation [11]. Nevertheless, the true effect of inverting the inspiration/expiration ratio is difficult to deduct from these studies, because mean airway pressure and inspiratory flow pattern were changed simultaneously.

However, main limitation of VCV, PCV, and IRV is the requirement of completely relaxed respiratory muscles to provide adequate ventilatory support. Any spontaneous efforts of the patients will cause fighting the ventilator and necessitate deep sedation and even neuromuscular blockade.

Partial versus full ventilatory support

Partial ventilatory support is used, not only to separate patients from mechanical ventilation, but also to provide stable ventilatory assistance of a desired degree [4, 12, 13]. Because excessive workload may lead to muscle fatigue, sufficient ventilatory support has to be provided to maintain work of breathing on a tolerable degree [14]. Increasing the level of ventilatory support beyond an adequate level of work of breathing and alveolar ventilation has not been demonstrated so far to be beneficial for the patient. Therefore, full ventilatory support has to be seen as an extreme level of ventilatory support. However, full ventilatory support may be justified in apneic patients, to provide artificial hyperventilation in patients with elevated intracranial pressure or in the presence of deep anaesthesia for invasive procedures.

Maintenance of spontaneous breathing during ventilatory support may avoid neuromuscular blockade, deep sedation, and immobility which has been claimed to contribute to impaired strength and dyscoordination of respiratory muscles and thereby may complicate weaning off the ventilator [15]. Partial ventilatory support when used as primary mechanical ventilatory support has been shown to reduce significantly the dose of analgesics and sedatives commonly used to adapt patients with mild pulmonary dysfunction [16, 17] or acute lung injury [18] to ventilatory support. Avoiding suppression of spontaneous breathing during ventilatory support in patients with acute lung injury seems to be associated with a shorter weaning period and admission to the intensive care unit (ICU), when compared to patients that were mechanically ventilated for three days and then weaned off with partial ventilatory support [18]. In addition, less sedation and a shorter ICU admission reduced significantly the costs for intensive care in patients that were allowed to breath spontaneously during ventilatory support (Fig. 1).

Full mechanical ventilatory support effects lung volume by an increase in airway and intrathoracic pressure and reduces the venous return to the right ventricle [19]. A decrease in right and left ventricular filling usually is associated with a decrease in stroke volume, cardiac output, and oxygen delivery in normo- and hypovolaemic patients [20]. In contrast, cardiac output and stroke volume should increase during sufficient partial ventilatory support because spontaneous inspirations cause periodic decreases in intrathoracic pressure and thus increased venous return [12, 21]. The concept is supported by an increase of right ventricular end-diastolic volume index (RVEDVI), right ventricular ejection fraction (RVEF), and cardiac output observed in patients with ARDS during spontaneous breathing with airway pressure release ventilation (APRV) or biphasic positive airway pressure (BIPAP) [22].

Radiographic studies have shown a significant difference in the distribution of ventilation between full ventilatory support and unsupported spontaneous breathing [23]. Unsupported spontaneous ventilation is preferably directed to well-perfused, dependent lung regions, whereas a mechanically delivered tidal

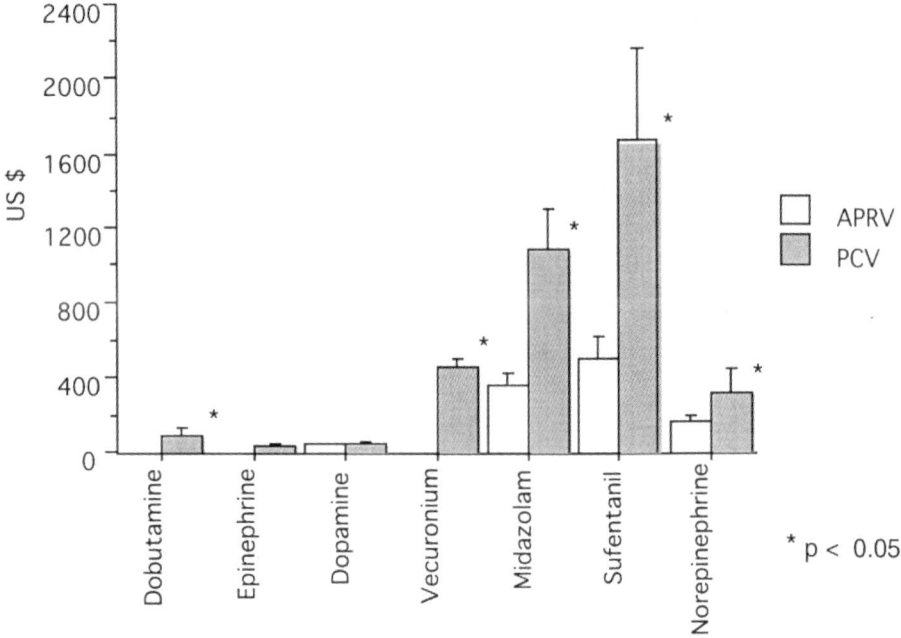

Fig. 1. Costs for analgesics and sedatives during spontaneous breathing with APRV/BIPAP and controlled mechanical ventilation with PCV

volume is directed primarily to nondependent lung areas, away from regions with maximal blood flow [23]. Presumably, diaphragmatic contraction augments the distribution of ventilation to dependent, well-perfused lung regions [23]. Therefore, an improvement in $\dot{V}_A/\dot{Q}$ matching has been claimed a major advantage of partial over full ventilatory support [13]. This assumption is supported by findings in animals with induced lung injury [12, 24] and patients with acute respiratory distress syndrome (ARDS) [22] demonstrating reduction in intrapulmonary shunting and improved arterial oxygenation during spontaneous breathing with APRV/BIPAP.

Partial ventilatory support

Techniques

Partial ventilatory support modalities provide either ventilatory assistance to every inspiratory effort and modulate tidal volume of the patient (e.g. pressure support ventilation, PSV; proportional assist ventilation, PAV) [25, 26] or modulate minute ventilation ($\dot{V}_E$) by adding mechanical insufflations to unsupported spontaneous breathing (e.g. IMV) [2]. Ventilatory support techniques, such as BIPAP [27, 28] which is equivalent to APRV [29, 30] allow unrestricted spontaneous breathing in any phase of the mechanical cycle.

Intermittent mandatory ventilation (IMV) allows unsupported and unrestricted spontaneous breathing to occur between mechanically delivered tidal volumes [2]. The mechanical breaths can be limited and cycled in any way and synchronized to be patient-triggered [13, 31]. Patient-triggered mechanical breaths have not been demonstrated to be advantageous for the patient [31]. The level of mechanical ventilatory support during IMV is primarily varied by the frequency of mandatory breaths. Consequently, higher mechanical ventilatory support during IMV requires an increase in the ventilatory rate and will unfortunately shorten the phase in which spontaneous breathing is possible. Therefore, controlled mechanical ventilation and IMV represent different levels of ventilatory support administered by using the same technique.

Biphasic positive airway pressure (BIPAP), *airway pressure release ventilation (APRV)* and PSV [27, 29] are similar in their pressure-limited delivery of tidal volume, but differ in their interfacing with spontaneous ventilation. Spontaneous breathing in any phase of the mechanical ventilator cycle may occur with APRV/BIPAP that ventilates by periodic switching between two pressure levels in a high flow or demand valve continuous positive airway pressure (CPAP) circuit [27, 29]. The degree of ventilatory support with APRV/BIPAP is determined by the duration of both CPAP levels (ventilator rate) and the delivered tidal volume (Fig. 2) [27-29, 32]. The tidal volume depends on the applied pressure difference between both CPAP levels and the respiratory impedance. By concept BIPAP is identical to APRV except that no restrictions are imposed on the duration of the low CPAP level (release pressure) [28]. Although, initially APRV studies in experimental induced lung injury and patients with mild pulmonary function favored a pressure release to near ambient pressure (5 to 10 cm H_2O) this may not be advantageous in patients with ARDS [22].

Two periods during the APRV/BIPAP cycle are particularly vulnerable to patient-ventilator asynchrony. Ventilation may be impaired, because spontaneous and ventilator efforts oppose each other when release of upper CPAP level occurs during spontaneous inspiration, and when restoration of the upper CPAP level occurs during spontaneous expiration. Asynchronous interferences between spontaneous and mechanical ventilation may increase the work of breathing and reduce effective ventilatory support during APRV/BIPAP [33]. Synchronization of the switching between the two CPAP levels to spontaneous inspiration or expiration has been used in commercial available demand valve APRV/BIPAP circuits of standard ventilators to avoid asynchronous interferences between spontaneous and mechanical breaths. Patient-triggered mechanical cycles during IMV have not been demonstrated to be advantageous for the patient and there is no reason why this should be different for APRV/BIPAP [31, 33]. In the absence of spontaneous breathing APRV/BIPAP is not different from a conventional pressure-controlled, time-cycled mechanical ventilation.

Airway Pressure Release Ventilation

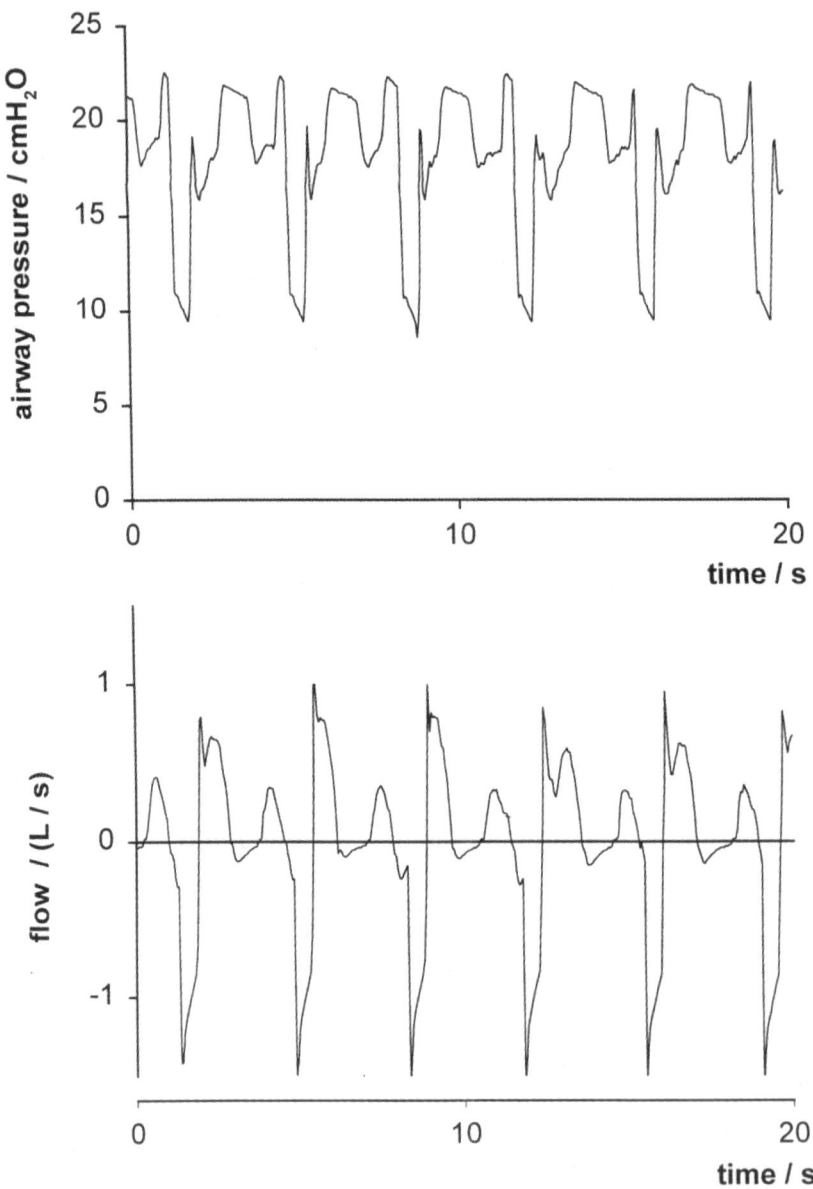

Fig. 2. Airway pressure (Paw), gas flow ($\dot{V}$), and volume (V) during ventilation with APRV/BI-PAP with and without spontaneous breathing. Note that when spontaneous breathing is absent, APRV/BIPAP is identical to a conventional, pressure-controlled mechanical ventilation

Pressure support ventilation (PSV) provides breath-to-breath synchronized insufflation to rapidly approach a preset pressure level, which in most available ventilators is terminated when inspiratory gas flow decreases to 25% of its peak flow value [26, 34, 35] (Fig. 3). Consequently, during PSV the degree of ventilatory support is determined by the pressure support, the respiratory rate, and the respiratory mechanics; the duration of inspiration by the interaction of spontaneous and mechanical ventilation and airway resistance [36]. Hence, an intact respiratory drive and a stable respiratory system impedance are required for the use of PSV as the sole ventilatory support. Because insufflation is not completed during PSV, equivalent low and high pressure levels are likely to result in a lower tidal volume during PSV compared to APRV/BIPAP [24].

In addition, insufflation is terminated when inspiratory gas flow decreases commonly to 25% of its peak flow value despite a continuing inspiratory effort which may result in a significant patient-ventilator asynchrony during PSV [37, 38]. Several modifications of PSV have been introduced. The fixed flow criterion for the ventilator to cycle off during PSV was lowered to 5% of the peak flow value or 5 l/min in some available ventilators to improve the patient synchrony [39]. To guarantee tidal volume, more recently introduced modifications of PSV provide instead of the flow-cycled a volume cycled insufflation [36]. However, potential advantages and disadvantages of different cycling criteria during PSV need still to be evaluated. The patient's breathing pattern and synchrony may also be affected by inspiratory flow delivery. Because an initial flow delivery matched to the patient's ventilatory demand and impedance will result in a maximal tidal volume and the lowest respiratory rate ventilator flow adjustment during PSV has been highly recommended [40].

Frequently, PSV has been used to guarantee a preset degree of ventilatory support for every spontaneous effort during IMV [41, 42]. Similarly, intermittent mandatory release ventilation (IMPRV) [43] uses PSV in conjunction with APRV. During IMPRV the airway pressure release occurs in the expiratory phase of a patient triggered pressure support insufflation [43]. Therefore, IMPRV is a breath-to-breath synchronized ventilatory support modality which requires an intact respiratory drive and stable respiratory system mechanics to be used as the sole ventilatory support [5, 28]. However, the advantage to use PSV in conjunction with other partial ventilatory modalities has not been proved.

Proportional assist ventilation (PAV) [25, 44] was recently introduced as a closed-loop ventilatory support with which the pressure generated by the ventilator is changed in proportion to the patient's inspiratory flow to overcome the resistive properties of the ventilatory system and airways (flow assist, FA), and the inspired volume to overcome the elastic properties of lung and thorax (volume assist, VA). Therefore, the generated pressure during PAV varies according to the patient's effort (Fig. 4). Unlike PSV, pressure during PAV is generated in conjunction with gas flow. Therefore, like PSV, PAV cannot be used in apneic patients.

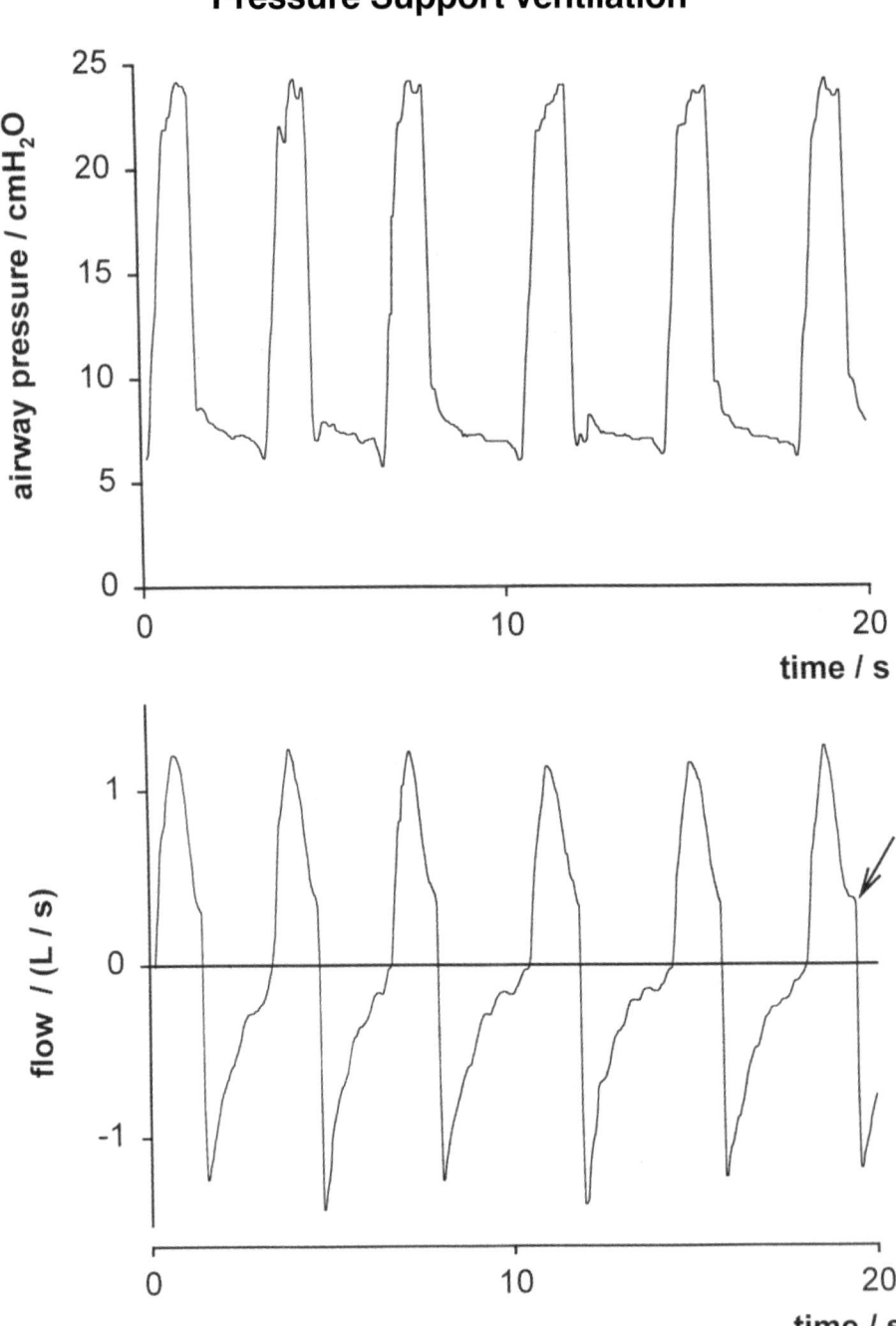

Fig. 3. Airway pressure (Paw) and gas flow (V̇) during PSV. Note that insufflation is cycled off at a flow of 25% of its peak flow value

Proportional Assist Ventilation

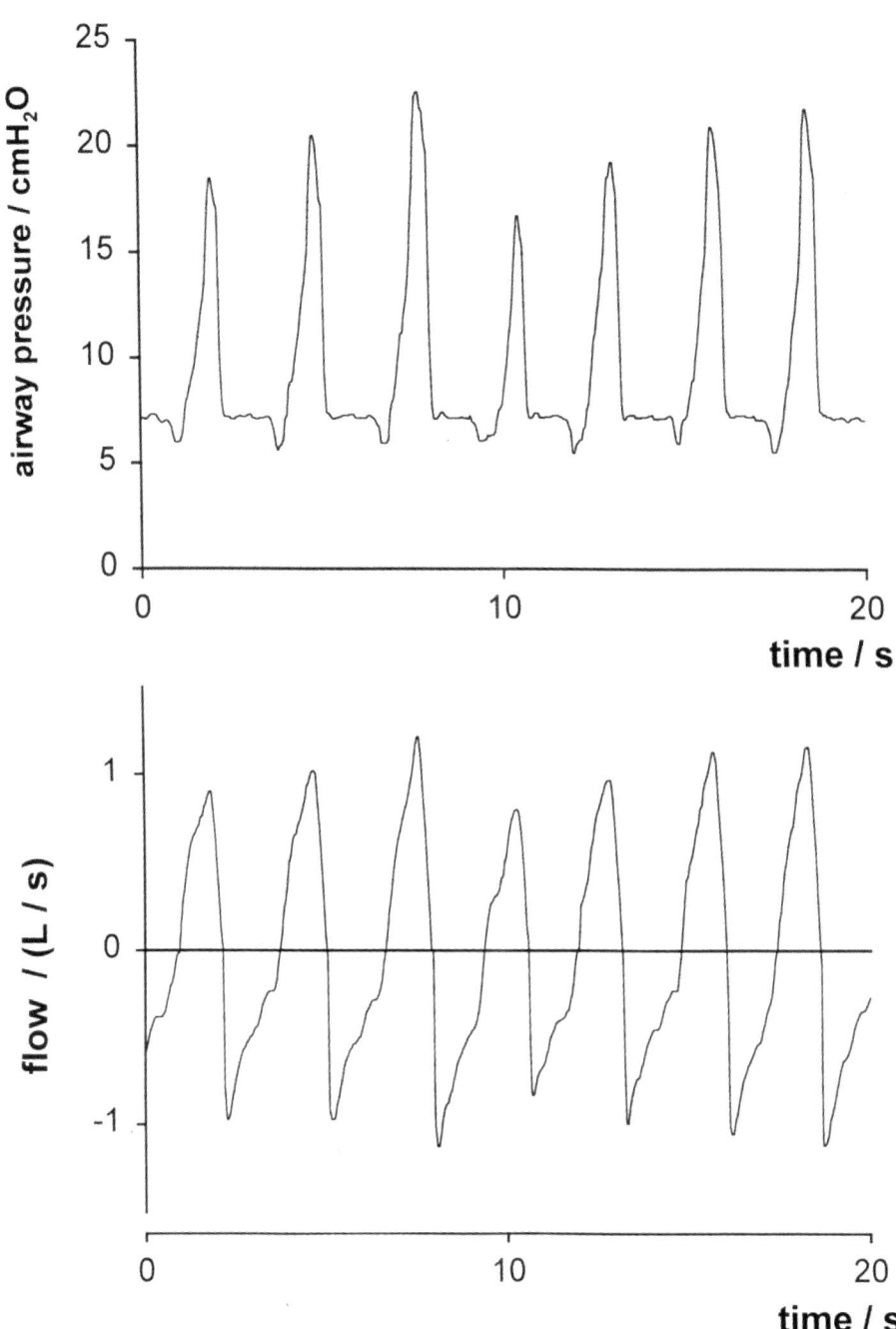

Fig. 4. Airway pressure (Paw) and gas flow (V̇) during PAV

During PAV not a target pressure but the amount of resistive and elastic un-loading and the proportion between the ventilator administered flow and volume and the patients inspiratory muscle effort is preset. Therefore, adequate adjust-ment of PAV would require at least periodic, better a continuous measurement of the patients elastance and resistance. If the level of volume assistance is cho-sen too high, a "runaway" will occur [45]. Then, the flow and volume generated by the ventilator exceeds the opposing elastic and resistive pressures and me-chanically insufflation is only terminated when the upper pressure threshold is reached. Unfortunately, up to now no continuous monitoring of the respiratory mechanics is available in ventilators providing PAV.

Physiologic effects

Pulmonary mechanics - work of breathing: If patients with respiratory failure breath spontaneously, work of breathing has to be maximally efficient. Any al-teration in the lung or thoracic mechanics will affect work of breathing. Poorly-designed ventilator circuits which add compliant or resistive components in the inspiratory limb, delay gas flow delivery, or create expiratory resistance and ar-tificial airway are also likely to cause inherent work of breathing. To allow effi-cient spontaneous breathing without imposing additional workload during par-tial ventilatory support requires well-designed breathing circuits.

Under normal conditions a small transpulmonary pressure change, allows normal tidal breathing from the end-expiratory lung volume along the steep slope of the pressure/volume relationship with minimal elastic work of breath-ing. When the end-expiratory lung volume is decreased in patients with acute respiratory failure, the pressure/volume relationship of the respiratory system is shifted to left, the compliance decreases, and an increased transpulmonary pres-sure change is required to generate the same tidal volume. Hence, work of breathing which corresponds to the area under the pressure/volume curve is in-creased (Fig. 5). As a result the patient will decrease tidal volume and increase respiratory rate to reduce the increased workload. Although, mechanical ventila-tory support is generally used to reduce work of breathing, an increase in the end-expiratory lung volume and the pulmonary compliance with CPAP may al-so effectively decrease work of breathing [46]. Partial ventilatory support modalities as IMV and APRV/BIPAP that do not provide ventilatory assistance to every inspiratory effort require the use of a proper CPAP level to allow effi-cient unsupported spontaneous breathing. In patients with ARDS CPAP levels adjusted to produce a tidal volume corresponding to the highest pulmonary compliance did not affect work of breathing and total oxygen consumption dur-ing APRV/BIPAP when compared to PCV [12, 24]. This observations are sup-ported by clinical observations indicating that total oxygen consumption is not measurably altered by spontaneous breathing during APRV/BIPAP [47] or SIMV [48].

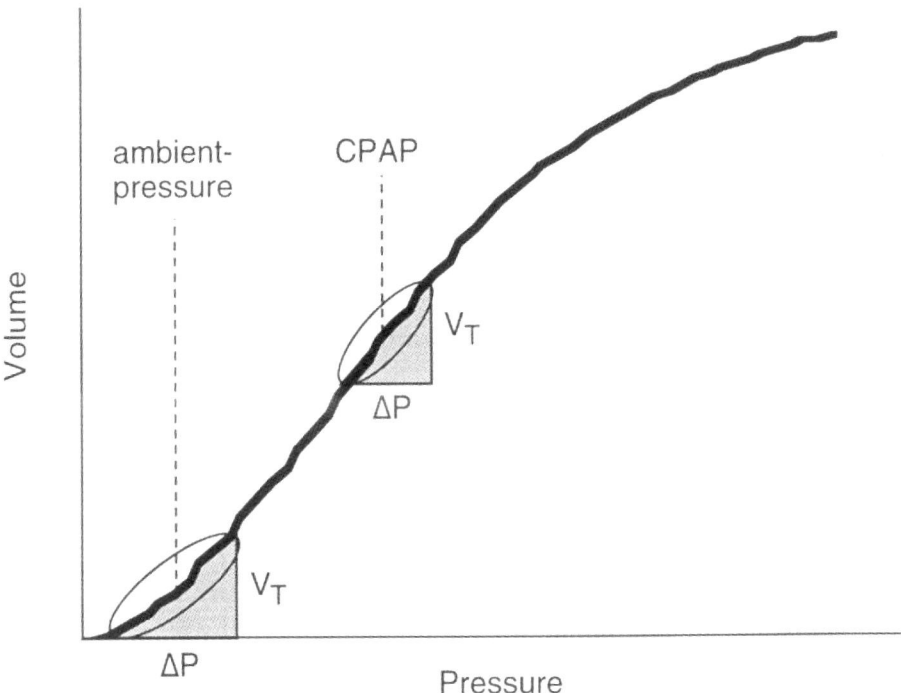

Fig. 5. Pressure/volume relationships of the respiratory system. When tidal breathing from the end-expiratory lung volume occurs along the flat slope of the pressure/volume relationship, the compliance is decreased, and an increased transpulmonary pressure change is required to generate the same tidal volume. The work of breathing which corresponds to the shaded area under the pressure/volume curve is increased. Application of CPAP increases end-expiratory lung volume and allows spontaneous breathing on a portion of the pressure/volume curve, where a small transpulmonary pressure change is required to produce the same tidal volume. Therefore, CPAP reduces the work of spontaneous breathing

To receive assistance of each spontaneous inspiration during PSV, the patient has to decrease intrapleural and airway pressure to open the demand-valve of the ventilator until a gas flow is delivered. Patients with obstructive lung disease may not be able to decrease sufficiently intrapleural pressure to overcome PEEPi and trigger a mechanical insufflation during PSV [37, 38]. Ineffective inspiratory efforts have been frequently observed during PSV, particularly when the pressure support level and the resulting tidal volumes were high [37, 38]. Then, an increasing pressure support level may cause a decrease in the ventilator rate, despite the patient's spontaneous respiratory rate is unchanged. Obviously, decrease in the ventilator rate cannot be interpreted in a reduction in work of breathing or an increase in patients comfort during PSV [37, 38]. Unfortunately, work of breathing supplied by the ventilator cannot be determined directly with PSV. However, studies have consistently demonstrated that PSV with pressure support levels of 10 cm H_2O or higher decreases work of breathing, oxygen consumption or the pressure time product when compared to CPAP in patients with mild pulmonary dysfunction [35, 49-51]. In patients recovering from acute respiratory failure that increasing levels of pressure support from 5 to 20 cm H_2O were observed to decrease work of breathing, oxygen consumption, and electromyographic activity of the diaphragm. Therefore, it was concluded that assistance of spontaneous inspiration with PSV may avoid diaphragmatic fatigue [35]. In patient with chronic obstructive pulmonary disease a decrease in oxygen consumption during PSV compared to IMV and CPAP was assumed to be the result of a decrease in the work of breathing. However, the circuit of the used ventilator may be in part responsible for the observed increase in the work of breathing during IMV and CPAP. Low pressure support levels of 5 cm H_2O reduced significantly the work of breathing when compared to a demand-valve CPAP, but not when compared to a continuous-flow CPAP [52]. Low-level PSV has been further advocated to reduce the work of spontaneous breathing through the tracheal tube or a breathing circuit [53].

Several trials have indicated a considerable reduction in work of breathing during PAV in patients with acute respiratory failure [54, 55]. At different levels of assist, the breathing patterns have been observed to be independent of the mechanical load during PAV [56]. Two studies compared breathing pattern and work of breathing during PAV and PSV [57, 58]. Patients respond with an increase respiratory rate to a higher ventilatory load during PSV when compared to PAV. The higher respiratory rate was associated with an increase in PEEPi, work of breathing, and respiratory discomfort during PSV. The higher variability of tidal volume might indicate an increased ability of the patients to change tidal volume in response to an altered respiratory demand during PAV.

Cardiopulmonary coupling: When cardiac function is normal, the filling of the right and left ventricle during diastole is the predominant determinant of the stroke volume and cardiac output. Spontaneous inspirations during sufficient partial ventilatory support cause periodic decreases in intrathoracic pressure and thus increase venous return towards the right ventricle without elevating the systemic venous pressure [21, 24]. Additionally, the outflow from the right ventricle which depends mainly on the lung volume which is the major determinant of pulmonary vascular resistance may benefit from a decrease in intrathoracic pressure during partial ventilatory support. As a consequence left ventricular filling can improve and subsequently left ventricular stroke volume will increase.

In contrast, a failing and dilated left ventricle may not benefit from an increase in preload and afterload [59]. Lemaire et al. [60] observed in a patient recovering from cardiopulmonary decompensation that an abrupt reduction in intrathoracic pressure due to a rapid weaning from mechanical ventilation to unsupported spontaneous breathing caused acute left ventricular failure. Similarly, Räsänen and coworkers [61, 62] reported the need of adequate ventilatory support and CPAP levels in patients with respiratory and cardiogenic failure. However, these studies also demonstrate that even patients with heart failure can tolerate adequate work of breathing and do not require full ventilatory support to improve cardiac function [59, 62].

Full mechanical ventilatory support effects lung volume by an increase in airway and intrathoracic pressure and reduces the venous return to the right ventricle [19]. A decrease in right and left ventricular filling usually results in a decrease in stroke volume, cardiac output, and oxygen delivery in normo- and hypovolaemic patients [20]. Cardiac output and stroke volume may be larger during partial than during full ventilatory support, because spontaneous breaths cause periodic decreases in intrathoracic pressure and an increase in abdominal pressure which may increase venous return [63, 64].

Not surprisingly, using similar mean airway pressure levels, no differences in the circulatory function have been observed between volume-controlled mechanical ventilation APRV/BIPAP without spontaneous breathing [29, 65, 66]. However, APRV/BIPAP was originally designed to allow unrestricted spontaneous breathing in any phase of the mechanical ventilation. Experimental investigations in dogs with experimental induced acute lung injury or bronchoconstriction revealed that stroke volume and cardiac output increased by 10%, and tissue oxygen delivery by 33% in the presence of spontaneous breathing during APRV/BIPAP. Sydow et al. [47] observed in patients with moderate to severe acute lung injury an increase in cardiac output and oxygen delivery by 11% with spontaneous breathing during APRV/BIPAP compared to volume controlled inverse ratio ventilation. A similar increase in cardiac output has been previously observed in clinical studies when IMV, which adds mechanical cycles to unsupported spontaneous breathing, was compared to volume-controlled mechanical ventilation [13, 67, 68]. Räsänen et al. [65] documented that a changeover from CPAP to spontaneous breathing with APRV/BIPAP did not affect cardiac output and tissue oxygen delivery. In contrast, a similar ventilatory support with a controlled mechanical ventilation reduced the stroke volume and oxygen delivery.

No change in stroke volume and cardiac output was observed during PSV when compared to APRV/BIPAP without spontaneous breathing (identical to PCV), using equal low and high CPAP levels [24, 69]. This finding is in agreement with previous clinical investigations reporting no change in cardiocirculatory variables during PSV compared to mechanical ventilation [34, 42, 70]. This indicates that cardiovascular function during ventilatory support with PSV was influenced by a lack of a sufficient decrease in mean intrathoracic pressure, as observed during mechanical ventilation. When comparing APRV/BIPAP to PSV in patients recovering from cardiac surgery Schirmer et al. [71] observed a small increase in the right ventricular ejection fraction from 47 to 51% with PSV. Ventilatory support in these patients with good cardiopulmonary function was provided with rather low airway pressure levels of 5 and 10 cm H_2O during APRV/BIPAP and PSV. Therefore, these data may not necessarily reflect the effect of interfacing of spontaneous and mechanical ventilation during APRV/BI-

PAP and PSV on the cardiocirculatory function in patients requiring ventilatory support during acute lung injury or cardiac failure.

Pulmonary and peripheral gas exchange: Several studies corroborated findings regarding the $\dot{V}_A/\dot{Q}$ matching between conventional controlled mechanical ventilation and breath-to-breath synchronized partial ventilatory support. Beydon et al. [72] observed no improvement in overall $\dot{V}_A/\dot{Q}$ matching during PSV compared to controlled mechanical ventilation. Intrapulmonary shunt remained unchanged, whereas dead space ventilation increased with PSV. Santak et al. [42] observed similar changes in the $\dot{V}_A/\dot{Q}$ distributions when comparing controlled mechanical ventilation with a combination of SIMV and PSV. Valentine et al. [73] who compared APRV/BIPAP and PSV at different pressure levels in patients recovering from open-heart operations found dead space to be considerably lower during APRV/BIPAP, whereas intrapulmonary shunt was not affected. Sydow et al. [47] who compared volume controlled inverse ratio ventilation with APRV/BIPAP found a significant improvement in the venous admixture with spontaneous breathing during APRV/BIPAP over time. Furthermore, it is difficult to evaluate the effect of different ventilatory support modalities on pulmonary gas exchange on the basis of previous non-randomized trials, because the degree of mechanical lung inflation or ventilatory support was altered considerably during the course of these investigations.

Experimental data suggest that interfacing between spontaneous breathing and mechanical ventilation is a critical determinant of the effects of ventilatory support on $\dot{V}_A/\dot{Q}$ matching [12, 24]. In an oleic-acid lung injury model, we observed better $\dot{V}_A/\dot{Q}$ matching during APRV/BIPAP with spontaneous breathing than during controlled mechanical ventilation or PSV when delivered with equal airway pressure limits [12, 24].

Recently, we randomly assigned patients with ARDS to receive APRV/BIPAP and PSV with equal airway pressure limits or $\dot{V}_E$. In both groups spontaneous breathing during APRV/BIPAP, accounting for 10% of $\dot{V}_E$ was associated with increases in right ventricular end-diastolic volume, stroke volume, cardiac index, PaO_2, oxygen delivery, and $P\bar{v}O_2$ and with reductions in oxygen extraction. PSV did not consistently improve cardiac index and PaO_2 when compared to APRV/BIPAP without spontaneous breathing. Spontaneous breathing during APRV/BIPAP with equal airway pressure limits or $\dot{V}_E$ accounted for a decrease in the blood flow to shunt units ($\dot{V}_A/\dot{Q} < 0.005$) and an increase in the fraction of cardiac output to units with a normal $\dot{V}_A/\dot{Q}$ ratio ($0.1 < \dot{V}_A/\dot{Q} < 10$). Pulmonary blood flow distribution to shunt and normal $\dot{V}_A/\dot{Q}$ units remained essentially unchanged during PSV, compared to APRV/BIPAP without spontaneous breathing in both groups (Fig. 6). Dead space ($\dot{V}_A/\dot{Q} > 100$) was lowest with spontaneous breathing during APRV/BIPAP (Fig. 6). Assisted spontaneous breathing with PSV produced no significant difference in dead space compared to APRV/BIPAP without spontaneous breathing. These findings strongly suggest that nonventilated lung units were completely recruited with spontaneous breathing. In addition, periodic decreases in intrathoracic pressure observed during sponta-

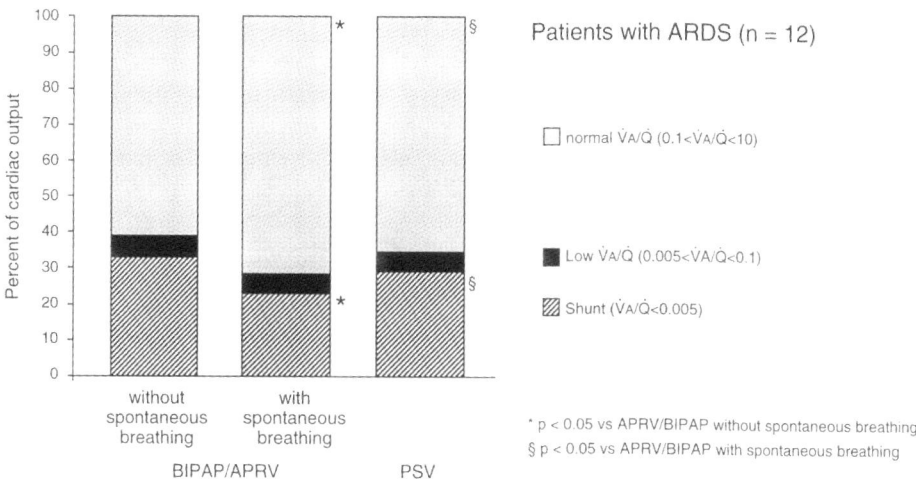

Fig. 6. Inert gas data derived by multiple inert gas elimination technique. Distribution of pulmonary blood flow to shunt units ($\dot{V}_A/\dot{Q} < 0.005$), low $\dot{V}_A/\dot{Q}$ units ($0.005 < \dot{V}_A/\dot{Q} < 0.1$), and normal $\dot{V}_A/\dot{Q}$ units ($0.1 < \dot{V}_A/\dot{Q} < 10$) during APRV/BIPAP with and without spontaneous breathing and PSV [22]. $* p < 0.05$

neous breathing with APRV/BIPAP, which are associated with an increase in cardiac output and may have supported perfusion of nondependent high $\dot{V}_A/\dot{Q}$ and dead space regions. In contrast, assisted spontaneous efforts with PSV, regardless of the pressure support, did not convert shunt to normal $\dot{V}_A/\dot{Q}$ units. Apparently the spontaneous contribution on a mechanically assisted breath was not sufficient to counteract the $\dot{V}_A/\dot{Q}$ maldistribution of positive pressure lung insufflation in patients with ARDS.

Decrease in dead space in the presence of a better $\dot{V}_A/\dot{Q}$ matching may indicate less hyperinflation during spontaneous breathing with APRV/BIPAP. Controlled mechanical ventilation and PSV appeared to worsen the $\dot{V}_A/\dot{Q}$ inequality in areas with ratios above normal. Ventilation during PSV was distributed in the presence of alveolar collapse mainly to poorly or non perfused lung units regardless of the level of ventilatory support. In agreement with previous experimental and clinical findings our observations indicate a lower inert gas dead space during spontaneous breathing with APRV/BIPAP when compared to PSV [24]. Wolff et al. [74] have shown that during synchronized IMV, the efficiency of alveolar carbon dioxide removal of an assisted breath is no better than that of a purely mechanical one. Therefore, the advantage of partial ventilatory support in ARDS may rest completely on the efficiency of the unsupported spontaneous breaths. Similarly, unsupported spontaneous breaths during APRV/BIPAP may have contributed to improved $\dot{V}_A/\dot{Q}$ matching and decreased dead space ventilation in the presence of ARDS [22, 24, 73].

No experimental or clinical data are available yet on the effect of PAV on $\dot{V}_A/\dot{Q}$ matching and gas exchange. Thus, it needs to be investigated if the effects on $\dot{V}_A/\dot{Q}$ matching and gas exchange during PAV are comparable to that during PSV.

Partial ventilatory support during weaning

Recently, two studies compared methods of gradual withdrawal of full ventilatory support [75, 76]. Based on these studies it has been concluded that three fourth of the patients can be discontinued effectively from controlled mechanical ventilation without using partial ventilatory support [75, 76]. Not surprisingly, these results only demonstrate that in patients with sufficient spontaneous breathing while cost-ineffective, gradual discontinuation with partial ventilatory support is not dangerous. In contrast, in patients with difficulties in tolerating unassisted spontaneous breathing PSV significantly reduced the duration of ventilatory support [75, 76]. However, it remains highly questionable if it was advantageous at all for these patients to receive controlled mechanical ventilation instead of an adequate mechanical ventilatory assistance of persisting spontaneous breathing. Modern respiratory care should consider partial ventilatory support as the primary ventilatory modality [4, 13, 18].

Conclusion

Recent development in mechanical ventilatory support has produced techniques that allow unrestricted breathing throughout mechanical ventilation. Investigations demonstrate that uncoupling of even minimal spontaneous and mechanical breaths during APRV/BIPAP contributes to improved $\dot{V}_A/\dot{Q}$ matching and increased systemic blood flow and thus oxygen supply and demand balance. In contrast during PAV flow and volume is generated by the ventilator in proportion to the patient's inspiratory effort to overcome the resistive properties and elastic properties of lung and thorax. Thus, PAV considerable reduces work of breathing. These data support the contention that mechanical ventilatory support techniques should allow unrestricted breathing throughout the mechanical cycle. Although these results are promising, more controlled clinical trials and long-term investigations are still warranted to evaluate the physiologic effects and allow a more rational application of the different partial ventilatory support modalities in critically ill patients. However, these observations already clearly demonstrate that partial ventilator support should not only be used to separate patients from mechanical ventilation, but to provide stable ventilatory assistance.

References

1. Marini JJ (1993) New options for the ventilatory management of acute lung injury. New Horiz 1:489-503
2. Downs JB, Klein EJ, Desautels D et al (1973) Intermittent mandatory ventilation: a new approach to weaning patients from mechanical ventilators. Chest 64:331-335
3. Downs JB, Block AJ, Vennum KB (1974) Intermittent mandatory ventilation in the treatment of patients with chronic obstructive pulmonary disease. Anesth Analg 53:437-443
4. Downs JB, Stock MC, Tabeling B (1982) Intermittent mandatory ventilation (IMV): A primary ventilatory support mode. Ann Chir Gynaecol 196:57-63
5. Räsänen J (1992) IMPRV-synchronized APRV, or more? Intensive Care Med 18:65-66
6. Räsänen J, Cane RD, Downs JB et al (1991) Airway pressure release ventilation during acute lung injury: A prospective multicenter trial. Crit Care Med 19:1234-41
7. Baum M, Hörmann C, Putensen C (1995) Inverse ratio ventilation (IRV): Only another form of PEEP. In: Rügheimer E (ed) Respiratorische Therapie nach operativen Eingriffen. Springer, Berlin, pp 147-155
8. Baum M, Benzer H, Mutz N et al (1980) Inversed ratio ventilation (IRV). Die Rolle des Atemzeitverhältnisses in der Beatmung des ARDS. Anaesthesist 29:592-597
9. Cole AGH, Weller SF, Sykes MK (1984) Inverse ratio ventilation compared with PEEP in adult respiratory failure. Intensive Care Med 10:227-232
10. Zavala E, Ferrer M, Polese G (1998) Effect of inverse I:E ratio ventilation on pulmonary gas exchange in acute respiratory distress syndrome. Anesthesiology 88:35-42
11. Mercat A, Diehl JL, Teboul JL et al (1998) Lengthening inspiratory time in the ARDS. Am J Respir Crit Care Med 157:A43
12. Putensen C, Räsänen J, López FA (1994) Ventilation-perfusion distribution during mechanical ventilation with and without superimposed spontaneous breathing in canine lung injury. Am J Respir Crit Care Med 150:101-108
13. Weisman IM, Rinaldo JE, Rogers RM et al (1983) Intermittent mandatory ventilation. Am Rev Respir Dis 127:641-647
14. Aubier M, Trippenbach T, Roussos C (1981) Respiratory muscle fatigue during cardiogenic shock. J Appl Physiol 51:499
15. Rossiter A, Souney PF, McGowan S et al (1991) Pancuronium-induced prolonged neuromuscular blockade. Crit Care Med 19:1583-1587
16. Wappler F, Scholz J, Prause A et al (1998) Stufenkonzept zur Analgosedierung in der Intensivmedizin mit Sufentanil. Anasthesiol Intensivmed Notfallmed Schmerzther 33:18-26
17. Rathgeber J, Schorn B, Falk V et al (1997) The influence of controlled mandatory ventilation (CMV), intermittent mandatory ventilation (IMV) and biphasic intermittent positive airway pressure (BIPAP) on duration of intubation and consumption of analgesics and sedatives. A prospective analysis in 596 patients following adult cardiac surgery. Eur J Anaesthesiol 14: 576-582
18. Putensen C, Zech S, Zinserling J (1998) Effect of early spontaneous breathing during airway pressure release ventilation on cardiopulmonary function. Am J Respir Crit Care Med 157:A45
19. Cournand A, Motley HL, Werkö L et al (1948) Physiologic studies of the effects of intermittent positive pressure ventilation on cardiac output in man. Am J Physiol 152:162-166
20. Jardin F, Delorme G, Hardy A et al (1990) Reevaluation of hemodynamic consequences of positive pressure ventilation: emphasis on cyclic right ventricular afterloading by mechanical lung inflation. Anesthesiology 72:966-970
21. Downs JB, Douglas ME, Sanfelippo PM et al (1977) Ventilatory pattern, intrapleural pressure, and cardiac output. Anesth Analg 56:88-96
22. Putensen C, Putensen G (1997) Effect of interfacing between spontaneous breathing and mechanical ventilation on gas exchange in acute lung injury. Am J Respir Crit Care Med 155:A771

23. Froese AB, Bryan AC (1974) Effects of anesthesia and paralysis on diaphragmatic mechanics in man. Anesthesiology 41:242-255
24. Putensen C, Räsänen J, López F et al (1994) Effect of interfacing between spontaneous and mechanical ventilation on the ventilation-perfusion distribution during in canine lung injury. Anesthesiology 81:921-930
25. Younes M (1992) Proportional assist ventilation, a new approach to ventilatory support. Theory. Am Rev Respir Dis 145:114-120
26. Hansen J, Wendt M, Lawin P (1984) Ein neues Weaning-verfahren (inspiratory flow assistance-IFA). Anaesthesist 33:428-432
27. Baum M, Benzer H, Putensen C et al (1989) Biphasic positive airway pressure (BIPAP) - a new form of augmented ventilation. Anaesthesist 38:452-458
28. Baum M, Mutz N, Hörmann C (1993) BIPAP, APRV, IMPRV: Methodological concept and clinical impact. In: Vincent JL (ed) Yearbook of intensive care and emergency medicine 5. Springer, Berlin, pp 514-526
29. Stock MC, Downs JB, Frolicher DA (1987) Airway pressure release ventilation. Crit Care Med 15:462-466
30. Downs JB, Stock MC (1987) Airway pressure release ventilation: a new concept in ventilatory support. Crit Care Med 15:459-461
31. Heenan TJ, Downs JB, Douglas ME et al (1980) Intermittent mandatory ventilation; is synchronization important? Chest 77:598-602
32. Putensen C, Lopez FA, Hörmann C (1995) Biphasic positive airway pressure (BIPAP) - Effects of spontaneous breathing during BIPAP on the ventilation-perfusion distribution. In: Rügheimer E (ed) Respiratory therapy following operative interventions. Springer, Berlin, pp 141-154
33. Putensen C, Leon M, Putensen-Himmer G (1994) Timing of pressure release affects power of breathing and minute ventilation during airway pressure release ventilation. Crit Care Med 22:872-878
34. Prakash O, Meij S (1985) Cardiopulmonary response to inspiratory pressure support during spontaneous ventilation versus conventional ventilation. Chest 88:403-408
35. Brochard L, Harf A, Lorino H et al (1989) Inspiratory pressure support prevents diaphragmatic fatigue during weaning from mechanical ventilation. Am Rev Respir Dis 139:513-521
36. MacIntyre NR (1986) Respiratory function during pressure support ventilation. Chest 89: 677-683
37. Fabry B, Guttmann J, Eberhard L et al (1995) An analysis desynchronization beween spontaneous breathing patients and ventilator during inspiratory pressure support. Chest 107: 1387-1394
38. Rossi A, Appendini L (1995) Wasted efforts and dyssynchrony: is the patient-ventilator battel back? Intensive Care Med 21:867-870
39. Bersten AD, Rutten AJ, Vedig AE (1993) Efficacy of pressure support in compensating for apparatus work. Anaesthesia Intensive Care 21:67-71
40. MacIntyre NR, Ho LI (1991) Effects of initial flow rate and breath termination criteria on pressure support ventilation. Chest 99:134-138
41. Jounieaux V, Duran A, Levi VP (1994) Synchronized intermittent mandatory ventilation with and without pressure support ventilation in weaning patients with COPD from mechanical ventilation. Chest 105:1204-1210
42. Santak B, Radermacher P, Sandmann W et al (1991) Influence of SIMV plus inspiratory pressure support on $\dot{V}_A/\dot{Q}$ distributions during postoperative weaning. Intensive Care Med 17: 136-140
43. Rouby JJ, Ben Ameur M, Jawish D et al (1992) Continuous positive airway pressure (CPAP) vs. intermittent mandatory release ventilation (IMPRV) in patients with acute respiratory failure. Intensive Care Med 18:69-75
44. Younes M, Puddy A, Roberts D et al (1992) Proportional assist ventilation. Results of an initial clinical trial. Am Rev Respir Dis 145:121-129

45. Younes M (1992) Proportional assist ventilation, a new approach to ventilatory support. Am Rev Respir Dis 145:114-120
46. Katz JA, Marks JD (1985) Inspiratory work with and without continuous positive airway pressure in patients with acute respiratory failure. Anesthesiology 63:598-607
47. Sydow M, Burchardi H, Ephraim E et al (1994) Long-term effect of two different ventilatory modes on oxygenation in acute lung injury. Am J Respir Crit Care Med 149:1550-1556
48. Räsänen J, Puhakka K, Leijala M (1992) Spontaneous breathing and total body oxygen consumption in children recovering from open-heart surgery. Chest 101:662-667
49. Brochard L, Pluskwa F, Lemaire F (1987) Improved efficiency of spontaneous breathing with inspiratory pressure support. Am Rev Respir Dis 136:411-415
50. Viale JP, Annat GJ, Bouffard YM et al (1988) Oxygen cost of breathing in postoperative patients. Pressure support ventilation vs continuous positive airway pressure. Chest 93:506-509
51. Annat GJ, Viale JP, Dereymez CP et al (1990) Oxygen cost of breathing and diaphragmatic pressure-time index. Measurement in patients with COPD during weaning with pressure support ventilation. Chest 98:411-414
52. Sassoon CS, Light RW, Lodia R et al (1991) Pressure-time product during continuous positive airway pressure, pressure support ventilation, and T-piece during weaning from mechanical ventilation. Am Rev Respir Dis 143:469-475
53. Brochard L, Rua F, Lorino H et al (1991) Inspiratory pressure support compensates for the additional work of breathing caused by the endotracheal tube. Anesthesiology 75:739-745
54. Ranieri VM, Grasso S, Mascia L et al (1997) Effects of proportional assist ventilation on inspiratory muscle effort in patients with chronic obstructive pulmonary disease and acute respiratory failure. Anesthesiology 86:79-91
55. Bigatello L, Nishimura M, Imanka H et al (1997) Unloading of the work of breathing by proportional assist ventilation. Crit Care Med 25:267-272
56. Navalesi P, Hernandez P, Wongsa A et al (1996) Proportional assist ventilation in acute respiratory failure: effects on breathing pattern and inspiratory effort. Am J Respir Crit Care Med 154:1330-1338
57. Wrigge H, Golisch W, Almeling G et al (1998) Proportional assist versus pressure support ventilation: Effects on breathing pattern and respiratory work of patients with chronic obstructive pulmonary disease. Intensive Care Med (in press)
58. Ranieri VM, Giuliani R, Mascia L et al (1996) Patient-ventilator interaction during acute hypercapnia: Pressure support vs proportional assist ventilation. J Appl Physiol 81:426-436
59. Räsänen J (1987) Conventional and high frequency controlled mechanical ventilation in patients with left ventricular dysfunction and pulmonary edema. Chest 91:225-229
60. Lemaire F, Teboul JL, Cinotti L et al (1988) Acute left ventricular dysfunction during unsuccessful weaning from mechanical ventilation. Anesthesiology 69:171-179
61. Räsänen J, Nikki P, Heikkila J (1984) Acute myocardial infarction complicated by respiratory failure. The effects of mechanical ventilation. Chest 85:21-28
62. Räsänen J, Heikkila J, Downs J et al (1985) Continuous positive airway pressure by face mask in acute cardiogenic pulmonary edema. Am J Cardiol 55:296-300
63. Kirby RR, Downs JB, Civetta JM et al (1975) High level positive end expiratory pressure (PEEP) in acute respiratory insufficiency. Chest 67:156-163
64. Douglas ME, Downs JB (1980) Cardiopulmonary effects of intermittent mandatory ventilation. Intern Anesthesiol Clin 18:97-121
65. Räsänen J, Downs JB, Stock MC (1988) Cardiovascular effects of conventional positive pressure ventilation and airway pressure release ventilation. Chest 93:911-915
66. Garner W, Downs JB, Stock MC et al (1988) Airway pressure release ventilation (APRV). A human trial. Chest 94:779-781
67. Räsänen J (1992) Supply-dependent oxygen consumption and mixed venous oxyhemoglobin saturation during isovolemic hemodilution in pigs. Chest 101:1121-1124
68. Räsänen J, Downs JB, Malec DJ et al (1987) Estimation of oxygen utilization by dual oximetry. Annals of Surgery 206:621-623

69. Putensen C, Räsänen J, López F (1995) Interfacing between spontaneous breathing and mechanical ventilation affects ventilation-perfusion distributions in experimental bronchoconstriction. Am J Respir Crit Care Med 151:993-999
70. Dries DJ, Kumar P, Mathru M et al (1991) Hemodynamic effects of pressure support ventilation in cardiac surgery patients. Am Surg 57:122-125
71. Schirmer U, Calzia E, Lindner KH et al (1994) Right ventricular function during weaning from respirator after coronary artery bypass grafting. Chest 105:1352-1356
72. Beydon L, Cinotti L, Rekik N et al (1991) Changes in the distribution of ventilation and perfusion associated with separation from mechanical ventilation in patients with obstructive pulmonary disease. Anesthesiology 75:730-738
73. Valentine DD, Hammond MD, Downs JB et al (1991) Distribution of ventilation and perfusion with different modes of mechanical ventilation. Am Rev Respir Dis 143:1262-1266
74. Wolff G, Brunner JX, Grädel E (1986) Gas exchange during mechanical ventilation and spontaneous breathing - intermittent mandatory ventilation after open heart surgery. Chest 90:11-17
75. Brochard L, Rauss A, Benito S et al (1994) Comparison of three methods of gradual withdrawal from ventilatory support during weaning from mechanical ventilation. Am J Respir Crit Care Med 150:896-903
76. Esteban A, Frutos F, Tobin MJ et al (1995) A comparison of four methods of weaning patients from mechanical ventilation. N Engl J Med 332:345-350

Proportional Assist Ventilation: Technique and Implementation

M. YOUNES

Proportional Assist Ventilation (PAV) is a form of partial ventilatory support with which the ventilator delivers pressure assist in proportion to instantaneous patient effort (Fig. 1). With PAV, the pressure delivered by the ventilator increases during inspiration so long as patient's effort is increasing. When the patient's effort ceases at the end of inspiration the pressure also decreases leading to a decrease in inspiratory flow and termination of the cycle (Fig. 1). If the patient makes a stronger effort, he/she receives more pressure support, and vice versa (Fig. 1). The main advantages of this approach, therefore, are the assured synchrony between the end of patient's inspiratory cycle and ventilator cycle and ability of the ventilator to adjust automatically the level of assist in response to changes in patient ventilatory demand. These technical advantages are expected to have some positive clinical implications [1, 2] although these clinical advantages are yet to be confirmed experimentally.

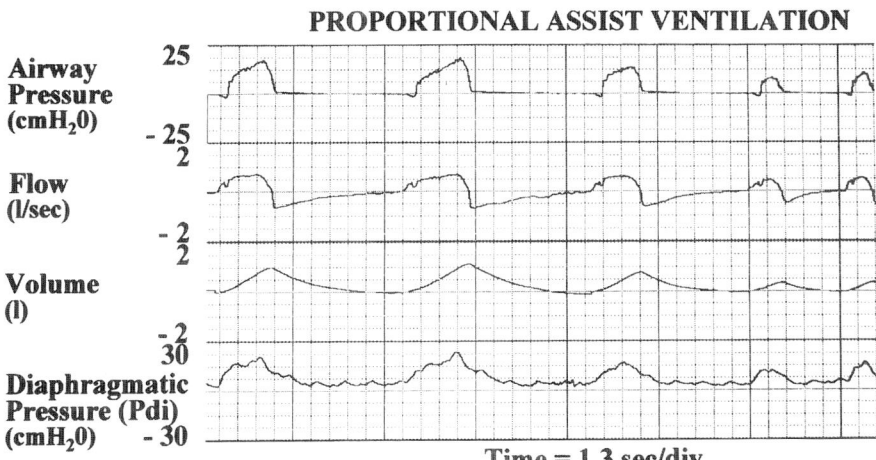

Fig. 1. Example of breathing on PAV. Note that level of assist (airway pressure) is proportional to patient's respiratory muscle output (Pdi in this case) and that the ventilator cycle is linked to the duration of inspiratory effort. Also note the substantial breath by breath variability in tidal volume and other variables typical of breathing on PAV particularly in alert patients

Technique

With PAV the ventilator continuously monitors the rate of airflow and the volume received by the patient from the beginning of inspiration. The PAV assist consists of a combination of pressure delivered in proportion to flow (referred to as flow assist, FA) and in proportion to instantaneous inspired volume (referred to as volume assist, VA). The theory of how such a combination results in the ventilator being able to track patient's effort has been described in detail elsewhere [1]. Briefly, if one wishes the proportionality between P_{aw} and the pressure generated by the patient's muscles (P_{mus}) to be 1:1, the flow assist is adjusted to be half the respiratory system resistance (R) and VA to be half the respiratory system elastance (E; elastance is the reciprocal of compliance). In this fashion the ventilator continuously delivers half the total pressure while the patient is producing the other half. The proportionality is then 1:1. Similarly, if the desired proportionality is 3 to 1, FA is adjusted to be 3/4 of R and VA is adjusted to be 3/4 of E. In this fashion the ventilator is responsible for 3/4 of the total pressure while the patient is responsible for 1/4 and the proportionality is 3 to 1. Clearly a whole range of proportionalities are possible between zero and near infinity. The general relation is given by:

$$\text{proportionality} = \% \text{ assist}/(1\text{-}\% \text{ assist})$$

Implementation

Ventilators equipped with the PAV mode will have one of two types of user interface:

1. The user inputs estimated values for the patient's resistance and elastance and the desired percent assist.
2. The user may simply input directly desired values of FA and VA.

The first type of user interface also allows the second application. To directly input a desired level of FA or VA without regard to the patient's R and E, the percent assist is selected at 100% and the desired FA is inputted as resistance while the desired VA is inputted as elastance. In this case the ventilator simply delivers an assist that equals the inputs relating to R and E without these actually representing the patient's R and E.

The major practical problem in properly implementing PAV is the need to know the patient's R and E. Reliable measurements of these parameters, using currently available techniques, require respiratory muscle relaxation (i.e. controlled mechanical ventilation, CMV). This is inconvenient. Furthermore, because respiratory mechanics can change quickly, and it is not practical to frequently determine R and E by CMV, changes in respiratory mechanics can be missed and this would result in a change in the level of support. Another implementation problem is the presence of non-linear behavior of the pressure-flow and pressure-volume relationships. Under these conditions there is no unique value for R and E and this may create some difficulties in setting the levels of support (for more details see [2]). The main technical problem in this regard occurs in patients in whom the respiratory system is stiffer in the low tidal volume range than in the higher volume. Here if the VA is set according to the higher elastance in the low volume range, overassist may develop when the patient decides to take a bigger volume. This results in the inflation cycle continuing until the cycle is terminated by one of the limiting variables (pressure limit, volume limit, or T_I limit). The occasional or frequent sounding of the alarm can be disruptive to the nursing personnel. Opposing these practical difficulties are the following considerations:

1. Precise knowledge of R and E is not really critical. So long as FA is less than R and VA is less than E, the ventilator continues to develop pressure in proportion to patient effort and will continue to terminate the cycle at the end of the patient's inspiratory effort. The main difference from the ideal situation is that the shape of the pressure wave form will differ somewhat from the shape of the patient's P_{mus} wave form. This is clearly not critical. The other consequence of errors in estimated R and E is that the patient may receive less assist than is intended. In the absence of any distress, this would have no consequence since the primary intent of mechanical ventilation is to avoid excessive work. On the other hand, if the underassist is below what can be tolerated by the patient, there will be evidence of respiratory distress. Under these conditions, the distress would be eliminated by increasing the level of assist.

2. Considerable progress has been made in developing automated systems for reliably monitoring R and E, including non-linearities, in the PAV mode [3, 4]. It is very likely that commercial ventilators will be equipped with similar systems in the near future. Once this occurs, the only variable to be set by the user will be the percent assist while the ventilator automatically monitors the patient's resistance and elastance on a continuous basis and adjusts the levels of FA and VA accordingly. In the meantime the following guidelines are recommended for implementation of PAV.

De novo implementation in the noninvasive setting

The main objective of noninvasive support is to reduce respiratory distress (reduce respiratory muscle work). The main practical problem of using PAV in the noninvasive mode is the presence of leaks. Unless the ventilator can estimate the amount of leak and subtract it from the flow leaving the ventilator, the ventilator will actually be providing assist in proportion to a greater flow than what the patient is actually receiving. Based on these considerations the following is the recommended approach:

a) use a good fitting nasal or facial mask;

b) where possible use a ventilator that can estimate leaks and subtract them from the flow signal;

c) set an expiratory pressure level to an initial value of 4 or 5 cm H_2O;

d) set the high pressure limit to 25 cm H_2O, the high volume limit to 1.5 l and the high T_I limit to 3 seconds;

e) set the initial FA to 2 and the initial VA to 5. This will cause substantial relief in most patients;

f) gradually increase the level of VA in small steps of 2 cm of H_2O/l with patient feedback. Continue increasing the level every minute or so until the patient indicates that he/she is getting too much assist. Reduce the level by one or two units;

g) after adjusting the VA, again increase the FA in small steps, one unit each, and getting patient feedback. With these titrations the patient usually indicates approval of the increase in assist until a point is reached at which he/she indicates that the assist is too much;

h) if the alarms sound off frequently, indicating the breaths are being terminated by one of the limiting factors, there are two basic possibilities. First the patient's respiratory drive has increased and he now requires greater tidal volumes with associated greater pressures. Second, respiratory mechanics have improved so that the settings that were appropriate before are now excessive and exceed the patient's R or E. The same would occur if new leaks develop that are not compensated for by the ventilator. To distinguish between these two possibilities the level of assist is decreased by 20 to 30%. In the event the problem was over assist, the frequent alarming by the ventilator will stop while the patient remains comfortable. In the event the cause was an increase in ventilatory drive, alarming may continue since the patient would still attempt to obtain the desired ventilation and some distress may redevelop. Under these conditions clinical assessment is necessary to identify the reasons for the increase in drive. If it is deemed advisable to continue with noninvasive support, then the pressure and/or volume limits may have to be increased.

Following the initial adjustment and disappearance of respiratory distress, the level of assist should at intervals be reduced in approximately 20 or 30% steps. If the patient tolerates the reduction for a reasonable amount of time, further reductions are implemented until the patient no longer requires support. The frequency at which reductions are tested will clearly depend on the progression of the clinical problem necessitating NIMV in the first place.

Implementation in intubated patients in the ICU

a) Adjustments of the PEEP level and FiO_2 are based on usual criteria independent of the mode.

b) If resistance and elastance are reliably known prior to institution of PAV, these values should be initially used. The percent support should depend on the status of the patient. In acute cases, a high level of 80% is recommended. In less acute patients 50 to 60% is usually quite adequate.

c) If R and E are not known in advance, initially enter default values for elastance of 12 cm H_2O/l. For initial estimated resistance, enter a value corresponding to the resistance of the ET tube at a flow of 40 l/min plus a value of 5 for an estimated patient resistance. The percent assist selected initially, in the case of using these default values, should be high (80%) since the likelihood of over assist with these default values is virtually non esistant.

d) Within a few minutes of instituting PAV at these default levels, perform an end expiratory occlusion (inspiratory hold). If the ventilator is provided with a graphic display, note the plateau pressure at approximately 0.25 seconds after flow has reached zero. We have found that this value provides an excellent substitute for passive elastic recoil [4]. Passive elastance in the tidal volume range can then be computed from this plateau pressure value at 0.25 sec less PEEP divided by the actual tidal volume that was occluded. This procedure may be repeated 2 or 3 times. Usually the results are consistent. If so then this new value of elastance should be inputted into the ventilator.

e) Until the automated mechanics system is implemented, there is currently no suitable way for determining, non-invasively, resistance in the PAV mode. Since in the majority of patients the ET tube is the main source of resistance, using the default values is usually quite acceptable. If, however, resistance values are available from a previous period of CMV, these should be used.

f) The percent assist is reduced in steps at intervals that are appropriate to the clinical course of the patient until a time is reached where the patient can function without assist. If respiratory distress appears within one hour of a step reduction, the level of assist should be increased to the level not associated with distress before.

Special issues

Breathing pattern on PAV

It is important to realize that with PAV the clinician does not set a target tidal volume, flow rate, respiratory rate or P_{aw}. What is set are the levels of FA and VA. Because P_{aw} is a function of patient's effort and, with properly adjusted PAV, the ventilator delivers always less than 100% of the total pressure, the patient remains entirely in control of all these ventilatory and pressure outputs. An increase in the level of support, therefore, need not (and usually does not) result in important increases in tidal volume, ventilation or flow rate. The patient usually chooses to reduce his own efforts in order to maintain these variables at approximately the same levels (5-7). One of the main challenges for the clinician while using PAV is the acceptance of the fact that he/she is no longer in control of ventilation or tidal volume. This becomes the responsibility of the patient. The clinician will simply have to decide whether the breathing pattern selected by the patient is acceptable to the clinician or not. If not, the clinician will simply have to switch the patient to another mode of ventilation. It must be pointed out that the formulas (rules of thumb) that many physicians use to set tidal volume are not based on any sound scientific evidence. In our experience on several hundred patients with PAV patient selected V_T is, on average, approximately 7 ml/kg and respiratory rate is, on average, 25 min^{-1}. There is, however, a very wide range of breathing patterns with some patients choosing to breathe with a rapid shallow pattern despite high levels of assist and with no apparent distress (e.g. see [6]). A rapid shallow pattern on PAV, therefore, need not be seen as necessarily an indication for switching to another mode. If there is no clinical evidence of distress by means other than respiratory rate (e.g. accessory muscle use, supraclavicular indrawing or chest wall paradox) a rapid shallow pattern may simply be the natural pattern the patient's control system desires. Even in normal people the preferred breathing pattern varies considerably [8].

Use of sedatives

With respect to the use of sedatives, a patient on a ventilator in the PAV mode is comparable to an unventilated person. The use of sedatives for the management of agitation or pain follows the same guidelines as in non-ventilated patients, namely they should be used enough to relieve the discomfort but without causing excessive central depression. Nonetheless, all ventilators providing the PAV mode should have a suitable back up system in the event an overdose of sedative is administered inadvertently and the patient becomes apneic or his ventilation or tidal volume decrease to unacceptable levels.

$PaCO_2$ on PAV

The ventilator in the PAV mode does not control PCO_2. Rather, it is the other way around; $PaCO_2$ and pH control ventilator output. If the patient's sensitivity to PCO_2 is low, PCO_2 may rise upon switching from a conventional mode to PAV but without any evidence of distress. An increase in PCO_2 without distress in the PAV mode, therefore, signifies low CO_2 response by the patient's respiratory control. This is not frequently seen and usually occurs only in patients who are very heavily sedated or in those patients with chronic CO_2 retention in the past whose PCO_2 was artificially kept low with other modes of ventilation. When this happens, the physician must decide whether to accept the increase in PCO_2 to a new and higher plateau or to switch the patient to another mode which forces a reduction in PCO_2. This decision will depend on clinical assessment of the possible reason for the depressed CO_2 sensitivity and the potential of allowing the CO_2 to rise to facilitate weaning. Clearly if the CO_2 rises to a point where the pH becomes unacceptable, the patient should be switched to another mode. Alternatively, if the patient is known to have chronic respiratory disease, his mechanics are poor, and the PCO_2 rises but with an acceptable pH (for example greater than 7.3) it may be appropriate to maintain the patient on PAV. This would in fact facilitate weaning by decreasing ventilatory requirements in a patient with very abnormal mechanics.

When PAV is instituted de novo in a patient with acute distress and associated acute hypercapnia (e.g. acute pulmonary oedema, status asthmaticus), $PaCO_2$ usually declines initially but some hypercapnia and acidaemia may remain, without distress, and gradually subside over a few hours [9]. This is likely related to residual effects of endogenous opiates released during the acute distress. In the absence of continued distress, slow normalization of PCO_2 and pH is not an indication of failure of PAV.

Continued distress despite seemingly adequate PAV support

Another scenario which occurs infrequently is the presence of clinical respiratory distress when the level of assist is deemed to be quite high (for example 80% or more). When this occurs the reasons are usually one of the following:

a) The presence of high level of dynamic hyperinflation that is not compensated by external PEEP. PAV only assists that portion of the patient's effort in excess of the pressure required to reverse flow from expiratory to inspiratory. In the presence of dynamic hyperinflation a portion of the patient's effort is unsupported. Accordingly, even if the assist to P_{mus} in excess of dynamic hyperinflation is high, the overall assist may be low. The presence of dynamic hyperinflation should be looked for in the flow tracing and if present, attempts should be made to offset it by increasing external PEEP (note that external PEEP does not always counteract dynamic hyperinflation).

b) The presence of a very high respiratory drive due to causes other than abnormal respiratory mechanics or respiratory muscle weakness. This occurs for example in the presence of severe metabolic acidosis, shock states and anxiety or agitation. Under such conditions it is preferable to switch the patient to another mode of ventilation which permits heavy sedation until the reasons for the excessive respiratory drive are corrected.

c) Ventilator malfunction (poor trigger sensitivity or very slow response). This would be evident from inspection of the graphic display if available. Poor trigger sensitivity would be evident from a substantial delay between the onset of inspiratory effort (decrease in expiratory flow or in P_{aw}) and the onset of the assist. Poor ventilator response would be evident from a slow rise in P_{aw} after triggering.

References

1. Younes M (1992) Proportional assist ventilation, a new approach to ventilatory support. Theory. Am Rev Respir Dis 145:114-120
2. Younes M (1994) Proportional assist ventilation. In: Tobin MJ (ed) Principles and practice of mechanical ventilation. McGraw-Hill, New York, pp 349-370
3. Younes M, Webster K, Kun J et al (1997) A method for determining the pressure-flow (P-V̇) relation during proportional assist ventilation. Am J Respir Crit Care Med 155:A525
4. Younes M, Webster K, Kun J et al (1997) A method for estimating pressure-volume (PV) relation during proportional assist ventilation (PAV). Am J Respir Crit Care Med 155:A525
5. Navalesi P, Hernandez P, Wongsa A et al (1996) Proportional assist ventilation in acute respiratory failure: effects on breathing pattern and inspiratory effort. Am J Respir Crit Care Med 154:1330-1338
6. Marantz S, Patrick W, Webster K et al (1996) Responses of ventilator dependent patients to different levels of proportional assist. J Appl Physiol 80:397-403
7. Meza S, Giannouli E, Younes M (1998) Control of breathing during sleep assessed by proportional assist ventilation. J Appl Physiol 84(1):3-12
8. Jammes Y, Auran Y, Gouvernet J et al (1979) The ventilatory pattern of conscious man according to age and morphology. Bull Eur Physiopathol Respir 15:527-540
9. Patrick W, Webster K, Ludwig L et al (1996) Noninvasive positive-pressure ventilation in acute respiratory distress without prior chronic respiratory failure. Am J Respir Crit Care Med 153:1005-1011

INDEX